Current Progress in Clinical Microbiology

Current Progress in Clinical Microbiology

Editor: Jessica Hoover

AMERICAN
MEDICAL PUBLISHERS
www.americanmedicalpublishers.com

AMERICAN
MEDICAL PUBLISHERS
www.americanmedicalpublishers.com

Cataloging-in-Publication Data

Current progress in clinical microbiology / edited by Jessica Hoover.
p. cm.
Includes bibliographical references and index.
ISBN 978-1-63927-260-0
1. Medical microbiology. 2. Diagnostic microbiology. 3. Microbiology. 4. Pathogenic microorganisms.
5. Medical sciences. I. Hoover, Jessica.
QR46 .C87 2022
616.904 1--dc23

American Medical Publishers,
41 Flatbush Avenue,
1st Floor, New York,
NY 11217, USA

ISBN 978-1-63927-260-0 (Hardback)

Contents

Preface

Clinical microbiology is the discipline of medical science that focuses on the prevention, diagnosis and treatment of infectious diseases. Numerous clinical applications of microbes for better health are studied in this domain. Clinical microbiology is also characterized as one of the primary sub-fields of microbiology that is applied to medicine. This field commonly focuses on the treatment of infections caused by various bacteria, fungi, viruses and parasites. The treatment of diseases caused by these pathogens is formulated after studying their characteristics such as mechanisms of infection, growth and modes of transmission. The field aims to focus on the presence and growth of microbial infections in individuals, their effects on the human body, and the methods of treating these infections. The most important part of clinical microbiology is epidemiology, which studies the patterns, causes and effects of health and disease in diverse populations. This book unravels the recent studies in the field of clinical microbiology. It traces the progress of this field and highlights some of its key concepts and applications. This book is a resource guide for experts as well as students.

After months of intensive research and writing, this book is the end result of all who devoted their time and efforts in the initiation and progress of this book. It will surely be a source of reference in enhancing the required knowledge of the new developments in the area. During the course of developing this book, certain measures such as accuracy, authenticity and research focused analytical studies were given preference in order to produce a comprehensive book in the area of study.

This book would not have been possible without the efforts of the authors and the publisher. I extend my sincere thanks to them. Secondly, I express my gratitude to my family and well-wishers. And most importantly, I thank my students for constantly expressing their willingness and curiosity in enhancing their knowledge in the field, which encourages me to take up further research projects for the advancement of the area.

Editor

1

Molecular characterization of selected multidrug resistant *Pseudomonas* from water distribution systems in southwestern Nigeria

Ayodele T. Adesoji[1*], Adeniyi A. Ogunjobi[2] and Isaac O. Olatoye[3,4]

Abstract

Background: Persistence of antibiotic resistant bacteria, including multidrug resistant (MDR) pseudomonads, is an important environmental health problem associated with drinking water distribution systems (DWDS) worldwide. There is paucity of data on the molecular characteristics of antibiotic resistance genes and their mode of transfer among pseudomonads from DWDS located in resource-challenged areas such as southwestern Nigeria.

Methods: MDR pseudomonads (n = 22) were selected from a panel of 296 different strains that were isolated from treated and untreated water in six DWDS located across southwest Nigeria. Primarily, the isolated pseudomonads strains were identified by 16S rDNA sequencing and antibiotic-resistance testing was completed using agar breakpoints assays. The final panel of strains of resistant to more than three classes of antibiotics (i.e. MDR), were further characterized by PCR genotyping, Sanger sequencing, and plasmid profiling.

Results: Pseudomonad resistance to gentamicin and streptomycin ranged from 22.7 to 54.6 % while resistance to tetracycline, ceftiofur and sulphamethoxazole ranged from 40.9 to 77.3 %. The most commonly detected antibiotic resistance genes were *tet*(A) (31.8 % of isolates), *sul1* (31.8 %), bla_{TEM} (40.9 %) and *aph(3″)*^{c} (36.4 %). Class 1 integron sequences were evident in 27.3 % of isolates and they harbored genes encoding resistance to aminoglycosides (*aadA2*, *aadA1*), trimethoprim (*dfrA15*, *dfr7*) and sulphonamide (*sul1*) while the plasmid ranged between 22 and 130 kb.

Conclusions: *Pseudomonas* spp, isolated from these DWDS possess resistance genes and factors that are of public and environmental health significance. Therefore, has the potential of contributing to the global scourge of resistance genes transfer in human, animals and environments, thereby, useful in the epidemiology of antimicrobial resistance.

Keywords: *Pseudomonas* spp, Antibiotic resistance genes, Multidrug resistance, Water distribution systems

Background

Pseudomonas spp, is a ubiquitous and diverse genus of Gram-negative bacteria that can be found in soil, water, decaying vegetation and animals. According to Craun et al. [1], *Pseudomonas* was one of the most frequently identified agents associated with waterborne outbreaks of dermatitis (rash or folliculitis), as well as conjunctivitis, otitis externa and other symptoms from recreational water in the US Pseudomonads are well adapted to survival in the warm temperatures found in whirlpools, hot tubs and indoor pools.

The most important and ubiquitous pathogenic pseudomonad is *P. aeruginosa.* It is medically significant and has a high intrinsic resistance to antibiotics while causing wide spectrum of opportunistic infections [2]. *P. aeruginosa* is best known for chronic lung infections among cystic fibrosis patients [3]. *P. aeruginosa* is also a cause of serious infections among immunocompromised cancer patients, burn patients, catheterized patients, and other hospitalized individuals [2].

Antibiotic resistance genes can be transferred between different microorganisms [4]. Mobile genetic elements

*Correspondence: timmyayus2002@yahoo.com
[1] Department of Biological Sciences, Federal University Dutsin-Ma, Dutsin-Ma, Katsina State, Nigeria
Full list of author information is available at the end of the article

such as plasmids, transposons and integrons contribute to *P. aeruginosa* multidrug resistance [5–8]. There is, however, a paucity of information about the molecular basis for antibiotic resistance for environmental *Pseudomonas* in southwestern Nigeria. Hence, we characterized selected multidrug resistant bacteria from water distribution systems from southwestern Nigeria using 16S rDNA sequencing and PCR genotyping.

Methods

Bacterial isolates

Independent multidrug resistant *Pseudomonas* isolates (n = 22) were selected between December 2010 and July 2011 from a pool of two hundred and ninety-one different bacteria genera from raw, treated and municipal taps of six selected water distribution systems in Ife, Ede, Asejire, Eleyele, Owena-Ondo and Owena-Idanre, in southwestern Nigeria. Methods for sampling and bacterial isolation were described previously [10]. Isolates were stored in freezing medium at −80 °C in 96-well plates until analysis.

Description of sample locations

The description of these dams' water distribution systems selected for this study is in our previous publications [9–11]. However, for clarity of this paper, raw water samples were taken from the untreated water from the dam at the point of entering the water treatment plants before passing through the plant. Treated water samples were taken from the final water after passing through all purification stages from the treatment plants before pumping to the municipal taps for public consumption while samples from the municipal taps were taking from the taps at the point of public consumption.

Extraction of DNA and molecular characterization of bacteria using 16S rDNA

The stock culture was streaked on Luria Betani (LB) agar and grown overnight. Afterwards, total genomic DNA was extracted by dispensing 200 μl of 5 % chelex in a tube. A loopful of the overnight grown colony of bacterium from LB agar was then inoculated into the solution. The mixture was then boiled at 100 °C for 10 min and centrifuge at 13 k×*g* for 1 min. Five microliter of the supernatant which consist of the extracted DNA was then used as template with 2 mM $MgCl_2$, 0.8 mM dNTPs, 0.2 μl of primer 1 and primer 2 and 1× PCR buffer. The reaction condition include 1 min denaturation (95 °C) followed by 30 cycles of 96 °C for 30 s, 60 °C for 30 s and 72 °C for 30 s and a final extension of 72 °C for 10 min. PCR products were then separated and visualized on 1 % agarose gel electrophoresis to confirm amplification. The 16S rDNA sequence was amplified using 16s-8F (AGAGTTTGATCMTGGCTCAG) and 16s-517 (ATTACCGCGGCTGCTGG) primers. PCR products were sequenced (Eurofins MWG, USA) and manual base calls and sequence trimming was completed by sequencer (5.0) BLAST [12] was used to identify close sequence matches (http://www.ncbi.nlm.nib.gov/BLAST/blast).

Phylogenetic tree construction

Phylogenetic relatedness of the 16s rDNA genes of these *Pseudomonas* was compared with 12 downloaded 16s rDNA sequences of other species from the gene bank. Sequences were aligned by multiple sequence alignment technique using CLUSTAL W [13] and a phylogenetic tree constructed by the neighbor joining method [14] using MEGA version 5 [15]. *Azotobacter chroococcum* (JQ692178)'s 16s rDNA was used as an outgroup.

Antimicrobial drug susceptibility and selection of multi-drug resistant *Pseudomonas* spp

Multi-drug resistant *Pseudomonas* was selected based on their resistance to over three classes of antibiotics. This was carried out after assessing antibiotic resistant properties of the *Pseudomonas* using break point assays on LB agar plates [9]. This involves autoclaving of LB agar and cooling down to 45 °C in a water bath and seeding with antibiotics of specific concentration (Table 1) based on Clinical Laboratory Standards Institute (CLSI) standard for gram negative bacteria [16]. Afterwards, the medium was then poured into Petri dishes (150 × 15 mm) and allowed to set. Overnight culture were then stabbed from 96-well plate onto agar plate using 96-well pin replicator and incubated overnight at 37 °C. Isolates were scored as '1' for growth and '0' for no growth on each antibiotics plate. It should be noted that *E. coli* strain K12 was used as negative control while *E. coli* strain H5N was used as positive control.

Table 1 Antibiotic concentrations tested against *Pseudomonas* spp

Code	Name	Concentration (μg/ml)
FF	Florfenicol	16
T	Tetracycline	16
S	Streptomycin	16
G	Gentamycin	16
K	Kanamycin	64
C	Chloramphenicol	32
N	Nalidixic acid	30
AMC	Amoxicillin/clavulanic acid	32/16
CEF	Ceftiofur	12
SU	Sulfamethoxazole	512
SXT	Sulfamethoxazole/trimethoprim	76/4

Assessing antibiotic resistance genes

In this study, six tetracycline, three sulfonamide, three extended β-lactamase and three streptomycin/spectinomycin resistance genes were amplified using specific primer specific for each gene and the annealing temperature as described in Table 2. The amplification of all the genes was carried out using 5 µl of the chelex extracted DNA as template for the PCR mixture with 5 µl of PCR buffer (1×), 2 µl of $MgCl_2$ (2 mM), 1 µl of dNTPs 0.8 mM and 1 µl (0.2 µl) each of the forward and reverse primers in a thermo cycler (Model: Bio Rad Laboratories, Richmond, CA, USA). The condition for the amplification of the genes include: 1 min of denaturation of 95 °C followed by 30 cycles of 96 °C for 30 s 60 °C for 30 s and

Table 2 Primers used in this study for amplification of class 1 and class 2 integrons and other antibiotic resistant genes

Primer pair	Target	Sequence (5′–3′)	Annealing temperature (oC)	Amplicon size (bp)	References
Primer 1 16s-8F	16S rDNA	AGAGTTTGATCMTGGCTCAG	60	456	[36]
Primer 2 16s-517	16S rDNA	ATTACCGCGGCTGCTGG	60	456	[37]
Intl1_F	Class 1 integrase gene	CCTCCCGCACGATGATC	55	270	[38]
Intl1_R		TCCACGCATCGTCAGGC			
Intl2_F	Class 2 integrase gene	TTATTGCTGGGATTAGGC	50	233	[39]
Intl2_R		ACGGCTACCCTCTGTTATC			
5′_CS	Class 1 integron variable region	GGCATCCAAGCAGCAAG	58.5	Variable	[40]
3′_CS		AAGCAGACTTGACCTGA			
Hep_F	Class 2 integron variable region	CGGGATCCCGGACGGCATGCACGATTTGTA	60	Variable	[41]
Hep_R		GATGCCATCGCAAGTACGAG			
Sul1-F	*sul*1	CGGCGTGGGCTACCTGAACG	60	433	[42]
Sul1-R		GCCGATCGCGTGAAGTTCCG			
Sul2-F	*sul*2	GCGCTCAAGGCAGATGGCATT	60	293	[42]
Sul2-R		GCGTTTGATACCGGCACCCGT			
pVP440sul3F	*sul*3	TCAAAGCAAAATGATATGAGC	55	787	[42]
pVP440sul3R		TTTCAAGGCATCTGATAAAGAC			
qacEΔ1F	*qacE*Δ1F	ATC GCA ATA GTT GGC GAA GT	58	800	[43]
sul1-B	*sul*1-B	GCA AGG CGG AAA CCC GCG CC	58		[44]
aph (3″)^c-F	*aph* (3″)^c	GCTCAAAGGTCGAGGTGTGG	55	515	[27]
aph (3″)^c-R		CCAGTTCTCTTCGGCGTTAG	55	515	[27]
ant (3″)^b-F	*ant* (3″)^b	CAGCGCAATGACATTCTTGC	55	295	[27]
ant (3″)^b-F		GTCGGCAGCGACA(C/T)CCTTCG	55	295	[27]
aph(6)-1d^d-F	*aph*(6)-1d^d	GACTCCTGCAATCGTCAAGG	55	560	[27]
aph(6)-1d^d-R		GCAATGCGTCTAGGATCGAG	55	560	[27]
tet(A)-F	*tet*(A)	TTGGCATTCTGCATTCACTC	60	494	[45]
tet(A)-R		GTATAGCTTGCCGGAAGTCG	60	494	[45]
tet(B)-F	*tet*(B)	CAGTGCTGTTGTTGTCATTAA	60	571	[45]
tet(B)-R		GCTTGGAATACTGAGTGTAA	60	571	[45]
tet(E)-F	*tet*(E)	TATTAACGGGCTGGCATTTC	55	544	[45]
tet(E)-R		AGCTGTCAGGTGGGTCAAAC	55	544	[45]
tet(M)-F		ACACGCCAGGACATATGGAT	55	536	[45]
tet(M)-R	*tet*(M)	ATTTCCGCAAAGTTCAGACG	55	536	[45]
tet(30)-F	*tet*(30)	CCGTCATGCAATTTGTGTTC	55	550	[45]
tet(30)-R		TAGAGCACCCAGATCGTTCC	55	550	[45]
SHV_F	bla_{SHV}	GCGAAAGCCAGCTGTCGGGC	62	538	[46]
SHV_R		GATTGGCGGCGCTGTTATCGC	62	538	[46]
CTX_F	bla_{CTX-M}	GTGCAGTACCAGTAAAGTTATGG	55	538	[46]
CTX_R		CGCAATATCATTGGTGGTGCC		538	[46]
TEM_F	bla_{TEM}	AAAGATGCTGAAGATCA	44	425	[46]
TEM_R		TTTGGTATGGCTTCATTC		425	[46]

72 °C for 30 s and final extension of 72 °C for 10 min. All these conditions remain the same during the amplification of the genes except the annealing temperature which is described in Table 2. PCR products were then separated and visualized on 1 % agarose gel electrophoresis to confirm amplification.

Assessing class 1 and 2 integrons

The integrase genes of class 1 and class 2 were amplified by the use of PCR using 5 µl of DNA template extracted by chelex method described above as template. Primer specific for the integrase gene and variable region was selected as described on Table 2. Condition for the PCR was also as described above except for the annealing temperature which was as described on Table 2. It should be noted that after amplification of gene cassette of both Class 1 and Class 2 integrons using 5′-CS/3′-CS and hep_F/hep_R, respectively. PCR products of the amplified genes were used for sequencing (Eurofins MWG, USA). The putative gene cassettes harboured on the integrase sequences were determined through online similarity searches using the BLAST software in the National Center for Biotechnology Information website (http://www.ncbi.nlm.nih.gov/).

Determination of presence of plasmid on bacteria isolates

Bacteria (*Pseudomonas* isolates) were grown on Luria–Bertani (LB) agar overnight and a single colony was picked and inoculated overnight as well in LB Broth. One hundred and fifty microliter of the culture was later pelleted from the culture by centrifugation for 10 min at 1000×*g*. The supernatant was removed and re-suspended in 100 µl of lysis buffer (3 % SDS, 50 mM Tris pH 12.6 with 50 mM Tris adjusted by 1.6 ml 2 N NaOH up to 100 ml final volume). The mixture was incubated at 55 °C for 1 h. The resulting plasmid was extracted with 150 µl of phenol:chloroform (1:1, v/v, pH 7.9) and mixed by inversion several times before spinning at highest speed for 10 min. Fifty microliter of the supernatant was transferred into a new tube and mixed with 10 µl of 10× loading dye (Invitrogen). The mixture containing the plasmid was run on 1 % agarose gel electrophoresis in 1× TAE (tris-acetate buffer).

Results

Bacteria isolates

In this study, 22 MDR *Pseudomonas* were identified by 16S rDNA out of a total of 296 different strains that were isolated from all sampled water as *P. putida*, *P. fluorescens* and *P. otitidis* (Table 3). Phylogenetic studies showed 10 of the Pseudomonads to be in single distinct cluster with *P. graminis* (KC790241.1) from leaf of *Wasabia japonica* from China, *P. putida* (JQ968690.1) from activated sludge in China, *Pseudomonas* spp (AB302400.1) from Japan and uncultured bacterium (HQ121069.1) from USA. Others such as *Pseudomonas* spp (JF683300) and *Pseudomonas* spp (FM161425.1) from Ede municipal tap and Asejire treated water, respectively belong to the same cluster (Fig. 1).

Antimicrobial susceptibility

Figure 2 and Table 3 showed the results of the percentage resistance of the studies bacteria and their phenotypic patterns of resistance, respectively. We observed among the studied *Pseudomonas* higher resistance to florfenicol (63.6 %), tetracycline (59.1 %), streptomycin (54.6 %), ceftiofur (59.1 %), amoxicillin/clavulanic acid (81.8 %), sulfamethoxazole (77.3 %) compared to chloramphenicol (40.9 %), gentamicin (31.8 %), kanamycin (31.8 %) and nalidixic acid (22.7 %). From these results, it was noticed that these isolates were more resistant to older generation antibiotics (such as sulfamethoxazole, tetracycline, streptomycin etc.) than new generation antibiotics such as (gentamicin, kanamycin and nalidixic acid). We also saw that out of 22 *Pseudomonas* spp isolated from all the sampled area 21 were multi-drug resistant (MDR) (Table 3). The MDR bacteria were selected based on resistant to over three classes of antibiotics.

Molecular characterization of antibiotic resistance genes

Beyond the phenotypic determination, we tested for the presence of some antibiotic resistance genes which could have been mediating the antibiotic resistance in the *Pseudomonas* spp. Among the tetracycline resistance gene tested i.e. *tet*(A), *tet*(B), *tet*(E) and *tet*30 encoding resistant by efflux pump mechanism and *tet*(O) and *tet*(M) encoding resistant by protection of the ribosome. We observed that *tet*(A) was the highest occurred (31.8 %) followed by *tet*(E) and *tet*30 (4.5 %) (Table 3). We did not detect *tet*(B), *tet*(M) and *tet*(O) among the *Pseudomonas* isolates. Among three sulphonamide resistance genes tested for in this study. It was observed that *sul 1* was the highest (31.8 %) detected followed by *sul 2* (27.3 %) (Table 3). *Sul 3* was not detected in any of the *Pseudomonas* while among the three extended beta lactamase (ESBL) genes: bla_{SHV}, bla_{CTX}, bla_{TEM}, we observed that bla_{TEM} was the highest (40.9 %) detected followed by bla_{SHV} (27.3 %) while bla_{CTX} was not detected at all (Table 3).

We also observed the presence of all three streptomycin resistance genes tested for in at least one of the isolates (Table 3). *Aph(3″)*[c] and *ant(3″)* was the most detected, each was observed to be present in 36.4 % of isolates tested while *aph (6)1d*[d] was the least (13.7) detected. Class 2 integron was not detected in any of the isolates

Table 3 Phenotypes, antibiotics resistance gene and integrons among MDR *Pseudomonas spp*

Source	Strain ID	Bacteria	Phenotype	*tet*(A)	*tet* (B)	*tet* (E)	*tet*(M)	*tet* (30)	*Sul 1*	*Sul 2*	*bla*SHV	*bla*CTX	*bla*TEM	*aph* (3″)[c]	*ant* (3″)[b]	*aph* (6)*1d*[d]	int 1	v 1	int 2	v 2
IRW	96b	*P. putida*	FF, T, CEF, SU, AMC	–	–	–	–	–	–	–	–	–	–	–	–	–	–	–	–	–
IFW	89	*P. putida*	T, S, G, K, C, SXT, AMC, SU	+	–	–	–	+	–	–	+	–	+	+	+	–	–	–	–	–
EDRW	299A	*P. otitidis*	FF, C, SXT, AMC, SU	–	–	–	–	–	–	–	–	–	–	–	–	–	–	–	–	–
EDRW	99A	*P. putida*	FF, SXT, AMC	–	–	–	–	–	–	+	–	–	–	–	–	–	–	–	–	–
EDRW	299B2	*P. otitidis*	FF, CEF, AMC, SU	–	–	–	–	–	–	–	–	–	–	–	+	–	–	–	–	–
EDM1	159B	*P. fluorescens*	T, S, G, N, CEF, SXT	–	–	–	–	–	–	–	–	–	+	–	–	–	–	–	–	–
EDM1	304A	*P. otitidis*	T, SU, SXT, AMC, S, G, CEF, FF	–	–	–	–	–	–	–	–	–	+	–	+	–	–	–	–	–
EDM1	306A	*P. otitidis*	FF, CEF, AMC, SU	–	–	–	–	–	–	–	–	–	–	–	–	–	–	–	–	–
EDM1	85B	*P. putida*	SXT, AMC, C, FF	–	–	–	–	–	–	+	+	–	–	–	–	–	–	–	–	–
EDM1	106	*P. putida*	T, SU, SXT, AMC, S, N	–	–	–	–	–	–	–	–	–	+	–	–	–	–	–	–	–
AFW	6B	*P. fluorescens*	T, S, G, K, CEF, SXT	–	–	–	–	–	–	+	–	–	–	–	–	–	–	–	–	–
AFW	6A	*P. fluorescens*	T, S, G, K, C, CEF, SXT, AMC, SU, FF	+	–	–	–	–	+	–	+	–	+	+	+	–	+	+	–	–
OWODFW	350	*P. otitidis*	SXT, SU	–	–	–	–	–	+	–	–	–	–	–	–	–	–	–	–	–
OWODM1	260	*P. putida*	FF, T, C, N, CEF, SXT, AMC, SU	–	–	–	–	–	–	–	–	–	+	–	+	–	–	–	–	–
OWODM2	251B	*P. putida*	T, S, C, SXT, SU	+	–	–	–	–	+	+	+	–	–	+	+	+	+	+	–	–
OWIRW	343B	*P. otitidis*	FF, T, S, N, CEF, AMC, SU	+	–	–	–	–	+	–	–	–	–	–	–	–	+	–	–	–
OWIRW	343A	*P. otitidis*	FF, K, C, SXT, N, CEF, AMC, SU	–	–	–	–	–	–	–	–	–	–	+	–	–	–	–	–	–
OWIRW	223	*P. otitidis*	FF, S, C, CEF, SXT, AMC, SU	–	–	–	–	–	–	–	–	–	–	+	–	–	–	–	–	–
OWRW	175B	*P. putida*	T, S, C, K, CEF, SXT, AMC, SU	+	–	–	–	–	+	+	–	–	+	+	–	+	+	+	–	–
OWIRW	342A	*P. otitidis*	FF, AMC, CEF, SU	–	–	–	–	–	–	–	–	–	–	–	–	–	–	–	–	–

Table 3 continued

Source	Strain ID	Bacteria	Phenotype	*tet*(A)	*tet* (B)	*tet* (E)	*tet*(M)	*tet* (30)	*Sul 1*	*Sul 2*	*bla*SHV	*bla*CTX	*bla*TEM	*aph* (3″)[c]	*ant* (3″)[b]	*aph* (6)1*d*[d]	int 1	v 1	int 2	v 2
OWIM1	196	*P. putida*	FF, T, S, G, K, AMC, SU	+	−	+	−	−	+	−	−	−	+	+	+	−	+	+	−	−
OWIM2	244B	*P. putida*	FF, T, S, G, K, C, SXT, AMC, SU	+	−	−	−	−	+	+	+	−	+	+	+	+	+	+	−	−
			Total	7	0	1	0	1	7	6	5	0	9	8	8	3	6			
			Percentages	31.8	0	4.6	0	4.6	31.8	27.3	27.3	0	40.9	36.4	36.4	13.6	27.3			

Antibiotics code: *FF* florfenicol, *T* tetracycline, *S* streptomycin, *G* gentamicin, *K* kanamycin, *C* chloramphenicol, *N* nalidixic acid, *AMC* amoxicillin/clavulanic acid, *CEF* ceftiofur, *SU* sulfamethoxazole, *SXT* sulfamethoxazole/trimethoprim

Source code: *IFW* Ife treated water, *EDM1* Ede municipal Tap 1, *AFW* Asejire treated water, *OWODM2* Owena Ondo Municipal Tap 2, *OWIRW* Owena-Idanre raw water, *OWIM1* Owena-Idanre Municipal Tap 1, *OWIM2* Owena-Idanre Municipal Tap 2

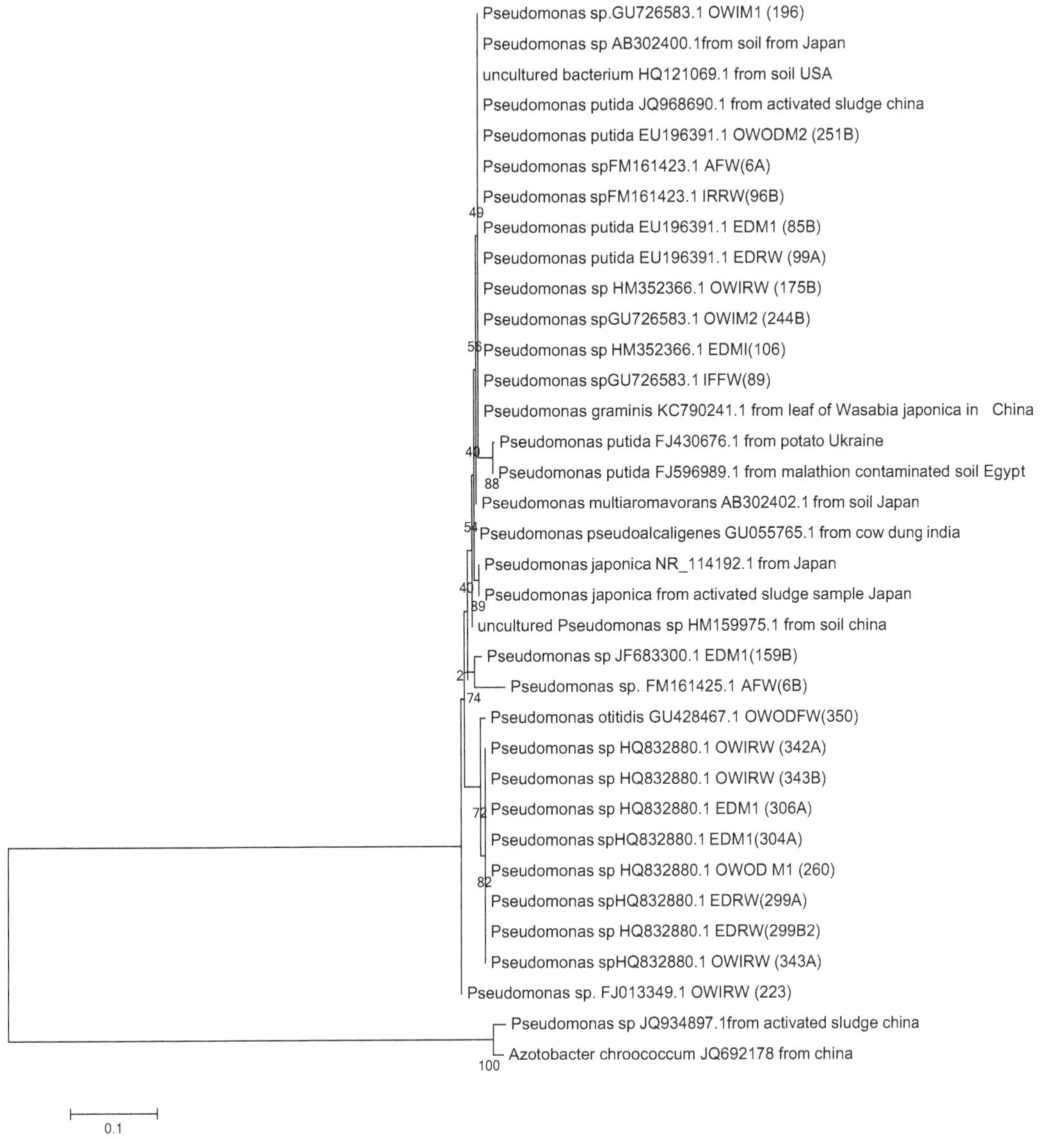

Fig. 1 Phylogenetic relationship of 16S rDNA of *Pseudomonas* spp from south western Nigeria water distribution system with sequence from gene bank

(Table 3). Whereas, 6 (27.3 %) of the isolates showed the occurrence of class 1 integron.

Plasmid profiling

The presence of plasmid was observed in 10 (45.5 %) out of 22 *Pseudomonas* studied (Table 4). Each of the bacteria was observed to be carrying 1 plasmid each ranging between 22 and 130 kb in size. None of the bacteria showed the occurrence of more than one plasmid.

Discussion

Pseudomonad is one of the most important and ubiquitous pathogen that is significantly important medically [17]. Aquatic ecosystems could serve as a reservoir of antibiotic resistant pathogen through transfer of resistant plasmid [18]. Many studies on antibiotic resistance in pseudomonads had been carried out using strains of clinical origin [19]. This study selected 22 MDR Pseudomonas from drinking water distribution systems from southwestern Nigeria. These selected MDR strains showed high resistant to amoxillin/clavulanic acid (81.8 %), sulfamethoxazole (77.3 %) and sulfamethoxazole/trimethoprim (72.7 %). Resistant to amoxillin/clavulanic acid is a little similar to the report of Mezue et al. [20] among *Pseudomonas* from urinary tract infection from Nigeria who reported 100 % resistant to the

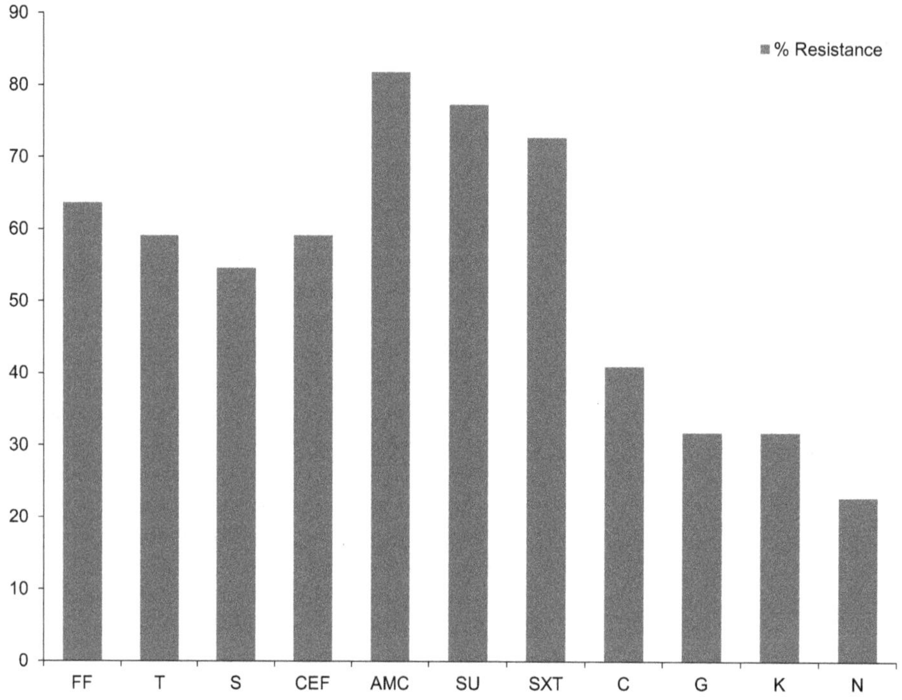

Fig. 2 Percentage resistance of *Pseudomonas* spp to various antibiotics. *FF* florfenicol, *T* tetracycline, *S* streptomycin, *G* gentamicin, *K* kanamycin, *C* chloramphenicol, *N* nalidixic acid, *AMC* amoxicillin/clavulanic acid, *CEF* ceftiofur, *SU* sulfamethoxazole, *SXT* sulfamethoxazole/trimethoprim

Table 4 Plasmid carrying *Pseudomonas* spp. isolated from selected water samples from southwestern Nigeria

Source	Bacteria/strain ID	Resistant phenotypes	No of plasmid and size
IFW	*Pseudomonas* sp (89)	T, S, G, K, C, SXT, AMC, SU	1 (95 kb)
EDM1	*Pseudomonas* sp (306A)	FF, CEF, AMC, SU	1 (95 kb)
AFW	*Pseudomonas* sp (6A)	T, S, G, K, C, CEF, SXT, AMC, SU, FF	1 (95 kb)
AFW	*Pseudomonas* sp (6B)	T, S, G, K, CEF, SXT	1 (95 kb)
OWODM2	*Pseudomonas putida* (251B)	T, S, C, SXT, SU	1 (22 kb)
OWIRW	*Pseudomonas* sp (175B)	T, S, C, K, CEF, SXT, AMC, SU	1 (55 kb)
OWIRW	*Pseudomonas* sp (342A)	FF, AMC, CEF, SU	1 (130 kb)
OWIRW	*Pseudomonas* sp (343B)	FF, T, S, N, CEF, AM, AMC, SU	1 (130 kb)
OWIM1	*Pseudomonas* sp (196)	FF, T, S, G, K, AM, AMC, SU	1 (120 kb)
OWIM2	*Pseudomonas* sp (244B)	FF, T, S, G, K, C, AM, SXT, AMC, SU	1 (130 kb)

Antibiotics code: *FF* florfenicol, *T* tetracycline, *S* streptomycin, *G* gentamicin, *K* kanamycin, *C* chloramphenicol, *N* nalidixic acid, *AMC* amoxicillin/clavulanic acid, *CEF* ceftiofur, *SU* sulfamethoxazole, *SXT* sulfamethoxazole/trimethoprim

Source code: *IFW* Ife treated water, *EDM1* Ede municipal Tap 1, *AFW* Asejire treated water, *OWODM2* Owena Ondo Municipal Tap 2, *OWIRW* Owena-Idanre raw water, *OWIM1* Owena-Idanre Municipal Tap 1, *OWIM2* Owena-Idanre Municipal Tap 2

antibiotics in their studies. Moderate resistant to florfenicol (63.6 %), tetracycline (59.1 %), streptomycin (54.6 %) and ceftiofur (59.1 %) was observed among these Pseudomonads. The tetracycline resistance obtained in our study is similar to what Akinpelu et al. [21] reported among *Pseudomonas* from another river in Nigeria. The author reported 50 % resistant to tetracycline among their pseudomonads while higher (100 %) resistant to streptomycin compare to what we obtained from the isolates in this study.

Molecular characterization of the antibiotic resistance gene showed high prevalence of *tet*(A) (31.8 %), *sul2* (27.8 %), bla_{TEM} (40.9) for tetracycline, sulfa drug and β-lactamase antibiotic resistance, respectively. There appears to be few studies on the molecular characterization of these genes among Nigeria environmental pseudomonads, therefore, making it difficult to compare with studies from Nigeria. However, among few of the studies, Chikwendu et al. [22] reported the presence of bla_{SHV} and bla_{TEM} among environmental pseudomonads from Nigeria while Odumosu et al. [23] reported $bla_{oxa\text{-}10}$, ampC β-lactamase in 50 and 70 % of *Pseudomonas aeruginosa*, respectively from Nigeria clinical source. The authors reported that only one of their isolates testing positive for bla_{SHV} and $bla_{CTXM\text{-}15}$. Studies have shown that due to overuse of β-lactam antibiotics, bla_{TEM} and bla_{SHV} enzyme that were originally found in enterobacteriaceae are now found in *Pseudomonas* [24]. Similarly, the authors also reported that bla_{SHV} enzyme that has been found in *Klebsiella, Escherichia* and *Salmonella* can also be found in *Pseudomonas.* Moreover, in this study we did not detect bla_{TEM} from any of the *Pseudomonas* studied from these water distribution systems.

We observed 36.36 % of our pseudomonas testing positive for each of *aph(3″)*^{c} and *ant(3″)*^{b} which are genes coding for enzymes that modifies aminoglycoside antibiotics. Odumosu et al. [23] also reported the presence of aminoglycoside modifying enzyme (AME) genes which include *aac(6′)-I* and *ant(2″)-I* in 50 and 45 %, respectively of their isolates from Nigeria clinical *Pseudomonas.* Publications on AME genes among Nigeria environmental *Pseudomonas* spp are also scarce. This could be the first time these genes will be described among pseudomonad from Nigeria environment. However, in Africa, Ndegwa et al. [25] reported the presence of AME in *E. coli, klebsiella, Pseudomonas* and *Acinetobacter* from clinical isolates from Kenya. Though in this study, at least one of the AME genes occurred in at least one of these environmental bacteria. It has been reported that the incidence of streptomycin resistance in pathogenic and commensal bacteria in clinical and agricultural habitats is often high. This is most likely caused by the use of streptomycin in these environments [26]. We observed *aph (3″)*^{c} and *ant (3″)* to be more frequently detected in this study than *aph (6)1d*^{d}. This is similar to the study of van Overbeek et al. [27] among bacterial populations in European habitat. The authors reported that out of 22 bacteria isolates whose genomic DNA was extracted and amplified for streptomycin resistance gene, *aph (3″)*^{c} was the highest occurred, showing its presence in 17 isolates, followed by *ant (3″)* and *aph* (6)-*1d* (both present in 13 isolates), whereas the incidence of *aph* (6)-*1c* and *ant* (6) genes was lowest (present in one and zero isolates, respectively). Occurrence of one bacteria carrying more than one of streptomycin resistance genes was observed in this study. This is also similar to the report of van Overbeek et al. [27].

Similarly, tetracycline resistance gene has also not been described in among Pseudomonads from Nigeria. Although our recent report [28] stated the occurrence of *tet*(E), *tet*(M), *tet*(30) among *Alcaligenes*, *tet*(E) in *Aeromonas* and *Klebsiella*, *tet*(B) in *Bacillus* and *Leucobacter* from these water distribution systems. Absence of *tet*(B) but highest occurrence of *tet*(A) which are both efflux pump genes in these pseudomonads is contrary to the report of Shababi et al. [29] who reported more prevalence of *tet*(B) than *tet*(A) in their studies among MDR *P. aeruginosa* from municipal sewage. However, a study had shown that *tet*(A) has a broad host range and is often carried by various environmental genera [4]. None of the isolates showed the presence of tetracycline resistance gene [*tet*(O) and *tet*(M)] that cause resistant by producing protein that modifies the ribosome.

Occurrence of class 1 integron among these bacteria showed their potential ability to shuttle antibiotic resistance between different bacteria species. This is because integrons are mobile DNA element with the ability to integrate and express gene cassettes by site-specific recombination [30, 31]. Integrase sequence can insert many cassettes coding for different antibiotic resistance, therefore, making a single bacterium possessing it to be resistant to multiple antibiotics. Therefore, emergence of these MDR bacteria with class 1 integron could lead to reduce antibiotic treatment option which could result to an increase possibility of treatment failure, if they infect user of these water. In fact, most of the genes like aminoglycoside resistance, β-lactam resistance and sulphadrug resistance have been reported as gene cassettes in association with class 1 integron [32]. Five of these pseudomonads were observed to test positive for the variable region of this class 1 integron. This implies the insertion of antibiotic resistant cassette in the integrase sequence and these resistance gene cassettes include aminoglycosides (*aadA2, aadA1*), trimethoprim (*dfrA15, dfr7*) and sulphonamide (*sul1*) resistance.

The size of plasmids observed from our study contradicts previous studies from Nigeria [6, 33] which reported low molecular weight plasmids (<2 kb) among bacteria from clinical isolates of *P. aeroginosa.* The relationship between plasmid profiles and MDR patterns observed in this study suggests that plasmids may have great role to play in the multidrug resistance of the *Pseudomonas.* Plasmids usually evolve as an integral part of the bacterial genome, consisting of several extra-chromosomal traits, one of which is their resistance genes, which can be exchanged among bacteria of different origins by conjugation [34]. Global dissemination of multiple antibiotic resistance and virulence traits by plasmids also poses an increasing threat to the successful treatment of bacterial infectious diseases in animals and humans alike [35].

Therefore, water sample containing these bacteria may be a source of transfer of antibiotic resistance genes to pathogenic bacteria of human, animal and environmental health significance.

Conclusion

In summary, the occurrence of MDR *Pseudomonas* harbouring various antibiotic resistance genes, class 1 integron and plasmid in drinking water systems signify that these environmental pseudomonads could significantly contribute to wide-scale transfer of resistance genes in these environments thereby posing health hazard to man and animals that depend on these water sources. This could play a major role in the epidemiology of antibiotic resistance in Nigeria and could also be responsible for prolong treatment of bacterial infection, the emergence of emerging and re-emerging infectious diseases. We hereby recommend integrated antibiotic resistant surveillance system and holistic one health approach as well as promoting prudent use of antibiotics both in clinical and agriculture settings in order to prevent and control multidrug resistant bacteria in southwestern Nigeria.

Authors' contributions

ATA and AAO planned this study. ATA performed the experiment in conjunction with IOO. ATA wrote the manuscript while IOO and AAO made significant contributions to the manuscript preparation. All authors read and approved the final manuscript.

Author details

[1] Department of Biological Sciences, Federal University Dutsin-Ma, Dutsin-Ma, Katsina State, Nigeria. [2] Department of Microbiology, University of Ibadan, Ibadan, Nigeria. [3] Department of Veterinary Public Health and Preventive Medicine, University of Ibadan, Ibadan, Oyo State, Nigeria. [4] Paul G. Allen School for Global Animal Health, Washington State University, Pullman, WA, USA.

Acknowledgements

We acknowledge Dr Call Douglas of Paul. G. Allen School of Global Animal Health, Washington State University, USA who allowed the Molecular Characterization of the bacteria isolates to be carried out in his Laboratory and also Lisa Lorfe who supplied the technical knowhow.

Competing interests

The authors declare that they have no competing interests.

References

1. Craun GF, Calderon RL, Craun MF. Outbreaks associated with recreational water in the United States. Int J Environ Health Res. 2005;15:243–62.
2. Pollack M. Principles and practice of infectious diseases, eds. In: Mandell, G. L., Bennet, J. E. and Dolin, R. (*Churchill Livingstone, Philadelphia*).2000 2: 2310-2335.
3. Lyczak JB, Cannon CL, Pier GB. Lung infection associated with cystic fibrosis. Clin Microbiol Rev. 2002;15:194–222.
4. Zhang XX, Zhang T, Fang HHP. Antibiotic resistance genes in water environment. Appl Microbiol Biotechnol. 2009;82:397–414.
5. Bonomo RA, Szabo D. Mechanisms of multidrug resistance in *Acinetobacter* species and *Pseudomonas aeruginosa*. Clin Infect Dis. 2006;43:49–56.
6. Yah SC, Eghafona NO, Enabulele IO. Prevalence of plasmids mediated *Pseudomonas aeruginosa* resistant genes from burn wound patients at the university of Benin teaching hospital Benin City. Nigeria J Biomed Sci. 2006;5:61–8.
7. Chen J, Su Z, Liu Y, Wang S, Dai X, Li Y, Peng S, Shao Q, Zhang H, Wen P, Yu J, Huang X, Xu H. Identification and characterization of class 1 integrons among *Pseudomonas aeruginosa* isolates from patients in Zhenjiang, China. Int J Infect Dis. 2009;13:717–21.
8. Ruiz-Martínez L, López-Jiménez L, Fusté E, Vinuesa T, Martínez JP, Viñas M. Class integrons in environmental and clinical isolates of *Pseudomonas aeruginosa*. Int J Antimicrob Agents. 2011;38:398–402.
9. Adesoji AT, Ogunjobi AA. Occurrence of multidrug-resistant bacteria in selected water distribution systems in Oyo State, Nigeria. Glob Vet. 2013;11:214–24.
10. Adesoji AT, Ogunjobi AA. Physicochemical properties and occurrence of antibiotic-resistant bacteria in Ife and Ede water distribution systems of southwestern Nigeria. World Appl Sci J. 2013;27:1098–110.
11. Adesoji AT, Ogunjobi AA, Olatoye IO. Drinking water distribution systems of dams in Ondo state, Nigeria as reservoir of multi-drug resistant bacteria. World Appl Sci J. 2014;32:403–14.
12. Altschul SF, Madden TL, Schäffer AA, Zhang J, Zhang Z, Miller W, Lipman DJ. Gapped BLAST and PSI-BLAST: a new generation of protein database search programs. Nucleic Acids Res. 2007;25:3389–402. http://www.ncbi.nlm.nih.gov/BLAST.
13. Thompson JD, Higgins DG, Gibson TJ. CLUSTAL W: improving the sensitivity of progressive multiple sequence alignment through sequence weighting, position-specific gap penalties and weight matrix choice. Nucleic Acids Res. 1994;22:4673–80.
14. Saitou N, Nei M. The neighbor-joining method: a new method for reconstructing phylogenetic trees. Mol Bio Evol. 1987;4:406–25.
15. Kumar S, Tamura K, Nei M. MEGA3: integrated software for molecular evolutionary genetics analysis and sequence alignment. Brief Bioinform. 2004;5:150–63.
16. CLSI (Clinical and Laboratory Standards Institute) Performance standards for antimicrobial susceptibility testing: 15th informational supplement M100-S15. Wayne: CLSI; 2005.
17. Pollack M. *Pseudomonas aeruginosa*. In: Mandell GL, Dolan R, Bennett JE, editors. Principles and practices of infectious diseases. New York: Churchill Livingstone; 1995. p. 1820–2003.
18. Baquero F, Martínez JL, Cantó N. Antibiotics and antibiotic resistance in water environments. Curr Opin Biotechnol. 2008;19:260–5.
19. Ndip RN, Dilonga HM, Ndip LM, Akoachere JF, Nkuo Akenji T. *Pseudomonas aeruginosa* isolates recovered from clinical and environmental samples in Buea, Cameroon: current status on biotyping and antibiogram. Trop Med Int Health. 2005;10:74–81.
20. Mezue K, Ofong C, Nmezi D, Ugochukwu-Obi G. Antibiotic Sensitivity patterns in urinary tract infection at Tertiary Hospital. Medikka J Univ Nigeria Med Stud. 2006. Available on http://www.medikkajournal.com/UTI.htm. Extracted on 7/01/2015.
21. Akinpelu AT, Akinloye OM, Olukemi BC, Adegoke AE, Olayinka S. Antibiotic resistant pattern of isolated bacteria from Obere River in Orile-Igbon, Oyo State Nigeria. Afr J Microbiol Res. 2014;8:1318–21.
22. Chikwendu CI, Ibe SN, Okpokwasili GC. Detection of bla_{SHV} and bla_{TEM} beta-lactamase genes in multi-resistant *Pseudomonas* isolates from environmental sources. Afr J Microbiol Res. 2011;5:2067–74.
23. Odumosu BT, Adeniyi BA, Chandra R. Analysis of integrons and associated gene cassettes in clinical isolates of multidrug resistant *Pseudomonas aeruginosa* from Southwest Nigeria. Ann Clin Microbiol Antimicrob. 2013;12:29–35.
24. Bradford PA. Extended-spectrum beta-lactamases in the 21st century: characterization, epidemiology, and detection of this important resistance threat. Clin Microbiol Rev. 2001;14:933–51.
25. Ndegwa DW, Budambula NLM, Kariuki G, Kiiru JN. Aminoglycoside modifying enzymes detected in strains of *Escherichia*, *Klebsiella*, *Pseudomonas* and *Acinetobacter* implicated in invasive infections in Nairobi, Kenya. In: Proceedings of 2010 JKUAT scientific technological and industrialization conference Centre for Microbiology. Nairobi, Kenya: Kenya Medical Research Institute; 2010.

26. Seveno NA, Kallifidas D, Smalla K, van Elsas JD, Collard JM, Karagouni AD, Wellington EMH. Occurrence of reservoirs of antibiotic resistance genes in the environment. Rev Med Microbiol. 2002;13:15–27.
27. van Overbeek LSV, Wellington EMH, Egan S, Smalla K, Heuer H, Collard JM, Guillaume G, Karagouni AD, Nikolakopoulou TL, Elsas JDVE. Prevalence of streptomycin-resistance genes in bacterial populations in European habitats. FEMS Microbiol Ecol. 2001;42:277–88.
28. Adesoji AT, Ogunjobi AA, Olatoye IO, Call DR. Prevalence of tetracycline resistance genes among multi-drug resistant bacteria from selected water distribution systems in southwestern Nigeria. Ann Clin Microbiol Antimicrob. 2015;14:35. doi:10.1186/s12941-015-0093-1.
29. Shehabi AA, Haider AA, Fayyad MK. Frequency of antimicrobial resistance markers among *Pseudomonas aeruginosa* and *Escherichia coli* isolates from municipal sewage effluent water and patients in Jordan. Int Arabic J Antimicrob Agents. 2011;1:1–5.
30. Mazel D. Integrons: agents of bacterial evolution. Nat Rev Microbiol. 2006;4:608–20.
31. Rowe-Magnus DA, Mazel D. The role of integrons in antibiotic resistance gene capture. Int J Med Microbiol. 2002;292:115–25.
32. Poonsuk K, Tribuddharat C, Chuanchuen R. Class 1 integrons in *Pseudomonas aeruginosa* and *Acinetobacter baumannii* isolated from clinical isolates. Southeast Asian J Trop Med Public Health. 2012;43:376–84.
33. Olayinka AT, Onile BA, Olayinka BO. Prevalence of multi-drug resistant (MDR) *Pseudomonas aeruginosa* isolates in surgical units of Ahmadu Bello University Teaching Hospital, Zaria, Nigeria: an indication for effective control measures. Afr Med. 2004;3:13–6.
34. Carattoli A. Plasmids in Gram negatives: molecular typing of resistance plasmids. Int J Med Microbiol. 2011;301:654–8.
35. Bush K. Bench-to-bedside review: the role of beta-lactamases in antibiotic-resistant Gram-negative infections. Crit Care. 2010;14:224.
36. Baker GC, Smith JJ, Cowan DA. Review and reanalysis of domain-specific 16S primers. J Microbiol Methods. 2003;55:541–55.
37. Muyzer G, de Waal EC, Uitterlinden AG. Profiling of complex microbial populations by denaturing gradient gel electrophoresis analysis of polymerase chain reaction-amplified genes coding for 16S rRNA. Appl Environ Microbiol. 1993;59:695–700.
38. Houang AT, Chu YW, Lo WS, Chu KY, Cheng AF. Epidemiology of rifampin ADP-ribosyltransferase (*arr-2*) and metallo-b-lactamase (bla_{IMP-4}) gene cassettes in class 1 integrons in *Acinetobacter* strains isolated from blood cultures in 1997 to 2000. Antimicrob Agents Chemother. 2003;47:1382–90.
39. Roe MT, Vega E, Pillai SD. Antimicrobial resistance markers of Class 1 and Class 2 integron bearing *Escherichia coli* from irrigation water and sediments. Emerg Infect Dis. 2003;9:822–6.
40. Hall RM, Collis CM. Mobile gene cassettes and integrons: capture and spread of genes by site-specific recombination. Mol Microbiol. 1995;15:593–600.
41. White PA, Mciver CJ, Rawlinson WD. Integrons and gene cassettes in the Enterobacteriaceae. Antimicrob Agents Chemother. 2001;45:2658–61.
42. Vinue L, Saenz Y, Rojo-Bezares B, Olarte I, Undabeitia E, Somalo S, Zarazaga M, Torres C. Genetic environment of *sul* genes and characterisation of integrons in *Escherichia coli* isolates of blood origin in a Spanish hospital. Int J Antimicrob Agents. 2010;35:492–6.
43. Stokes HW, Hall RM. A novel family of potentially mobile DNA elements encoding site-specific gene-integration functions: integrons. Mol Microbiol. 1989;3:1669–83.
44. Sundstrom L. The potential of integrons and connected programmed rearrangements for mediating horizontal gene transfer. APMIS. 1998;84:37–42.
45. Call DR, Brockman FJ, Chandler DP. Detecting and genotyping *Escherichia coli* O157:H7 using multiplexed PCR and nucleic acid microarrays. Int J Food Microbiol. 2003;67:71–80.
46. Henriques IS, Fonseca F, Alves A, Saavedra MJ, Correia A. Occurrence and diversity of integrons and β-lactamase genes among ampicillin-resistant isolates from estuarine waters. Res Microbiol. 2006;157:938–47.

2

Occurrence of *bla*$_{DHA-1}$ mediated cephalosporin resistance in *Escherichia coli* and their transcriptional response against cephalosporin stress

Birson Ingti[1], Deepjyoti Paul[1], Anand Prakash Maurya[1], Debajyoti Bora[3], Debadatta Dhar Chanda[2], Atanu Chakravarty[2] and Amitabha Bhattacharjee[1*]

Abstract

Background: Treatment alternatives for DHA-1 harboring strains are challenging as it confers resistance to broad spectrum cephalosporins and may further limit treatment option when expressed at higher levels. Therefore, this study was designed to know the prevalence of DHA genes and analyse the transcription level of DHA-1 against different β-lactam stress.

Methods: Screening of AmpC β-lactamase phenotypically by modified three dimensional extract method followed by Antimicrobial Susceptibility and MIC determination. Genotyping screening of β-lactamase genes was performed by PCR assay followed by their sequencing. The *bla*$_{DHA-1}$ transcriptional response was evaluated under different cephalosporin stress by RT PCR. Transferability of *bla*$_{DHA}$ gene was performed by transformation and conjugation and plasmid incompatibility typing, DNA fingerprinting by enterobacterial repetitive intergenic consensus sequences PCR.

Results: 16 DHA-1 genes were screened positive from 176 *Escherichia coli* isolates and primer extension analysis showed a significant increase in DHA-1 mRNA transcription in response to cefotaxime at 8 μg/ml (6.99×10^2 fold), ceftriaxone at 2 μg/ml (2.63×10^3 fold), ceftazidime at 8 μg/ml (7.06×10^3 fold) and cefoxitin at 4 μg/ml (3.60×10^4 fold) when compared with untreated strain. These transcription data were found significant when analyzed statistically using one way ANOVA. Four different ESBL genes were detected in 10 isolates which include CTX-M (n = 6), SHV (n = 4), TEM (n = 3) and OXA-10 (n = 1), whereas, carbapenemase gene (NDM) was detected only in one isolate. Other plasmid mediated AmpC β-lactamases CIT (n = 9), EBC (n = 2) were detected in nine isolates. All DHA-1 genes detected were encoded in plasmid and incompatibility typing from the transformants indicated that the plasmid encoding *bla*$_{DHA-1}$ was carried mostly by the FIA and L/M Inc group.

Conclusion: This study demonstrates the prevalence of DHA-1 gene in this region and highlights high transcription of DHA-1 when induced with different β-lactam antibiotics. Therefore, cephalosporin treatment must be restricted for the patients infected with pathogen expressing this resistance determinant.

Background

Escherichia coli (E. coli) possess a chromosomal cephalosporinase gene, which is regulated by a weak promoter and a transcriptional attenuator. The gene confers resistance only to narrow-spectrum cephalosporins [1, 2]. However, spontaneous mutations in the promoter, as well as transcriptional attenuator region of the AmpC gene may induce constitutive overproduction of the cephalosporinase resulting in resistance to penicillins and broad-spectrum cephalosporins (e.g. cefotaxime, ceftazidime, ceftriaxone, aztreonam etc.) [3, 4]. Besides hyper-production of the chromosomally encoded enzyme, the presence of one or more plasmid-mediated AmpC β-lactamases along with other intrinsic mechanisms in *E. coli* leads to resistance

*Correspondence: ab0404@gmail.com
[1] Department of Microbiology, Assam University, Silchar 788011, India
Full list of author information is available at the end of the article

against multiple antimicrobial agents, compromising the efficacy of treatment [5–7]. Six families of plasmid-encoded AmpC β-lactamases were described based on their sequence similarities as CIT, FOX, MOX, DHA, EBC, and ACC [8]. The most commonly recognized plasmid-mediated AmpC among the strains of *E. coli* includes the CMY-2 type which belongs to the CIT family [9, 10].

DHA-1, another plasmid-mediated AmpC β-lactamase, belonging to DHA family was found increasingly among Enterobacteriaceae in many parts of the world and was a growing concerned in the medical world as it leads to treatment failure [7]. It was first characterized in a *Salmonella enteritidis* which has the ability to hydrolyze penicillins, cephamycin, including broad spectrum cephalosporin leaving physicians with limited antibiotic choices. It was also the first plasmid-encoded β-lactamase found to be inducible and can be expressed in high levels [11, 12]. So far a total of 24 gene types of DHA family have been reported (http://www.ncbi.nlm.nih.gov/projects/pathogens/submit_beta_lactamase). The regulation of this β-lactamase expression is closely linked to cell wall recycling and involves at least three genes: *ampR* (codes for a transcriptional regulator of the LysR family), *ampG* (codes for a transmembrane permease) and *ampD* (codes for a cytosolic *N*-acetyl-anhydromuramyl- L-alanine amidase) [13].

Though it was well established that β-lactam antibiotics are potent inducers of class C in most of the members of the family Enterobacteriaceae [7], there is no relevant information on the level of AmpC expression taking place when the strains with incomplete regulatory elements were under antibiotic stress. Therefore, this study was undertaken to investigate the transcriptional response of DHA-1 under various cephalosporin's stresses.

Methods

Bacterial strains

A total of 176 consecutive, non-duplicate *Escherichia* isolates were collected from different clinical specimens (mostly from urine followed by pus) obtained from different Wards/OPD of Silchar Medical College and Hospital, India from October 2012 to March 2013. The isolates were identified by cultural characteristics, biochemical reactions and further confirmed by 16S rDNA sequencing using primers, a forward primer 5′-AGAGTTTGATCMTGGCTCAG-3′ and a reverse primer 5′-TACGGYTACCTTGTTACGACTT-3′.

Screening of AmpC β-lactamase by cefoxitin disc test and modified three dimensional extract method

Preliminary screening of AmpC β-lactamase was carried out on Mueller–Hinton Agar plates containing cefoxitin (30 μg) (Hi Media, Mumbai). Isolates with inhibition zones of less than 18 mm, were considered as screen positives [14]. The suspected AmpC β-lactamase producers were further confirmed by modified three dimensional extract test (M3DET) [15]. *Escherichia coli* ATCC 25922 and *Enterobacter cloacae* P99 were used as negative and positive control respectively.

Antimicrobial susceptibility and minimum inhibitory concentrations (MIC's) determination

Antimicrobial susceptibility was determined by Kirby Bauer disc diffusion method on Mueller–Hinton Agar plates. Following antibiotics were used: amikacin (30 μg), gentamicin (10 μg), ciprofloxacin (30 μg), trimethoprim/sulphamethoxazole (1.25/23.75 μg), tigecycline (15 μg) (Hi Media, Mumbai). MIC's of various antibiotics were also determined on Mueller–Hinton Agar plates by agar dilution method according to CLSI and EUCAST guidelines [16, 17]. Following antibiotics were used: cefotaxime, ceftazidime, ceftriaxone, cefepime, imipenem, meropenem, ertapenem and aztreonam (Hi-Media, Mumbai, India).

Detection of DHA gene by polymerase chain reaction

Polymerase chain reaction (PCR) was performed targeting all the DHA genes by using a pair of primers as listed in Table 1. Isolates positive for DHA genes were further investigated for the presence of other AmpC gene families, namely: CIT, ACC, FOX and EBC [18]. PCR amplification was performed using 30 μl of total reaction volume. Reactions were run under the following conditions: initial denaturation at 95 °C for 2 min, 34 cycles of 95 °C for 15 s, 51 °C for 1 min, 72 °C for 1 min and final extension at 72 °C for 7 min.

PCR products were purified by QIAquick Gel Extraction Kit (QIAGEN, Germany) and sequenced. Sequence results were analysed using a BLAST suite program of NCBI (http://blast.ncbi.nlm.nih.gov/Blast.cgi).

Molecular characterization of ESBL and carbapenemase genes by multiplex PCR

For amplification and characterization of ESBL genes, a set of five primers were used, namely: TEM, CTX-M, SHV, OXA-2, and PER [19]. Reactions were run under the following conditions: initial denaturation at 94 °C for 5 min, 33 cycles of 94 °C for 35 s., 51 °C for 1 min, 72 °C for 1 min and a final extension at 72 °C for 7 min.

For amplification and characterization of carbapenemase genes, a set of seven primers were used, namely: KPC, IMI, NMC, SME, VIM, IMP, and NDM (Table 1). Reactions were run as described previously.

Transcriptional expression analysis of bla_{DHA-1} by quantitative realtime PCR

Expression of the bla_{DHA-1} gene was studied in response to cefoxitin, cefotaxime, ceftriaxone and ceftazidime

Table 1 List of oligonucleotide primers for amplification of β-lactamase genes

Serial no.	Targets	Primers pairs	Sequence (5′→3′)	Product size (bp)	Reference
1	DHA-1 and DHA-2	DHA F DHA R	TGATGGCACAGCAGGATATTC GCTTTGACTCTTTCGGTATTCG	997	[18]
2	KPC	KPC F KPC R	5′-CATTCAAGGGCTTTCTTGCTGC-3′ 5′-ACGACGGCATAGTCATTTGC-3′	538	[20]
3	IMI/NMC	IMI/NMC F IMI/NMC R	5′-CCATTCACCCATCACAAC-3′ 5′-CTACCGCATAATCATTTGC-3′	440	[21]
4	SME	SME F SME R	5′-AACGGCTTCATTTTTGTTTAG-3′ 5′-GCTTCCGCAATAGTTTTATCA-3′	831	[22]
5	VIM	VIM F VIMR	5′-GATGGTGTTTGGTCGCATA-3′ 5′-CGAATGCGCAGCACCAG-3′	390	[23]
6	IMP	IMP F IMP R	5′-TTGACACTCCATTTACDG-3′ 5′-GATYGAGAATTAAGCCACYCT-3′	139	[23]
7	NDM	NDM F NDM R	5′-GGGCAGTCGCTTCCAACGGT-3′ 5′-GTAGTGCTCAGTGTCGGCAT-3′	476	[24]
8	DHA-1	DHA-RT F DHA-RT R	5′-TGATGGCACAGCAGGATATTC-3′ 5′-TACTTACAGATCCGAGCTCAA-3′	144	This study

stress at different concentrations (2, 4, 8 μg/ml) and was determined by inoculating the organisms harboring $bla_{\text{DHA-1}}$ in Luria–Bertani broth (Hi-media, Mumbai, India). Isolate without any antibiotic pressure was used as a control. A total RNA was isolated using Qiagen RNase Mini Kit (Qiagen, Germany), immediately reverse transcribed into cDNA by using QuantiTect® reverse transcription kit (Qiagen, Germany). The cDNA was quantified by Picodrop (Pico 200, Cambridge, UK) and quantitative real time PCR was performed using Power Sybr Green Master Mix (Applied Biosystem, Warrington, UK) in step one plus real time detection system (Applied Biosystem, USA). The house keeping gene *rpsel* of *E. coli* was used as an internal standard [25]. DHA-1 positive isolates showing resistance to broad spectrum cephalosporins and also devoid of other β-lactamases was selected for this study. The primer used for amplification of DHA-1 is listed in Table 1. PCR reactions were performed in triplicates for the isolate. The reaction was run under the following conditions: 95 °C for 2 min, 32 cycles of 95 °C for 20 s, 48 °C for 40 s and 72 °C for 1 min. The relative expression of $bla_{\text{DHA-1}}$ at a different antibiotics pressure was determined by the $\Delta\Delta C_t$ method. Relative quantification was compared with strain grown for 16 h without any antibiotic pressure.

Statistical analysis

The changes in DHA-1 mRNA expression in response to different β-lactam antibiotic stresses at different concentration were analyzed using one-way ANOVA followed by Tukey–Kramer (Tukey's W) multiple comparison test using SPSS version 17.0. Differences were considered statistically significant at both 5 and 1% level when $p < 0.05$. Data are presented as mean fold change + standard error of the mean.

Plasmid preparation

The bacterial isolates were cultured in Luria–Bertani broth (LB broth) containing 0.25 μg/ml of cefotaxime. Cultures were incubated on shaker incubator overnight at 37 °C, 160 rpm. Plasmids were purified by QIA prep Spin Miniprep Kit (QIAGEN, Germany).

Transferability of bla_{DHA} gene by transformation and conjugation

The transformation experiments were carried out by heat shock method [26] using *E. coli* DH5α as the recipient. Transformants were selected on cefotaxime (0.5 μg/ml) containing LB Agar plates.

Conjugation experiments were carried out between clinical isolates as donors and a streptomycin resistant *E. coli* strain B (Genei, Bangalore) as the recipient. An overnight culture of the bacteria was diluted in Luria–Bertani broth (Hi-Media, Mumbai, India) and was grown at 37 °C till the O.D. of the recipient and donor culture reached 0.8–0.9 at A_{600}. Donor and recipient cells were mixed at 1:5 donor-to-recipient ratios and transconjugants were selected L.B Agar plates supplemented with cefotaxime (0.5 μg/ml) and streptomycin (600 μg/ml).

Plasmid incompatibiltiy typing

For detection of incompatibility group type of plasmid carrying bla_{DHA}, PCR based replicon typing was carried out, targeting 18 different replicon types, to perform five multiplex and three simplex PCRs to amplify the FIA,

FIB, FIC, HI1, HI2, I1-Ig, L/M, N, P, W, T, A/C, K, B/O, X, Y, F and FIIA replicons [27].

DNA fingerprinting by enterobacterial repetitive intergenic consensus sequences PCR

Typing of all $bla_{\text{DHA-1}}$ producing *E. coli* isolates was done by enterobacterial repetitive intergenic consensus (ERIC) PCR as described previously [28]. Isolates were put into cluster based on banding pattern and dendogram was prepared by NTSYS software.

Results

During the study period, a total of 176 *E. coli* isolates were obtained from different clinical samples. Among these, 110 (62.5%) were resistant to cefoxitin and 63 (35.8%) isolates were found to show AmpC activity by M3DET. By performing PCR, 16 isolates were detected for DHA genes and showed a sequence identical to that of DHA-1 (Table 1). These isolates harboring DHA-1 gene were selected for further study. Among DHA-1 positive isolates four different ESBL genes were detected in 10 isolates which include CTX-M (n = 6), SHV (n = 4), TEM (n = 3) and OXA-10 (n = 1). Carbapenemase gene (NDM-1) was detected only in one isolate. Other plasmid mediated AmpC β-lactamase CIT (n = 9), EBC (n = 2) were detected in nine isolates that carried either CTX-M (n = 3),SHV (n = 1), TEM (n = 1), NDM (n = 1) alone or CTX-M plus SHV(n = 2), CTX-M plus TEM (n = 1) and OXA-10 plus SHV (n = 1) (Table 2). These isolates harboring AmpC β-lactamase were mostly obtained from Surgery and medicine ward. To demonstrate whether DHA-1 expression would take place in the presence of different cephalosporins at a different concentration, an *E.coli* strain BM-567 (Table 2) harboring only DHA-1 β-lactamase and showing resistance to broad spectrum cephalosporins was selected. The fold increase in mRNA production was measured using primer extension analysis. It was observed that there was a significant increase in the expression of DHA-1 gene in response to cefotaxime, ceftriaxone, ceftazidime but not as high as those for cefoxitin when compared with the basal level without antibiotic pressure (Fig. 1). Though increased in transcription was observed in response to these β-lactam antibiotics, high transcript level were achieved when induced by cefotaxime at 8 μg/ml (6.99×10^2 fold), ceftriaxone at 2 μg/ml (2.63×10^3 fold), ceftazidime at 8 μg/ml (7.06×10^3 fold) and cefoxitin at 4 μg/ml (3.60×10^4 fold) (Fig. 1). The ANOVA and Tukey–Kramer (Tukey's W) multiple comparison test for checking the differences in the expression of DHA-1 was found to be significant (*p* value is less than 0.05; Table 3).

Typing by ERIC-PCR confirmed 16 different haplotypes (Fig. 2) indicating the diversity of the isolates. The susceptibility pattern of these $bla_{\text{DHA-1}}$ harboring isolates showed resistance towards β-lactam including broad spectrum cephalosporin but most of them were susceptible against a carbapenem group of drugs. They also show susceptibility to tigecycline and moderate to high resistance against amikacin, gentamycin, co-trimoxazole, ciprofloxacin. The MICs of selected β-lactam antibiotics for all the parental strains harboring DHA-1 were found to be above breakpoint level (Table 2). The transformation experiment could establish that DHA-1 was encoded in plasmid however, conjugation experiment revealed that only 4 isolates could conjugatively transfer DHA-1 gene in *E. coli* strain B which was confirmed by PCR analysis. On performing incompatibility typing it was established that most of the transformants with DHA-1 were associated with K, FIA, L/M, FIB, HI1, B/O & I1 *Inc* group (Table 2).

Discussion

The first plasmid mediated AmpC β-lactamase, to be reported was CMY-1, in 1989 [29]. Since then, several plasmid-encoded AmpC β-lactamases (ACC, FOX, MOX, CMY, ACT, etc.) have been reported in several genera of bacteria, including *Salmonella* spp., *Pseudomonas* spp., *Proteus mirabilis* and *Klebsiella pneumoniae* [7]. Among them plasmid encoded DHA-1; a clinically important AmpC β-lactamase was the first β-lactamase found to be inducible and can be expressed at higher levels in strains having AmpR regulatory gene [11, 30]. This plasmid- mediated β-lactamase is now being increasingly detected in a strain of *E. coli* worldwide [31–33] and early detection of this β-lactamase (DHA-1) is mandatory for better antibiotic therapy and also to prevent further spread. The present study reports the prevalence of DHA-1 (9%) among *E. coli* strains in this region which is quite high compared to other studies [30, 32, 33] and typing of these DHA-1 harboring isolates by ERIC PCR revealed diverse haplotypes, indicating the spread of the DHA-1 gene through horizontal transfer. Based on the present susceptibility data (Table 2) and previous studies [11, 12], carbapenem and other non-β-lactam antibiotics such as tigecycline could be better drugs of choice for the treatment of infections caused by *E. coli* producing DHA-1.

From the earlier study, it appears that *E. coli* lack one of the regulatory component (AmpR gene), which leads to the lower level, non-inducible expression of AmpC [34]. However, inducible cephalosporinase ($bla_{\text{CMY-13}}$) found associated with an AmpR gene was detected recently in a strain of *E. coli* [35]. Several broad spectrum cephalosporins were believed to increase the expression of AmpC β-lactamase [36], although the concentration which leads to increase in the expression of AmpC β-lactamase was not established.

Table 2 Clinical history, their molecular details and resistance profile of DHA-1 gene-positive *E. coli* isolates

Sl. No.	Sample ID	Age (years)	Sex	Ward/clinics	Type of clinical specimen	[a]ESBL genes detected	Carbapenemase genes detected	Other plasmid AmpC genes	(Inc type)	Resistance profile	MIC of β-lactam (mg/l)							
											CTX	CAZ	CRO	FEP	ATM	IMP	MEM	ETP
1	BM12	35	Male	Surgery	Pus	–	–	–	K	AMK, GEN, SXT	>512	>512	256	>512	64	16	8	8
2	BM26	107	Female	Pediatrics	Urine	TEM	–	–	FIA,	CIP, AMK, GEN, SXT	64	128	64	8	64	<2	<2	<2
3	BM59	55	Female	Medicine	Urine	–	–	–	FIA	CIP, AMK, GEN, SXT	128	64	64	16	128	<2	<2	<2
4	BM63	60	Female	Surgery	Pus	CTX-M	–	CIT	–	CIP, AMK, GEN, SXT	128	128	256	16	64	<2	<2	<2
5	BM130	27	Female	Surgery	Pus	TEM	–	CIT, EBC	HI1, L/M	CIP, AMK, GEN, SXT	>512	512	>512	64	256	16	4	4
6	BM138	45	Male	Surgery	Pus	CTX-M	–	–	–	CIP, GEN, SXT	64	128	128	32	128	<2	<2	<2
7	BM197	30	Female	Surgery	Pus	–	–	CIT	L/M	CIP, AMK, GEN, SXT	512	>512	256	64	512	2	<2	<2
8	BM230	43	Female	Surgery	Pus	CTX-M, SHV	–	CIT	L/M	CIP, AMK, GEN, SXT	64	128	256	32	256	16	8	16
9	BM252	7	Female	Paediatrics	Urine	SHV	–	CIT, EBC	F1B, FIA	CIP, AMK, GEN, SXT	>512	>512	>512	128	256	8	<2	<2
10	BM355	10	Male	Paediatrics	Urine	–	NDM	CIT	FIA	CIP, AMK, SXT	>512	512	>512	8	256	<2	<2	<2
11	BM409	61	Male	Medicine	Urine	CTX-M	–	CIT	K	CIP, AMK, GEN, SXT	64	64	32	16	128	<2	<2	<2
12	BM441	40	Male	Medicine	Stool	CTX-M, SHV	–	–	FIA	CIP, AMK, GEN, SXT	32	64	128	32	256	<2	<2	<2
13	BM508	48	Male	Surgery	Pus	–	–	CIT	I1	CIP, AMK, GEN	32	32	32	16	256	<2	<2	<2
14	BM520	55	Female	Surgery	Pus	OXA-10, SHV	–	–	–	CIP, GEN, SXT	16	128	128	32	32	<2	<2	<2
15	BM567	30	Male	Medicine	Urine	–	–	–	–	CIP, AMK, GEN, SXT	128	256	256	32	256	<2	<2	<2
16	BM576	40	Female	Medicine	Urine	CTX-M, TEM	–	CIT	K, B/O	AMK, GEN, SXT	>512	>512	>512	128	>512	16	16	32

AMK amikacin; *GEN* gentamycin; *CIP* ciprofloxacin; *SXT* cottrimoxazole; *CTX* cefotaxime; *CAZ* ceftazidime; *CRO* ceftriaxone; *FEP* cefepime; *ATM* aztreonam; *IMP* imipenem; *MEM* meropenem; *ETP* ertapenem

[a] Extended spectrum β-lactamase

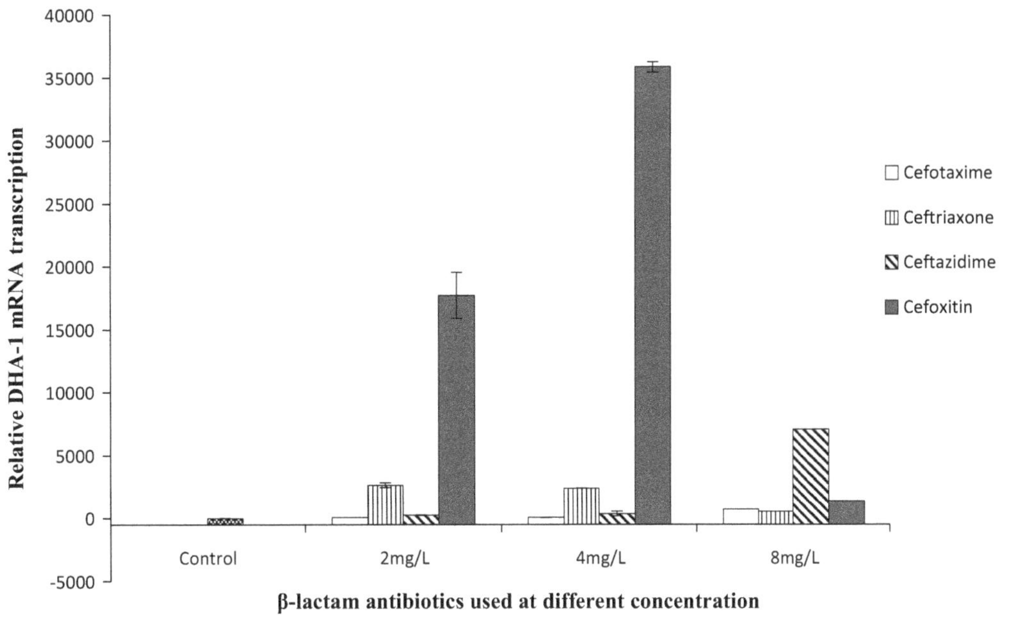

Fig. 1 Transcriptional analysis of DHA-1 espression by RT-PCR. Total bacterial RNA was isolated from mid-log- phase cultures of *E. coli*. The *error bars* represent the standard deviations of the means of triplicate samples

Table 3 Statistical analysis of changes in DHA-1 mRNA expression in response to different-lactam antibiotic stress at different concentration using one way ANOVA

Sl no.	β-lactam antibiotics	Value (Mean ± SEM)				p value
		NA	2 mg/l	4 mg/l	8 mg/l	
1	Cefotaxime	1.00 ± 0	56.66 ± 1.18	58.10 ± 0.58	699.25 ± 5.27	0.001*
2	Ceftriaxone	1.00 ± 0	2634.69 ± 16.58	2383.97 ± 20.73	510.70 ± 6.04	
3	Ceftazidime	1.00 ± 0	249.50 ± 11.63	356.27 ± 14.20	7059.48 ± 60.91	
4	Cefoxitin	1.00 ± 0	17721.31 ± 608.47	35855.21 ± 1050.38	1363.69 ± 237.37	

NA no antibiotic; *SEM* standard error of the mean

* Significant ($p < 0.05$)

This study demonstrates higher transcription of DHA-1 when induced with different cephalosporins. These differences in the relative amounts of RNA transcription of DHA-1 gene, when induced with different cephalosporins at a concentration below MIC level suggest that the transcription varies depending on the level of antibiotics stress. Higher AmpC production was supported by another finding, where *bla*MIR-1, a plasmid-encoded *AmpC* gene exhibited a 95-fold increase in expression relative to WT *AmpC* [37]. Concentration dependent expression of AmpC cephalosporinase was also observed in a strain of *Pseudomonas aeruginosa,* when the strain was induced with cefoxitin or clavulanic acid at 8, 16 and 50 μg/ml [38]. So far, the factors behind the quantitative differences of AmpC expression in *E.coli* strain when exposed to different β-lactam concentration is unknown. A transformation experiment could establish that all the DHA-1 gene were encoded in a plasmid which is in agreement with the previous study [12, 30–33] and Incompatibility typing from the transformants indicated that the plasmid encoding $bla_{\text{DHA-1}}$ was carried mostly by FIA and L/M Inc group as found in another study [39]. Although detection of other Inc group, namely HI1, FIB, I1, K in the present study was mostly associated with CMY-2 and ACC harboring strains [39]. Plasmids carrying genes for AmpC β-lactamases often carry ESBL genes such as CTX-M [40, 41] as found in the present study, where most of these DHA-1 harboring isolates co-harbour ESBL genes (Table 2). Co-existence of New Delhi metallo-β-lactamase (NDM) gene was also observed in one isolate as the high prevalence of the *E. coli* harboring a metallo-β-lactamase known as the NDM has been increasingly observed in the Indian subcontinent [42].

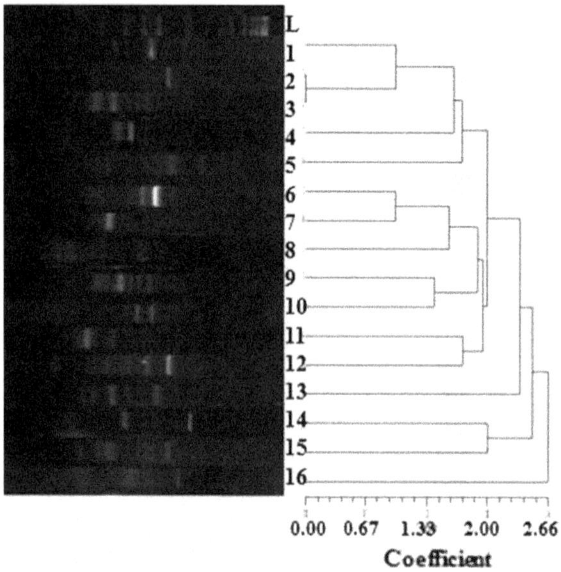

Fig. 2 ERIC PCR analysis of *E. coli* producing DHA-1 β-lactamase. *Lane* L: molecular weight marker; *lanes* 1–16: isolates harboring DHA-1 β-lactamase

Conclusion

Strains harboring plasmid mediated AmpC (DHA-1) genes are often resistant to multiple antimicrobial agents and the overexpression of this resistant determinant when induced with different cephalosporins stress will further limit treatment option. The present study demonstrates that higher expression of DHA-1 takes place when induced with specific concentrations of β-lactam antibiotics, although further research is required to understand the factors behind the upregulation of DHA-1 gene in the future. Therefore, revision in cephalosporin usage policy is required for effective treatment of patients infected with pathogen harboring this mechanism.

Authors' contributions

BI performed the experimental work, data collection and analysis and prepared the manuscript. AB supervised the research work and participated in designing the study and drafting the manuscript. DP and APM participated in sample collection and part of experiments. DB participated in statistical analysis. DD and AC Participated in experiment designing and manuscript correction. All authors read and approved the final manuscript.

Author details

[1] Department of Microbiology, Assam University, Silchar 788011, India. [2] Department of Microbiology, Silchar Medical College and Hospital, Silchar 788014, India. [3] Department of Statistics, Dibrugarh University, Dibrugarh, India.

Acknowledgements

The authors would like to acknowledge the help of HOD, Microbiology, Assam University for providing infrastructure. The authors sincerely acknowledge the financial support provided by University Grants Commissions (UGC-MRP) Government of India. Authors also acknowledge the help from Assam University Biotech Hub for providing laboratory facility to complete this work.

Competing interests

The authors declared that they have no competing interests.

Funding

University grants commission (UGC-MRP) and (UGC-RGNF) to Birson Ingti Vide letter no. F1-17.1/2013-14/RGNF-2013-14-ST-ASS-38069/(SAIII/Website).

References

1. Jaurin B, Grundstrom T. AmpC cephalosporinase of *Escherichia coli* K-12 has a different evolutionary origin from that of β-lactamases of the penicillinase type. Proc Natl Acad Sci USA. 1981;78:4897–901.
2. Bergstrom S, Normark S. β-Lactam resistance in clinical isolates of *Escherichia coli* caused by elevated production of the *ampC* mediated chromosomal β-lactamase. Antimicrob Agents Chemother. 1979;16:427–33.
3. Caroff N, Espaze E, Gautreau D, Richet H, Reynaud A. Analysis of the effects of −42 and −32 ampC promoter mutations in clinical isolates of *Escherichia coli* hyperproducing ampC. J Antimicrob Chemother. 2000;45:783–8.
4. Jaurin B, Grundstrom T, Edlund T, Normark S. The *E. coli* β-lactamase attenuator mediates growth rate-dependent regulation. Nature. 1981;290:221–5.
5. Deshpande LM, Jones RN, Fritsche TR, Sader HS. Occurrence of plasmidic AmpC type β-lactamase-mediated resistance in *Escherichia coli*: report from the SENTRY Antimicrobial Surveillance Program (North America, 2004). Int J Antimicrob Agents. 2006;28:578–81.
6. Mammeri H, Nordmann P, Berkani A, Eb F. Contribution of extended-spectrum AmpC (ESAC) β-lactamases to carbapenem resistance in *Escherichia coli*. FEMS Microbiol Lett. 2008;282:238–40.
7. Jacoby GA. *AmpC* β-lactamases. Clin Microbiol Rev. 2009;22:161–82.
8. Pérez-Pérez FJ, Hanson ND. Detection of plasmid-mediated AmpC β-lactamase genes in clinical isolates by using multiplex PCR. J Clin Microbiol. 2002;40:2153–62.
9. Naseer U, Haldorsen B, Simonsen GS, Sundsfjord A. Sporadic occurrence of CMY-2-producing multidrug-resistant *Escherichia coli* of ST-complexes 38 and 448, and ST131 in Norway. Clin Microbiol Infect. 2010;16:171–8.
10. Pavez M, Neves P, Dropa M, et al. Emergence of carbapenem resistant *Escherichia coli* producing CMY-2-type AmpC β-lactamase in Brazil. J Med Microbiol. 2008;57:1590–2.
11. Gaillot O, Clement C, Simonet M, Philippon A. Novel transferable β-lactam resistance with cephalosporinase characteristics in *Salmonella enteritidis*. J Antimicrob Chemother. 1997;39:85–7.
12. Barnaud G, Arlet G, Verdet C, Gaillot O, Lagrange PH, Philippon A. *Salmonella enteritidis*: AmpC plasmid-mediated inducible β-lactamase (DHA-1) with an *ampR* gene from *Morganella morganii*. Antimicrob Agents Chemother. 1998;42:2352–8.
13. Hanson ND, Sanders CC. Regulation of inducible AmpC β-lactamase expression among Enterobacteriaceae. Curr Pharm Des. 1999;5:881–94.
14. Lorian V. Antibiotics in laboratory medicine. 5th ed. Philadelphia: Lippincott Williams and Wilkins; 2005.
15. Coudron PE, Moland ES, Thomson KS. Occurrence and detection of AmpC β-lactamases among *Escherichia coli*, *Klebsiella pneumoniae*, and *Proteus mirabilis* isolates at a Veterans Medical Center. J Clin Microbiol. 2000;38:1791–6.
16. Clinical and Laboratory Standards Institute. Performance standards for antimicrobial susceptibility testing; twenty-third informational supplement. M100-S23. Wayne: CLSI; 2013.
17. European committee on antimicrobial susceptibility testing. Breakpoint tables for interpretation of MICs and zone diameters, version 6.0; 2016.
18. Caroline D, Anaelle DC, Dominique D, Christine F, Guillaume A. Development of a set of multiplex PCR assays for the detection of genes encoding important β-lactamases in Enterobacteriaceae. J Antimicrob Chemother. 2010;65:490–5.
19. Lee S, Park YJ, Kim M, Lee HK, Han K, Kang CS. Prevalence of Ambler class A and D β-lactamases among clinical isolates of *Pseudomonas aeruginosa* in Korea. J Antimicrob Chemother. 2005;56:122–7.
20. Nass T, Cuzon G, Villegas MV, Lartigue MF, Quinn JP, Nordmann P. Genetic structures at the origin of acquisition of the β-lactamase blaKPC gene. Antimicrob Agents Chemother. 2008;52:1257–63.

21. Rasmussen BA, Bush K, Keeney D, Yang Y, Hare R, Gara CO, et al. Characterization of IMI-1 betalactamase, a class A carbapenem-hydrolyzing enzyme from Enterobacter cloaceae. Antimicrob Agents Chemother. 1996;40:2080–6.
22. Nass T, Vandel L, Sougakoff W, Livermore DM, Nordmann P. Cloning and sequence analysis of the gene for a carbapenem hydrolyzing class A β-lactamase, SME-1, from Serratia marcescens S6. Antimicrob Agents Chemother. 1994;38:1262–70.
23. Jh Y, Yi K, Lee H, Yong D, Lee K, Kim JM, et al. Molecular characterization of metallo-β-lacatamaseproducing Acinetobacter baumannii and Acinetbacter genomospecies 3 from Korea: identification of two new integrons carrying the blaVIM-2 gene cassettes. J Antimicrob Chemother. 2002;49:837–40.
24. Yong D, Toleman MA, Giske CG, Cho HS, Sundman K, Lee K, et al. Characterization of a New Metallo-β-Lactamase Gene, blaNDM-1, and a Novel Erythromycin Esterase Gene Carried on a Unique Genetic Structure in Klebsiella pneumoniae Sequence Type 14 from India. Antimicrob Agents Chemother. 2009;53:5046–54.
25. Swick MC, Morgan-Linnell SK, Carlson KM, et al. Expression of multidrug efflux pump genes *acrAB-tolC*, *mdfA* and *norE* in *Escherichia coli* clinical isolates as a function of fluroquinolone and multidrug resistance. Antimicrob Agents Chemother. 2011;55:921–4.
26. Sambrook J, Fritsch EF, Maniatis T. Molecular cloning: a laboratory manual. 2nd ed. New York: Cold Spring Harbor Laboratory Press; 1989.
27. Carattoli A, Bertini A, Villa L, Falbo V, et al. Identification of plasmids by PCR-based replicon typing. J Microbiol Methods. 2005;63:219–28.
28. Versalovic J, Koeuth T, Lupski JR. Distribution of repetitive DNA sequences in eubacteria and application to fingerprinting of bacterial genomes. Nucleic Acids Res. 1995;19:6823–31.
29. Bauernfeind A, Chong Y, Schweighart S. Extended broad spectrum β-lactamase in *Klebsiella pneumoniae* including resistance to cephamycins. Infection. 1989;17:316–21.
30. Yong D, Limc Y, Song W, et al. Plasmid-mediated, inducible AmpC β-lactamase (DHA-1)-producing Enterobacteriaceae at a Korean hospital: wide dissemination in *Klebsiella pneumoniae* and *Klebsiella oxytoca* and emergence in *Proteus mirabilis*. Diagn Microbiol Infect Dis. 2005;53:65–70.
31. Pham JN, Chambers I, Poirel L, Nordmann P, Bell SM. Detection of a plasmid-mediated inducible cephalosporinase DHA-1 from *Escherichia coli*. Pathology. 2010;42(2):196–7.
32. Giakkoupi P, Tambic-Andrasevic A, Vourli S, et al. Transferable DHA-1 ceph alosporinase in *Escherichia coli*. Int J Antimicrob Agents. 2006;27:77–80.
33. Song W, Kim JS, Kim HS, et al. Emergence of *Escherichia coli* isolates producing conjugative plasmid-mediated DHA-1 β-lactamase in a Korean University Hospital. J. Hospital Infection. 2006;63:459–64.
34. Honore N, Nicolas MH, Cole ST. Inducible cephalosporinase production in clinical isolates of *Enterobacter cloacae* is controlled by a regulatory gene that has been deleted from *Escherichia coli*. EMBO J. 1986;5(13):3709–14.
35. Miriagou V, Tzouvelekis LS, Villa L, Lebessi E, Vatopoulos AC, Carattoli A, et al. CMY-13, a novel inducible cephalosporinase encoded by an *Escherichia coli* plasmid. Antimicrob Agents Chemother. 2004;48:3172–4.
36. Livermore DM. Clinical significance of β-lactamase induction and stable derepression in gram-negative rods. Eur. J. Clin. Microbiol. 1987;6:439–45.
37. Reisbig MD, Ashfaque H, Nancy DH. Factors influencing gene expression and resistance for gram-negative organisms expressing plasmid-encoded *ampC* genes of *Enterobacter* origin. J Antimicrob Chemother. 2003;2003(51):1141–51.
38. Lister PD, Gardner VM, Sanders CC. Clavulanate induces expression of the *Pseudomonas aeruginosa* AmpC cephalosporinase at physiologically relevant concentrations and antagonizes the antibacterial activity of ticarcillin. Antimicrob Agents Chemother. 1999;43:882–9.
39. Mata C, Miro E, Alvarado A, et al. Plasmid typing and genetic context of AmpC β-lactamases in Enterobacteriaceae lacking inducible chromosomal ampC genes: findings from a Spanish hospital 1999–2007. J Antimicrob Chemother. 2012;67:115–22.
40. Migma DT, Hyang NM, Geum CJ, Su RK, Myung HC, Suk CJ, et al. Molecular characterization of extended-spectrum-β-lactamase- producing and plasmid-mediated AmpC β-lactamase-producing *Escherichia coli* isolated from stray dogs in South Korea. Antimicrob Agents Chemother. 2012;56:2705–12.
41. Lee CH, Liu JW, Li CC, Chien CC, Tang YF, Su LH. Spread of IS*CR1* elements containing *bla*$_{DHA-1}$ and multiple antimicrobial resistance genes leading to increase of flomoxef resistance in extended-spectrum-β-lactamase producing *Klebsiella pneumoniae*. Antimicrob Agents Chemother. 2011;55:4058–63.
42. Kumarasamy KK, Toleman MA, Walsh TR, Bagaria J, Butt F, Balakrishnan R, et al. Emergence of a new antibiotic resistance mechanism in India, Pakistan, and the UK: a molecular, biological, and epidemiological study. Lancet Infect. Dis. 2012;10:597–602.

3

VacA, cagA, iceA and *oipA* genotypes status and antimicrobial resistance properties of *Helicobacter pylori* isolated from various types of ready to eat foods

Behsan Hemmatinezhad[1], Hassan Momtaz[2] and Ebrahim Rahimi[3*]

Abstract

Background: Despite the high clinical standing of *Helicobacter pylori*, its exact routes of transmission and origin have not been determined. Based on the contentious hypothesis, foods play an important roles in the transmission of *H. pylori* to humans. The present study was carried out to investigate the *vacA, cagA, oipA* and *iceA* genotypes status of *H. pylori* isolated from the various types of ready to eat foods.

Methods: A total of 550 ready to eat food samples were cultured and tested. *H. pylori*-positive strains were analyzed for the presence of various genotypes and antimicrobial resistance pattern.

Results: Seventy four out of 550 (13.45 %) samples were positive for *H. pylori*. Olvie salad (36 %), restaurant salad (30 %), fruit salad (28 %) and soup (22 %) were the most commonly contaminated. *H. pylori* strains harbored the highest levels of resistance against amoxicillin (94.59 %), ampicillin (93.24 %), metronidazole (89.18 %) and tetracycline (72.97 %). The most commonly detected genotypes were *vacA s1a* (78.37 %), *vacA m2* (75.67 %), *vacA m1a* (51.35 %) and *cagA* (41.89 %). The prevalence of *iceA1, iceA2* and *oipA* genotypes were 13.51, 4.05 and 18.91 %, respectively. *S1am2* (70.27 %), *s1am1a* (39.18 %) and *m1am2* (31.08 %) were the most commonly detected combined genotypes. Of 40 different genotypic combinations, s1a/cagA+/iceA1/oipA− (12.16 %), s1a/cagA+/iceA1/oipA+ (10.81 %) and s1a/cagA−/iceA1/oipA+ (10.81 %) were the most prevalent.

Conclusions: The present investigation showed that some types of ready to eat food samples maybe the sources of resistant and virulent strains of *H. pylori*. Warily use of antibiotics with respect to the results of disk diffusion method and careful health monitoring on food and staffs of food producing companies maybe reduce the risk of *H. pylori* in foods.

Keywords: *Helicobacter pylori*, Genotypes, Genotyping, Ready to eat foods

Background

Ready to eat foods play an important roles in the nutrition of Iranian people. Every day millions of people use from ready to eat foods in their main meals. Therefore, hygienic quality of ready to eat foods is extremely important regarding public health hazards.

Helicobacter pylori (*H. pylori*) is a microaerophilic gram-negative bacterium which is known as the causative agent of peptic ulcer disease, type B gastritis, gastric adenocarcinoma and mucosa-associated lymphoid tissue lymphoma [1]. It has been estimated that 17–86 % of hospitalized patients with peptic ulcers were infected with *H. pylori* [1–3].

The role of foods in the transmission of *H. pylori* is still unknown but there were several investigations which focused on the identification of this bacterium in various types of food samples [4–8]. Good conditions for the

*Correspondence: Ebrahimrahimi55@yahoo.com
[3] Department of Food Hygiene and Public Health, College of Veterinary Medicine, Islamic Azad University, Shahrekord, Iran
Full list of author information is available at the end of the article

growth of bacteria in various types of foods cause it to be survive [6, 8].

To appraise the pathogenicity of *H. pylori*, evaluation of latent virulence factors and genotypes is essential. The most commonly important virulence factors among *H. pylori* strains of different clinical outcomes of human and animal beings are the vacuolating cytotoxin (*vacA*), induced by contact with the epithelium antigen (*iceA*), cytotoxin associated gene (*cag*) and outer inflammatory protein (*oip*) [6, 9, 10]. These genes are usually induced adhesion and invasion to the gastric epithelial cells [11, 12]. The *vacA* belongs to the group of genes with variable genotypes or structures. This gene is associated with injury to epithelial cells. The *vacA* gene is polymorphic, comprising variable signal regions (type *s1* or *s2*) and mid-regions (type *m1* or *m2*). The *s1* type is further subtyped into *s1a*, *s1b* and *s1c* subtypes and the *m1* into *m1a* and *m1b* subtypes. The mosaic combination of s and m-region allelic types determines the particular cytotoxin and consequently, the pathogenicity of the bacterium [11, 13]. The *iceA* gene has two main allelic variants *iceA1* and *iceA2* but their functions are not yet clear. *Cag* pathogenicity island (PAI) has been shown to be involved in persuading inflammation, ulceration and carcinogenesis [12]. The *cagA* gene has been detected in the specimens taken from the severe cases of peptic ulcer [8–12]. The *oipA* gene plays a significant role in effective colonization of mucosa [8–12]. Genotyping using these virulence markers is considered as one of the best approaches for study of correlations between *H. pylori* isolates from different samples.

Data on the epidemiology and transmission of *H. pylori* is extremely significant in order to prevent its distribution and to identify high-risk populations, especially in areas that have high rates of gastritis, peptic ulcers and gastric cancer such as Iran [6–10, 13]. Considering the unclear epidemiological aspects of *H. pylori* in ready to eat foods and according to the high prevalence of *H. pylori* all-around the world, the present investigation was carried out in order to study the exact status of *vacA*, *cagA*, *iceA* and *oipA* genotypes and antibiotic resistance pattern of *H. pylori* isolated from various types of ready to eat food samples.

Methods

Sample collection

From December 2013 to May 2014, overall 550 ready to eat food samples including cream-candy (n = 50), traditional bread (n = 50), sausage (n = 50), salami (n = 50), hamburger (n = 50), soup (n = 50), restaurant salad (n = 50), falafel (n = 50), olvie salad (n = 50), chicken nugget (n = 50) and fruit salad (n = 50) were purchased from the supermarkets of Isfahan province, Iran. Samples (100 mL, in sterile glass containers) were transported to the laboratory at 4 °C. All samples were kept under refrigeration in plastic bags; information about dates of production and of assigned shelf lives was not presented.

Isolation of *Helicobacter pylori*

Twenty five milliliters of each homogenized sample were added to 225 mL of Wilkins Chalgren anaerobe broth (Oxoid, UK) supplemented with colistin methanesulfonate (30 mg/L) and 5 % of horse serum (Sigma, St. Louis, MO, USA) and nalidixic acid (30 mg/L), vancomycin (10 mg/L) cycloheximide (100 mg/L) and trimethoprim (30 mg/L) (Sigma, St. Louis, MO, USA) and incubated for 7 days at 37 °C with shaking under microaerophilic conditions. Then, 0.1 mL of the enrichment selective broth was plated onto Wilkins Chalgren anaerobe agar (Oxoid, UK) supplemented with 5 % of defibrinated horse blood and 30 mg/L colistin methanesulfonate, 100 mg/L cycloheximide, 30 mg/L nalidixic acid, 30 mg/L trimethoprim, and 10 mg/L vancomycin (Sigma, St. Louis, MO, USA) and incubated for 7 days at 37 °C under microaerophilic conditions. For comparison, a reference strain of *H. pylori* (ATCC 43504) was employed.

DNA extraction and *Helicobacter pylori* 16S rRNA gene amplification

Suspected colonies were identified as *H. pylori* based on the PCR technique. Genomic DNA was extracted from the colonies with typical characters of *H. pylori* using a DNA extraction kit for cells and tissues (Roche Applied Science, Germany, 11814770001) according to the manufacturer's instructions and its density was assessed by optic densitometry. Extracted DNA was amplified for the *16S rRNA* gene (primers: HP-F: 5′-CTGGAGAGACTAAGCCCTCC-3′ and HP-R: 5′-ATTACTGACGCTGATTGTGC-3′) [14]. PCR reactions were performed in a final volume of 50 µL containing 5 µL 10 × buffer + $MgCl_2$, 2 mM dNTP, 2 unit Taq DNA polymerase, 100 ng genomic DNA as a template, and 25 pmol of each primer. PCR was performed using a thermal cycler (Eppendorf Co., Germany) under the following conditions: an initial denaturation for 2 min at 94 °C; 30 cycles of 95 °C for 30 s, 60 °C for 30 s, and 72 °C for 30 s and a final extension at 72 °C for 8 min.

Antimicrobial susceptibility testing

Pure cultures of *H. pylori* were applied for antibiotic susceptibility test. One strain from each *H. pylori*-positive sample was selected for this aim. Antimicrobial susceptibility test was accomplished by the Kirby-Bauer disc diffusion method using Mueller–Hinton agar (Merck, Germany) supplemented with 5 % defibrinated sheep blood and 7 % fetal calf serum, according to the Clinical Laboratory Standards Institute [15]. The antimicrobial resistance of *H. pylori* was measured against the widely used antibiotics in cases of *H. pylori* gastric ulcer. The following antimicrobial disks (HiMedia Laboratories, Mumbai, India) were used: ampicillin (10 μg), metronidazole (5 μg), erythromycin (5 μg), clarithromycin (2 μg), amoxicillin (10 μg), tetracycline (30 μg), levofloxacin (5 μg), streptomycin (10 μg), rifampin (30 μg), cefsulodin (30 μg), trimethoprim (25 μg), furazolidone (1 μg) and spiramycin (100 μg). After incubation at 37 °C for 48 h in a microaerophilic atmosphere, the susceptibility of the *H. pylori* was measured against each antimicrobial agents. Results were construed in accordance with interpretive criteria provided by CLSI (2012) [15]. The *H. pylori* ATCC 43504 was used as quality control organisms in antimicrobial susceptibility determination.

Genotyping of vacA, cagA, iceA and oipA genes of *Helicobacter pylori*

Presence of the *oipA*, *cagA* and the genotypes of *vacA* (*s1a*, *s1b*, *s1c*, *m1a*, *m1b* and *m2*) and *iceA* (*iceA1* and *iceA2*) alleles were determined using PCR technique. List of primers is shown in Table 1 [12, 16–21].

The PCR were performed in a total volume of 50 μl containing 1 μM of each primers, 1 μL of genomic DNA (approximately 200 ng), 1 mM of dNTPs mix (invitrogen), 2 mM of Mgcl2, and 0.05 U/μL Taq DNA polymerase (invitrogen). PCR amplifications were performed in an automated thermal cycler (Biometra Co., Germany). The following cycle conditions were used for PCR amplification: for *vacA*: 32 cycles of 45 s at 95 °C, 50 s at 64 °C, and 70 s at 72 °C; for *cagA*: 1 min at 94 °C, 1 min at 56 °C, and 1 min at 72 °C; for *iceA*: 1 min at 94 °C, 1 min at 56 °C, and 1 min at 72 °C and finally, for *oipA*: 1 min at 94 °C, 1 min at 56 °C and 1 min at 72 °C. All runs included one negative DNA control consisting of PCR grade water and two or more positive controls (26695, J99, SS1, Tx30, 88–23 and 84–183).

Table 1 Oligonucleotide primers used for genotyping of *Helicobacter pylori* strains isolated from ready to eat food samples

Genes name	Primer Sequence (5′–3′)	Size of product (bp)
vacA s_1a	F: CTCTCGCTTTAGTAGGAGC R: CTGCTTGAATGCGCCAAAC	213
vacA s_1b	F: AGCGCCATACCGCAAGAG CTGCTTGAATGCGCCAAAC	187
vacA s_1c	F: CTCTCGCTTTAGTGGGGYT R: CTGCTTGAATGCGCCAAAC	213
vacA s_2	F: GCTAACACGCCAAATGATCC R: CTGCTTGAATGCGCCAAAC	199
vacA m_1A	F: GGTCAAAATGCGGTCATGG R: CCATTGGTACCTGTAGAAAC	290
vacA m_1B	F: GGCCCCAATGCAGTCATGGA R: GCTGTTAGTGCCTAAAGAAGCAT	291
vacA m_2	F: GGAGCCCCAGGAAACATTG R: CATAACTAGCGCCTTGCA	352
cag A	F: GATAACAGCCAAGCTTTTGAGG R: CTGCAAAAGATTGTTTGGCAGA	300
$iceA_1$	F: GTGTTTTTAACCAAAGTATC R: CTATAGCCASTYTCTTTGCA	247
$iceA_2$	F: GTTGGGTATATCACAATTTAT R: TTRCCCTATTTTCTAGTAGGT	229/334
oip A	F: GTTTTTGATGCATGGGATTT R: GTGCATCTCTTATGGCTTT	401

Gel electrophoresis

The PCR amplification products (10 μl) were subjected to electrophoresis in a 1.5 % agarose gel in 1X TBE buffer at 80 V for 30 min, stained with ethidium bromide, and images were obtained in a UVIdoc gel documentation systems (UK). The PCR products were identified by 100 bp DNA size marker (Fermentas, Germany).

Statistical analysis

Data were transferred to Microsoft Excel spreadsheet (Microsoft Corp., Redmond, WA, USA) for analysis. Using SPSS 16.0 statistical software (SPSS Inc., Chicago, IL, USA), Chi square test and Fisher's exact two-tailed test analysis was performed and differences were considered significant at values of $P < 0.05$. Distribution of *H. pylori* genotypes isolated from food stuffs were statistically analyzed.

Results

Prevalence of *Helicobacter pylori* in various types of ready to eat food samples

All of the ready to eat food samples were examined using the culture and PCR techniques. Table 2 shows

Table 2 Distribution *of Helicobacter pylori* in various types of ready to eat food samples

Types of samples	No. samples collected	Positive results for *H. pylori* (%)
Cream-candy	50	9 (18)
Traditional bread	50	3 (6)
Sausage	50	–
Salami	50	–
Hamburger	50	1 (2)
Soup	50	11 (22)
Restaurant salad	50	15 (30)
Falafel	50	3 (6)
Olvie salad	50	18 (36)
Chicken nugget	50	–
Fruit salad	50	14 (28)
Total	550	74 (13.45)

the total distribution of *H. pylori* in the ready to eat food samples. Of 550 ready to eat food samples, 74 (13.45 %) were positive for *H. pylori*. The most commonly contaminated samples were olvie salad (36 %), restaurant salad (30 %), fruit salad (28 %) and soup (22 %). There were no positive results for sausage, salami and chicken nugget. There were statistically significant differences amongst the incidence of bacteria in hamburger and olvie salad ($P = 0.027$), traditional bread and restaurant salad ($P = 0.033$) and soup and falafel ($P = 0.041$).

Antimicrobial susceptibility pattern

Antimicrobial susceptibility of *H. pylori* isolates of ready to eat food samples is shown in Table 3. *H. pylori* strains showed the highest levels of resistance against amoxicillin (94.59 %), ampicillin (93.24 %), metronidazole (89.18 %) and tetracycline (72.97 %) antibiotics. There were significant difference between the levels of antibiotic resistance and sources of *H. pylori* strains ($P = 0.039$). There were statistically significant differences in the levels of antibiotic resistance between amoxicillin and spiramycin ($P = 0.015$), ampicillin and spiramycin ($P = 0.018$), metronidazole and furazolidone ($P = 0.023$), tetracycline and furazolidone ($P = 0.027$), amoxicillin and furazolidone ($P = 0.025$), metronidazole and rifampin ($P = 0.031$), ampicillin and erythromycin ($P = 0.026$) and amoxicillin and cefsulodin ($P = 0.022$).

Distribution of *Helicobacter pylori* genotypes

Distribution of *vacA*, *cagA*, *iceA* and *oipA* genotypes of the *H. pylori* strains of ready to eat food samples is shown in Table 4. We found that the most commonly detected genotypes were *vacA s1a* (78.37 %), *vacA m2* (75.67 %), *vacA m1a* (51.35 %) and *cagA* (41.89 %). Total prevalence of *iceA1*, *iceA2* and *oipA* genotypes were 13.51, 4.05 and 18.91 %, respectively. Significant differences were found between the incidence of *s1a* and *s1c* ($P = 0.028$) and also between *s1a* and *s2* ($P = 0.021$), *s1a* and *m1b* ($P = 0.019$), *m2* and *s1c* ($P = 0.023$), *m1a* and *m1b* ($P = 0.024$), *m2* and *s2* ($P = 0.030$), *m2* and *m1b* ($P = 0.036$), *iceA1* and *iceA2* ($P = 0.042$) and *cagA* and *oipA* ($P = 0.037$) genotypes. Fifteen different genotypic combinations were detected in the *H. pylori* isolates of ready to eat food samples (Table 5). The most commonly detected combined genotypes were *s1am2* (70.27 %), *s1am1a* (39.18 %) and *m1am2* (31.08 %). There were no positive results for *m1bs2* genotype. Significant differences were found between the incidence of *s1am2* and *s1am1b* ($P = 0.025$), *s1am2* and *s1cm1b* ($P = 0.039$), *s1am1a* and *s2m2* ($P = 0.041$), *s1am2* and *m1bm2* ($P = 0.043$), *m2s1a* and *iceA1iceA2* ($P = 0.025$).

Distribution of combined genotypes

Forty different genotypic combinations were detected in the *H. pylori* strains of food stuffs (Table 6). The most commonly detected combined genotypes were s1a/cagA+/iceA1/oipA− (12.16 %), s1a/cagA+/iceA1/oipA+ (10.81 %), s1a/cagA−/iceA1/oipA+ (10.81 %), s1b/cagA+/iceA1/oipA− (9.45 %), m2/cagA+/iceA1/oipA+ (9.45 %), m2/cagA+/iceA1/oipA− (9.45 %), m2/cagA−/iceA1/oipA+ (9.45 %) and m2/cagA−/iceA1/oipA− (9.45 %).

Discussion

The results of our study showed that 13.45 % of ready to eat food samples were contaminated with *H. pylori* which was entirely high. In comparison with other investigations which were conducted on food staffs, the prevalence of *H. pylori* in our study was higher than those of milk (12.5 %) [22] and vegetable and salad (10.86 %) [7] but was lower than dairy products (19.2 %) [6], vegetable (13.68 %) [8] and restaurant salad (14 %) [8]. To date, various studies have been conducted on the prevalence of *H. pylori* in foods with animal origin [22–25]. In a study accompanied in Italy [23], the *H. pylori* was detected in more than 25 % of foods with animal origin. Japanese researchers reported the higher levels of contamination in foods with animal origin (72.2 %) [26]. In despite of other foods with animal origin [22–26], prevalence of *H. pylori* in the hamburger, olvie salad and soup (meat based ready to eat food stuffs) of our study were 2, 36 and 22 %, respectively. Prevalence of bacterium in Greek [24] and USA [25] were 20 % and 60 %, respectively which was higher than our results.

One of the most important substances in the preparation of sausage, salami, hamburger, olvie salad, chicken nugget and soup is meat. There were no positive results for chicken nugget, sausage and salami samples of our study. It is maybe related to the application of high temperature during processing of these products. In addition, observation of hygienic conditions in the preparation and packaging of these products maybe another reason for lack of *H. pylori*. In comparison with sausage, salami and chicken nugget samples, the *H. pylori* had significant prevalence in hamburger (2 %), olvie salad (36 %) and soup (22 %) samples. High amount of water activity (Aw) in these food samples, optimum pH and salt levels, presence of appropriate levels of amino acids including arginine, histidine, isoleucine, leucine, methionine, phenylalanine, alanine, valine, proline, serine, and tryptophan which are necessary for growth of *H. pylori* [27], presence of vegetables in some of these foods (olvie salad and soup) which are maybe reservoir for *H. pylori* [7, 8], unsanitary conditions in their preparation and finally

Table 3 Antimicrobial resistance pattern of *Helicobacter pylori* isolates of ready to eat food samples

Types of samples (no. positive results)	Pattern of antibiotic resistance (%)												
	AM10	Met5	ER5	CLR2	AMX 10	Tet30	Lev5	S10	RIF30	Cef30	TRP25	FZL1	Spi100
Cream-candy (9)	8 (88.88)	9 (100)	6 (66.66)	4 (44.44)	8 (88.88)	7 (77.77)	3 (33.33)	3 (33.33)	2 0	3 (33.33)	5 (55.55)	1 (11.11)	1 (11.11)
Traditional bread (3)	3 (100)	3 (100)	2 (66.66)	1 (33.33)	3 (100)	2 (66.66)	1 (33.33)	1 (33.33)	1 (33.33)	1 (33.33)	1 (33.33)	–	–
Hamburger (1)	1 (100)	–	1 (100)	–	1 (100)	1 (100)	–	1 (100)	–	–	1 (100)	–	–
Soup (11)	10 (90.90)	10 (90.90)	6 (54.54)	5 (45.45)	10 (90.90)	8 (72.72)	4 (36.36)	3 (27.27)	3 (27.27)	3 (27.27)	6 (54.54)	2 (18.18)	1 (9.09)
Restaurant salad (15)	13 (86.66)	13 (86.66)	8 (53.33)	6 (40)	14 (93.33)	10 (66.66)	5 (33.33)	4 (26.66)	4 (26.66)	4 (26.66)	7 (46.66)	4 (26.66)	2 (13.33)
Falafel (3)	3 (100)	3 (100)	2 (66.66)	1 (33.33)	3 (100)	2 (66.66)	2 (66.66)	1 (33.33)	1 (33.33)	1 (33.33)	2 (66.66)	1 (33.33)	–
Olvie salad (18)	16 (88.88)	16 (88.88)	10 (55.55)	9 (50)	17 (94.44)	13 (72.22)	6 (33.33)	5 (27.77)	5 (27.77)	6 (33.33)	10 (55.55)	6 (33.33)	3 (16.66)
Fruit salad (14)	13 (92.85)	12 (85.71)	8 (57.14)	11 (78.57)	14 (100)	11 (78.57)	6 (42.85)	5 (35.71)	5 (35.71)	4 (28.57)	8 (57.14)	5 (35.71)	2 (14.28)
Total (74)	69 (93.24)	66 (89.18)	43 (58.10)	34 (45.94)	70 (94.59)	54 (72.97)	27 (36.48)	23 (31.08)	21 (28.37)	22 (29.72)	40 (54.05)	19 (25.67)	9 (12.16)

AM10 ampicillin (10 μg), *Met5* metronidazole (5 μg), *ER5* erythromycin (5 μg), *CLR2* clarithromycin (2 μg), *AMX10* amoxicillin (10 μg), *Tet30* tetracycline (30 μg), *Lev5* levofloxacin (5 μg), *S10* streptomycin (10 μg), *RIF30* rifampin (30 μg), *Cef30* cefsulodin (30 μg), *TRP25* trimethoprim (25 μg), *FZL1* furazolidone (1 μg) and *Spi100* spiramycin (100 μg)

Table 4 Distribution of various genotypes in *Helicobacter pylori* strains of ready to eat food samples

Types of samples (no. positive results)	Distribution of *vacA, cagA, iceA and oipA* genotypes (%)										
	S1a	*S1b*	*S1c*	*S2*	*M1a*	*M1b*	*M2*	*CagA*	*IceA1*	*IceA2*	*OipA*
Cream-candy (9)	7 (77.77)	3 (33.33)	1 (11.11)	–	4 (44.44)	2 (22.22)	7 (77.77)	1 (11.11)	2 (22.22)	–	3 (33.33)
Traditional bread (3)	2 (66.66)	–	–	–	1 (33.33)	–	2 (66.66)	1 (33.33)	–	–	–
Hamburger (1)	1 (100)	–	–	–	–	–	–	1 (100)	–	–	–
Soup (11)	11 (100)	4 (36.36)	2 (18.18)	1 (9.09)	4 (36.36)	3 (27.27)	10 (90.90)	9 (81.81)	3 (27.27)	1 (9.09)	4 (36.36)
Restaurant salad (15)	10 (66.66)	4 (26.66)	3 (20)	2 (13.33)	8 (53.33)	1 (6.66)	11 (73.33)	2 (13.33)	2 (13.33)	1 (6.66)	3 (20)
Falafel (3)	2 (66.66)	1 (33.33)	–	–	1 (33.33)	–	1 (33.33)	1 (33.33)	–	–	–
Olvie salad (18)	16 (88.88)	5 (27.77)	4 (22.22)	2 (11.11)	13 (72.22)	2 (11.11)	15 (83.33)	15 (83.33)	2 (11.11)	1 (5.55)	2 (11.11)
Fruit salad (14)	9 (64.28)	3 (21.42)	3 (21.42)	1 (7.14)	7 (50)	–	10 (71.42)	1 (7.14)	1 (7.14)	–	2 (14.28)
Total (74)	58 (78.37)	20 (27.02)	13 (17.56)	6 (8.10)	38 (51.35)	8 (10.81)	56 (75.67)	31 (41.89)	10 (13.51)	3 (4.05)	14 (18.91)

Table 5 Distribution of combined genotypes of *Helicobacter pylori* isolated from ready to eat foods

Genotypes	Prevalence (%)[a]
M1as1a	29 (39.18)
M1as1b	12 (16.21)
M1bs1a	4 (5.40)
M1bs1b	2 (2.70)
M1as1c	3 (4.05)
M1bs1c	1 (1.35)
M2s1a	52 (70.27)
M2s1b	11 (14.86)
M2s1c	6 (8.10)
M2s2	1 (1.35)
M1as2	1 (1.35)
M1bs2	–
M1am2	23 (31.08)
M1bm2	2 (2.70)
CagA+	31 (41.89)
CagA−	43 (58.10)
IceA1	10 (13.51)
IceA2	3 (4.05)
IceA1 IceA2	1 (1.35)
OipA+	14 (18.91)
OipA−	60 (81.08)

[a] From a total of 74 positive strains of *H. pylori*

cross contamination of these foods due to handling by factory and food units staffs are the main reasons for the high prevalence of *H. pylori* in these samples. The results of Mhaskar et al. [28] confirmed the finding of our study about the risk of meat products for *H. pylori* infection. They reported that the prevalence of peptic ulcer and *H. pylori* infection were entirely higher in those patients which were used from meat and meat products [odds ratio (OR) 2.35, 95 % confident interval (CI): 1.30–4.23] and restaurant foods (OR 3.77, 95 % CI 1.39–10.23) than vegans.

Preparation of some kinds of these food samples including falafel (pea based fast food with some kinds of vegetables), cream-candy, restaurant salad, traditional bread, fruit salad and olvie salad need moderate levels of water. Roles of contaminated water and even drinking water in transmission of *H. pylori* have been confirmed previously [29–32]. Probably, the water sources used for production and processing of these foods samples were contaminated. Finally, using from unsanitary conditions, handling contamination, use of contaminated equipment and lack of public and individual hygiene are the main reasons for the high prevalence of *H. pylori* in food samples of our study. Food safety regulations as well as quality standards—including good agricultural practices (GAPs), good manufacturing practices (GMPs) and hazard analysis and critical control points (HACCP)—should be introduced in Iranian food units and factories in order to control contamination and proliferation of pathogenic bacteria.

Another part of our investigation focused on the distribution of *vacA*, *cagA*, *oipA* and *iceA* genotypes. Results showed that *vacA s1a* (78.37 %), *vacA m2* (75.67 %), *vacA m1a* (51.35 %) and *cagA* (41.89 %) were the most commonly detected genotypes in *H. pylori* strains of ready to eat foods. Our results showed that the *cagA* gene had the highest prevalence in the hamburger (100 %), soup (81.81 %) and olvie salad (83.33 %). As we said, these are a meat based ready to eat food samples and the high prevalence of *cagA* gene in these samples maybe showed the high presence of *cagA* positive strains of *H. pylori* in the meat used for production of these food stuffs. Yahaghi et al. [8] reported that the *oipA* (86.44 %), *cagA* (57.62 %), *vacA s1a* (37.28 %) and *vacA m1a* (30.50 %) were the most commonly detected genotypes in the *H. pylori* isolates of vegetable and salad. They showed that *vacA s1c*

Table 6 Combined *vacA, cagA, iceA* and *oipA* genotypes of *Helicobacter pylori* isolated from ready to eat food samples

Combined genotypes	Total distribution (%)[a]
s1a/cagA+/iceA1/oipA+	8 (10.81)
s1b/cagA+/iceA1/oipA+	5 (6.75)
s1c/cagA+/iceA1/oipA+	2 (2.70)
s1a/cagA+/iceA2/oipA+	1 (1.35)
s1b/cagA+/iceA2/oipA+	-
s1c/cagA+/iceA2/oipA+	-
s1a/cagA−/iceA1/oipA+	8 (10.81)
s1b/cagA−/iceA1/oipA+	6 (8.10)
s1c/cagA−/iceA1/oipA+	2 (2.70)
s1a/cagA−/iceA2/oipA+	1 (1.35)
s1b/cagA−/iceA2/oipA+	-
s1c/cagA−/iceA2/oipA+	-
s1a/cagA+/iceA1/oipA−	9 (12.16)
s1b/cagA+/iceA1/oipA−	7 (9.45)
s1c/cagA+/iceA1/oipA−	3 (4.05)
s2/cagA+/iceA1/oipA+	3 (4.05)
s2/cagA+/iceA2/oipA+	-
s2/cagA−/iceA1/oipA+	4 (5.40)
s2/cagA−/iceA2/oipA+	-
s2/cagA−/iceA2/oipA−	-
s2/cagA+/iceA2/oipA−	1 (1.35)
s2/cagA+/iceA1/oipA−	2 (2.70)
m1a/cagA+/iceA1/oipA+	5 (6.75)
m1b/cagA+/iceA1/oipA+	2 (2.70)
m1a/cagA+/iceA2/oipA+	1 (1.35)
m1b/cagA+/iceA2/oipA+	-
m1a/cagA−/iceA1/oipA+	6 (8.10)
m1b/cagA−/iceA1/oipA+	3 (4.05)
m1a/cagA−/iceA2/oipA+	-
m1b/cagA−/iceA2/oipA+	-
m1a/cagA+/iceA1/oipA−	5 (6.75)
m1b/cagA+/iceA2/oipA−	2 (2.70)
m2/cagA+/iceA1/oipA+	7 (9.45)
m2/cagA+/iceA2/oipA+	1 (1.35)
m2/cagA+/iceA2/oipA−	1 (1.35)
m2/cagA+/iceA1/oipA−	7 (9.45)
m2/cagA−/iceA1/oipA+	7 (9.45)
m2/cagA−/iceA2/oipA+	1 (1.35)
m2/cagA−/iceA2/oipA−	1 (1.35)
m2/cagA−/iceA1/oipA−	7 (9.45)

[a] From a total of 74 positive strains of *H. pylori*

(10.16 %) had low prevalence which was similar to our findings. *VacA s1a*, *m2* and *m1a* and *cagA* were the most commonly detected genotypes in the clinical samples of human beings [9, 10, 13, 33], foods [6, 8]) and those of animal sources [9]. Close association of *vacA* and *cagA* genotypes with interleukin 8 (IL-8) production, cytotoxin production, gastric epithelial cells adhesion, inflammatory effects, vacuolization and apoptosis in gastric epithelial cells has been observed previously [34, 35]. Since *H. pylori* isolates in our study harbored *vacA* and *cagA* genotypes, consumption of ready to eat foods contaminated with virulent strains may provoke duodenal ulceration, gastric mucosal atrophy and gastric cancer.

Another important finding of our investigation is about the presence of high antibiotic resistance in the *H. pylori* strains of ready to eat food samples. Our results revealed that the *H. pylori* strains of ready to eat food samples had the high levels of antibiotic resistance against ampicillin, metronidazole, erythromycin, amoxicillin, tetracycline and trimethoprim. Similar findings have been reported previously by Yahaghi et al. [8], Thyagarajan et al. [36], Secka et al. [37] and Bang et al. [38]. Low levels of antibiotic resistance in the *H. pylori* strains against spiramycin, furazolidone, cefsulodin, rifampin, streptomycin and levofloxacin is may be due to the regular and low prescription of these antibiotics. Epidemiological investigations of Nigeria, Senegal, Iran, India, China, Taiwan, Saudi-Arabia, Thailand, Egypt, Brazil, Colombia and Argentina showed that the *H. pylori* isolates of human clinical specimens had the highest levels of resistance against metronidazole, amoxicillin, quinolones and tetracycline [39] which was similar to our results.

The results of antimicrobial resistance pattern had indirectly confirmed that the *H. pylori* strains of hamburger, soup and olvie salad (meat based ready to eat foods) were transferred from the meat samples of infected animals. It is because of the *H. pylori* strains of these food stuffs were relatively resistant to the antibiotics used especially in the veterinary medicine. Prescription of metronidazole, clarithromycin, levofloxacin, rifampin, cefsulodin, furazolidone and spiramycin antimicrobial agents is not routine in the cases of diseases in animals. Therefore, the prevalence of resistance against these antibiotics in the *H. pylori* strains of hamburger, soup and olvie salad samples which are relatively made from meat is low and this finding can indirectly confirm the primary infections of meat used from production of hamburger, soup and olvie salad.

Conclusions

In conclusion, ready to eat foods in Iran harbor *H. pylori* strains with high prevalence of *vacA*, *cagA*, *iceA* and *oipA* genotypes. High prevalence of *H. pylori* in our samples suggest that contaminated ready to eat foods maybe the sources of the bacteria and that it entered the human population in period of time. Diversity of *H. pylori* genotypes between various types of ready to eat food samples maybe showed that there were various sources of contamination for these food stuffs. Bacterial strains had the lowest levels of resistance against spiramycin and furazolidone which was quite interesting. The most important finding of this study is that the ready to eat food stuffs harbored virulent and resistant strains of *H. pylori*. Carefully prescription of antibiotics with respect to the results of disk diffusion method and cautious health monitoring on food and staffs of food producing companies maybe reduce the risk of virulent and resistant strains of *H. pylori* in Iranian food samples.

Abbreviations

H. pylori: *Helicobacter pylori*; *VacA*: vacuolating cytotoxin; *IceA*: induced by contact with the epithelium antigen; *Cag*: cytotoxin associated gene; *Oip*: outer inflammatory protein; PCR: polymerase chain reaction.

Authors' contributions

BH and ER contributed to study design. BH collected the samples, DNA extraction and culture examinations. ER contributed to PCR analysis and data interpretation. BH and ER wrote and drafted the manuscript. HM contributed on the statistical analysis.

Author details

[1] Graduated Student of Veterinary Medicine, College of Veterinary Medicine, Islamic Azad University, Shahrekord, Iran. [2] Department of Microbiology, College of Basic Sciences, Islamic Azad University, Shahrekord, Iran. [3] Department of Food Hygiene and Public Health, College of Veterinary Medicine, Islamic Azad University, Shahrekord, Iran.

Acknowledgements

The authors would like to thank Dr. Farhad Safarpoor Dehkordi at the Department of Food Hygiene and Quality Control, University of Tehran, his important technical support. This work was supported by the Azad University, Shahrekord, Iran, grant n. 94/90215.

Competing interests

The authors declare that they have no competing interests

References

1. Shrestha S, Paudel P, Pradhan GB, Shrestha L, Bhattachan CL. Prevalence study of *H. pylori* infection in dyspeptic patients coming to Nepal Medical College Teaching Hospital, Jorpati, Kathmandu. Nepal Med Coll J. 2012;14:229–33.
2. Mastromarino P, Conti C, Donato K, Strappini PM, Cattaruzza MS, Orsi GB. Does hospital work constitute a risk factor for *Helicobacter pylori* infection. J Hosp Infect. 2005;60:261–8.
3. Vu C, Ng YY. Prevalence of *Helicobacter pylori* in peptic ulcer disease in a Singapore hospital. Singapore Med J. 2000;41:478–81.
4. Webberley MJ, Webberley JM, Newell DG, Lowe P, Melikian V. Seroepidemiology of *Helicobacter pylori* infection in vegans and meat-eaters. Epidemiol Infect. 1992;108:457–62.
5. Stevenson TH, Bauer N, Lucia LM, Acuff GR. Attempts to isolate *Helicobacter* from cattle and survival of *Helicobacter pylori* in beef products. J Food Protect. 2000;63:174–8.
6. Mousavi S, Safarpoor Dehkordi F, Rahimi E. Virulence factors and antibiotic resistance of *Helicobacter pylori* isolated from raw milk and unpasteurized dairy products in Iran. J Venom Anim Toxins Incl Trop Dis. 2014;20:51.
7. Atapoor S, Safarpoor Dehkordi F, Rahimi E. Detection of *Helicobacter pylori* in various types of vegetables and salads. Jundishapur J Microbiol. 2014;7:e10013.
8. Yahaghi E, Khamesipour F, Mashayekhi F, Safarpoor Dehkordi F, Sakhaei MH, Masoudimanesh M, Khameneie MK. *Helicobacter pylori* in vegetables and salads: genotyping and antimicrobial resistance properties. Biomed Res Int. 2014;2014:757941.
9. Momtaz H, Dabiri H, Souod N, Gholami M. Study of *Helicobacter pylori* genotype status in cows, sheep, goats and human beings. BMC Gastroenterol. 2014;14:61.
10. Momtaz H, Souod N, Dabiri H, Sarshar M. Study of *Helicobacter pylori* genotype status in saliva, dental plaques, stool and gastric biopsy samples. World J Gastroenterol. 2012;18:2105–11.
11. Torres LE, Melián K, Moreno A, Alonso J, Sabatier CA, Hernández M, Bermúdez L, Rodríguez BL. Prevalence of *vacA*, *cagA* and *babA2* genes in Cuban *Helicobacter pylori* isolates. World J Gastroenterol. 2009;15:204–10.
12. Yamazaki S, Yamakawa A, Okuda T, Ohtani M, Suto H, Ito Y, Yamazaki Y, Keida Y, Higashi H, Hatakeyama M, Azuma T. Distinct diversity of *vacA*, *cagA*, and *cagE* genes of *Helicobacter pylori* associated with peptic ulcer in Japan. J Clin Microbiol. 2005;43:3906–16.
13. Momtaz H, Souod N, Dabiri H. Comparison of the virulence factors of *Helicobacter pylori* isolated in stomach and saliva in Iran. Am J Med Sci. 2010;340:345–9.
14. Ho SA, Hoyle JA, Lewis FA. Direct polymerase chain reaction test for detection of *Helicobacter pylori* in humans and animals. J Clin Microbiol. 1991;29:2543–9.
15. Clinical and Laboratory Standards Institute (CLSI). Performance standards for antimicrobial susceptibility testing. Twenty-second informational supplement M100-S21, Wayne Pa, 2012.
16. Wang J, Chi DS, Laffan JJ, Ferguson DA Jr, Litchfield P, Thomas E. Comparison of cytotoxin genotypes of *Helicobacter pylori* in stomach and saliva. Dig Dis Sci. 2002;47:1850–6.
17. Kauser F, Hussain MA, Ahmed I, Ahmad N, Habeeb A, Khan AA, Ahmed N. Comparing genomes of *Helicobacter pylori* strains from the high-altitude desert of Ladakh, India. J Clin Microbiol. 2005;43:1538–45.
18. Thirumurthi S, Graham DY. *Helicobacter pylori* infection in India from a western perspective. Ind J Med Res. 2012;136:549–62.
19. Tumurru MK, Cover TL, Blaser MJ. Cloning and expression of a highmolecular mass major antigen of *Helicobacter pylori*: evidence of linkage to cytotoxin production. Infect Immun. 1993;61:1799–809.
20. Peek RM, Thompson SA, Donahue JP, Tham KT, Atherton JC, Blaser MJ, Miller GG. Adherence to gastric epithelial cells induces expression of a *Helicobacter pylori* gene, iceA, that is associated with clinical outcome. Proc Assoc Am Physicians. 1998;110:531–44.
21. Versalovic J, Koeuth T, Lupski JR. Distribution of repetitive DNA sequences in Eubacteria and application to fingerprinting of bacterial genomes. Nucleic Acids Res. 1991;19:6823–31.
22. Rahimi E, Kheirabadi EK. Detection of *Helicobacter pylori* in bovine, buffalo, camel, ovine, and caprine milk in Iran. Foodborne Pathog Dis. 2012;9:453–6.
23. Quaglia NC, Dambrosio A, Normanno G, Parisi A, Patrono R, Ranieri G, Rella A, Celano GV. High occurrence of *Helicobacter pylori* in raw goat, sheep and cow milk inferred by glmM gene: a risk of food-borne infection. Int J Food Microbiol. 2008;124:43–7.
24. Angelidis AS, Tirodimos I, Bobos M, Kalamaki MS, Papageorgiou DK, Arvanitidou M. Detection of *Helicobacter pylori* in raw bovine milk by fluorescence in situ hybridization (FISH). Int J Food Microbiol. 2011;151:252–6.
25. Dore MP, Sepulveda AR, El-Zimaity H, Yamaoka Y, Osato MS, Mototsugu K, Nieddu AM, Realdi G, Graham DY. Isolation of *Helicobacter pylori* from sheep-implications for transmission to humans. Am J Gastroenterol. 2001;96:1396–401.
26. Fujimura S, Kawamura T, Kato S, Tateno H, Watanabe A. Detection of *Helicobacter pylori* in cow's milk. Lett Appl Microbiol. 2002;35:504–7.
27. van Duynhoven YT, de Jonge R. Transmission of *Helicobacter pylori*: a role for food. Bull World Health Organ. 2001;79:455–60.
28. Mhaskar RS, Ricardo I, Azliyati A, Laxminarayan R, Amol B, Santosh W, Boo K. Assessment of risk factors of *Helicobacter pylori* infection and peptic ulcer disease. J Glob Infect Dis. 2013;5:60–7.
29. Queralt N, Bartolomé R, Araujo R. Detection of *Helicobacter pylori* DNA in human faeces and water with different levels of faecal pollution in the north-east of Spain. J Appl Microbiol. 2005;98:889–95.

30. Dube C, Tanih NF, Ndip RN. *Helicobacter pylori* in water sources: a global environmental health concern. Rev Environ Health. 2009;24:1–14.
31. Samra ZQ, Javaid U, Ghafoor S, Batool A, Dar N, Athar MA. PCR assay targeting virulence genes of *Helicobacter pylori* isolated from drinking water and clinical samples in Lahore metropolitan, Pakistan. J Water Health. 2011;9:208–16.
32. Amirhooshang A, Ramin A, Ehsan A, Mansour R, Shahram B. High frequency of *Helicobacter pylori* DNA in drinking water in Kermanshah, Iran, during June–November 2012. J Water Health. 2014;12:504–12.
33. Havaei A, Mohajeri P, Khashei R, Salehi R, Tavakoli H. Prevalence of *Helicobacter pylori vacA* different genotypes in Isfahan, Iran. Adv Biomed Res. 2014;3:48.
34. Yamaoka Y, Reddy R, Graham DY. *Helicobacter pylori* virulence factor genotypes in children in the United States: clues about genotype and outcome relationships. J Clin Microbiol. 2010;48:2550–1.
35. Siddique I, Al-Qabandi A, Al-Ali J, Alazmi W, Memon A, Mustafa AS, Junaid TA. Association between *Helicobacter pylori* genotypes and severity of chronic gastritis, peptic ulcer disease and gastric mucosal interleukin-8 levels: evidence from a study in the Middle East. Gut Pathog. 2014;6:41.
36. Thyagarajan SP, Ray P, Das BK, Ayyagari A, Khan AA, Dharmalingam S, Rao UA, Rajasambandam P, Ramathilagam B, Bhasin D, Sharma MP, Naik SR, Habibullah CM. Geographical difference in antimicrobial resistance pattern of *Helicobacter pylori* clinical isolates from Indian patients: multicentric study. J Gastroenterol Hepatol. 2003;18:1373–8.
37. Secka O, Berg DE, Antonio M, Corrah T, Tapgun M, Walton R, Thomas V, Galano JJ, Sancho J, Adegbola RA, Thomas JE. Antimicrobial susceptibility and resistance patterns among *Helicobacter pylori* strains from The Gambia, West Africa. Antimicrob Agents Chemother. 2013;57:1231–7.
38. Bang SY, Han DS, Eun CS, Kim JE, Ahn SB, Sohn JH, Jeon YC, Kang JO. Changing patterns of antibiotic resistance of *Helicobacter pylori* in patients with peptic ulcer disease. Korean J Gastroenterol. 2007;50:356–62.
39. World Gastroenterology Organization (WGO). Global guideline. *Helicobacter pylori* in developing countries, 2010.

4

Phenotypic and genotypic characteristics of carbapenem-resistant *Enterobacteriaceae* in a tertiary-level reference hospital in Turkey

Irmak Baran[1,2*] and Neriman Aksu[1]

Abstract

Background: *Enterobacteriaceae* are among the most common pathogens that are responsible for serious community-acquired, hospital-acquired, and health-care associated infections. The emergence and spread of carbapenem-resistant *Enterobacteriaceae* (CRE) have become an increasing concern for healthcare services worldwide. Infections caused by these bacteria have been associated with significant morbidity and mortality and treatment options have been limited. The rapid and accurate detection of carbapenem resistance in these bacteria is important for infection control. The aim of this study was to investigate the phenotypic and genotypic features of CRE strains isolated in a tertiary-level reference hospital in Turkey.

Methods: A total of 181 CRE strains were included in the study. Antimicrobial susceptibility rates were tested using Vitek 2 system. Modified Hodge test (MHT) was performed using meropenem and ertapenem discs. Metallo-β-lactamase antimicrobial gradient test (E-test MBL strips) were used for evaluation of metallo-β-lactamase production. A multiplex PCR was used for detection of carbapenems resistance genes (IMP, VIM, KPC, NDM-1 and OXA-48).

Results: The OXA-48 gene was detected in 86 strains, NDM-1 gene in six strains, VIM gene in one strain. IMP and KPC genes were not identified. Three strains produced both OXA-48 and NDM-1 and one strain produced both OXA-48 and VIM. In two patients more than one genus of OXA-48 positive CREs was isolated. Ninety-two of the isolates were multidrug-resistant. One hundred and ten isolates were MHT with meropenem (MEM-MHT) positive and 109 isolates were MHT with ertapenem (ERT-MHT) positive. Nine of the isolates were positive with E-test MBL strips. The sensitivity of MEM-MHT and ERT-MHT for detection of OXA-48 was 70.9 and 70.6 %, respectively. MEM-MHT was found highly discriminative for OXA-48 *Escherichia coli* ($p < 0.001$). The sensitivity of E-test MBL for NDM-1 was 66.7 %. A statistically significant correlation was observed between OXA-48 gene and MHT positivity and between NDM-1, VIM gene and E-test MBL positivity ($p < 0.001$).

Conclusions: OXA-48 gene is spreading rapidly to many different species of *Enterobacteriaceae* in the hospital environment. While OXA-48 is still the most common source of carbapenem resistance in *Enterobacteriaceae* in our country, NDM-1 is increasingly being isolated from patients without a history of foreign contact.

Keywords: *Enterobacteriaceae*, Carbapenem resistance, OXA-48, NDM-1, VIM, Modified Hodge test, Multiplex PCR, Multidrug resistance

*Correspondence: irmakmor@yahoo.com
[1] Department of Microbiology, Ankara Numune Training and Research Hospital, Talatpaşa Bulvarı No:5 Altındağ, 06100 Ankara, Turkey
Full list of author information is available at the end of the article

Background

Enterobacteriaceae are common human pathogens and colonizers of the human intestinal tract which can cause a broad range of diseases including urinary tract infections, pneumonia, bloodstream infections, intra-abdominal, skin and soft tissue infections in both community and hospital settings [1–4]. Antibiotic resistance in *Enterobacteriaceae* is an important public health problem. Because these microorganisms are associated with increased length of hospital stay, the cost of treatment, mortality and morbidity [5–8].

Dissemination of infections caused by extended-spectrum β-lactamases (ESBL) and AmpC β-lactamases-producing *Enterobacteriaceae* has compromised susceptibility to cephalosporins in many areas of the world and has led to increased use of carbapenems which are stable antibiotics against these enzymes. However widespread use of carbapenems resulted in the emergence of carbapenem-resistant *Enterobacteriaceae* (CRE) [3, 4, 6, 9, 10].

Mainly two different mechanisms are responsible for carbapenem resistance in *Enterobacteriaceae*: (i) hyper production of ESBL or AmpC enzymes combined with porin loss or alteration or upregulated efflux pump and/or (ii) production of carbapenem-hydrolyzing carbapenemases [1, 6, 11–13].

In 1993, NmcA in *Enterobacter cloacae* was identified as the first carbapenemase enzyme in *Enterobacteriaceae* [4, 10]. Since then, outbreaks caused by carbapenemase-producing *Enterobacteriaceae* (CPE) have been reported from various regions of the world [1, 4, 14].

Carbapenemases are categorized in Ambler classification system as follows, the class A carbapenemases (GES, KPCs) which are inhibited by clavulanic acid; the class B or metallo-β-lactamases (VIM, IMP, NDMs) which are inhibited by ethylene diamine tetra-acetic acid (EDTA); and the class D oxacillinases which are not affected by clavulanic acid or EDTA [3, 7, 8, 14, 15].

Plasmid-mediated carbapenemase production is the most important and common cause of carbapenem resistance in CRE [3, 7, 9, 12, 16]. The emergence of plasmids containing carbapenemase genes was considered as a serious health threat because it may ease the spread of carbapenem resistance [17]. Also, carbapenem-resistant isolates frequently carry additional antimicrobial resistance genes to other classes of antibiotics including fluoroquinolones, aminoglycosides, trimethoprim—sulfamethoxazole, and this limits the treatment options [1, 6, 9, 10, 13, 18].

A limited number of published data from our country about carbapenem resistance in *Enterobacteriaceae* other than carbapenem-resistant *Klebsiella pneumonia* (CRKP) are available.

The aim of this study was to investigate phenotypic and genotypic characteristics of carbapenem resistance in CRE isolated from patients in our hospital.

Methods

Setting and study design

This prospective study was conducted over a period of 13 months between January 31st 2013–February 14th 2014 in Medical Microbiology Laboratory of Ankara Numune Research and Training Hospital which is a 1200 bed capacity tertiary-level reference hospital with surgical, medical, orthopaedic and intensive care units and serves not only a population of 4,000,000 inhabitants but also the surrounding cities.

In this period, a total of 6426 *Enterobacteriaceae* species were isolated from different clinical specimens (blood, urine, wound, tracheal aspirate, abscess, etc.) sent to our laboratory. Clinical samples were analysed with standard laboratory techniques.

Bacterial strains and antimicrobial susceptibility testing

All *Enterobacteriaceae* isolates at the time of isolation were identified using Vitek 2 automated system (bioMérieux, France) with ID-GNB card and then confirmed by MALDI Biotyper (Bruker, Germany). Antibiotic susceptibility tests were done using vitek AST-GN cards. Susceptibilities to ampicillin (AMP), amoxicillin-clavulanic acid (AMC), piperacillin-tazobactam (TZP), cefuroxime (CXM), cefuroxime-axetil (CAE), cefoxitin (FOX), ceftazidime (CAZ), ceftriaxone (CRO), cefepime (FEP), ertapenem (ERT), imipenem (IPM), meropenem (MEM), amikacin (AMK), gentamicin (GEN), ciprofloxacin (CIP), colistin (CST), trimethoprim-sulfamethoxazole (SXT) were tested. CLSI 2013 M100-S23 breakpoint values were used [19]. For colistin the CLSI recommendation for *Acinetobacter* spp. were used [19, 20]. *Escherichia coli* ATCC 25922 and *Pseudomonas aeruginosa* ATCC 27853 were used as quality control strains.

Isolates were considered as CRE if they were found resistant or intermediate to one or more of the carbapenems (ERT, IPM and MEM). A total of 181 (2.82 %) isolates were identified as CRE and were included in this study. Minimal inhibitory concentration (MIC) of ERT, IPM and MEM were also tested by E-test. E-test results were interpreted according to the CLSI 2013 criteria [19].

Phenotypic methods for detecting carbapenemase activity testing and ESBL production

Modified Hodge test (MHT) was used for screening carbapenemase production using ERT and MEM according to CLSI guidelines [19]. Metallo-β-lactamase production was investigated with metallo-β-lactamase antimicrobial gradient test which is IPM and IPM/EDTA E-test MBL strips (bioMérieux, France). A ratio of $MIC_{IPM}/MIC_{IPM/EDTA} \geq 8$ considered presumptive of metallo-β-lactamase. ESBL production was evaluated by CLSI screening and confirmatory test methods [19].

Molecular analysis of carbapenemase genes

For investigation of carbapenemases genes a multiplex PCR (hyplex® SuperBug ID, Amplex, Germany) was used. This system can identify metallo-β-lactamase genes such as $bla_{VIM(1-13)}$, $bla_{IMP(1-22)}$ and bla_{NDM-1}, oxacillinase genes such as bla_{OXA-48}-like encoding genes (including. $bla_{OXA-162, OXA-181, OXA.204}$ and $bla_{OXA-244}$) and all variants of $bla_{KPC(1-10)}$ genes.

DNA was extracted from bacteria grew in 24-h culture. After PCR reactions, amplification products were heat-denaturated to obtain single-stranded DNA and loaded to microtiter plates coated with specific probes. Hybridization reaction principle was used to investigate carbapenemase gene loci in loaded DNA. Hybridization of complementary sequences was then detected using ELISA principle. The colour formed by the chromogenic reaction was then measured by a photometer at a wavelength of 450 nm.

Statistical analysis

All data were evaluated by using SPSS for Windows version 11.5. We used Chi square test and Fischer's exact test to relate genes and MHTs for categorical data, and we also calculated screening test results. Descriptive statistics, frequencies and percentages were given. The statistical significance level was set to 0.05.

Results

CRE isolates

During the study period 181 CRE were identified from 6426 *Enterobacteriaceae* isolates. The most common species were *Klebsiella pneumoniae* (69, 38.12 %), followed by *Serratia marcescens* (33, 18.23 %), *Morganella morganii* (17, 9.39 %), *Proteus mirabilis* (17, 9.39 %), *E. coli* (13, 7.18 %), *Enterobacter cloacae* (13, 7.18 %), *Enterobacter aerogenes* (10, 5.52 %), *Citrobacter freundii* (2, 1.1 %), *Raoultella planticola* (2, 1.1 %), *Proteus vulgaris* (1, 0.55 %), *Providencia rettgeri* (1, 0.55 %), *Providencia stuartii* (1, 0.55 %), *Cronobacter sakazakii* (1, 0.55 %), *Klebsiella oxytoca* (1, 0.55 %).

The majority of strains were isolated from internal medicine intensive care unit (ICU) (49, 27.07 %). This was followed by post anesthesia care unit (PACU) (18, 9.94 %), surgical ICU (10, 5.52 %), general surgery unit (10, 5.52 %), burn unit (9, 4.97 %), urology (9, 4.97 %), and emergency internal medicine (9, 4.97 %). Remaining isolates were isolated from other clinics. Most of the 181 isolates were collected from blood (59 isolates, 32.6 %), from urine (49, 27.07 %), and from wounds (31, 17.13 %). The remaining isolates were from tracheal aspirates (21, 11.6 %), abscess culture (9, 4.97 %), catheter (4, 2.21 %), pleural fluid (3, 1.66 %), peritoneal fluid (1, 0.55 %), bile (1, 0.55 %), sputum (1, 0.55 %), rectal swab (1, 0.55 %), cerebrospinal fluid (CSF) (1, 0.55 %). Table 1 shows distribution of *Enterobacteriaceae* species according to clinical samples.

Phenotypic tests for carbapenemase production and carbapenemase genes identified by multiplex PCR

When 181 CRE isolates were analyzed with MHT with MEM (MEM-MHT) and MHT with ERT (ERT-MHT) for carbapenemase production; 110 (60.8 %) isolates were found positive with MEM-MHT and 109 (60.2 %) isolates were positive with ERT-MHT. Only nine (5 %) of the isolates were tested positive with E-test MBL strips for metallo-β-lactamase production.

In 86 (47.51 %) of the isolates, the bla_{OXA-48} gene was detected by multiplex PCR. Six isolates (3.33 %) were bla_{NDM-1} gene positive. In one strain (0.56 %) bla_{VIM} gene was found positive. A breakdown of carbapenemase positive isolates is presented in Table 2. At least one carbapenemase-encoding gene was found positive in 90 (49.72 %) of the isolates. In four of the strains, multiple carbapenemase genes were identified. Three of the bla_{NDM-1} positive *K. pneumoniae* also possessed bla_{OXA-48} gene. In one of the *K. pneumoniae,* bla_{VIM} gene was detected alongside bla_{OXA-48} gene. The bla_{IMP} and bla_{KPC} genes were not detected in any of the isolates.

MEM-MHT was positive in 78 of the 86 (90.69 %) bla_{OXA-48} positive isolates. ERT-MHT was positive in 77 of the 86 (89.53 %) bla_{OXA-48} positive isolates. All NDM and VIM positive isolates were positive with MHT and E-test MBL. NDM-1-positive *E. cloacae* were both MHT and E-test MBL positive. MEM-MHT, ERT-MHT results according to different OXA-48 positive CRE isolates was shown in Table 3. Sensitivity, specificity, negative predictive value (NPV) and positive predictive value (PPV) of MEM-MHT and ERT-MHT for bla_{OXA-48} positive isolates were given in Table 4.

There was a statistically significant correlation between bla_{OXA-48} gene positivity and MEM-MHT positivity ($p < 0.001$). There was also a statistically significant correlation between bla_{OXA-48} gene positivity and ERT-MHT positivity ($p < 0.001$). MEM-MHT was found highly discriminative for bla_{OXA-48}-positive *E. coli* ($p < 0.001$). Accuracy rate of MEM-MHT and ERT-MHT were not good for other CRE species. High rate of false positive and negative results were observed.

The sensitivity of E-test MBL for bla_{NDM-1} positive isolates was 66.7 %, specificity was 100 %, NPV 98.3 %, PPV 100 %. There was a statistically significant correlation

Table 1 Species and specimen distribution of 181 carbapenem-resistant *Enterobacteriaceae*

Species	Specimen type (n)								
	Blood	Urine	Wound	Trachael aspirate	Abscess	Catheter	Pleural fluid	Other*	Total
K. pneumoniae	18	25	8	10	3	4		1	69
S. marcescens	29	1	1	1	1				33
M. morganii	2	3	9	2				1	17
P. mirabilis	3	7	5	2					17
E. coli	3	5	1		3			1	13
E. cloacae	1	4	4				3	1	13
E. aerogenes	1	2		4	2			1	10
C. freundii	1	1							2
R. planticola		1		1					2
P. vulgaris			1						1
P. rettgeri			1						1
P. stuartii			1						1
C. sakazakii	1								1
K. oxytoca				1					1
Total	59	49	31	21	9	4	3	5	181

*Bile, sputum, rectal swab, peritoneal fluid, cerebrospinal fluid

Table 2 Distribution of positive carbapenemase gene loci according to bacteria types

Genes	Type of bacteria n (%)											Total
	K. pneumoniae	*S. marcescens*	*M. morganii*	*P. mirabilis*	*E. coli*	*E. cloacae*	*E. aerogenes*	*C. freundii*	*R. planticola*	*P. stuartii*	*K. oxytoca*	
OXA-48	52 (75.36)	5 (15.15)	3 (17.65)	6 (35.29)	8 (61.54)	3 (23.08)	5 (50)	1 (50)	1 (50)	1 (100)	1 (100)	86 (47.51)
NDM-1	5 (7.25)	0	0	0	0	1 (7.69)	0	0	0	0	0	6 (3.31)
VIM	1 (1.45)	0	0	0	0	0	0	0	0	0	0	1 (0.55)

between bla_{NDM-1} positivity and E-test MBL positivity ($p < 0.001$). When bla_{NDM-1} positive and bla_{VIM} positive isolates were considered together sensitivity of E-test MBL was 77.8 %, specificity was 100 %, NPV 98.9 %, PPV 100 %.

Carbapenemase genes were detected in 31 (36.05 %) strains isolated from urine samples, 21 (24.42 %) strains isolated from blood samples, 16 (18.60 %) strains isolated from tracheal aspirate samples, 11 (12.79 %) strains isolated from wound samples, 4 (4.65 %) strains from abscess samples, 3 (3.49 %) strains isolated from catheter samples, 1 (1.16 %) strain from sputum, 1 (1.16 %) strain from peritoneal fluid, 1 (1.16 %) strain from isolated from bile.

Carbapenemase genes were detected mostly in 18 (20.93 %) samples isolated from patients from internal ICU. This was followed by 13 (15.12 %) samples isolated from PACU patients, 9 (10.47 %) samples from surgical ICU, 6 (6.77 %) samples from urology patients, 5 (5.81 %) samples from emergency internal medicine patients, 4 (4.65 %) samples from neurosurgery patients 4 (4.65 %) samples from general surgery patients, 4 (4.65 %) samples from emergency medicine patients and 23 samples from other hospital units.

Isolation of multiple CRE from the same patient

In two patients more than one genus of CREs was isolated, and the bla_{OXA-48} gene was positive in all these isolates. First was a patient from surgical ICU. OXA-48-positive *K. pneumoniae* was isolated from wound sample then 2 days later OXA-48-positive *K. oxytoca* was isolated from tracheal aspirate and then 4 days later OXA-48-positive *E. coli* was isolated from an abscess. The second was a patient from bone marrow transplantation (BMT) unit. An OXA-48-positive *E. cloacae* was isolated from urine and 9 days later OXA-48-positive *E. coli* was isolated from blood.

Antimicrobial susceptibility results of carbapenemase negative and positive CRE

When all 181 CRE isolates were considered; 95.58 % were resistant to AMP, 91.16 % were resistant to AMC, 80.11 %

Table 3 Distribution of MEM-MHT, ERT-MHT results according to carbapenem- resistant *Enterobacteriaceae* isolates

	Total number	Number of MEM-MHT (+) isolates	Number of MEM-MHT (−) isolates	Number of ERT-MHT(+) isolates	Number of ERT-MHT(−) isolates
All isolates	181	110	71	109	72
OXA-48 positive isolates	86	78	8	77	9
K. pneumoniae	69	56	13	55	14
OXA-48 positive *K. pneumoniae*	52	50	2	51	1
S. marcescens	33	10	23	6	27
OXA-48 positive *S. marcescens*	5	2	3	1	4
M. morganii	17	8	9	9	8
OXA-48 positive *M. morganii*	3	3	0	3	0
P. mirabilis	17	9	8	10	7
OXA-48 positive *P. mirabilis*	6	4	2	4	2
E. coli	13	8	5	10	3
OXA-48 positive *E. coli*	8	8	0	8	0
E. cloacae	13	8	5	8	5
OXA-48 positive *E. cloacae*	3	3	0	3	0
E. aerogenes	10	7	3	7	3
OXA-48 positive *E. aerogenes*	5	5	0	5	0
C. freundii	2	0	2	1	1
OXA-48 positive *C. freundii*	1	0	1	0	1
R. planticola	2	1	1	0	2
OXA-48 positive *R. planticola*	1	1	0	0	1
P. stuartii	1	1	0	1	0
OXA-48 positive *P. stuartii*	1	1	0	1	0
K. oxytoca	1	1	0	1	0
OXA-48 positive *K. oxytoca*	1	1	0	1	0

MEM-MHT modified Hodge test with meropenem, *ERT-MHT* modified Hodge test with ertapenem

were resistant to TZP, 80.11 % were resistant to CXM, 82.32 % were resistant to CAE, 76.80 % were resistant to FOX, 60.22 % were resistant to CAZ, 68.51 % were resistant to CRO, 51.38 % were resistant to FEP, 55.80 % were resistant to ERT, 94.47 % were resistant to IPM, 44.75 % were resistant to MEM, 23.20 % were resistant to AMK, 39.23 % were resistant to GEN, 46.96 % were resistant to CIP, 46.41 % were resistant to CST, 38.67 % were resistant to SXT. Antimicrobial resistance results of each species were shown in Table 5.

Ninety-two of the 181 isolates (50.8 %) were multidrug-resistant which was defined as being resistant to three or more functional classes of drugs simultaneously by Magiorakos et al. [21]. Fifty-one of the 69 *K. pneumoniae* isolates were found to be multidrug-resistant, and four of them were found to be resistant to all tested antibiotics. Eight of the 13 *E. coli,* 10 of 17 *P. mirabilis*, eight of 17 *M. morganii*, eight of the 13 *E. cloacae*, one the 10 *E. aerogenes,* two of the two *C. freundii*, one the two *R. planticola,* one of one *P. rettgeri*, one of one *P. stuartii*, and only one of the 33 *S. marcescens* were multidrug-resistant. Fifty three (61.62 %) of 86 OXA-48 positive isolates and 39 (41.05 %) of the 95 OXA-48 negative isolates were multidrug-resistant. There were more multidrug-resistant isolates in OXA-48 positive isolates than OXA-48 negative ones, and this difference was statistically significant ($p < 0.01$). All metallo-β-lactamase (NDM-1, VIM) positive isolates were found to be multidrug-resistant ($p < 0.01$). There was a statistically significant correlation between having one of the carbapenemase genes and being multidrug-resistant ($p < 0.001$).

Most of the *K. pneumoniae, E. coli* and *E. cloacae* isolates were resistant to carbapenems, beta-lactam/beta-lactamase inhibitor combinations, third and fourth generation cephalosporins, CIP and SXT. Thirty-seven out of 69 *K.pneumoniae* were found to be susceptible to AMK, and 25 were susceptible to GEN. Ten of the *K. pneumoniae* were found to be resistant to CST. One *E.cloacae* and one *E.coli* isolate were found to be resistant to CST. Twenty-three of *K. pneumoniae* isolates were identified as ESBL producers.

Fifty-four of the 69 *K. pneumoniae* (78.26 %) had a least a carbapenemase gene. Eighteen of the carbapenemase-positive *K. pneumoniae* were also ESBL positive. Both

Table 4 Sensitivity, specificity, negative predictive value, positive predictive value of MEM-MHT, ERT-MHT and correlation with OXA-48 gene positivity

		Sensitivity %	Specificity %	NPV %	PPV %	Correlation with OXA-48 gene positivity
All OXA-48 positive isolates	MEM-MHT	70.9	88.7	66.3	90.7	$p < 0.001$
	ERT-MHT	70.6	87.5	66.3	89.5	$p < 0.001$
OXA-48 positive *K. pneumoniae*	MEM-MHT	89.3	84.6	64.7	96.2	$p < 0.001$
	ERT-MHT	92.7	92.9	76.5	98.1	$p < 0.001$
OXA-48 positive *S. marcescens*	MEM-MHT	20	86.9	71.4	40	$p > 0.05$
	ERT-MHT	16.7	85.2	82.1	20	$p > 0.05$
OXA-48 positive *M. morganii*	MEM-MHT	37.5	100	64.3	100	$p > 0.05$
	ERT-MHT	33.3	100	57.1	100	$p > 0.05$
OXA-48 positive *P. mirabilis*	MEM-MHT	44.4	75	54.6	66.7	$p > 0.05$
	ERT-MHT	40	71.4	45.5	66.7	$p > 0.05$
OXA-48 positive *E. coli*	MEM-MHT	100	100	100	100	$p < 0.001$
	ERT-MHT	80	100	60	100	$p < 0.05$
OXA-48 positive *E. cloacae*	MEM-MHT	37.5	100	50	100	$p > 0.05$
	ERT-MHT	37.5	100	50	100	$p > 0.05$
OXA-48 positive *E. aerogenes*	MEM-MHT	71.43	100	60	100	$p > 0.05$
	ERT-MHT	71.43	100	60	100	$p > 0.05$

MEM-MHT modified Hodge test with meropenem, *ERT-MHT* modified Hodge test with ertapenem, *NPV* negative predictive value, *PPV* positive predictive value

Table 5 Antibiotic resistance rates of most commonly isolated carbapenem-resistant *Enterobacteriaceae* species in our study

Species	Antibiotic resistance rate (%)																
	AMP	AMC	TZP	CXM	CAE	FOX	CAZ	CRO	FEP	ERT	IPM	MEM	AMK	GEN	CIP	CST	SXT
K. pneumoniae	100	100	100	88.41	88.41	85.51	86.96	86.96	86.96	100	92.75	78.26	46.38	63.77	78.26	14.49	55.07
S. marcescens	100	100	30.30	100	100	100	30.30	100	6.06	0	100	0	3.03	0	0	100	0
M. morganii	100	100	52.94	100	100	52.94	58.82	41.18	58.82	0	100	11.76	17.65	11.76	29.41	100	47.06
P. mirabilis	52.94	29.41	17.65	0	0	0	23.53	0	17.65	0	100	5.88	0	29.41	35.29	100	41.18
E. coli	100	92.31	92.31	92.31	84.62	76.92	69.23	76.92	76.92	84.62	84.62	76.92	15.38	53.85	61.54	7.69	61.54
E. cloacae	100	100	69.23	76.92	100	100	61.54	61.54	38.46	84.62	92.31	61.54	30.77	61.54	61.54	7.96	53.85
E. aerogenes	100	100	50	50	60	100	40	30	0	50	90	30	0	0	10	10	0

AMC amoxicillin-clavulanic acid, *AMK* amikacin, *AMP* ampicillin, *CAE* cefuroxime-axetil, *CAZ* ceftazidime, *CIP* ciprofloxacin, *CRO* ceftriaxone, *CST* colistin, *CXM* cefuroxime, *ERT* ertapenem, *FEP* cefepime, *FOX* cefoxitin, *GEN* gentamicin, *IPM* imipenem, *MEM* meropenem, *SXT* trimethoprim-sulfamethoxazole, *TZP* piperacillin-tazobactam

carbapenemase-negative and carbapenemase-positive *K. pneumoniae* were found to be 100 % resistant to AMP, AMC, TZP and ERT. Carbapenemase-positive *K. pneumoniae* was found to be slightly more resistant to FOX (87.04 vs 80 %), CAZ (87.04 vs 86.67 %), CRO (87.04 vs 86.67 %), FEP (87.04 vs 86.67 %), IPM (96.30 vs 86.67 %), MEM (79.63 vs 73.33 %), GEN (64.81 vs 60 %), CST (16.67 vs 6.67 %) than carbapenemase-negative *K. pneumoniae.* On the other hand carbapenemase-negative *K. pneumoniae* were more resistant to CXM (93.33 vs 88.89 %), CAE (93.33 vs 88.89 %), AMK (66.67 vs 40.74 %), CIP (80 vs 77.78 %), and SXT (73.33 vs 50 %) than carbapenemase-positive *K. pneumoniae.* However, these differences were not statistically significant ($p > 0.05$).

One of the OXA-48 and NDM-1 positive *K.pneumoniae* was found resistant to all of the tested antibiotics.

Three *E.coli* isolates were ESBL positive. Eight of the OXA-48 positive isolates were found to be multidrug-resistant. Both OXA-48 positive and negative isolates were found to be 100 % resistant to AMP. *E. coli* which posses $bla_{OXA\text{-}48}$ gene were found to be more resistant to antibiotics than $bla_{OXA\text{-}48}$ negative *E. coli*: AMC (100 vs 80 %), TZP (100 vs 80 %), CXM (100 vs 80 %), CAE (100 vs 60 %), FOX (100 vs 40 %), CAZ (100 vs 20 %), CRO (100 vs 40 %), FEP (100 vs 40 %), ERT (100 vs 60 %), IPM (100 vs 60 %), MEM(100 vs 40 %), AMK (25 vs 0 %), GEN (62.5 vs 20 %), CIP (75 vs 40 %), SXT (62.5 vs 60 %) except for CST (0 vs 20 %). Only the differences for FOX, CAZ, CRO, FEP, MEM were statistically significant ($p < 0.05$).

One isolate of *E. cloacae* was found to produce bla_{NDM-1}. This isolate was found to be highly resistant to tested antibiotics with high MICs and found to be susceptible to only to CST. It was isolated from the urine sample of a patient who was residing at internal medicine unit. When patient's history was examined, there was no history of foreign travel. This patient had a previous history of use of cephalosporins and carbapenems. Similarly, none of the other patients with bla_{NDM-1} gene positive CRE infections had records of foreign travel.

S. marcescens isolates were mostly resistant to beta-lactam/beta-lactamase inhibitor combinations, second and third generation cephalosporins. All were resistant to IMP, and all were resistant to CST. All were susceptible to ERT, MEM, GEN, CIP and SXT.

M. morganii isolates were mostly resistant to beta-lactam/beta-lactamase inhibitor combinations, IMP and CST. Nearly half of the *M. morganii* isolates were resistant to FOX, CAZ, CRO, FEP and SXT. All *M. morganii* isolates were susceptible to ERT. Two of the isolates were resistant to MEM. Three of the isolates were resistant to AMK, two were resistant to GEN, and five were resistant to CIP.

P. mirabilis isolates were mostly susceptible to beta-lactam/beta-lactamase inhibitor combinations, cephalosporins and aminoglycosides. All *P. mirabilis* isolates were found to be susceptible to ERT, and only one was resistant to MEM. All *P. mirabilis* isolates were resistant to IMP and CST.

All *E. aerogenes* isolates were susceptible to FEP, aminoglycosides (AMK and GEN) and SXT. Only one *E. aerogenes* was found to be resistant to CST, and one was resistant to CIP.

In our study *K. pneumoniae, E. coli, E. cloacae* isolates were found highly resistant to ERT, IPM and MEM. *S. marcescens, M. morganii, P. mirabilis* were mostly susceptible to ERT but highly resistant to IPM. CST was found to be most effective antibiotic against *K. pneumoniae, E. coli, E. cloacae.* On the other hand, *S. marcescens, M. morganii, P. mirabilis, P. vulgaris, P. stuartii, P. rettgeri, C. sakazakii* were found to be 100 % resistant to CST. When 181 CRE are considered AMK (23.20 % resistant) and SXT (38.67 % resistant) were found as most effective antibiotics. Resistance to CST was 46.41 % overall but when the resistance of species with intrinsic resistance were excluded (*Serratia, Morganella, Proteus*, etc.) it was 12.61 %.

Discussion

CRE are increasingly isolated from community-acquired and nosocomial infections [6]. CRE can spread clonally from person to person or genes which encode carbapenemases can spread horizontally between isolates [2]. This is an important health concern because plasmid-encoded and easily transferable carbapenemases are involved [10]. The most important carbapenemases are KPC, VIM, NDM and OXA-48 [6]. CRE infections are highly mortal, and treatment options are narrow [7, 10]. Rapid identification of carbapenemase-producing strains is crucial for preventing hospital infections and outbreaks [7].

Certain risk factors were found to be related to the acquirement of CRE infections. These situations are being admitted to ICU, central venous catheter presence, usage of antibiotic such as cephalosporins, having diabetes mellitus, having surgical procedures, long stay in the hospital and being a transplant patient [7]. In our study majority of our CRE strains were isolated from ICUs.

The rate of CRE in our hospital during the study period was found as 2.82 %. In the United States prevalence of CRE was found to be between 1.4–4.2 % [2]. Similar CRE isolation rates to our study have been reported from many Asian countries: 1.2 % in Lebanon, 4.05 % from Malaysia, <1 in Singapore, 1.2 % in Taiwan, 1.17 % in Saudi Arabia [4, 5].

The most common CRE species isolated in the US and European countries are *K. pneumoniae* followed by *E. aerogenes* and *E. coli* [2, 18]. In accordance to this in our study, the most common isolated species was *K. pneumoniae.* But our second most was *S. marcescens* and third most were *M. morganii* and *P. mirabilis.*

Our country has a geographical importance for isolation of carbapenemase-producing bacteria. However molecular studies regarding carbapenemase resistance are limited especially for CRE other than CRKP [7].

After its initial identification from a *K. pneumoniae* strain in 2001 in Turkey, OXA-48 producers have become increasingly important causes of nosocomial outbreaks in our country [22, 23]. Today OXA-48 producing *Enterobacteriaceae* have spread to Middle East (Lebanon, Israel), and North African countries (Morocco, Tunisia, Egypt, Libya, Algeria), Mediterranean countries (Greece, Spain, Italy, France, Slovenia, Croatia), and European countries (Germany, Belgium, Switzerland, the Netherlands, the UK), North America (USA), South America (Argentina) and Asia (India, Taiwan) [7, 10, 17, 20, 22, 23]. The bla_{OXA-48} gene in *Enterobacteriaceae* is located between two identical copies of IS*1999*, which altogether forms composite transposon Tn*1999* on a mobilizable, self-conjugative plasmid [4, 7, 8, 10, 14, 17, 22–25] In previous studies it was shown that bla_{OXA-48}-carrying plasmids can transfer both clonally and horizontally [25].

Initially and most commonly bla_{OXA-48} gene was identified in *K. pneumoniae*. But currently, many other species of *Enterobacteriaceae* are known to possess them, such as *E. coli, Enterobacter* spp., *K. oxytoca, C. freundii, S. marcescens, M. morganii, P. mirabilis* [17, 25]. In our study majority of OXA-48 producing isolates were *K. pneumoniae*. There is an ongoing epidemic of bla_{OXA-48} positive *K. pneumoniae* nosocomial infections in our hospital since 2010 (personal data). We guess spread to other *Enterobacteriaceae* species was occurred from these *K. pneumoniae* isolates. Interestingly, during our study period more than one genus of bla_{OXA-48} gene positive CRE were isolated in two patients. This suggests horizontal interspecies dissemination. The bla_{OXA-48}-like genes were known to be located on conjugative plasmids of IncL/M incompatibility group which can transfer between different species of *Enterobacteriaceae* [25]. The bla_{OXA-48} can successfully spread to different enterobacterial species with the help of high transfer efficiency of the plasmids that carry this gene [23]. This explains the interspecies transmission of the bla_{OXA-48} gene.

Arana et al. have reported they have recovered four different CRE species (*K. pneumoniae, E. coli, S. marcescens, C. freundii*) from a patient hospitalized for 4 months. These bacteria all had the bla_{OXA-48} gene. They mentioned the great ability of OXA-48 carbapenemase to spread among different enterobacterial species [26].

In our country, the bla_{OXA-48} genes were identified previously in *K. pneumoniae, E. aerogenes, E. coli, C. freundii, E. cloacae, S. marcescens, P. rettgeri, K. oxytoca* [24, 27, 28]. To our knowledge, this is the first report of bla_{OXA-48} genes identified in *P. mirabilis, M. morganii, P. stuartii, R. planticola* in Turkey.

The OXA-48 enzyme can successfully hydrolyze penicillins but have poor or no activity against extended-spectrum cephalosporins and aztreonam. They also have a weak carbapenemase activity and cannot show a high level of carbapenem resistance. The contribution of other factors such as the production of ESBLs or cell wall permeability defects are necessary for the increased level of resistance to cephalosporins and carbapenems [10, 20, 22–26]. In other studies, a close association was found between OXA-48 enzyme production and expression of ESBLs (CTX-M-15, SHV) [8, 10, 13, 17, 20, 24]. Co-expression of OXA-48 and AmpC enzymes in CRE were demonstrated, previously [1].

In our study majority of OXA-48 positive isolates were resistant to extended-spectrum cephalosporins and had high levels of resistance to carbapenems. These findings suggest that other mechanisms of resistance are present in our isolates.

On the other hand, metallo-β-lactamases (IMP, VIM, and NDM) can yield high levels of resistance to carbapenems. But they cannot hydrolyze aztreonam. They can be inhibited by EDTA [1, 10, 12]. E-test MBL strips use the principle of inhibition of metallo-β-lactamases by EDTA when IPM is used as a substrate. Doyle et al. said that it is often difficult to interpret E-test MBL for investigation of metallo-β-lactamases in *Enterobacteriaceae* because MIC values of IPM are low in metallo-β-lactamases -producing *Enterobacteriaceae*. They found that sensitivity of metallo-β-lactamases was low, but specificity was high [15]. However, in our study, we found nine isolates positive with E-test MBL and seven of these isolates had a metallo-β-lactamases gene. The sensitivity and specificity of E-test MBL for metallo-β-lactamases in our study was 77.8 and 100 %, respectively. The false positive results may be due to increased outer membrane permeability caused by EDTA used in the test [29].

Verona integron encoded metallo-β-lactamase (VIM) was first reported from Italy in 1997 [23]. *Enterobacteriaceae* producing VIM enzymes are found prevalently in Mediterranean countries. VIM -1- producing *Enterobacteriaceae* are endemic in Greece [10, 22, 23]. In Turkey the first detection of VIM-1 was from a *K. pneumoniae* isolate from the urine of three-year-old girl in 2005 by Yıldırım et al. [30]. In our study, we identified bla_{VIM} in a *K. pneumoniae* isolate which also had the bla_{OXA-48} gene. This strain was resistant to all tested antibiotics (including CST) except SXT. VIM enzymes are found to be associated with class1 integrons that carry gene cassettes which encode resistance genes to various antibiotics [22].

Another plasmid-mediated metallo-β-lactamases, New Delhi metallo-β-lactamase-1 (NDM-1) was first discovered in a *K. pneumoniae* strain isolated from the urine sample of a Swedish patient who was previously hospitalized in India in 2009 [3, 10, 22, 23]. Later it spread to Balkans and Middle East [1]. NDM-producing *Enterobacteriaceae* are widespread in India, Pakistan, and Bangladesh [22]. The first report of NDM-1 from Turkey was in 2011 by Poirel et al. from a *K. pneumoniae* strain isolated from an allogenic stem cell-transplanted leukemia patient who was previously hospitalized in Iraq [7]. The second case report in Turkey was from our laboratory in 2013 from a *K. pneumoniae* isolated from the blood culture of a Syrian patient [31]. In the present study, we detected bla_{NDM-1} gene in six of the CRE isolates (five *K. pneumoniae* and one *E. cloacae*). Three of the bla_{NDM-1} positive *K. pneumoniae* isolates were also positive for the bla_{OXA-48} gene. We have found that all six bla_{NDM-1} positive isolates were resistant to all β-lactam antibiotics, AMK, GEN, CIP, and SXT. Two of the bla_{NDM-1} positive *K. pneumoniae* isolates were found to be resistant to CST.

In previous studies, similar to our findings NDM-1 producing *Enterobacteriaceae* are found to be often broadly resistant to many other drug classes besides β-lactams. NDM-1 producing isolates may carry a diversity of other resistance mechanisms such as β-lactamases (AmpC cephalosporinases, CTX-M, CMY), other types of carbapenemases (OXA-48, KPC and VIM), enzymes that cause resistance to aminoglycosides (16S RNA methylase), to quinolones (Qnr), to macrolids (esterases), to rifampicin (rifampicin-modifying enzymes), to chloramphenicol and SXT, to CST [2, 10, 22, 23].

NDM-1 was most commonly identified in *K. pneumoniae* and *E. coli* isolates but has been increasingly reported in other species of *Enterobacteriaceae* including *C. freundii, M. morganii, E. cloacae, K. oxytoca* [2, 3, 6, 22]. This may be because NDM enzymes are encoded on highly mobile, conjugative plasmids which facilitate horizontal inter- and intraspecies transfer between bacteria rather than clonal spread [2, 3, 10]. We have found one NDM-1 producing *E. cloacae* in our study. Previously Poirel et al. reported an NDM-1-producing *E. cloacae* outbreak in a neonatal ICU in Turkey [32]. NDM-1 producing *E. cloacae* previously have been defined as one of the most commonly reported CRE species and known to cause hospital outbreaks in many other parts of the world [3]. In another study from our country, Demir et al. isolated NDM-1 positive *S. marcescens* and *K. oxytoca* [6]. This is particularly concerning because NDM isolates are highly resistant to many classes of antibiotics and have the potential to spread rapidly to many members of *Enterobacteriaceae* and cause nosocomial outbreaks.

The first identified cases of NDM-producing CRE in our country had histories of foreign country travel [7, 31]. None of the NDM cases in our study had a history of foreign travel. Similar to our findings in two studies from our country conducted by Alp *et al.* and Sahin *et al.* no international contact history was found in patients with NDM-1-producing CRE [7, 33]. This is important because it means NDM-1 carbapenem resistance is spreading in Turkey.

The development of methods for rapid and accurate identification of CRE is necessary for appropriate selection of antibiotic treatment and prevention of hospital outbreaks [7, 9]. Automated antibiotic susceptibility systems were found to be unreliable for detection of carbapenem resistance. These automated systems either over or under reported carbapenem resistance [2, 12]. More practical molecular methods are needed. In this study, we used a hybridization-based multiplex PCR method which was reported to have 99 % specificity for OXA-48 and 100 % for other enzymes [34]. Two other studies from our country reported to use this multiplex PCR method and get accurate results [6, 7]. Demir et al. analyzed 95 *Enterobacteriaceae* spp. isolates with this system and found bla_{OXA-48} in 49 isolates, bla_{NDM-1} in six isolates and bla_{VIM} in two isolates. They did not find any carbapenemase genes in carbapenemase susceptible strains [6]. Sahin et al. found seven bla_{OXA-48} positive strain and one bla_{NDM-1} positive strain when they studied 43 CRE isolate [7].

MHT is known be reliable for detection of KPCs and OXA-48-like enzymes but perform poorly for metallo-β-lactamases (NDMs, VIMs, and IMPs) [2, 9, 12, 15, 24]. In a study Doyle et al. found MHT had the sensitivity of 98 % for detection of KPC-producers, 93 % for OXA-48-like producers and only 12 % for metallo-β-lactamase producers [15]. However, we found that all metallo-β-lactamase (NDM-1 and VIM) positive bacteria in our study were MHT positive.

Another shortcoming of MHT is it can give false-positive results for carbapenem-resistant but noncarbapenemase-producing strains [15]. Also, there is limited data on MHT's performance for CRE other than carbapenem-resistant *K. pneumoniae* and *E. coli*. Hammoud et al. showed MHT gave false-positive results in *E. cloacae* [4]. In this regard, our study was the first study that analyzed performance of MHT on many different CRE species. The sensitivity of MEM-MHT for bla_{OXA-48} positive isolates was found 70.9 %; specificity was 88.7 %, sensitivity of ERT-MHT for bla_{OXA-48} positive isolates was 70.6 %, specificity was 87.5 %. A good correlation was found between bla_{OXA-48} and MHT positivity.

In our study MHT performed gave best results for OXA-48-producing *E. coli*. MHT's results for *K. pneumoniae* were acceptable. However, MHT performed poorly for *S. marcescens, M. morganii, P. mirabilis, E. cloacae, E. aerogenes.*

MHT gave false positive and negative results for OXA-48-producing *K. pneumoniae, S. marcescens, P. mirabilis, and C. freundii.* MHT gave false positive results for OXA-48-producing *M. morganii, E. cloacae, E. aerogenes.*

In many studies, tigecycline and CST were found as most effective antimicrobial agents against CRE [1, 5, 24, 25]. In our study when antibiotic resistance profiles of all isolates were considered together, AMK (23.20 %) was found as most effective antibiotic, followed by SXT (38.67 %). Similar to our findings Wang et al. found that AMK susceptibility was very high among the CRE in their study [1]. Pollet et al. found that AMK and GEN were the most effective antibiotics followed by SXT when cumulative antibiogram of 115 CRE isolates was studied. In that study, CST and tigecycline were not tested [2]. CST resistance rate was high in our study because of the strains with intrinsic CST resistance were included in cumulative antibiotic resistance profile. On the other hand, CST was found as the most effective antibiotic against non-intrinsically CST resistant CRE strains (*K. pneumoniae, E. coli, E. cloacae, E. aerogenes, R. planticola, K. oxytoca*).

We have found that 92 of the 181 isolates were multidrug-resistant. The number of multidrug-resistant strains in OXA-48 producing isolates were slightly more than OXA-48 negative ones, and this difference was statistically significant. All metallo-β-lactamase positive isolates were multidrug-resistant. In previous studies, it was shown that the same plasmids that carry carbapenemase genes can often carry resistance genes to other antibiotics, and the rate of multidrug resistance among CRE is high [14, 24, 25].

Hammoudi et al. in their study found that OXA-48 positive *S. marcescens* remained susceptible to most tested aminoglycosides and fluoroquinolones while all the remaining CRE that they studied were multidrug-resistant [14]. Similar to this *S. marcescens* isolates in our study were found susceptible to AMK, GEN, CIP, and SXT. Only one *S. marcescens* in our study was multidrug-resistant. Similar to this *E. aerogenes* strains in our study were mostly susceptible to AMK, GEN, CIP, SXT and CST and only one of *E. aerogenes* strains was multidrug-resistant.

Fursova et al. showed that most of the CRE strains they studied were multidrug-resistant (98.9 % of *K. pneumoniae* and 100 % of *P. mirabilis*). They found that most active antibiotic against *K. pneumoniae* was CST and most effective antibiotics against *P. mirabilis* were cefoperazone/sulbactam, ERT, and CAZ [25]. Similar to this we found most effective antibiotics against carbapenem-resistant *P. mirabilis* were CXM, CAE, FOX, CRO, ERT, and AMK.

Conclusions

The findings of our study indicate that OXA-48 resistance is spreading rapidly throughout many *Enterobacteriaceae* species in Turkey. Also, NDM-1 isolates without a history of foreign contact are increasingly being found in our country. This is alarming. Therefore, carbapenem resistance mechanisms in *Enterobacteriaceae* should be rapidly determined and infection control precautions should be immediately taken.

Abbreviations

AMC: amoxicillin-clavulanic acid; AMK: amikacin; AMP: ampicillin; AmpC: AmpC beta-lactamases; ATCC: American Type Culture Collection; BMT: bone marrow transplantation; CAE: cefuroxime-axetil; CAZ: ceftazidime; CIP: ciprofloxacin; CLSI: Clinical and Laboratory Standards Institute; CPE: carbapenemase-producing *Enterobacteriaceae*; CRE: carbapenem-resistant *Enterobacteriaceae*; CRKP: carbapenem-resistant *Klebsiella pneumonia*; CRO: ceftriaxone; CSF: cerebrospinal fluid; CST: colistin; CXM: cefuroxime; DNA: deoxyribonucleic acid; EDTA: ethylene diamine tetra-acetic acid; ELISA: enzyme linked immunosorbent assay; ERT: ertapenem; ERT-MHT: modified Hodge test with ertapenem; ESBL: extended-spectrum β-lactamases; E-test: epsilometer test; FEP: cefepime; FOX: cefoxitin; GEN: gentamicin; GES: Guiana extended spectrum; ICU: intensive care unit; IMP: IMP type metallo-beta-lactamase; IPM: imipenem; KPC: Klebsiella pneumoniae carbapenemase; MALDI: matrix assisted laser desorption ionisation; MBL: metallo-β-lactamase; MEM: meropenem; MEM-MHT: modified Hodge test with meropenem; MHT: modified Hodge test; MIC: minimal inhibitory concentration; NDM-1: New Delhi metallo-β-lactamase-1; NmcA: not metalloenzyme carbapenemase; NPV: negative predictive value; OXA: oxacillinase; PACU: post anesthesia care unit; PCR: polymerase chain reaction; PPV: positive predictive value; RNA: ribonucleic acid; SXT: trimethoprim-sulfamethoxazole; TZP: piperacillin-tazobactam; VIM: Verona integron encoded metallo-β-lactamase.

Authors' contributions

IB and NA planned the study, collected bacterial isolates,performed bacterial identification, antimicrobial susceptibility, PCR, MHT, E-test MBL tests, analyzed information, did statistical analysis. IB wrote the manuscript, NA made significant contributions to manuscript preparation. Both authors read and approved the final manuscript.

Author details

[1] Department of Microbiology, Ankara Numune Training and Research Hospital, Talatpaşa Bulvarı No:5 Altındağ, 06100 Ankara, Turkey. [2] Present Address: Esat Caddesi 101/3 Küçükesat, 06660 Ankara, Turkey.

Competing interests

The authors declare that they have no competing interests.

References

1. Wang JT, Wu UI, Lauderdale TL, Chen MC, Li SY, Hsu LY, et al. Carbapenem-nonsusceptible *Enterobacteriaceae* in Taiwan. PLoS One. 2015;10:e0121668.
2. Pollett S, Miller S, Hindler J, Uslan D, Carvalho M, Humphries RM. Phenotypic and molecular characteristics of carbapenem-resistant *Enterobacteriaceae* in a health care system in Los Angeles, California, from 2011 to 2013. J Clin Microbiol. 2014;52:4003–9.
3. Wang X, Chen G, Wu X, Wang L, Cai J, Chan EW, et al. Increased prevalence of carbapenem resistant *Enterobacteriaceae* in hospital setting due to cross-species transmission of the bla NDM-1 element and clonal spread of progenitor resistant strains. Front Microbiol. 2015;6:595.
4. Hammoudi D, Ayoub Moubareck C, Aires J, Adaime A, Barakat A, Fayad N, et al. Countrywide spread of OXA-48 carbapenemase in Lebanon: surveillance and genetic characterization of carbapenem-non-susceptible *Enterobacteriaceae* in 10 hospitals over a one-year period. Int J Infect Dis. 2014;29:139–44.
5. Hamzan NI, Yean CY, Rahman RA, Hasan H, Rahman ZA. Detection of blaIMP4 and blaNDM1 harboring Klebsiella pneumoniae isolates in a university hospital in Malaysia. Emerg Health Threats J. 2015;8:26011.
6. Demir Y, Zer Y, Karaoglan I. Investigation of VIM, IMP, NDM-1, KPC AND OXA-48 enzymes in *Enterobacteriaceae* strains. Pak J Pharm Sci. 2015;28:1127–33.
7. Sahin K, Tekin A, Ozdas S, Akin D, Yapislar H, Dilek AR, et al. Evaluation of carbapenem resistance using phenotypic and genotypic techniques in *Enterobacteriaceae* isolates. Ann Clin Microbiol Antimicrob. 2015;14:44.
8. Pecora ND, Li N, Allard M, Li C, Albano E, Delaney M, et al. Genomically informed surveillance for carbapenem-resistant *Enterobacteriaceae* in a health care system. MBio. 2015;6:e01030.
9. Bae IK, Kang HK, Jang IH, Lee W, Kim K, Kim JO, et al. Detection of carbapenemases in clinical *Enterobacteriaceae* isolates using the VITEK AST-N202 card. Infect Chemother. 2015;47:167–74.
10. Djahmi N, Dunyach-Remy C, Pantel A, Dekhil M, Sotto A, Lavigne JP. Epidemiology of carbapenemase-producing *Enterobacteriaceae* and acinetobacter baumannii in Mediterranean countries. Biomed Res Int. 2014;2014:305784.
11. Rajabnia R, Asgharpour F, Ferdosi Shahandashti E, Moulana Z. Nosocomial emerging of (VIM1) carbapenemase-producing isolates of Klebsiella pneumoniae in North of Iran. Iran J Microbiol. 2015;7:88–93.
12. Solanki R, Vanjari L, Subramanian S, B A, E N, Lakshmi V. Comparative

evaluation of multiplex PCR and routine laboratory phenotypic methods for detection of carbapenemases among gram negative bacilli. J Clin Diagn Res. 2014;8:DC23–6.
13. Del Franco M, Paone L, Novati R, Giacomazzi CG, Bagattini M, Galotto C, et al. Molecular epidemiology of carbapenem resistant *Enterobacteriaceae* in Valle d'Aosta region, Italy, shows the emergence of KPC-2 producing Klebsiella pneumoniae clonal complex 101 (ST101 and ST1789). BMC Microbiol. 2015;15:260.
14. Hammoudi D, Moubareck CA, Kanso A, Nordmann P, Sarkis DK. Surveillance of carbapenem non-susceptible gram negative strains and characterization of carbapenemases of classes a, b and d in a Lebanese hospital. J Med Liban. 2015;63:66–73.
15. Doyle D, Peirano G, Lascols C, Lloyd T, Church DL, Pitout JD. Laboratory detection of *Enterobacteriaceae* that produce carbapenemases. J Clin Microbiol. 2012;50:3877–80.
16. Karuniawati A, Saharman YR, Lestari DC. Detection of carbapenemase encoding genes in *Enterobacteriace*, *Pseudomonas aeruginosa*, and *Acinetobacter baumanii* isolated from patients at Intensive Care Unit Cipto Mangunkusumo Hospital in 2011. Acta Med Indones. 2013;45:101–6.
17. Ma L, Wang JT, Wu TL, Siu LK, Chuang YC, Lin JC, et al. Emergence of OXA-48-producing Klebsiella pneumoniae in Taiwan. PLoS One. 2015;10:e0139152.
18. Glasner C, Albiger B, Buist G, Tambić Andrasević A, Canton R, Carmeli Y, et al. Carbapenemase-producing *Enterobacteriaceae* in Europe: a survey among national experts from 39 countries, February 2013. Euro Surveill. 2013;18(28). doi:10.2807/1560-7917.
19. Performance Standards for antimicrobial susceptibility testing, 23rd informational supplement. CLSI document M100-S23. Clinical and Laboratory Standards Institute. 2013.
20. Tsakris A, Poulou A, Bogaerts P, Dimitroulia E, Pournaras S, Glupczynski Y. Evaluation of a new phenotypic OXA-48 disk test for differentiation of OXA-48 carbapenemase-producing *Enterobacteriaceae* clinical isolates. J Clin Microbiol. 2015;53(4):1245–51.
21. Magiorakos AP, Srinivasan A, Carey RB, Carmeli Y, Falagas ME, Giske CG, et al. Multidrug-resistant, extensively drug-resistant and pandrug-resistant bacteria: an international expert proposal for interim standard definitions for acquired resistance. Clin Microbiol Infect. 2012;18:268–81.
22. van der Bij AK, Pitout JD. The role of international travel in the worldwide spread of multiresistant *Enterobacteriaceae*. J Antimicrob Chemother. 2012;67:2090–100.
23. Nordmann P, Poirel L. The difficult-to-control spread of carbapenemase producers among *Enterobacteriaceae* worldwide. Clin Microbiol Infect. 2014;20:821–30.
24. Poirel L, Potron A, Nordmann P. OXA-48-like carbapenemases: the phantom menace. J Antimicrob Chemother. 2012;67:1597–606.
25. Fursova NK, Astashkin EI, Knyazeva AI, Kartsev NN, Leonova ES, Ershova ON, et al. The spread of bla OXA-48 and bla OXA-244 carbapenemase genes among Klebsiella pneumoniae, proteus mirabilis and enterobacter spp. isolated in Moscow, Russia. Ann Clin Microbiol Antimicrob. 2015;14:46.
26. Arana DM, Saez D, García-Hierro P, Bautista V, Fernández-Romero S, Ángel de la Cal M, et al. Concurrent interspecies and clonal dissemination of OXA-48 carbapenemase. Clin Microbiol Infect. 2015;21:148.
27. Balkan II, Aygün G, Aydın S, Mutcalı SI, Kara Z, Kuşkucu M, et al. Blood stream infections due to OXA-48-like carbapenemase-producing *Enterobacteriaceae*: treatment and survival. Int J Infect Dis. 2014;26:51–6.
28. Nazik H, Aydin S, Albayrak R, Bilgi EA, Yildiz I, Kuvat N, et al. Detection and spread of oxa-48-producing Klebsiella oxytoca isolates in Istanbul, Turkey. Southeast Asian J Trop Med Public Health. 2014;45:123–9.
29. Chu YW, Cheung TK, Ngan JY, Kam KM. EDTA susceptibility leading to false detection of metallo-beta-lactamase in *Pseudomonas aeruginosa* by Etest and an imipenem-EDTA disk method. Int J Antimicrob Agents. 2005;26:340–1.
30. Yildirim I, Ceyhan M, Gur D, Mugnaioli C, Rossolini GM. First detection of VIM-1 type metallo-beta-lactamase in a multidrug-resistant Klebsiella pneumoniae clinical isolate from Turkey also producing the CTX-M-15 extended-spectrum beta-lactamase. J Chemother. 2007;19:467–8.
31. Aksu N, Baran I. New Delhi metallo beta laktamaz (NDM-1) oluşturan bir Klebsiella pneumoniae olgusu. 1. Klimud Günleri Gap İllerinde Yaygın Görülen Enfeksiyonlar Sempozyum Kitabı. Şanlıurfa, Türkiye. 2013;27.
32. Poirel L, Yilmaz M, Istanbullu A, Arslan F, Mert A, Bernabeu S, et al. Spread of NDM-1-producing *Enterobacteriaceae* in a neonatal intensive care unit in Istanbul, Turkey. Antimicrob Agents Chemother. 2014;58:2929–33.
33. Alp E, Perçin D, Colakoğlu S, Durmaz S, Kürkcü CA, Ekincioğlu P, et al. Molecular characterization of carbapenem-resistant Klebsiella pneumoniae in a tertiary university hospital in Turkey. J Hosp Infect. 2013;84:178–80.
34. Kaase M, Szabados F, Wassill L, Gatermann SG. Detection of carbapenemases in *Enterobacteriaceae* by a commercial multiplex PCR. J Clin Microbiol. 2012;50:3115–8.

5

Evaluation of the SLOMYCO Sensititre® panel for testing the antimicrobial susceptibility of *Mycobacterium marinum* isolates

Marion Chazel[1], Hélène Marchandin[1,2], Nicolas Keck[3], Dominique Terru[1], Christian Carrière[1,5,6], Michael Ponsoda[4], Véronique Jacomo[4], Gilles Panteix[4], Nicolas Bouzinbi[1], Anne-Laure Bañuls[7], Marc Choisy[7], Jérôme Solassol[6,8,9], Alexandra Aubry[10,11,12,13†] and Sylvain Godreuil[1,5,6*†]

Abstract

Background: The agar dilution method is currently considered as the reference method for *Mycobacterium marinum* drug susceptibility testing (DST). As it is time-consuming, alternative methods, such as the E-test, were evaluated for *M. marinum* DST, but without success. The SLOMYCO Sensititre® panel, recently commercialized by TREK Diagnostic Systems (Cleveland, OH), can be used for DST in slow-growing mycobacteria and for antimicrobial agents recommended by the Clinical and Laboratory Standards Institute (CLSI) for *M. marinum* DST. The main goal of this work was to evaluate the SLOMYCO Sensititre® panel method for DST in *M. marinum* isolates from human patients and fish relative to the reference agar dilution method.

Methods/Results: The reproducibility of the minimum inhibitory concentration (MIC) determination (± 1 $\log_2$ dilution) was very good for both the agar dilution method and SLOMYCO Sensititre® panel (>90 % agreement). The percentage essential agreement between methods varied, depending on the drug: between 97 and 75 % for ciprofloxacin, moxifloxacin, linezolid, isoniazid, clarithromycin, amikacin, rifabutin and rifampin, 74 % for trimethoprim, 72 % for doxycycline, 70 % for sulfamethoxazole, 59 % for streptomycin, 33 % for ethambutol and only 2.2 % for ethionamide. When the agar dilution and SLOMYCO Sensititre® panel results were converted into interpretive criteria, the category agreement was 100 % for amikacin, ciprofloxacin, clarithromycin, moxifloxacin, rifabutin, sulfamethoxazole and trimethoprim, 98 % for ethambutol and 96 % for rifampin and no agreement for doxycycline.

Conclusions: The SLOMYCO Sensititre® panel method could provide a potential alternative to the reference agar dilution method, when DST in *M. marinum* is required, except for doxycycline.

Keywords: *Mycobacterium marinum*, SLOMYCO Sensititre® panel, Agar dilution method, Antimicrobial susceptibility testing, Human and fish isolates

Background

Mycobacterium marinum, a slow-growing nontuberculous photochromogenic mycobacteria, is an ubiquitous waterborne organism [9, 10, 17] that causes diseases in many fish species from cold or warm, fresh or salted water, and also in many other aquatic animals, such as amphibians, mammals and oysters [9, 10, 17]. In humans, *M. marinum* infection is commonly limited to the skin, but it can spread to deeper structures, resulting in tenosynovitis, arthritis and osteomyelitis [1, 8, 13] and, rarely, in disseminated infection in immunocompromised patients [13].

Mycobacterium marinum is naturally multi-drug resistant and there is no standardized antimicrobial treatment for *M. marinum* infections [7]. As the wild-type

*Correspondence: s-godreuil@chu-montpellier.fr
†Alexandra Aubry and Sylvain Godreuil contributed equally to this work
[5] Department of Bacteriology-Virology, INSERM U1058 "Pathogenesis and Control of Chronic Infections", Université Montpellier-EFS, CHU Arnaud de Villeneuve 371 avenue du Doyen Gaston Giraud, 34295 Montpellier, France
Full list of author information is available at the end of the article

susceptibility pattern of *M. marinum* is well known [2] and acquired resistance has not been described so far, antimicrobial susceptibility testing is not recommended except in the case of treatment failure and relapse [16].

The Clinical and Laboratory Standards Institute (CLSI) recommends microdilution for *M. marinum* drug susceptibility testing (DST) [16], but the agar dilution method is currently considered to be the reference method [2, 4, 19]. As this method is time-consuming, alternative methods, such as the E-test, were evaluated, but showed poor agreement with the reference method and therefore are not suitable for DST in *M. marinum* [2, 11, 19]. Recently, the SLOMYCO Sensititre® panel was commercialized by TREK Diagnostic Systems (Cleveland, OH) [3]. This is a standard-order broth microdilution panel that can be used to evaluate the susceptibility of slow growing mycobacteria to 14 antimicrobial agents, including those recommended by CLSI for *M. marinum* DST [3].

The main goal of this work was to evaluate the SLOMYCO Sensititre® panel method for DST in *M. marinum* strains from humans and fish relative to the reference agar dilution method.

Methods

Bacterial strains and growth conditions

The origin and other information concerning the tested *M. marinum* isolates are described in Broutin et al. [5]. The 35 *M. marinum* isolates from human patients and nine from fish were collected in France between 1995 and 2007. None was from patients who experienced treatment failure or relapse. *M. marinum* identification was performed using GenoType Mycobacterium AS/CM, a commercial multiplex line-probe assay (Hain Lifescience GmbH, Nehren, Germany). Isolates were stored at −80 °C in Middlebrook 7H9 broth (DIFCO, Detroit, MI, USA) containing 5 % OADC (DIFCO, Detroit, MI, USA) until determination of the Minimum inhibitory concentrations (MICs). Mycobacteria were then cultured in Löwenstein-Jensen (LJ) slants (bioMérieux, Marcy l'Etoile, France) and in Middlebrook 7H10 agar (DIFCO, Detroit, MI, USA). The *M. marinum* ATCC 927 strain (from fish) and the *M. marinum* ATCC BAA-535/M strain isolated from an infected patient were used as controls for MIC determination.

Antimicrobial agents

Amikacin, ciprofloxacin, clarithromycin, doxycycline, ethambutol, ethionamide, isoniazid, rifampin, rifabutin, streptomycin and trimethoprim (Sigma-Aldrich, Lyon, France), linezolid (Pfizer, France) and moxifloxacin (Bayer, Wuppertal, Germany) were tested in this study. Stock solutions of each drug were prepared using the appropriate solvent and were filter-sterilized before storage at −80 °C. To prior testing, each drug was freshly diluted in sterile deionized water. The concentration ranges of the tested antimicrobial agents are indicated in Table 1.

MIC determination by using the agar dilution method

The agar dilution method was performed on Müller-Hinton agar (Becton–Dickinson, France) supplemented with 5 % OADC according to CLSI [16]. Twofold dilutions of the antibiotics to be tested were added to obtain the required final concentrations. Confluent colonies of the different bacteria in LJ slants were swept with a loop and emulsified in sterile water and the concentration was adjusted to the McFarland n. 1 standard turbidity. A 1/100 dilution of each suspension adjusted to the McFarland n. 1 standard was inoculated using a Steers replicator to deliver approximately 10^4 colony-forming units (CFU) per spot. Plates were incubated at 30 °C [16]. The MICs (i.e., the lowest concentration of antibiotic resulting in complete inhibition of growth) of the tested antibiotics were determined after 7 and 14 days of growth of the different *M. marinum* isolates/controls.

MIC determination using the SLOMYCO Sensititre® panel (broth micro-dilution method)

Inocula for the SLOMYCO Sensititre® panel were prepared according to the CLSI and the manufacturer's instructions [16]. SLOMYCO plates were incubated in a non-CO_2 incubator at 30 °C until the controls showed sufficient growth (7–14 days). The MICs were determined visually using an inverted mirror and read as the lowest concentration of the antibiotic showing 100 % growth inhibition.

Analysis of the results

The reproducibility of both methods was evaluated by performing two independent tests for each method and for each of the 44 isolates (a total of 176 tests) and five independent tests for the *M. marinum* ATCC 927 and ATCC BAA-535/M strains (a total of 30 tests). Each test result was independently interpreted by two blinded readers. The reproducibility value was defined as the percentage of strains with the same MIC value $\pm 1 \log_2$ dilution at each test. The essential agreement between the agar dilution and SLOMYCO Sensititre® panel results was expressed as the percentage of isolates that showed the same MIC value $\pm 1 \log_2$ dilution with the two methods. Category agreement was evaluated using the breakpoints for determining the susceptibility and resistance categories recommended by CLSI [16]. For this study only very major errors (i.e., an isolate resistant [R] by the reference method, but susceptible [S] by the tested method) and major errors (S by the reference method

Table 1 MIC (μg/mL) of the 14 antibiotics tested in 46 *M. marinum* isolates (35 clinical, 9 fish and 2 references strains), determined by using the agar dilution method

Antimicrobial agent [breakpoints (μg/mL)][a]	MIC_{50}			MIC_{90}			Range
	Total (n = 46)	Human (n = 35)	Fish (n = 9)	Total (n = 46)	Human (n = 35)	Fish (n = 9)	
Amikacin (>32)	2	2	2	4	4	2	2–4
Ciprofloxacin (>2)	2	2	2	2	2	2	2
Clarithromycin (>16)	2	2	2	2	2	2	1–2
Doxycycline (>4)	4	4	4	4	4	4	1–4
Ethambutol (>4)	2	2	2	4	4	2	1–8
Ethionamide (NA)	5	5	5	10	10	10	2.5–10
Isoniazid (NA)	8	8	8	8	8	8	2–8
Linezolid (NA)	1	1	1	2	2	2	0.5–4
Moxifloxacin (>2)	1	1	1	1	1	1	0.12–1
Rifabutin (>2)	0.12	0.12	0.12	0.12	0.12	0.12	0.12
Rifampin (>1)	0.5	0.5	0.5	1	1	1	0.5–2
Streptomycin (NA)	16	16	16	16	16	16	4–32
Sulfamethoxazole (>38)	9.5	9.5	9.5	19	19	19	4.75–19
Trimethoprim (>2)	0.5	0.5	0.5	1	1	1	0.25–1

[a] Concentration range of the tested drugs by using the agar dilution method (ADM) and the SLOMYCO Sensititre® panel method (SSPM): amikacin (0.25–32 mg/L, ADM; 1–64 μg/mL, SSPM); ciprofloxacin (0.12–16 μg/mL, ADM, SSPM); clarithromycin (0.06–32 μg/mL, ADM, SSPM); doxycycline (0.12–16 μg/mL, ADM, SSPM); ethambutol (0.5–16 μg/mL, ADM, SSPM); ethionamide (0.3–20 μg/mL, ADM, SSPM); isoniazid (0.25–16 μg/mL, ADM; 0.25–8 μg/mL, SSPM); linezolid (0.12–32 μg/mL, ADM; SSPM, 1–64 μg/mL); moxifloxacin (0.06–8 μg/mL, ADM; 0.12–8 μg/mL, SSPM); rifabutin (0.06–16 μg/mL, ADM; 0.25–8 mg/L, SSPM); rifampin (0.12–8 mg/L, ADM; 0.25–8 μg/mL, SSPM); streptomycin (0.5–32 μg/mL, ADM; 0.5–64 μg/mL, SSPM); sulfamethoxazole (2.38–152 μg/mL, ADM, SSPM); trimethoprim (0.12–8 μg/mL, ADM, SSPM); *NA* not available

and R by the test method) were considered. Minor errors (intermediate [I] by one method and S or R by the other method) were not considered because the CLSI breakpoints allow only two characterization categories (R or S) [16].

Results

The reproducibility of the results obtained with the agar dilution method (reference method) was very good (Table 2) for all antibiotics. The MICs of the 14 antimicrobial agents determined by using the agar dilution method were distributed in a narrow range (Table 1). Comparison of the MICs for the *M. marinum* isolates from infected humans and fish did not reveal any difference.

The MICs for the two reference *M. marinum* strains (ATCC 927 and ATCC BAA-535/M) were within 0–1 dilution of the MICs of the 44 tested isolates and within the expected range.

The MICs at which 90 % of isolates were inhibited (MIC_{90}) of amikacin (4 μg/mL), clarithromycin (2 μg/mL) and rifabutin (0.12 μg/mL) were below the CSLI breakpoint, whereas the MIC_{90} of ciprofloxacin (2 μg/mL), doxycycline (4 μg/mL), ethambutol (4 μg/mL), moxifloxacin (1 μg/mL), rifampin (1 μg/mL) and sulfamethoxazole (19 μg/mL) were close to the breakpoint [16]. The MIC_{90} of rifampin, rifabutin, moxifloxacin and trimethoprim (between 0.1 and 1 μg/mL) were lower than those of the other tested antibiotics.

The relatively high MIC_{90} of ethionamide (10 μg/mL), isoniazid (8 μg/mL) and streptomycin (16 μg/mL), for which breakpoints are not available, suggests that they are not good candidates for the treatment of *M. marinum* infection. In contrast, linezolid (MIC_{90}: 2 μg/mL) was very effective against the different *M. marinum* isolates with MIC values among the lowest in our study.

The SLOMYCO Sensititre® panel method (tested method) produced remarkably consistent and reproducible results (Table 3). Reproducibility with this method was 100 % in the case of ethionamide, isoniazid, moxifloxacin, rifampin, trimethoprim and sulfamethoxazole, and between 98 and 87 % for amikacin, ciprofloxacin, clarithromycin, doxycycline, ethambutol, linezolid, rifabutin and streptomycin (Table 3). The percentage essential agreement (±1 $\log_2$ dilution) between the MICs obtained with the tested and the reference methods (Table 4) greatly varied depending on the drug: from 98 % for ciprofloxacin and linezolid to 2.2 % for ethionamide. Good agreement percentages were obtained for moxifloxacin (91.3 %), isoniazid (87 %) and clarithromycin (85 %); whereas, agreement was lower for amikacin (76.1 %), rifampin (76.1 %), rifampin (76 %), trimethoprim (74 %), doxycycline (72 %), sulfamethoxazole

Table 2 Reproducibility of the results (i.e., MIC, expressed in μg/mL, of the tested antibiotics in the 46 *M. marinum* isolates) obtained with the agar dilution method

Antimicrobial agents	No. of results within $\log_2$ concentration difference of							% agreement (confidence interval)
	>−2	−2	−1	0	1	2	>2	
Amikacin	0	0	0	45	1	0	0	100 (89–100)
Ciprofloxacin	0	0	4	33	7	2	0	96 (84.3–99.3)
Clarithromycin	0	0	10	23	13	0	0	100 (88–99)
Doxycycline	0	0	6	38	1	1	0	98 (87–100)
Ethambutol	0	0	2	43	0	1	0	98 (87–100)
Ethionamide	0	0	7	29	10	0	0	100 (90.4–100)
Isoniazid	0	0	5	21	20	0	0	100 (86–99.3)
Linezolid	0	1	12	20	12	1	0	96 (87–100)
Moxifloxacin	0	0	10	33	3	0	0	100 (90.4–100)
Rifabutin	0	1	3	28	14	0	0	98 (87–100)
Rifampin	0	0	12	30	4	0	0	100 (90.4–100)
Streptomycin	0	1	5	29	11	0	0	98 (87–100)
Sulfamethoxazole	0	0	10	25	11	0	0	100 (90.4–100)
Trimethoprim	0	0	10	26	10	0	0	100 (90.4–100)

Table 3 Reproducibility of the results (i.e., MIC, expressed in μg/mL, of the tested antibiotics in the 46 *M. marinum* isolates) obtained with the SLOMYCO Sensititre® panel method

Antimicrobial agents	No. of results within $\log_2$ concentration difference of							% agreement (confidence interval)
	>−2	−2	−1	0	1	2	>2	
Amikacin	0	0	0	45	0	1	0	98 (87–100)
Ciprofloxacin	0	1	4	33	7	1	0	96 (84.3–99.3)
Clarithromycin	0	0	10	23	10	3	0	93.5 (81.1–98.3)
Doxycycline	0	0	6	38	1	1	0	97 (87–100)
Ethambutol	0	1	1	43	0	1	0	95.6 (84–99.2)
Ethionamide	0	0	4	29	13	0	0	100 (90.4–100)
Isoniazid	0	0	7	19	20	0	0	100 (86–99.3)
Linezolid	0	1	12	20	12	1	0	96 (87–100)
Moxifloxacin	0	0	7	36	3	0	0	100 (90.4–100)
Rifabutin	0	0	3	28	14	1	0	98 (87–100)
Rifampin	0	0	8	34	4	0	0	100 (90.4–100)
Streptomycin	0	1	5	29	11	0	0	98 (87–100)
Sulfamethoxazole	0	0	5	30	11	0	0	100 (90.4–100)
Trimethoprim	0	0	7	28	11	0	0	100 (90.4–100)

(70 %), streptomycin (59 %) and particularly ethambutol (33 %). In the case of ethambutol and ethionamide, the SLOMYCO Sensititre® panel method underestimated the MICs by 2–3 dilutions compared with the reference method. When the agar dilution and SLOMYCO Sensititre® panel results were converted into interpretive categories (resistance/susceptibility) using the CLSI breakpoints, the category agreement was 100 % for amikacin, ciprofloxacin, clarithromycin, moxifloxacin, rifabutin and sulfamethoxazole–trimethoprim (SMT-TMP), 98 % for ethambutol and 96 % for rifampin (Table 5). Two very major discrepancies were observed for rifampin (2/46) and one for ethambutol (1/46). No agreement was observed between the two methods for doxycycline, with 46 (100 %) major discrepancies. The SLOMYCO Sensititre® method overestimated the doxycycline MIC by 1 dilution; however, with this method, doxycycline MIC_{90} (8 μg/mL) was close to the susceptibility breakpoint obtained by using the agar dilution method (4 μg/mL).

Table 4 Comparison of the MIC values obtained by using the SLOMYCO Sensititre® panel and the agar dilution methods for 46 *M. marinum* isolates

Antimicrobial agents	No. of results within log_2 concentration difference of							% essential agreement (confidence interval)
	>−2	−2	−1	0	1	2	>2	
Amikacin	0	11	34	1	0	0	0	76.1 (70–87)
Ciprofloxacin	0	1	32	11	2	0	0	98 (87–100)
Clarithromycin	4	3	23	15	1	0	0	85 (70.5–93.2)
Doxycycline	0	0	0	0	33	12	1	72 (56.3–83.5)
Ethambutol	12	19	14	1	0	0	0	33 (20–48.1)
Ethionamide	36	9	1	0	0	0	0	2.2 (0.1–13)
Isoniazid	0	6	27	11	2	0	0	87 (73–95)
Linezolid	0	0	10	20	15	1	0	98 (87–100)
Moxifloxacin	0	4	20	18	3	0	1	91.3 (87–100)
Rifabutin	0	0	0	0	35	11	0	76.1 (61–87)
Rifampin	0	11	20	15	0	0	0	76.1 (61–87)
Streptomycin	2	17	22	5	0	0	0	59 (43.3–72.7)
Sulfamethoxazole	2	10	15	13	4	1	1	70 (54.1–82)
Trimethoprim	3	9	26	6	2	0	0	74 (59–85.2)

Table 5 Comparison of the susceptibility testing results (resistance/susceptibility) and category errors (very major or major error) by using the SLOMYCO Sensititre® panel (SSPM) and the agar dilution method (ADM) for 46 *M. marinum* isolates following the CLSI guidelines

Antimicrobial agents [breakpoints (μg/mL)]	% resistant ADM	% resistant SSPM	Category errors (N°)	% agreement
Amikacin (32)	0	0	None	100
Ciprofloxacin (2)	0	0	None	100
Clarithromycin (16)	0	0	None	100
Doxycycline (4)	0	100	Major (46)	0
Ethambutol (4)	2.2	0	Very major (1)	98
Moxifloxacin (2)	0	0	None	100
Rifabutin (2)	0	0	None	100
Rifampin (1)	4.3	0	Very major (2)	96
SMT-TMP (2/38)	0	0	None	100

SMT–TMP sulfamethoxazole–trimethoprim

Discussion

The manufacturer's guidelines (TREK Diagnostic Systems, Cleveland, OH) recommend the SLOMYCO Sensititre® method for antibiotic susceptibility testing in *M. marinum*, but studies evaluating the concordance with the reference agar dilution method have not been published yet. As the SLOMYCO Sensititre® panel technique presents several advantages (commercial availability; standardization; easy to set up and to interpret; and amenable to automation [2, 19] compared to the time-consuming and cumbersome agar dilution method, our objective was to compare the performance of these two methods.

The lack of difference between the MICs for the *M. marinum* isolates from infected humans and fish could be explained by the fact that most of the clinical samples were from patients who handled infected fish (from aquarium tanks or fish-related work) and, therefore, the antibiotic susceptibility profiles of the human isolates reflected those of the fish isolates.

Our results show that the reproducibility of the SLOMYCO Sensititre® results for the reference strains and the *M. marinum* isolates (from human and fish) was very good. All results of the independent tests were within the ± 1 log_2 dilution acceptable level of variation. Moreover, the level of agreement (± 1 log_2 dilution) between the results (MICs and interpretive categories) obtained with the SLOMYCO Sensititre® panel and the agar dilution methods was good for most of the antibiotics recommended by CLSI and ATS [12] for the treatment of (rifampin, rifabutin, amikacin, clarithromycin and sulfamethoxazole–trimethoprim) or with therapeutic potential (linezolid, isoniazid) for *M. marinum* infections. It should be noted that two very major errors were observed for rifampin in isolates in which the MIC for rifampin was just above the breakpoint (2 μg/mL) and that still belong to the wild type population [2]. The clinical significance of these data is unclear. Moreover, the MIC of the only rifampin-resistant *M. marinum* reported until now [14] was clearly above the breakpoint (>16 μg/

mL). Unfortunately, we could not evaluate the ability of the SLOMYCO Sensititre® panel to detect resistant strains, because none of the isolates tested in this study was considered as antibiotic-resistant.

Conversely, poor agreement was observed for ethambutol. The MICs for ethambutol obtained with the SLOMYCO Sensititre® panel were 2–3 dilutions lower than those obtained with the reference method. However, this poor agreement resulted in only one very major error, when MICs were converted into interpretive categories. This discrepancy corresponds to a strain with a MIC just above the breakpoint (16 μg/mL) (Table 1).

In the case of doxycycline, no agreement was observed between methods resulting in 46 major errors. This could be explained by (i) the overestimation of doxycycline MICs by the SLOMYCO Sensititre® panel that could be due to the medium or pH, and (ii) the fact that the MIC_{50} and MIC_{90} were similar to the breakpoint value. Among the antibiotics recommended by CLSI and on the basis of in vitro susceptibility testing, our results confirm that rifampin, rifabutin, amikacin, clarithromycin and sulfamethoxazole–trimethoprim are good options for the treatment of *M. marinum* infections, as reported in previous studies [2, 4, 11, 14, 15, 19]. Sulfamethoxazole and trimethoprim showed good in vitro activity against *M. marinum* and could be considered as an alternative treatment [19]. The present study brings new data on *M. marinum* susceptibility pattern to ethionamide, streptomycin and linezolid. The American Thoracic Society recommendations for the treatment of some nontuberculous mycobacteria (NTM) infections include the use of streptomycin (for rifampin-resistant *M. kansassii* infection) and ethionamide (for *M. malmoense* infection) [7, 12]. However, the lack of clinical experience in *M. marinum* infections and the absence of breakpoints for NTM susceptibility and resistance to these two antibiotics did not allow predicting their potential efficiency in *M. marinum* infections [16]. Linezolid has been reported to be effective against mycobacteria (*M. chelonae* and *M. marinum*) [6, 7] and for treating skin and soft tissue infections [6, 7]. In our study, linezolid was one of the most active antimicrobial agents in agreement with the low MIC determined in a previous study [4]. Despite the lack of breakpoint values for *M. marinum*, linezolid may be an interesting alternative therapeutic agent due to its pharmacological properties. This study confirmed that *M. marinum* is resistant to isoniazid and ethambutol [7] and the observed *M. marinum* susceptibility pattern corresponded to the wild type phenotype, as previously reported [2, 7, 14, 18, 19]. As the ethambutol MIC_{90} was close to the breakpoint and clear evidence on the clinical efficacy of this antibiotic are lacking, it should not be recommended as a first-line drug for *M. marinum* infection treatment.

Conclusion

In this study, we evaluated the SLOMYCO Sensititre® panel method for susceptibility testing in 44 *M. marinum* isolates (from humans and fish) relative to the reference agar dilution method. Our results indicate that the SLOMYCO Sensititre® panel method could provide a potential alternative to the reference agar dilution method, when DST in *M. marinum* is required, except for doxycycline. If doxycycline susceptibility needs to be tested, the use of another method (broth microdilution) is more appropriate.

Consent

Written informed consent was obtained from the patients for the publication of this report.

Authors' contributions

MC, HM, NK, DT, SG designed this study and did most of the writing, supported by CC, MP, VJ, GP, NB, ALB, MC, JS, AA and SG who have been involved in drafting the manuscript and have made substantial contributions to data acquisition. All authors read and approved the final manuscript.

Author details

[1] Département de Bactériologie-Virologie, CHRU Montpellier, Montpellier, France. [2] UMR 5119 ECOSYM, Equipe Pathogènes et Environnements, Laboratoire de Bactériologie, U.F.R. des Sciences Pharmaceutiques et Biologiques, Montpellier, France. [3] Laboratoire Départemental Vétérinaire de l'Hérault, Montpellier, France. [4] Laboratoire Biomnis, Lyon, France. [5] Department of Bacteriology-Virology, INSERM U1058 "Pathogenesis and Control of Chronic Infections", Université Montpellier-EFS, CHU Arnaud de Villeneuve 371 avenue du Doyen Gaston Giraud, 34295 Montpellier, France. [6] Université Montpellier, Montpellier, France. [7] MIVEGEC (Laboratoire Maladies Infectieuses et Vecteurs, Ecologie, Génétique, Evolution et Contrôle), UMR CNRS 5290/IRD 224, Université de Montpellier, Montpellier, France. [8] Department of Biopathology, CHRU Montpellier, Montpellier, France. [9] Department of Clinical Oncoproteomic, Montpellier Cancer Institute, Montpellier, France. [10] Centre National de Référence des Mycobactéries et de la Résistance aux Antituberculeux, Paris, France. [11] Laboratoire de Bactériologie-Hygiène Paris, AP-HP, Hôpital Pitié-Salpêtrière, 75013 Paris, France. [12] Centre for Immunology and Microbial Infections, team 13, Sorbonne Universités, UPMC Univ Paris 06, U1135, 75013 Paris, France. [13] INSERM, U1135, Paris, France.

Acknowledgements

This study was supported by the Montpellier University Teaching Hospital (CHU Montpellier, "Equipe Performante Recherche" contract). We would like to thank INSERM, IRD and CNRS for technical support. We thank Elisabetta Andermarcher for assistance in preparing and editing the manuscript, and Nicolas Veziris for helpful discussions. The authors declare they have no conflict of interest.

Competing interests

The authors declare that they have no competing interests.

References

1. Aubry A, Chosidow O, Caumes E, Robert J, Cambau E. Sixty-three cases of *Mycobacterium marinum* infection: clinical features, treatment, and antibiotic susceptibility of causative isolates. Arch Intern Med. 2002;162:1746–52.
2. Aubry A, Jarlier V, Escolano S, Truffot-Pernot C, Cambau E. Antibiotic susceptibility pattern of *Mycobacterium marinum*. Antimicrob Agents Chemother. 2000;44:3133–6.

3. Babady NE, Hall L, Abbenyi AT, Eisberner JJ, Brown-Elliott BA, Pratt CJ, McGlasson MC, Beierle KD, Wohlfiel SL, Deml SM, Wallace RJ Jr, Wengenack NL. Evaluation of *Mycobacterium avium* complex clarithromycin susceptibility testing using SLOMYCO Sensititre panels and JustOne strips. J Clin Microbiol. 2010;48:1749–52.
4. Braback M, Riesbeck K, Forsgren A. Susceptibilities of Mycobacterium marinum to gatifloxacin, gemifloxacin, levofloxacin, linezolid, moxifloxacin, telithromycin, and quinupristin-dalfopristin (Synercid) compared to its susceptibilities to reference macrolides and quinolones. Antimicrob Agents Chemother. 2002;46:1114–6.
5. Broutin V, Banuls AL, Aubry A, Keck N, Choisy M, Bernardet JF, Michel C, Raymond JC, Libert C, Barnaud A, Stragier P, Portaels F, Terru D, Belon C, Dereure O, Gutierrez C, Boschiroli ML, Van De Perre P, Cambau E, Godreuil S. Genetic diversity and population structure of *Mycobacterium marinum*: new insights into host and environmental specificities. J Clin Microbiol. 2012;50:3627–34.
6. Brown-Elliott BA, Crist CJ, Mann LB, Wilson RW, Wallace RJ Jr. In vitro activity of linezolid against slowly growing nontuberculous Mycobacteria. Antimicrob Agents Chemother. 2003;47:1736–8.
7. Brown-Elliott BA, Nash KA, Wallace RJ Jr. Antimicrobial susceptibility testing, drug resistance mechanisms, and therapy of infections with nontuberculous mycobacteria. Clin Microbiol Rev. 2012;25:545–82.
8. Eberst E, Dereure O, Guillot B, Trento C, Terru D, van de Perre P, Godreuil S. Epidemiological, clinical, and therapeutic pattern of *Mycobacterium marinum* infection: a retrospective series of 35 cases from southern France. J Am Acad Dermatol. 2012;66:e15–6.
9. Falkinham JO 3rd. Epidemiology of infection by nontuberculous mycobacteria. Clin Microbiol Rev. 1996;9:177–215.
10. Falkinham JO 3rd. Nontuberculous mycobacteria in the environment. Clin Chest Med. 2002;23:529–51.
11. Flynn CM, Kelley CM, Barrett MS, Jones RN. Application of the Etest to the antimicrobial susceptibility testing of *Mycobacterium marinum* clinical isolates. J Clin Microbiol. 1997;35:2083–6.
12. Griffith DE, Aksamit T, Brown-Elliott BA, Catanzaro A, Daley C, Gordin F, Holland SM, Horsburgh R, Huitt G, Iademarco MF, Iseman M, Olivier K, Ruoss S, von Reyn CF, Wallace RJ Jr, Winthrop K. An official ATS/IDSA statement: diagnosis, treatment, and prevention of nontuberculous mycobacterial diseases. Am J Respir Crit Care Med. 2007;175:367–416.
13. Lahey T. Invasive *Mycobacterium marinum* infections. Emerg Infect Dis. 2003;9:1496–8.
14. Parrish N, Luethke R, Dionne K, Carroll K, Riedel S. Case of *Mycobacterium marinum* infection with unusual patterns of susceptibility to commonly used antibiotics. J Clin Microbiol. 2011;49:2056–8.
15. Rhomberg PR, Jones RN. In vitro activity of 11 antimicrobial agents, including gatifloxacin and GAR936, tested against clinical isolates of *Mycobacterium marinum*. Diagn Microbiol Infect Dis. 2002;42:145–7.
16. Standards., N. C. C. C. L. S. Susceptibility testing of mycobacteria, nocardia, and other aerobic actinomycetes; approved standard- second edition. NCCLS documented M24-A2. National Committee for Clinical Laboratory Standards, Wayne; 2011.
17. Vincent V, Gutierrez C. *Mycobacterium marinum*. Antibiotiques. 2005;7:133–7.
18. Wallace RJ Jr, Brown-Elliott BA, Crist CJ, Mann L, Wilson RW. Comparison of the in vitro activity of the glycylcycline tigecycline (formerly GAR-936) with those of tetracycline, minocycline, and doxycycline against isolates of nontuberculous mycobacteria. Antimicrob Agents Chemother. 2002;46:3164–7.
19. Werngren J, Olsson-Liljequist B, Gezelius L, Hoffner SE. Antimicrobial susceptibility of *Mycobacterium marinum* determined by E-test and agar dilution. Scand J Infect Dis. 2001;33:585–8.

6

Evaluation of carbapenem resistance using phenotypic and genotypic techniques in *Enterobacteriaceae* isolates

Kazım Sahin[1*], Ayse Tekin[2], Sule Ozdas[3], Demet Akin[4], Hande Yapislar[5], Aziz Ramazan Dilek[1] and Emine Sonmez[6]

Abstract

Background: Bacterial resistance to antibiotics is increasing worldwide. Antibiotic-resistant strains can lead to serious problems regarding treatment of infection. Carbapenem antibiotics are the final treatment option for infections caused by serious and life-threatening multidrug-resistant gram-negative bacteria. Therefore, an understanding of carbapenem resistance is important for infection control. In the study described herein, the phenotypic and genotypic features of carbapenem-resistant *Enterobacteriaceae* strains isolated in our hospital were evaluated.

Methods: In total, 43 carbapenem-resistant strains were included in this study. Sensitivity to antibiotics was determined using the VITEK®2 system. The modified Hodge test (MHT) and metallo-β-lactamase (MBL) antimicrobial gradient test were performed for phenotypic identification. Resistance genes IMP, VIM, KPC, NDM-1, and OXA-48 were amplified by multiplex PCR.

Results: The OXA-48 gene was detected in seven strains, and the NDM-1 gene in one strain. No resistance genes were detected in the remainder of strains. A significant correlation was observed between the MHT test and OXA-48 positivity, and between the MBL antimicrobial gradient test and positivity for resistance genes ($p < 0.05$).

Conclusion: The finding of one NDM-1-positive isolate in this study indicates that carbapenem resistance is spreading in Turkey. Carbapenem resistance spreads rapidly and causes challenges in treatment, and results in high mortality/morbidity rates. Therefore, is necessary to determine carbapenem resistance in Enterobacteriaceae isolates and to take essential infection control precautions to avoid spread of this resistance.

Keywords: *Enterobacteriaceae*, Carbapenemase, Carbapenem resistance, OXA-48, NDM-1, Modified Hodge test, Metallo-β-lactamase antimicrobial gradient test

Background

The increase in antibiotic resistance in the *Enterobacteriaceae* family has become a major threat to public health. Especially in recent years, *Enterobacteriaceae* family members have been identified as important nosocomial pathogens; infection can lead to severe morbidity and mortality, particularly in intensive care units (ICU), internal medicine and surgical units, and pediatric units [1].

Within the *Enterobacteriaceae* family, carbapenem-resistant *Klebsiella pneumoniae* strains have recently been noted in many parts of the world [2, 3]. Carbapenemase, an enzyme belonging to the *K. pneumoniae* carbapenemase (KPC) gene family, causes resistance by breaking down carbapenems. This enzyme was first isolated from a *K. pneumoniae* strain in 1996 and is included in the Ambler classification of β-lactamases. Although KPC β-lactamases are mostly found in *K. pneumoniae*, they can also be found in *Enterobacter* and *Salmonella* species. While metallo-β-lactamase (MBL) enzymes

*Correspondence: ksahin3@mynet.com
[1] Department of Microbiology, Medical Faculty, Recep Tayyip Erdogan University, Islampasa mah., 53000 Rize, Turkey
Full list of author information is available at the end of the article

(which belong to Ambler class B) are frequently observed in non-fermentative bacteria, they can also be found in enteric bacteria. The most frequently described MBLs are Verona integron encoded metallo-*β-lactamase* (VIM), imipenem-hydrolyzing β-lactamase (IMI), Seoul imipenemase (SIM), and German imipenemase (GIM) enzymes.

The Clinical and Laboratory Standards Institute (CLSI) has increased the minimum inhibitory concentration (MIC) value or reduced the disk diffusion zones and recommended confirmation of carbapenemase production by the modified Hodge test (MHT) of *Enterobacteriaceae* in order to facilitate the detection of *Enterobacteriaceae* [4].

While resistance of chromosomal-mediated (intrinsic) carbapenemases is limited, some plasmid-mediated carbapenemases have emerged in recent years. These enzymes have primarily been described in *Klebsiella* spp. and *Serratia marcescens*, and throughout different countries [5, 6]. Plasmid-mediated (extrinsic) carbapenemases can hydrolyse other β-lactam antibiotics in addition to carbapenems. These are the members of Ambler class A, B and D β-lactamases. The SME, NMC, IMI, KPC, and GES enzymes comprise class A carbapenemases. Moreover, IPM, VIM, GIM, SPM, SIM, and NDM-1 enzymes comprise class B, and OXA enzymes that hydrolyse oxacillins comprise class D [7].

In Turkey, resistance mediated by KPC and New Delhi metallo-β-lactamase (NDM-1) enzymes in gram-negative enteric bacilli have been reported [8, 9]. Class D OXA carbapenemase-mediated carbapenem resistance has also been observed among gram-negative enteric bacilli in the context of nosocomial infections.

However, there are a limited number of studies related to carbapenem resistance mechanisms. In the study described herein, the characteristics of phenotypic and genotypic resistance of the carbapenem-resistant *Enterobacteriaceae* (*Escherichia coli* and *Klebsiella* spp.) strains isolated from patients in our hospital were evaluated. The clinical importance of this resistance was also determined.

Methods

Our study was conducted on isolates derived from the following clinical samples: blood, rectal swab, urine, peritoneal fluid, sputum, tracheal aspirate, wounds, bronchoalveolar lavage (BAL) and pleural fluid, etc. Samples were isolated from patients in intensive care, internal intensive care, the surgical clinic, the internal medicine clinic, and the bone marrow transplantation (BMT) unit at Istanbul Bilim University Europe Florence Nightingale Hospital between January 7th 2012 to January 7th 2013, and subsequently transferred to the microbiology laboratory. The experiments were conducted on 43 carbapenem-resistant *Enterobactericeae* isolates. Only one strain from each patient was included in the study. *Enterobactericeae* strains were detected as carbapenem-resistant by using the VITEK®2 automated system (bioMérieux, France). Bacterial suspensions were stored in freezing tubes including beads at −40 °C. Sensitivities to IMP (imipenem), MEM (meropenem) and ERT (ertapenem) were confirmed by the antimicrobial gradient test in collected isolates. Carbapenemase production was determined by the MHT. Metallo-β-lactamase (MBL) production was evaluated using IMP and IMP/EDTA antimicrobial gradient test strips (E-test, bioMérieux, France). When the rate of IMP/IMP + EDTA was ≥ 8, isolates considered MBL-positive. When the rate of IMP/IMP + EDTA was <8, isolates were considered MBL-negative [10].

Multiplex PCR (Hyplex® SuperBug ID, Germany) was used to search for genes affecting carbapenemase production. DNA extraction was conducted using the AxyPrep Microbial DNA Isolation Kit (Axygen Biosciences, USA) that lysed microorganisms by heating, use of detergents and mechanical techniques. The Hyplex® SuperBug ID system was used to detect VIM, IPM, NDM-1, OXA-48, and KPC. No additional control strains were used.

Mean, standard deviation, minimum–maximum, rate, and frequency values were used to determine statistical significance. A kappa test was used for compliance analysis. The SPSS 22.0 program was used for statistical analyses.

Results

A total of 43 patients were registered for the study, whose mean age was 53.8 (range 3–86). 28 (65.1 %) were male and 15 (34.9 %) male.

Of 43 strains, 38 were *K. pneumoniae* (88.4 %), four were *E. coli* (9.3 %), and one was *K. oxytoca* (2.3 %). According to antimicrobial gradient test and VITEK®2 test results, the greatest resistance to these 43 isolates was to ERT among the carbapenems (97.7 and 100 %, respectively), followed by MEM (93 and 90.7 % resistance, respectively) and IMP (79.1 and 88.4 % resistance, respectively).

Forty percent of these patients were followed up in the internal ICU, 36 % were followed up in the surgery ICU, 12 % were followed up in the BMT unit, and 12 % were followed up in the internal medicine unit. Of these 25 patients, bacterial growth was observed in blood cultures (eight patients), respiratory isolates (six), rectal swabs (five), urine cultures (three), wound cultures (two), and peritoneal fluid culture (one). Additionally, 19 of 43 patients had a history of stem cell-solid organ transplantation.

According to the MHT, of 43 strains, 35 (85 %) were carbapenemase-positive. According to MBL antimicrobial gradient test results, only two were MBL-positive (4.7 %).

Seven of the isolates (16.3 %) were positive for the OXA-48 gene, as determined by multiplex PCR. The NDM-1 gene was detected only in one strain (2.3 %). VIM, IPM and KPC resistance genes were not detected in any isolate (Table 1).

There was no significant correlation between OXA-48 resistance gene positivity and the ERT antimicrobial gradient test, MEM antimicrobial gradient test or IMP antimicrobial gradient test, nor was there a correlation between OXA-48 resistance gene positivity and ERT VITEK®2 or MEM VITEK®2 results ($p > 0.05$). Additionally, no correlation was detected between OXA-48 resistance gene positivity and IMP VITEK®2 results (Table 2).

A correlation was observed between OXA-48 resistance gene positivity and MHT positivity ($p = 0.004$). A significant relationship between the MBL antimicrobial gradient test and NDM-1 was also observed ($p = 0.000$) (Table 3).

Discussion

Carbapenem antibiotics are the last treatment option for severe, life-threatening infections caused by gram negative enteric bacilli with multiple drug resistance. Therefore, an understanding of carbapenem resistance is important. The emergence of resistant strains, as well as those with the potential to become resistant, can differ according to geographical region.

The source of microorganisms leading to hospital outbreaks and determination of the transmission path, as well as the identification of control methods, create a basis for epidemiological studies. Rapid identification of strains is important whether or not there is an outbreak and provides crucial information regarding the control of hospital outbreaks. Antibiotic susceptibility tests have become fundamental tools in the identification of many hospital outbreaks due to their common usage. Moreover, these tests are standardized and can be applied to many other factors. However, as for other phenotypic methods, antibiotic susceptibility profiles are not ideal because they can be affected by growth medium, phase of reproduction and rate of spontaneous mutations. Therefore, genotyping techniques are preferentially used worldwide. With regard to determining the relationship between bacterial isolates, the techniques of serotyping, biotyping, antibiotyping, and bacteriophage typing have been replaced by others, including plasmid analysis and PCR-based typing methods, such as ribotyping [11].

In Turkey, molecular studies focusing on carbapenem resistance mechanisms are limited [8, 12]. Some regional studies have shown an association between the OXA-48 gene and carbapenem resistance in gram-negative enteric bacilli [13, 14]. It was recently reported that carbapenem resistance may be associated with certain situations, such as being transferred between hospitals or from long-term care centers, stay in the ICU, the presence of a central venous catheter, usage of antibiotics, and having diabetes mellitus [15, 16]. In this study, 27 of 43 patients were monitored in the ICU. Since our hospital was the reference hospital for units such as cardiovascular surgery and transplantation of stem cells and solid organs, most of our patients had follow-up or hospitalization histories prior to being admitted to our hospital.

In our study, of 43 patients infected with carbapenem-resistant *Enterobacteriaceae* strains, 25 patients died (58.1 %). Patel et al. [2] demonstrated that the mortality rates of carbapenem-resistant *K. pneumoniae* infected

Table 1 Results of multiplex PCR for carbapenem-resistance genes in *Enterobacteriaceae* isolates

Genes	Positive		Negative	
	n	%	n	%
OXA-48	7	16.3	36	83.7
VIM	0	0.0	43	100.0
IPM	0	0.0	43	100.0
NDM-1	1	2.3	42	97.7
KPC	0	0.0	43	100.0

Table 2 Relationship between susceptibility to carbapenems and OXA-48 gene positivity

Antibiotics	E-TEST and OXA-48					VITEK® 2 and OXA-48				
	Positive		Negative		*p*	Positive		Negative		*p*
	S	R	S	R		S	R	S	R	
ERT	7	0	36	0	0.655	7	0	36	0	–
MEM	5	2	34	2	0.407	6	1	35	1	0.055
IMP	5	2	33	3	0.587	4	3	32	4	0.126

ERT ertapenem, *MEM* meropenem, *IMP* imipenem, *S* sensitive, *R* resistance

Table 3 Relationship between MHT and MBL E-test results with OXA-48 and NDM-1 genes positivity

Test	Positive		Negative		*p*
	n	%	n	%	
OXA-48					
MHT					
Positive	3	43	32	88.9	0.004
Negative	4	57	4	11.1	
NDM-1					
MBL E-test					
Positive	1	100	1	2.4	0.000
Negative	0	0	41	97.6	

MHT modifiye Hodge test, *MBL E-test* metallo-beta-lactamase E-test

in-patients were significantly higher compared to patients infected with carbapenem-sensitive strains (48 and 20 %, respectively; $p = 0.001$). In this study, it was noted that receiving a transplant was an independent factor in carbapenem-resistant *K. pneumoniae* infection. In another study, the mortality rate was 60 % in a heterogeneous patient population that included carbapenem-resistant *K. Pneumoniae*-infected transplant recipients [17]. In addition, staying in the ICU, surgical procedures, using catheter, length of hospitalization and using of cephalosporins and aminoglycosides are risk factors for carbapenem-resistant *K. pneumoniae* infections [18, 19].

In our study, sensitivity was determined using the automated VITEK®2 Compact system and the antimicrobial gradient test. Of the 43 strains, all were ertapenem-resistant, 95.3 % were meropenem-resistant and 83.7 % were imipenem-resistant. A resistance rate of 97.7 % to ertapenem was detected using antimicrobial gradient test techniques, whereas the resistance rate was 100 % according to the VITEK®2 automated system. Additionally, meropenem resistance was calculated using the antimicrobial gradient test (93 %) and the automated system (90.7 %).

The MHT is one of the simplest techniques used to indicate carbapenemase activity. In this test, carbapenem inhibition zone diameter and MIC values are considered sufficient [4] and valuable for the determination of KPC, OXA and MBL enzymes in laboratories in which dilution techniques cannot be performed [2, 20]. Herein, a correlation was found between MHT technique results and OXA-48 gene positivity ($p = 0.004$) (Table 3). Raghunathan et al. conducted studies in which they determined the carbapenem resistance of *Enterobacteriaceae* strains by comparing PCR and MHT techniques. The authors revealed a 96 % correlation between PCR positivity and MHT positivity in terms of KPC genes (causing carbapenem resistance) [21]. MHT is not sufficient to detect OXA-48 or other carbapenemase producing isolates. Combining carbapenemase inhibitor test, using phenylboronic acid, with MHT is a good indicator fort the detection of carbapenemase producing isolates [22].

In the present study, the MBL antimicrobial gradient test was used to detect class B metallo-β-lactamases. Of the 43 isolates, MBL positivity was found in two. Of these two isolates, only one was NDM-1 positive according to PCR results. A correlation was observed between MBL antimicrobial gradient test results and NDM-1 positivity/negativity by multiplex PCR (Table 3). NDM-1 resistance has been described in several case reports in recent years [14, 23]. However, class D OXA carbapenemase-mediated carbapenem resistance has become prevalent, especially among *Enterobacteriaceae* strains causing nosocomial infections. In our country, an OXA-48 type β-lactamase belonging to class D carbapenemases was detected for the first time at the Istanbul University Faculty of Medicine Hospital. This carbapenemase enzyme was isolated from *K. pneumoniae* strains obtained from a urine culture of an in-patient [24]. The OXA-48 carbapenemase enzyme has mostly been identified in *K. pneumoniae* strains in Turkey, Lebanon and Belgium [14, 25, 26]. Two studies evaluated carbapenem resistance in ESBL-producing carbapenem-resistant *K. pneumoniae* strains using disc diffusion and antimicrobial gradient test techniques [27, 28]. Of the 14 strains examined, the OXA-1 gene was detected in all, the OXA-48 gene in two, and the NDM-1 gene in two [27]. In addition, the IS1999 location was shown in strains expressing OXA-48, indicating that ERT resistance was higher in OXA-48 positive strains compared to other carbapenems [29]. According to studies performed in Greece and Spain, all carbapenem-resistant *K. pneumoniae* strains were positive for the OXA-48 gene. The OXA-48 gene was associated with the IS1999 element [30, 31]. In Turkey, the first NDM-1 resistance gene was identified in 2011 by Poirel et al. [14]. This gene was isolated from an allogeneic stem cell-transplanted leukemia patient from Iraq. From this isolated case, NDM-1 was identified as the first resistance gene detected from an international origin [14]. Yanik et al. [12] conducted a study in Samsun-Turkey in which the carbapenemase enzyme was detected using the MHT technique in gram-negative strains resistant to at least one of the antibiotics (imipenem, meropenem or doripenem). PCR was performed to detect NDM-1, but no NDM-1 gene resistance was found in any of the 210 clinical isolates. These results indicate that NDM-1 is not yet common in Turkey. The NDM-1 resistance gene with no history of foreign contacts was firstly determined by Alp et al. [23], in which 137 carbapenem-resistant *K. pneumoniae* strains were examined for resistance genes. Of 127 strains, OXA-48 was detected in 91.5 %, IMP in 3.2 %, NDM-1 in 4.3 %, and both OXA-48 and NDM-1 in 1 %. This study described herein has added Turkey to the list of countries in which NDM-1 has been isolated. According to our results, *K. pneumoniae* isolates were found to be NDM-1-positive (Table 3). This *K. pneumoniae* was isolated from a rectal swab of a patient who did not have any foreign origin.

It has been reported that carbapenem-producing *Enterobactericeae* strains lead to both infection and colonisation, and these microorganisms cause nosocomial outbreaks as well as epidemics. Additionally, it is known that OXA carbapenemase-mediated carbapenem resistance in particular is increasing [20]. Therefore, if there are high MIC values against carbapenems in *Klebsiella* strains, other accompanying resistance mechanisms should also be examined. In addition to phenotypic tests, genotypic investigations should be commonly used in order to decrease mortality and morbidity due to infections with *Enteobactericeae* spp.

Conclusion

The finding of one NDM-1-positive isolate in this study indicates that carbapenem resistance is spreading in Turkey. The finding of one NDM-1-positive isolate in this study indicates that carbapenem resistance is spreading in Turkey. Carbapenem resistance spreads rapidly and causes challenges in treatment, and results in high mortality/morbidity rates. Therefore, is necessary to determine carbapenem resistance in *Enterobacteriaceae* isolates and to take essential infection control precautions to avoid spread of this resistance.

Authors' contributions

KS and AT carried out the study and participated in drafting the manuscript. AT and ARD participated in statistical analysis and procedures. SO, DA and HY carried out the laboratory work. KS and ES coordinated and participated in designing the study. All the authors read and approved the final version.

Author details

[1] Department of Microbiology, Medical Faculty, Recep Tayyip Erdogan University, Islampasa mah., 53000 Rize, Turkey. [2] Department of Infectious Diseases, Cengiz Gökcek Women and Obstetrics Hospital, Osmangazi mah., 27010 Gaziantep, Turkey. [3] Department of Molecular Biology and Genetics, Medical Faculty, Istanbul Bilim University, Buyukdere cad., No: 120, Esentepe-Sisli-Istanbul, Turkey. [4] Department of Pharmacology, Medical Faculty, Istanbul Bilim University, Buyukdere cad., No: 120, 34394 Esentepe-Sisli-Istanbul, Turkey. [5] Department of Physiology, Medical Faculty, Istanbul Bilim University, Buyukdere cad., No: 120, 34394 Esentepe-Sisli-Istanbul, Turkey. [6] Department of Infectious Diseases, Medical Faculty, Recep Tayyip Erdogan University, Islampasa mah., 53000 Rize, Turkey.

Competing interests

The authors declare that they have no competing interests.

References

1. Nordmann P, Naas T, Poirel L. Global spread of carbapenemase-producing *Enterobacteriaceae*. Emerg Infect Dis. 2011;17:1791–8.
2. Patel JB, Rasheed JK, Kitchel B. Carbapenemases in *Enterobacteriaceae*: activity, epidemiology, and laboratory detection. Clin Microbiol Newsl. 2009;31:55–62.
3. Shah PM. Parenteral carbapenems. Clin Microbiol Infect. 2008;14(Suppl 1):175–80.
4. Performance standards for antimicrobial susceptibility testing, 21st informational supplement. Clinical and Laboratory Standards Institute; 2013.
5. Tsakris A, Kristo I, Poulou A, Markou F, Ikonomidis A, Pournaras S. First occurrence of KPC-2-possessing *Klebsiella pneumoniae* in a Greek hospital and recommendation for detection with boronic acid disc tests. J Antimicrob Chemother. 2008;62:1257–60.
6. Wei ZQ, Du XX, Yu YS, Shen P, Chen YG, Li LJ. Plasmid-mediated KPC-2 in a *K. pneumoniae* isolate from China. Antimicrob Agents Chemother. 2007;51:763–5.
7. Queenan AM, Bush K. Carbapenemases: the versatile beta-lactamases. Clin Microbiol Rev. 2007;20:440–58 **(table of contents)**.
8. Gür D, Hasçelik G, Aydın N, Telli M, Gültekin M, Ogul D. Antimicrobial resistance in gram-negative hospital isolates: results of the Turkish HITIT-2 Surveillance Study of 2007. J Chemother. 2009;21:383–9.
9. Korten V, Ulusoy S, Zarakolu P, Mete B. Antibiotic resistance surveillance over a 4-year period (2000–2003) in Turkey: results of the MYSTIC Program. Diagn Microbiol Infect Dis. 2007;59:453–7.
10. Yan JJ, Wu JJ, Tsai SH, Chuang CL. Comparison of the double-disk, combined disk, and E test methods for detecting metallo-beta-lactamases in gram-negative bacilli. Diagn Microbiol Infect Dis. 2004;49:5–11.
11. Us E, Tekeli A, Arıkan Akan O, Dolapçı I, Şahin F, Karahan ZC. Molecular epidemiology of carbapenem-resistant *Klebsiella pneumoniae* strains isolated between 2004–2007 in Ankara University Hospital, Turkey. Mikrobiyol Bul. 2010;44(1):1–10.
12. Yanık K, Emir D, Eroglu C, Karadag A, Guney AK, Gunaydin M. Investigation of the presence of New Delhi metallo-beta-lactamase-1 (NDM-1) by PCR in carbapenem-resistant gram-negative isolates. Mikrobiyol Bul. 2013;47(2):382–4.
13. Aktas Z, Kayacan CB, Schneider I, Can B, Midilli K, Bauernfeind A. Carbapenem-hydrolyzing oxacillinase, OXA-48, persists in *Klebsiella pneumoniae* in Istanbul, Turkey. Chemotherapy. 2008;54:101–6.
14. Poirel L, Özdamar M, Ocampo-Sosa AA, Türkoğlu S, Ozer UG, Nordmann P. NDM-1-producing *Klebsiella pneumoniae* now in Turkey. Antimicrob Agents Chemother. 2012;56:2784–5.
15. Perez F, Van Duin D. Carbapenem-resistant *Enterobacteriaceae*: a menace to our most vulnerable patients. Cleve Clin J Med. 2013;80:225–33.
16. Saidel-Odes L, Borer A. Limiting and controlling carbapenem-resistant. Infect Drug Resist. 2013;7:9–14.
17. Nguyen M, Eschenauer GA, Bryan M, O'Neil K, Furuya EY, Della-Latta P, et al. Carbapenem-resistant *Klebsiella pneumoniae* bacteremia: factors correlated with clinical and microbiologic outcomes. Diagn Microbiol Infect Dis. 2010;67:180–4.
18. Dizbay M, Tunccan OG, Karasahin O, Aktas F. Emergence of carbapenem-resistant *Klebsiella* spp infections in a Turkish university hospital: epidemiology and risk factors. J Infect Dev Ctries. 2014;8:044–9.
19. Teo J, Cai Y, Tang S, Lee W, Tan TY, Tan TT, et al. Risk factors, molecular epidemiology and outcomes of ertapenem-resistant, carbapenem-susceptible *Enterobacteriaceae*: a case–case–control study. PLoS One. 2012;7:e34254.
20. Yigit H, Queenan AM, Rasheed JK, Biddle JW, Domenech-Sanchez A, Alberti S, et al. Carbapenem-resistant strain of *Klebsiella oxytoca* harboring carbapenem-hydrolyzing beta-lactamase KPC-2. Antimicrob Agents Chemother. 2003;47:3881–9.
21. Raghunathan A, Samuel L, Tibbetts RJ. Evaluation of a real-time PCR assay for the detection of the *Klebsiella pneumoniae* carbapenemase genes in microbiological samples in comparison with the modified Hodge test. Am J Clin Pathol. 2011;135:566–71.
22. Song W, Hong SG, Yong D, Jeong SH, Kim HS, et al. Combined use of the modified Hodge test and carbapenemase inhibition test for detection of carbapenemase-producing *Enterobacteriaceae* and metallo-β-lactamase-producing *Pseudomonas* spp. Ann Lab Med. 2015;35:212–9.
23. Alp E, Percin D, Colakoglu S, Durmaz S, Kurkcu CA, Ekincioglu P, et al. Molecular characterization of carbapenem-resistant *Klebsiella pneumoniae* in a tertiary university hospital in Turkey. J Hosp Infect. 2013;84:178–80.
24. Carrer A, Poirel L, Yılmaz M, Akan OA, Feriha C, Cuzon G, et al. Spread of

OXA-48 encoding plasmid in Turkey and beyond. Antimicrob Agents Chemother. 2010;54:1369–73.

25. Cuzon G, Naas T, Bogaerts P, Glupczynski Y, Huang TD, Nordmann P. Plasmid-encoded carbapenem hydrolyzing beta-lactamase OXA-48 in an imipenem susceptible *Klebsiella pneumoniae* strain from Belgium. Antimicrob Agents Chemother. 2008;52:3463–4.
26. Matar GM, Cuzon G, Araj GF, Naas T, Corkill J, Kattar MM, et al. Oxacillinase-mediated resistance to carbapenems in *Klebsiella pneumoniae* from Lebanon. Clin Microbiol Infect. 2008;14:887–8.
27. Baroud M, Dandache I, Araj GF, Wakim R, Kanj S, Kanafani Z, et al. Underlying mechanisms of carbapenem resistance in extended spectrum beta-lactamase producing *Klebsiella pneumoniae and Escherichia coli* isolates at a tertiary care centre in Lebanon: role of OXA-48 and NDM-1 carbapenemases. Int J Antimicrob Agents. 2013;41:75–9.
28. Eser Koseoglu O, Uludag Altun H, Ergin A, Boral B, Sener B, Hascelik G. Carbapenem resistance in ESBL positive *Enterobacteriaceae* isolates causing invasive infections. Mikrobiyol Bul. 2014;48(1):59–69.
29. Voulgari E, Zarkotou O, Ranellou K, Karageorgopoulos DE, Vrioni G, Mamali V, et al. Outbreak of OXA-48 carbapenemase-producing *Klebsiella pneumoniae* in Greece involving an ST11 clone. J Antimicrob Chemother. 2013;68:84–8.
30. Pano-Pardo JR, Ruiz-Carrascoso G, Navarro-San Francisco C, Gomez-Gil R, Mora- Rillo M, et al. Infections caused by OXA-48-producing *Klebsiella pneumoniae* in a tertiary hospital in Spain in the setting of a prolonged, hospital-wide outbreak. J Antimicrob Chemother. 2013;68:89–96.
31. Adler A, Shklyar M, Schwaber MJ, Navon-Venezia S, Dhaher Y, Edgar R, et al. Introduction of OXA-48-producing *Enterobacteriaceae* to Israeli hospitals by medical tourism. J Antimicrob Chemother. 2011;66:2763–6.

7

Recurrent *Scedosporium apiospermum* mycetoma successfully treated by surgical excision and terbinafine treatment

Eszter J. Tóth[1,2], Géza R. Nagy[3], Mónika Homa[1,2], Marianna Ábrók[4], Ildikó É. Kiss[4], Gábor Nagy[1,2], Zsuzsanna Bata-Csörgő[3], Lajos Kemény[3], Edit Urbán[4], Csaba Vágvölgyi[2] and Tamás Papp[1,2*]

Abstract

Background: *Scedosporium apiospermum* is an emerging opportunistic filamentous fungus, which is notorious for its high levels of antifungal-resistance. It is able to cause localized cutaneous or subcutaneous infections in both immunocompromised and immunocompetent persons, pulmonary infections in patients with predisposing pulmonary diseases and invasive mycoses in immunocompromised patients. Subcutaneous infections caused by this fungus frequently show chronic mycetomatous manifestation.

Case report: We report the case of a 70-year-old immunocompromised man, who developed a fungal mycetomatous infection on his right leg. There was no history of trauma; the aetiological agent was identified by microscopic examination and ITS sequencing. This is the second reported case of *S. apiospermum* subcutaneous infections in Hungary, which was successfully treated by surgical excision and terbinafine treatment. After 7 months, the patient remained asymptomatic. Considering the antifungal susceptibility and increasing incidence of the fungus, *Scedosporium* related subcutaneous infections reported in the past quarter of century in European countries were also reviewed.

Conclusions: Corticosteroid treatment represents a serious risk factor of *S. apiospermum* infections, especially if the patient get in touch with manure-enriched or polluted soil or water. Such infections have emerged several times in European countries in the past decades. The presented data suggest that besides the commonly applied voriconazole, terbinafine may be an alternative for the therapy of mycetomatous *Scedosporium* infections.

Keywords: Filamentous fungi, Cutaneous infection, Antifungal susceptibility, Immunosuppression, Corticosteroid therapy, *Scedosporium apiospermum*

Background

Scedosporium apiospermum is a ubiquitous, saprophytic filamentous fungus, which can be isolated mainly from environments affected by human activity (i.e. manure-enriched or polluted soils and water) [1]. It is an emerging opportunist that can cause trauma-associated, localized infections, colonization of pulmonary cavities in patients with predisposing pulmonary disorders (such as cystic fibrosis) and systemic invasive diseases in immunocompromised patients [2]. This mould is notorious for its therapy-refractory nature and resistance for several antifungal agents [1, 3]. Traumatic localized infections can occur in both immunocompromised and immunocompetent persons and are most frequently manifested as mycetomatous, chronic progressive subcutaneous infections, which may also reach the muscles and the bones [1]. *Scedosporium*-caused mycetomas can be found

*Correspondence: pappt@bio.u-szeged.hu
[2] Department of Microbiology, Faculty of Science and Informatics, University of Szeged, Közép fasor 52, Szeged 6726, Hungary
Full list of author information is available at the end of the article

worldwide but most cases have been reported in western Europe, Australia and North America [4–6]. Here, we report a Hungarian patient with recurrent mycetomatous *S. apiospermum* infection successfully treated by surgical excision and terbinafine treatment and review the similar cases reported during the past 2 decades in Europe.

Case presentation

A 70-year-old man, who worked at a vegetable plantation in previous years, was admitted to our institution with severe edema on the lower right leg and foot, accompanied by pain, fever (38.3 °C), erythema, numerous small-sized papules and abscesses. There was no medical history of notable trauma, however the patient did undergo a prosthesis implantation surgery of the right knee, 10 years ago.

In the previous year, he was hospitalized because of melena and anemia. The patient was given 8 units of red blood cell transfusions and underwent gastroscopy, colonoscopy and abdominal computed tomography angiography. Comprehensive gastrointestinal examination found no source of bleeding, however, laboratory tests showed significant proteinuria (10 g/day), low albumin (22 g/L) and IgG (5.24 g/L) levels. A kidney biopsy was performed, which revealed focal segmental glomerulosclerosis. Owing to the possibility of myeloma multiplex and amyloidosis, additional tests were also carried out with negative results. Based on these findings, the patient was diagnosed with nephrotic syndrome and received corticosteroid pulse therapy (3 × 750 mg) intravenously, which was then switched to oral administration. In the following weeks, the corticosteroid dose was gradually reduced from 80 to 16–8 mg, without any complications.

Three months later, he developed fever (38.3 °C), swelling and erythema on both legs. In addition, small petechiae could also be observed on his arms, torso and right knee, which was interpreted as vasculitis caused by the patient's septic state. Laboratory results displayed profoundly high C-reactive protein (CRP; 354.9 mg/L) level and erythrocyte sedimentation rate (94 mm/h). Based on the clinical symptoms, erysipelas and sepsis were considered to be the initial diagnoses and the patient was put on a course of antibiotic treatment (3 × 1.2 g amoxicillin and clavulanic acid). After 4 days, subsequent laboratory values for CRP and erythrocyte sedimentation rate showed 76.8 mg/L and 84 mm/h, respectively.

After 2 weeks, however, the patient was referred to our clinic, owing to the progression in his cutaneous symptoms. The patient then presented with a severely oedemic and painful lower right leg, with slight erythema and multiple small soft papules (Fig. 1). In addition, the whole skin of this extremity had a sponge-like feel to the touch. No notable symptoms were present on the left leg.

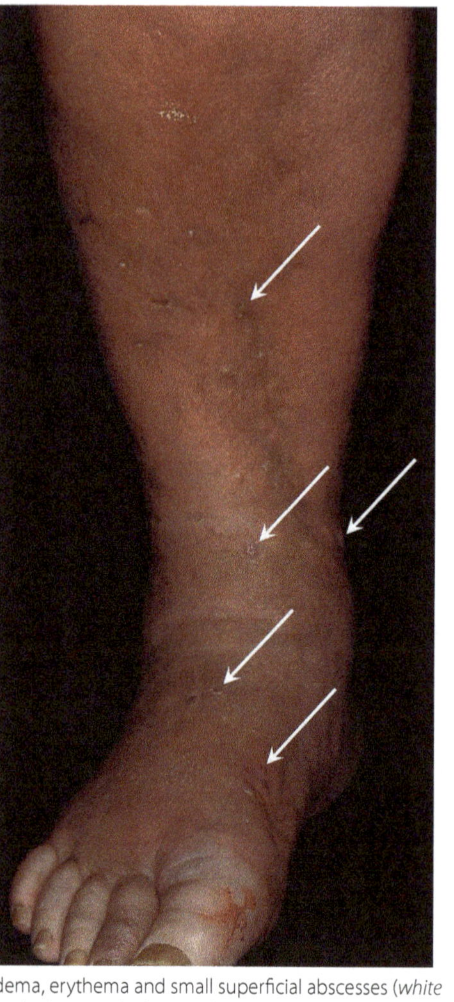

Fig. 1 Edema, erythema and small superficial abscesses (*white arrows*) on the lower right leg and foot

Laboratory tests showed elevated CRP (38 mg/L) and high white blood cell count (12.85 × 10^9/L). Ultrasound revealed four 10–13 mm-sized subcutaneous collections of echogenic fluid in the right leg. After incision and drainage of these lesions, swabs were sent to the microbiological laboratory for culturing. Only *Scedosporium apiospermum* grew in culture after 3 days of incubation at normal atmosphere at 30 °C. After accurate morphological assessment, the sample was sent for additional identification by DNA sequencing.

Considering this finding, instead of the initially administered penicillin-type antibiotic, the patient was given fluconazole (200 mg) intravenously on six occasions, to which his symptoms markedly improved. Subsequently, taking the patient's low glomerular filtration rate (56 mL/min) into account, he was prescribed a synthetic allylamine antifungal medication (250 mg terbinafine) to take every second day with the aim of minimizing potential side effects and underwent several other abscess drainages in the following weeks, in addition to the local antimicrobial agents (i.e. betadine, hydrogen peroxide, and boric acid powder). Parallel with his treatment for the mycotic infection, his steroid therapy dose was gradually decreased and his nephrotic syndrome improved. Two months into his treatment, he experienced a recurrent infection on the right leg. At this time, no mycotic infection could be proven, as only *Staphylococcus aureus* was cultured from multiple small superficial abscesses, thus the patient received a combination antibiotic of piperacillin and tazobactam (3 × 4.5 g) for a week, followed by amoxicillin and clavulanic acid (4 × 1.2 g) for another week, to which his symptoms regressed.

Though edema of the right leg persisted even after many months, there were no longer any clinical signs of inflammation and the patient did not experience any pain. Leukocyte scintigraphy displayed increased activity around the right ankle, suggesting the development of a new abscess, but it was successfully managed with antibiotic and local treatment. After 7 months, the patient remained asymptomatic and currently maintains a low dose of corticosteroid (4 mg/day) therapy. In addition to occupational exposure, low serum IgG levels and the immunosuppressive effect of the corticosteroid treatment were most likely compelling factors in further substantiating the likelihood of this rare fungal infection in our patient's case.

Mycological investigations

The isolate was deposited in the Szeged Microbiology Collection (SZMC; http://www.wfcc.info/ccinfo/collection/by_id/987) with the strain number SZMC 23374 and was sub-cultured on malt extract agar (MEA; 5% malt extract, 1% glucose, 2% agar) plates at 37 °C for further morphological and molecular examinations. It formed greyish–white, cotton-like colonies on MEA (Fig. 2a). Microscopic examination revealed branched hyphae with clavate or ovoid conidia born singly on simple or branched conidiophores or laterally on the hyphae (Fig. 2b).

For molecular identification, genomic DNA was extracted from 10 mg of mycelium ground to a fine powder in liquid nitrogen and purified by using the MasterPure Yeast DNA purification kit (Epicentre, USA) according to the instructions of the manufacturer. The complete ITS (internal transcribed spacer, including ITS1-5.8S rRNA-ITS2) region was amplified by PCR, using the primers ITS1 and ITS4 [7]. The resulting amplicons were sequenced at LGC Genomics (Germany). The determined sequence was deposited in the European Nucleotide Archive (ENA, http://www.ebi.ac.uk/ena) database (Accession number: LT703449) and used for similarity searches in the NCBI database using the BLASTN algorithm (http://blast.ncbi.nlm.nih.gov/Blast.cgi), which confirmed the fungus as *S. apiospermum* (identities for the whole ITS region, 99%).

In vitro susceptibility of the *S. apiospermum* isolate to amphotericin B (AMB), fluconazole (FLC), itraconazole (ITC), voriconazole (VRC), caspofungin (CSP), natamycin (NTM) and terbinafine (TRB) (Sigma-Aldrich, USA) was tested using the broth microdilution method according to the CLSI guideline M38-A2 [8]. Minimal inhibitory concentration (MIC) values were determined in 96-well microtiter plates by visual inspection of the cultures after 72 h incubation at 37 °C in standard RPMI-1640 medium (Sigma-Aldrich, USA). Inocula were prepared from 14-day cultures grown on MEA; the final conidial suspensions contained 10^4 CFU/mL. Final concentrations of the drugs ranged from 0.5 to 256 μg/mL. Each plate contained a sterile control (containing medium alone) and a growth control (containing inoculated medium without the drugs). Each experiment was performed in triplicates;

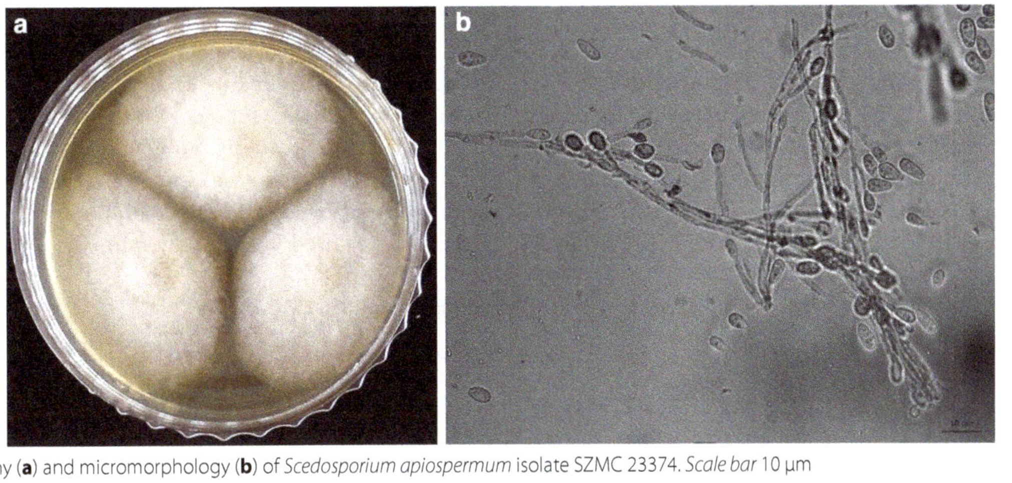

Fig. 2 Colony (**a**) and micromorphology (**b**) of *Scedosporium apiospermum* isolate SZMC 23374. *Scale bar* 10 μm

Paecilomyces variotii ATCC 22319 was used as the quality control strain. Table 1 shows the antifungal susceptibility of the case isolate to the most frequently used antifungal agents. The strain showed low susceptibility to AMB, CSP, ITC and TRB. FLC and NTM proved to be ineffective against the isolate in the investigated concentration range (MIC >128 μg/mL). It was the most susceptible to VRC (MIC 2 μg/mL).

Discussion

Mycetoma (syn. Madura foot) is the infection of the skin and subcutaneous tissues, which usually develops after a traumatic event of the leg or the foot. It is endemic in tropical and subtropical countries, but rarely reported from temperate regions, as well. Based on the causative agents, the disease can be divided into two categories: actinomycetoma or actinomycosis is caused by Actinomycetes, while eumycetoma or maduramycosis is caused by filamentous fungi [2].

Scedosporium apiospermum was first isolated in 1909 as the aetiological agent of a white grain mycetoma in Sardinia by Tarozzi [9, 10]. This species was considered to be the anamorph of *Scedosporium boydii* (previously known as *Pseudallescheria boydii*) until 2005, when they proved to be two distinct species based on molecular, physiological and biochemical data [11]. According to the latest molecular studies *S. apiospermum* is a species complex, comprising five distinct species: *S. apiospermum*, *Scedosporium aurantiacum*, *S. boydii*, *Scedosporium minutisporum*, and *Scedosporium dehoogii*. Out of them, *S. apiospermum*, *S. aurantiacum* and *S. boydii*, are regularly isolated from human infections [12]. Their incidence seems to be increasing, especially among immunocompromised patients. After *Aspergillus fumigatus*, *S. apiospermum* and *S. boydii* are the second most frequently isolated moulds in cystic fibrosis patients [13].

Based on the available case reports in English and Spanish in the PubMed (http://www.ncbi.nlm.nih.gov/pubmed) and Google Scholar (https://scholar.google.hu/) databases, 20 cases of mycetoma or subcutaneous infections were reported due to *Scedosporium* species between 1992 and 2015 from ten European countries: 4–4 from Germany and the UK, 2–2 from The Netherlands, Spain, France, and Turkey and 1–1 from Italy, Serbia, Slovenia, and Hungary [14–32] (Table 2; Fig. 3). Two additional cases have been diagnosed in France, but these patients arrived from outside of Europe (Ivory Coast and Martinique) for hospitalization [33, 34] (not included in Table 2). Of the 20 European cases, 15 were registered in immunosuppressed patients having different underlying conditions, such as organ transplantations, acute myeloid leukemia (AML) or chronic obstructive pulmonary disease (COPD). Similarly to the presented case, out of these patients, 12 had been given a corticosteroid treatment. Although it was not yet proven that these drugs would play a role in the development of *Scedosporium* infections not just as immunosuppressants but as fungal growth stimulators as well, hydrocortisone has previously proven to enhance the growth of Aspergilli [35]. Taking into account that the patient in the present case had worked with manured garden soil during the corticosteroid therapy, characteristic preference of the fungus for such eutrophic and manure-enriched environments [1] could also represent a serious risk factor for the patient besides the corticosteroid treatment.

The causative agents were identified as *S. apiospermum* and *S. boydii* in 15 and 7 cases, respectively. While, coinfections of Scedosporia and bacteria (i.e. *Nocardia abscessus* or unidentified Gram+ and Gram− bacteria) were recorded in two cases [15, 30]. However, the real incidence of the two species is unknown, since much of the case reports have been published before 2005 and mention *S. boydii* and *S. apiospermum* as the sexual and asexual form of the same organism. It is also worth to mention that according to a recent case study of Chen et al. [13], the discrimination of *S. apiospermum* and *S. boydii* does not result in a different therapeutic approach.

Sixteen of the cases identified in our literature review had positive outcome, one patient did not show up for follow-up examinations, while in another case, the infected limb has been amputated. In addition to these, two fatal cases have also been recorded, however they could not be connected to the infections caused by Scedosporia. Based on the summarized literature data in Table 2, the most common successfully applied medical therapy involved azole antifungals, i.e. voriconazole or itraconazole. Reimann et al. [16] achieved improvement using miconazole combined with vacuum seal and suction technique. Combination antifungal therapy was reported in one case, when after a failed treatment with fluconazole and liposomal amphotericin B, the patient was cured successfully with the combination of

Table 1 MIC values (μg/mL) of antifungal drugs to the *S. apiospermum* isolate SZMC 23374

Aetiological agent	MIC (μg/mL)						
	AMB	CSP	FLC	ITC	NTM	TRB	VRC
S. apiospermum	16	32	>256	32	>128	64	2

AMB amphotericin B, *CSP* caspofungin, *FLC* fluconazole, *ITC* itraconazole, *NTM* natamycin, *TRB* terbinafine, *VRC* voriconazole

Table 2 Subcutaneous infections caused by *Scedosporium* species in Europe since 1990

Age, gender	Immune status	Predisposing conditions	Signs, symptoms	Aetiological agent	Site of infection	Therapy	Outcome	References
The Netherlands								
59, M	Immunosupp.	Renal transplantation, IV catheter	Purple nodules, slight desquamation	*S. apiospermum*	Left hand and lower arm	VRC	Recovered	[14]
84, M	Immunosupp.	COPD, Periprosthetic fracture	Inflammation with bullae	*S. apiospermum*	Right elbow	VRC	Death after good initial response	[14]
Germany								
24, M	Immunocomp.	Fracture of the tibia	Edematous swellings	*S. boydii, Nocardia abscessus*	Lower left leg	ITC	Recovered	[15]
58, M	Immunosupp.	Chronic glomerulonephritis, Renal transplantation, Insect sting	Painful, swollen induration	*S. apiospermum*	Right forefoot	MCZ, Vacuum seal and suction technique	Recovered	[16]
15, M	Immunosupp.	Lupus erythematodes, Tibia and fibula fracture	Swelling, impaired wound healing	*S. boydii*	Lower leg	VRC	Recovered	[17]
53, F	Immunosupp.	AML	Reddish, inflammatory, painless tumor with central necrosis	*S. apiospermum*	Right forearm	CSP, VRC	Recovered	[18]
Spain								
58, M	Immunosupp.	Chronic glomerulonephritis	Fever, cutaneous lesions	*S. apiospermum*	Both legs	VRC	Recovered	[19]
51, M	Immunosupp.	Renal transplantation	Nodular lesions	*S. apiospermum*	Left heel	ITC, SI	Recovered	[20]
France								
79, M	Immunosupp.	Bronchospasm	Fever, bullous and necrotic purpura	*S. apiospermum*	n.a.	ITC	Death (due to *Pseudomonas* lung infection)	[21]
65, M	Immunosupp.	COPD, IV catheter	Purple nodules, slight desquamation	*S. apiospermum*	Left wrist and lower arm	VRC	Recovered	[22]
UK								
51, M	Immunocomp.	Stepped in a dung fork	Swollen, painful foot	*S. boydii*	Foot (bone involvement)	ITC	Recovered	[23]
71, M	Immunosupp.	AML	Painful, swollen, erythematous foot, necrotic ulcer between toes	*S. apiospermum*	Right foot	ITC	Recovered	[24]
81, M	Immunosupp.	Renal impairment, Pulmonary fibrosis, Scratch from a bush.	Tender subcutaneous nodules	*S. apiospermum*	Left forearm (joint involvement)	ITC	No follow up	[25]
35, M	Immunocomp.	na	Painless swelling	*S. apiospermum*	Right ankle	VRC	Recovered	[26]
Italy								
59, F	Immunosupp.	Renal transplantation	Pain, Achilles tendonitis	*S. apiospermum*	Skin, knee, and Achilles tendon of the left leg	VRC	Recovered	[27]

Table 2 continued

Age, gender	Immune status	Predisposing conditions	Signs, symptoms	Aetiological agent	Site of infection	Therapy	Outcome	References
Serbia								
50, F	Immunocomp.	na	Pain, indurations, local redness	*S. boydii*	Soft tissue and bone involvement	SI	Recovered	[28]
Slovenia								
64, M	Immunosupp.	Microscopic polyangiitis	Swelling, pain	*S. boydii*	Left leg and foot	VRC	Recovered	[29]
Turkey								
48, M	Immunocomp.	na	Swelling	Bacteria, *S. boydii*	Right hand	Amputation	Recovered	[30]
62, F	Immunosupp.	Renal transplantation	Edema, erythema, painful, indurated lesion	*S. boydii*	Left leg	ITC	Recovered	[31]
Hungary								
63, M	Immunosupp.	AML	Swelling, tenderness	*S. apiospermum*	Lower left leg	ITC	Recovered	[32]
70, M	Immunosupp.	Nephrotic syndrome	Pain, edema, fever, erythema	*S. apiospermum*	Lower right leg and foot	TRB, SI	Recovered	Present case

AML acute myeloid leukemia, *COPD* chronic obstructive pulmonary disease, *CSP* caspofungin, *F* female, *Immunocomp.* immunocompetent, *Immunosupp.* immunosuppressed, *ITC* itraconazole, *IV* intravenous, *M* male, *MCZ* miconazole, *na* not available, *SI* surgical intervention, *TRB* terbinafine, *VRC* voriconazole

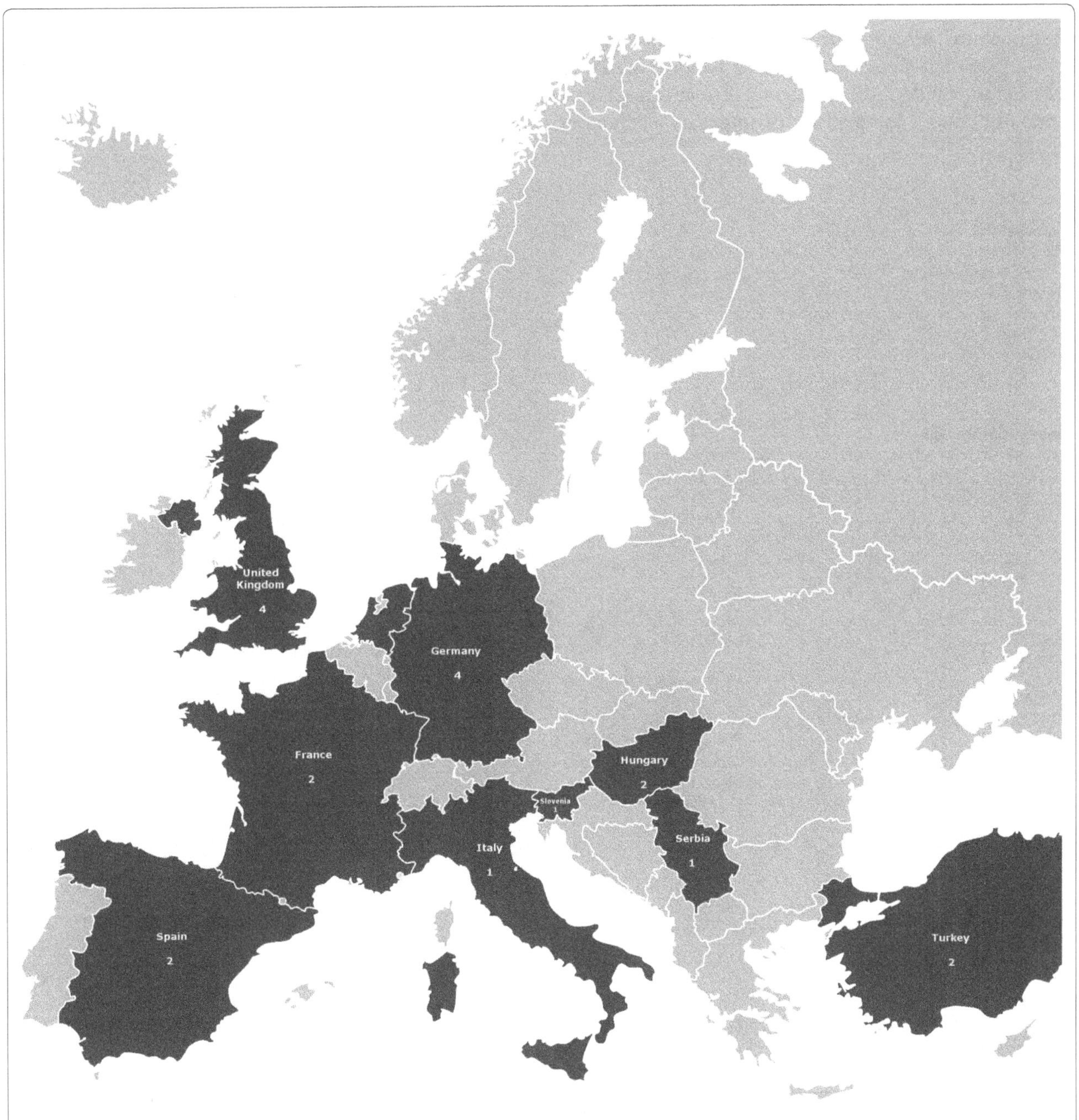
United Kingdom
4
Germany
4
France
2
Hungary
2
Slovenia
1
Italy
1
Serbia
1
Spain
2
Turkey
2

Fig. 3 Distribution of subcutaneous *Scedosporium* infections in Europe since 1990

voriconazole and caspofungin [18]. Surgical excision alone without antifungal therapy was applied in one case [28], while amputation without attempting any antifungal treatment was performed once in Turkey [30]. Medical therapy (itraconazole) plus surgery was used in the case reported by Montero et al. [20]. Amphotericin B has been applied several times, but it has always been replaced by other antifungals due to its toxicity or ineffectiveness. Based on these data, the treatment applied in the present case is unique in the European literature, since terbinafine alone or in combination with other antifungals or surgical intervention has not been applied successfully for the treatment of *S. apiospermum* mycetoma before. Although, an *S. apiospermum* skin infection has been successfully treated by terbinafine combined with voriconazole and surgical excision in Spain [36].

We also would like to highlight here that the patient responded well to terbinafine treatment, despite the relatively high in vitro MIC of the drug. A similar phenomenon was observed by Cunningham and Mitchell [24] in case of amphotericin B. These findings underline the need to handle with care the in vitro antifungal susceptibility data in the clinical treatment of filamentous fungi.

Abbreviations

AMB: amphotericin B; AML: acute myeloid leukemia; COPD: chronic obstructive pulmonary disease; CRP: C-reactive protein; CSP: caspofungin; ENA: European nucleotide archive; FLC: fluconazole; ITC: itraconazole; ITS: internal transcribed spacer; MEA: malt extract agar; MIC: minimal inhibitory concentration; NTM: natamycin; TRB: terbinafine; VRC: voriconazole; SZMC: Szeged microbiology collection.

Authors' contributions

TP coordinated the study and participated in design and writing of the manuscript. ET, GN, MH and VC participated in the morphological and molecular identification, antifungal susceptibility testing and drafting the manuscript. MÁ, IÉK, and EU isolated the fungus and participated in its microbiological characterization. GRN, LK and ZB-C performed the management of the patient and participated in the isolation of the aetiological agent. All authors read and approved the final manuscript.

Author details

[1] MTA-SZTE "Lendület" Fungal Pathogenicity Mechanisms Research Group, Hungarian Academy of Sciences, University of Szeged, Közép fasor 52, Szeged 6726, Hungary. [2] Department of Microbiology, Faculty of Science and Informatics, University of Szeged, Közép fasor 52, Szeged 6726, Hungary. [3] Department of Dermatology and Allergology, Albert Szent-Györgyi Medical Centre, University of Szeged, Szeged, Hungary. [4] Institute of Clinical Microbiology, Albert Szent-Györgyi Medical Centre, University of Szeged, Szeged, Hungary.

Competing interests

The authors declare that they have no competing interests.

Funding

This study was supported by the "Momentum" Grant of the Hungarian Academy of Sciences (LP2016-8/2016) and the project GINOP-2.3.2-15-2016-00035.

References

1. Guarro J, Kantarcioglu AS, Horré R, Rodriguez-Tudela JL, Cuenca Estrella M, Berenguer J, et al. *Scedosporium apiospermum*: changing clinical spectrum of a therapy-refractory opportunist. Med Mycol. 2006;44:295–327.
2. Cortez KJ, Roilides E, Quiroz-Telles F, Meletiadis J, Antachopoulos C, Knudsen T, et al. Infections caused by *Scedosporium* spp. Clin Microbiol Rev. 2008;21:157–97.
3. Tammer I, Tintelnot K, Braun-Dullaeus RC, Mawrin C, Scherlach C, Schlüter D, et al. Infections due to *Pseudallescheria/Scedosporium* species in patients with advanced HIV disease—a diagnostic and therapeutic challenge. Int J Infect Dis. 2011;15:e422–9.
4. Harun A, Perdomo H, Gilgado F, Chen SC, Cano J, Guarro J, et al. Genotyping of *Scedosporium* species: a review of molecular approaches. Med Mycol. 2009;47:406–14.
5. Heath CH, Slavin MA, Sorrell TC, Handke R, Harun A, Phillips M, et al. Population-based surveillance for scedosporiosis in Australia: epidemiology, disease manifestations and emergence of *Scedosporium aurantiacum* infection. Clin Microbiol Infect. 2009;15:689–93.
6. Chiang CH, Hsu CK, Lee JYY, Chang TC, Hsueh YY, Shieh SJ, et al. Recurrent *Scedosporium apiospermum* mycetoma successfully treated by surgical excision and voriconazole. Dermatol Sin. 2014;32:29–32.
7. White TJ, Bruns T, Lee S, Taylor JW. Amplification and direct sequencing of fungal ribosomal RNA genes for phylogenetics. In: Innis MA, Gelfand DH, Sninsky JJ, White TJ, editors. PCR protocols: a guide to methods and applications. New York: Academic Press; 1990. p. 315–22.
8. Clinical and Laboratory Standards Institute. Reference method for broth dilution antifungal susceptibility testing of filamentous fungi. Approved standard-2nd ed. CLSI document M38-A2. Wayne: Clinical and Laboratory Standards Institute; 2008.
9. Ajello L. The isolation of *Allescheria boydii* shear, an etiologic agent of mycetomas, from soil. Am J Trop Med Hyg. 1952;1:227–38.
10. Tarozzi G. Ricerche anatomo-patologiehe, baceriologiehet e sperimentali sopra un caso di actinomicosi del piede. Arch Perle Sc Med. 1909;33:553–632.
11. Gilgado F, Cano J, Gené J, Guarro J. Molecular phylogeny of the *Pseudallescheria boydii* species complex: proposal of two new species. J Clin Microbiol. 2005;43:4930–42.
12. Giraud S, Bouchara JP. *Scedosporium apiospermum* complex: diagnosis and species identification. Curr Fungal Infect Rep. 2014;8:211–9.
13. Chen M, Zeng J, De Hoog GS, Stielow B, Gerrits Van Den Ende AH, Liao W, et al. The 'species complex' issue in clinically relevant fungi: a case study in *Scedosporium apiospermum*. Fungal Biol. 2016;120:137–46.
14. Bosma F, Voss A, van Hamersvelt HW, de Sévaux RG, Biert J, Kullberg BJ, et al. Two cases of subcutaneous *Scedosporium apiospermum* infection treated with voriconazole. Clin Microbiol Infect. 2003;9:750–3.
15. Horré R, Schumacher G, Marklein G, Stratmann H, Wardelmann E, Gilges S, et al. Mycetoma due to *Pseudallescheria boydii* and co-isolation of *Nocardia abscessus* in a patient injured in road accident. Med Mycol. 2002;40:525–7.
16. Reimann D, Büssemaker E, Gross P. Successful treatment due to vacuum seal technique of a severe *Scedosporium apiospermum* skin infection in a renal transplant recipient. Nephrol Dial Transplant. 2004;19:245–8.
17. Tammer I, Seibold M, Krause H, Tintelnot K, König W, König B. Successful topical therapy with voriconazole: pseudallescheriasis after injury. J Trauma. 2007;62:1295–7.
18. Beier F, Kittan N, Holzmann T, Schardt K, Andreesen R, Holler E, et al. Successful treatment of *Scedosporium apiospermum* soft tissue abscess with caspofungin and voriconazole in a severely immunocompromised patient with acute myeloid leukemia. Transpl Infect Dis. 2010;12:538–42.
19. Montejo M, Muñiz ML, Zárraga S, Aguirrebengoa K, Amenabar JJ, López-Soria L, et al. Infection due to *Scedosporium apiospermum* in renal transplant recipients: a report of two cases and literature review of central nervous system and cutaneous infections by *Pseudallescheria boydii/Sc. apiospermum*. Mycoses. 2002;45:418–27.
20. Montero LA, Cid A, Fernández CM, Calzadad JM. Lesiones nodulares en retropié en un paciente con trasplante renal. Enferm Infecc Microbiol Clin. 2004;22:551–2.
21. Lemerle E, Bastien M, Demolliens-Dreux G, Forest JL, Boyer E, Chabasse D, et al. Scédosporiose cutanée révélée par un purpura bullo-nécrotique. Ann Dermatol Venereol. 1998;125:711–4.
22. Eldin C, Chiche L, Thomas G, Dicostanzo MP, Durand JM, Harle JR, et al. *Scedosporium apiospermum* catheter-related soft-tissue infection: a case report and review of the literature. Med Mycol. 2012;50:627–30.
23. Pether JV, Jones W, Greatorex FB, Bunting W. Acute pyogenic *Pseudallescheria boydii* foot infection sequentially treated with miconazole and itraconazole. J Infect. 1992;25:335–6.
24. Cunningham R, Mitchell DC. Amphotericin B responsive *Scedosporium apiospermum* infection in a patient with acute myeloid leukaemia. J Clin Pathol. 1996;49:93–4.
25. Bower CP, Oxley JD, Campbell CK, Archer CB. Cutaneous *Scedosporium apiospermum* infection in an immunocompromised patient. J Clin Pathol. 1999;52:846–8.
26. Gulati V, Bakare S, Tibrewal S, Ismail N, Sayani J, Baghla DPS. A rare presentation of concurrent *Scedosporium apiospermum* and *Madurella grisea* eumycetoma in an immunocompetent host. Case Rep Pathol. 2012;2012:154201.

27. Rogasi PG, Zanazzi M, Nocentini J, Fantoni E, Trotta M, Faggi E, et al. Disseminated *Scedosporium apiospermum* infection in renal transplant recipient: long-term successful treatment with voriconazole: a case report. Transplant Proc. 2007;39:2033–5.
28. Sopta J, Atanacković M, Raspopović V, Marković L, Kranjcić-Zec I, Lesić A. *Pseudoallescheria boydii* (*Scedosporium apiospermum*), cause of mycotic granulomatous osteomyelitis—case diagnosis. Srp Arh Celok Lek. 2005;133:366–9.
29. Lainščak M, Hočevar A, Logar D, Beović B, Matos T, Tomšič M. Subcutaneous infection with *Pseudallescheria boydii* in an immunocompromised patient. Clin Rheumatol. 2007;26:1023–4.
30. Kantarcioğlu SA, Yücel A. Pseudallescheriasis cases identified at department of microbiology and clinical microbiology, Cerrahpasa Medical Faculty and European Confederation of Medical Mycology (ECMM) Pseudallescheriasis Study Group. Cerrahpaşa J Med. 2005;36:90–6.
31. Taşbakan MI, Önal U, Metin DY, Pullukçu H, Yamazhan T, Çeltik A, et al. A rare cause of soft tissue infections: *Pseudallescheria boydii*. J Microbiol Infect Dis. 2015;5:176–9.
32. Török L, Simon G, Csornai A, Tápai M, Török I. *Scedosporium apiospermum* infection imitating lymphocutaneous sporotrichosis in a patient with myeloblastic-monocytic leukaemia. Br J Dermatol. 1995;133:805–9.
33. Béraud G, Desbois N, Coyo C, Quist D, Rozé B, Savorit L, et al. Paradoxical response preceding control of *Scedosporium apiospermum* mycetoma with posaconazole treatment. Infect Dis. 2015;47:830–3.
34. Porte L, Khatibi S, Hajj LE, Cassaing S, Berry A, Massip P, et al. *Scedosporium apiospermum* mycetoma with bone involvement successfully treated with voriconazole. Trans R Soc Trop Med Hyg. 2006;100:891–4.
35. Ng TT, Robson GD, Denning DW. Hydrocortisone-enhanced growth of *Aspergillus* spp.: implications for pathogenesis. Microbiology. 1994;140:2475–9.
36. Valenzuela Salas I, Martinez Peinado C, Fernandez Miralbell A, Soto Diaz A, Nogueras Morillas P, Martin Castro A, et al. Skin infection caused by *Scedosporium apiospermum* in immunocompromised patients. Report of two cases. Dermatol Online J. 2013;19:20022.

8

Sphingobacterium spiritivorum infection in a patient with end stage renal disease on haemodialysis

Amit Gupta[1*], Julie Logan[2], Nada Elhag[1,2] and Mike Almond[1]

Abstract

Background: *Sphingobacterium spiritivorum* is a microorganism that is ubiquitously found in the environment. However, it is rarely isolated from human clinical specimens. There are few reports to date of *Sphingobacterium spiritivorum* causing disease in humans.

Case report: We describe a case of *Sphingobacterium spiritivorum* infection in a patient on haemodialysis, which to our knowledge, has not been described before. Further testing revealed this strain was sensitive to multiple antimicrobials.

Conclusion: Despite interrupted courses of several antibiotics, our patient clinically made a good recovery and continued to receive haemodialysis.

Background

An 80 year old woman with end stage renal failure, secondary to type 2 diabetes mellitus, was established on long term unit based haemodialysis via a tunneled central venous dialysis catheter. She experienced symptoms of a generalised infection with no specific signs on examination to identify a potential source. Her past medical history included *treated* hypertension and calcified valvular heart disease.

Initial blood tests showed: haemoglobin 8.0 g/dL; white cell count 7.9×10^9/L (neutrophils 5×10^9/L); platelet 198×10^9/L; C-reactive protein 58 ml/L. A set of blood cultures from the dialysis line and haemodialysis circuit both grew gram negative rods from the aerobic bottle only. The microorganism, as identified by the "bioMérieux API® 20 NE ID kit", was determined to be *Sphingobacterium spiritivorum* (with 98.7 % certainty).

The same organism grew from two subsequent blood cultures which were referred to the Public Health England AMRHAI reference laboratory (ARMRL) for confirmation of identification and antibiotic sensitivities. Matrix-assisted laser desorption/ionization time of flight (MALDI-TOF) mass spectrometry, using Microflex LT with Biotyper v3.1 database (Bruker Daltonics, Bremen, Germany), provided identification for both isolates, with log score values of 2.273 and 2.265 matching with *S. spiritovorum* type strain DSM 11722^T. Partial (~1100 bp) 16S rRNA gene sequencing for both isolates were 100 % identical to each other and matched at 99.9 % to the *S. spiritivorum* type strain NCTC 11386^T (GenBank accession no KU759703) [1].

Sensitivity testing by ARMRL revealed no MBL activity. Further analyses showed that this strain was sensitive to co-trimoxazole, meropenem, ceftazidime, ciprofloxacin and trimethoprim. This strain was tested resistant to aminoglyclosides, amoxicillin and piperacillin–tazobactam (Table 1). Carbapenemase detection was also sought by polymerase chain reaction technique for the reference lab's current catalogue of genes for class A (KPC, IMI, NMC, GES and SME), class B (IMP, VIM, GIM, NDM, KHM, TMB, SIM and SPM) and class D (OXA-48 like) carbapenemases.

The patient was initially commenced on trimethoprim for 5 days, followed by a 7 day course of meropenem. The patient did not tolerate either of these antibiotics due to

*Correspondence: amit.gupta9@nhs.net
[1] Southend University Hospital, Prittlewell Chase, Westcliff-on-Sea SS0 0RY, UK
Full list of author information is available at the end of the article

Table 1 ARMRL antibiotic sensitivity testing for *Sphingobacterium spiritivorum*

Antibiotic	Minimum inhibitory concentration (mg/L)	Sensitive/inhibitory/resistant
Amikacin	>64	Resistant
Gentamicin	16	Resistant
Tobramycin	>32	Resistant
Aztreonam	>64	Resistant
Ceftazidime	8	Sensitive
Imipenem	8	Inhibitory
Meropenem	1	Sensitive
Piperacillin	32	Resistant
Piperacillin/tazobactam	32	Resistant
Co-trimoxazole	0.064	Sensitive
Colistin	>32	Resistant
Ciprofloxacin	1	Inhibitory
Minocycline	0.5	Undetermined

Minocycline activity could not be determined

severe side effects. A subsequent course of ciprofloxacin, was not well tolerated either for similar reasons.

Despite incomplete courses of antibiotics, the patient clinically made a good recovery. However, subsequent blood cultures a month later persistently grew *S. spiritivorum*. The source of infection was presumed to be the dialysis line as cultures from here were also positive, although this was not confirmed. After discussion with the patient, it was established that she would not consent for an elective dialysis line exchange. As a result of her well clinical status, plans were made to monitor her for signs of further infection and intervene with further antibiotics only if necessary.

No other patient on the dialysis unit was identified as having a similar infection.

Discussion

After cardiovascular disease, infections are the second most common cause of morbidity and mortality in patients with end stage renal disease on haemodialysis. Other co-factors such as older age, diabetes, low serum albumin and dialysis through temporary venous catheters are all independent risk factors for infection and sepsis [2]. Peritoneal dialysis and haemodialysis through a fistula have lower rates of septicaemia than haemodialysis via intravenous catheters [3]. Interestingly, the incidence of pneumonia is also higher in patients on haemodialysis compared to those receiving peritoneal dialysis [4].

End stage renal disease imposes higher rates of infection due to a multitude of factors that may be associated with either one of impaired host immunity, enhanced bacterial virulence properties or risks inherent within haemodialysis [5]. In vitro and in vivo data demonstrates that uraemia impairs polymorphonuclear cell chemotaxis, phagocytosis and cytotoxic activities [6]. Uraemic retention solutes such as parathyroid hormone, polyamines, angiongenin and complement factor D may all impair neutrophil activity by causing inappropriate expression of cell adhesion molecules that result in a transient leukopenia. Degranulation and release of reactive oxygen species can also lead to "cell exhaustion," impairing any anti-microbial capabilities [7].

Abundant iron stores or iron overload are also associated with impaired immune cell function. Parkinnen et al. showed that routine intravenous iron injections in haemodialysis patients may enhance bacterial virulence properties and contribute to bacterial spread [8].

The process of haemodialysis may expose patients to bacterial infections through the repeated breaching of the protective skin barrier during needle insertion, colonisation of indwelling dialysis catheters or contamination of the dialysate [5]. Catheter tips may become infected as bacteria grow along the tract within skin or improper handling of the catheter ports. Intraluminal infection and indirect haematogenous spread from another infection focus may also cause catheter infection [9]. Internal jugular lines carry a lower risk of bacteraemia compared to femoral vein lines [10]. Catheters made from polyvinyl chloride or polyethylene are perhaps more susceptible to bacterial adherence when compared to those catheters made out of polytetralfuoroethylene, silicone elastomer or polyurethane [11].

Sphingobacterium, first classified as a distinct species of bacteria in 1983, are characterised by the high sphingophospholipid content within their cell walls [12]. Sphingobacterium species are non-fermentative, non-motile, non-spore-forming aerobic gram-negative bacilli. They are also oxidase and catalase positive. The organism produces yellow colonies on blood agar plate [13].

Infections caused by the then named "*Flavobacterium*" species were first described in 1980 [14]. Infection and septicaemia caused by *Sphingobacterium* have since been well described in a variety of settings, including peritonitis, nectrotising fasciitis and respiratory tract infections [15]. Although 15 species of *Sphingobacterium* have been identified to date, literature describes *Sphingobacterium multivorum/spiritivorum* as the only species that have been isolated from human clinical specimens [16]. Results here show that *S. spiritivorum* can reliably be identified by MALDI-TOF mass spectrometry and 16S rRNA gene sequencing.

Sphingobacterium are usually found within soil, stagnant water and vegetation. They are described as opportunistic pathogens, however, they may cause infections in immunocompetent hosts. Four cases of *S. spiritivorum* associated infection have been described thus far. Two of these cases were of cellulitis, one of extrinsic allergic alveolitis, and the most recent case of septicaemia in a patient with acute myeloid leukaemia [15, 17–19]. Death only occurred in the patient with leukaemia, whereas the other cases resolved after antibiotic therapy. The source of infection was only determined in the patient with extrinsic allergic alveolitis, as the strain of bacteria isolated from patient sputum was isolated from a water reservoir within his steam iron [18].

Sphingobacterium multivorum septicaemia was originally described in a haemodialysis patient in 1984 [20]. There are, however, no cases of *S. spiritivorum* infections in the context of chronic kidney or end stage renal disease or dialysis. The source of haemodialysis catheter colonisation in this case was not determined. It is assumed that the patient was susceptible to opportunistic pathogens as a result of her comorbidities and her dialysis status.

The mainstay of treatment in previous cases has been antibiotic therapy with either combination cephalosporins with either penicillins or ciprofloxacin. *Sphingobacterium* are generally intrinsically resistant to aminoglycosides and polymyxin B [21]. Antibiotic sensitivity testing by multiple sources suggests Sphingobacterium are sensitive to quinolones and trimethoprim–sulfamethoxazole with *S. spiritivorum* having further sensitivities to carbapenems and some cephalosporins [15].

Data suggests that there are always inherent and unavoidable risks with implantable dialysis catheters, however, fully implanted devices such as Lifesite® HD Access System have shown to cause fewer infective complications [10].

There has been some interest over the past decade in the prophylactic application of topical antibiotics at the dialysis catheter site. A meta-analysis covering 2445 patients revealed that when treated with topical mupirocin, there is a 78 and 66 % risk reduction in *Staphylococcus aureus* infection in patients on haemodialysis and peritoneal dialysis respectively [22]. Furthermore, a randomised controlled trial comparing the use of topical triple agent products such as polysporin, (bacitracin, gramicidin and polymyxin B), versus placebo showed a 60–65 % risk reduction in bacteraemia over a 6 month period [23]. With comparable results to that of mupirocin use, further studies are required to determine superiority and appropriate regimens.

Other potential infection preventative measures that are undergoing trials include catheter lock therapies, pneumonococcal and influenza vaccinations and pre-emptive recombinant human granulocyte colony stimulating factor.

Conclusions

This report describes the first case of *S. spiritivorum* in a patient undergoing regular haemodialysis. Despite our patient not tolerating a wide range of antibiotics, she seemed to respond clinically and currently remains well on haemodialysis.

Authors' contribution

AG authored the main text and conducted the literature review. JL helped with the microorganism identification process and kindly authored the description of this methodology in this script. NE was the lead clinical microbiologist that assisted us in proper treatment of the patient. MA, as the consultant physician in charge oversaw the management of this patient and provided guidance on the literature review. All authors read and approved the final manuscript.

Author details

[1] Southend University Hospital, Prittlewell Chase, Westcliff-on-Sea SS0 0RY, UK. [2] Antimicrobial Resistance and Healthcare Associated Infections (AMRHAI) Reference Unit, Public Health England, London NW9 5EQ, UK.

Acknowledgements

Thanks to staff in the Bacterial Identification Services (BIDS) and Antimicrobial Susceptibility Testing (AST) services in AMRHAI for the reference laboratory identification and antibiotic sensitivities services provided.

Competing interests

The authors declare that they have no competing interests.
Written informed consent was obtained from the patient for publication of this case report. It has not been included as it contains patient indentifying information.

References

1. Edwards KJ, et al. Utility of real-time amplification of selected 16S rRNA gene sequences as a tool for detection and identification of microbial signatures directly from clinical samples. J Med Microbiol. 2012;61(Pt 5):645–52.
2. Powe NR, et al. Septicemia in dialysis patients: incidence, risk factors, and prognosis. Kidney Int. 1999;55(3):1081–90.
3. Foley RN. Infectious complications in chronic dialysis patients. Perit Dial Int. 2008;28(Suppl 3):S167–71.
4. Guo H, et al. Pneumonia in incident dialysis patients–the United States renal data system. Nephrol Dial Transplant. 2008;23(2):680–6.
5. Jaber BL. Bacterial infections in hemodialysis patients: pathogenesis and prevention. Kidney Int. 2005;67(6):2508–19.
6. Horl WH. Neutrophil function and infections in uremia. Am J Kidney Dis. 1999;33(2):xlv–xlviii.
7. Jaber BL, et al. Effect of biocompatibility of hemodialysis membranes on mortality in acute renal failure: a meta-analysis. Clin Nephrol. 2002;57(4):274–82.
8. Parkkinen J, et al. Catalytically active iron and bacterial growth in serum of haemodialysis patients after i.v. iron-saccharate administration. Nephrol Dial Transplant. 2000;15(11):1827–34.
9. Eleftheriadis T, et al. Infections in hemodialysis: a concise review—Part 1: bacteremia and respiratory infections. Hippokratia. 2011;15(1):12–7.
10. Oliver MJ, et al. Risk of bacteremia from temporary hemodialysis catheters by site of insertion and duration of use: a prospective study. Kidney Int. 2000;58(6):2543–5.
11. Ashkenazi S, Weiss E, Drucker MM. Bacterial adherence to intravenous catheters and needles and its influence by cannula type and bacterial surface hydrophobicity. J Lab Clin Med. 1986;107(2):136–40.

12. Yabuuchi E, Kaneko T, Yano I, Moss CW, Miyoshi N. *Sphingobacterium* gen. nov., *Sphingobacterium spiritivorum* comb. nov., *Sphingobacterium multivorum* comb. nov., *Sphingobacterium mizutae* sp. nov., and *Flavobacterium indologenes* sp. nov.: glucose-nonfermenting gram-negative rods in CDC groups IIK-2 and IIb. Int J Syst Bacteriol. 1983;33(3):18.
13. Holmes B, Owen RJ, Hollis DG. *Flavobacterium spiritittorum*, a new species isolated from human clinical specimens. Int J Syst Bacteriol. 1982;32:7.
14. Dhawan VK, et al. Spontaneous bacterial peritonitis due to a group IIk-2 strain. J Clin Microbiol. 1980;11(5):492–5.
15. Koh YR, et al. The first Korean case of *Sphingobacterium spiritivorum* bacteremia in a patient with acute myeloid leukemia. Ann Lab Med. 2013;33(4):283–7.
16. Yabuuchi E, Kaneko T, Yano I, Moss CW, Miyoshi N. *Sphingobacterium* gen. nov., *Sphingobacterium spiritivorum* comb. nov., *Sphingobacterium multivorum* comb. nov., *Sphingobacterium mizutae* sp. nov., and *Flavobacterium indologenes* sp. nov.: glucose-nonfermenting gram-negative rods in CDC groups IIK-2 and IIb. Int J Syst Bacteriol. 1983;33:580–98.
17. Marinella MA. *Cellulitis and sepsis due to sphingobacterium*. JAMA. 2002;288(16):1985.
18. Tronel H, et al. *Bacteremia caused by a novel species of Sphingobacterium*. Clin Microbiol Infect. 2003;9(12):1242–4.
19. Kampfer P, et al. Extrinsic allergic alveolitis (hypersensitivity pneumonitis) caused by *Sphingobacterium spiritivorum* from the water reservoir of a steam iron. J Clin Microbiol. 2005;43(9):4908–10.
20. Potvliege C, et al. *Flavobacterium multivorum* septicemia in a hemodialyzed patient. J Clin Microbiol. 1984;19(4):568–9.
21. Lambiase A, et al. Sphingobacterium respiratory tract infection in patients with cystic fibrosis. BMC Res Notes. 2009;2:262.
22. Tacconelli E, et al. Mupirocin prophylaxis to prevent *Staphylococcus aureus* infection in patients undergoing dialysis: a meta-analysis. Clin Infect Dis. 2003;37(12):1629–38.
23. Lok CE, et al. Hemodialysis infection prevention with polysporin ointment. J Am Soc Nephrol. 2003;14(1):169–79.

9

Molecular characteristic of *mcr*-1 producing *Escherichia coli* in a Chinese university hospital

Qing-wen He[1,2†], Xiao-hong Xu[1†], Fang-jun Lan[1,2], Zhi-chang Zhao[3], Zhi-yun Wu[1,2], Ying-ping Cao[1] and Bin Li[1*]

Abstract

Background: Colistin has been considered as a last-line treatment option in severe infections caused by multidrug-resistant (MDR) gram-negative pathogens. However, the emergence of the mobile colistin resistance gene (*mcr*-1) has challenged this viewpoint. The aim of this study is to explore the prevalence of *mcr*-1 in *Escherichia coli* (*E. coli*) in a Chinese teaching hospital, and investigate their molecular characteristics.

Methods: A total of 700 *E. coli* isolates were used to screen *mcr-1* by PCR and sequencing in a Chinese university hospital from August 2014 to August 2015. Susceptibility test of *mcr*-1-producing isolates was determined by Vitek -2 Compact system. 26 virulence factors (VFs), phylogenetic groups, Multi-locus sequence typing (MLST), and DNA Fingerprinting (ERIC-PCR) of strains were investigated by PCR.

Results: Four (0.6%) *mcr*-1 producing *E. coli* isolates were found in this study. The results of antibiotic susceptibility test showed that all four isolates were resistant to colistin, ciprofloxacin, levofloxacin, cefazolin, and trimethoprim/sulfamethoxazole, and were susceptible to amikacin, ertapenem and imipenem. In addition, all 4 isolates exhibited high-level resistance to aztreonam, cefotaxime and gentamicin. The numbers of VFs contained in *mcr*-1 positive isolates were no more than 4 in our study. MLST result demonstrated that these isolates were assigned to two sequence types: ST156 and ST167. The result of phylogenetic analysis showed that four *mcr*-1-positive isolates belong to two phylogenetic groups: A and B1 group. ERIC-PCR showed that four *mcr*-1 positive strains were categorized into three different genotypes.

Conclusions: Our study demonstrated a low prevalence of *mcr*-1 in *E. coli* clinical isolates in a Chinese teaching hospital, and we have gained insights into the molecular characteristics of these *mcr*-1-positive strains. Increasing the surveillance of these infections, as well as taking effective infection control measures are urgently needed to take to control the transmission of *mcr*-1 gene.

Keywords: *E. coli*, *mcr*-1, Colistin, Multidrug-resistant

Background

In recent years, colistin has been considered as an effective therapeutic option for the rapid increasing of multidrug-resistant (MDR) gram-negative pathogens [1, 2]. However, the prevalence of the mobile colistin resistance gene (*mcr*-1) in animals and human beings worldwide has challenged this viewpoint [3, 4]. Resistance to polymyxins is mainly caused by the modification to bacterial outer membrane, which was usually considered as chromosomally mediated resistance [5, 6].

Since it was initially found, plasmid-mediated *mcr*-1 has been detected widely [3, 7]. Nowadays, *mcr*-1-producing bacteria have been reported in many regions in China [4, 8]. *Mcr*-1 was firstly found in *Escherichia coli* (*E. coli*), and now it has been spreading to other *Enterobacteriaceae* [9]. Several reports showed that the *mcr*-1 gene could coexist with other resistance genes (such as

*Correspondence: leonlee307@hotmail.com
†Qing-wen He and Xiao-hong Xu contributed equally to this work
[1] Department of Clinical Laboratory, Fujian Medical University Union Hospital, 29# Xinquan Road, Fuzhou 350001, Fujian, China
Full list of author information is available at the end of the article

CRE/ESBL) in *E. coli* and *Klebsiella pneumoniae*, which probably lead to the emergence pan-drug resistant and increase the difficulty of treatment [8, 10]. Therefore, the emergence and spread of *mcr*-1 gene among human beings should be given close attention. The aim of this study was to evaluate the prevalence of *mcr*-1 in *E. coli* clinical isolates in a Chinese teaching hospital, and to investigate the molecular characteristics of these strains.

Methods

Bacterial strains

A total of 700 *E. coli* clinical isolates were collected from the clinical laboratory of Fujian Medical University Union Hospital (Fuzhou, Fujian province, China) from August 2014 to August 2015. It is a 2200-bed tertiary care teaching hospital with approximately 95,000 hospital admissions per year, located in southeastern China. All isolates were identified by GNI card of the Vitek system (BioMèrieux, Missouri, France).

Antibiotic susceptibility testing

Antimicrobial susceptibility testing was performed using the AST-GN16 of Vitek-2 Compact system (Bio Mérieux, France). The antimicrobial agents tested included: tigecycline (glycycline); ertapenem and imipenem (carbapenems); cefazolin; cefoxitin; cefepime, and cefotaxime (cephalosporins); aztreonam (monobactam); amikacin and gentamicin (aminoglycosides); ciprofloxacin and levofloxacin (quinolone); piperacillin/tazobactam; trimethoprim/sulfamethoxazole. The results were interpreted by the Clinical and Laboratory Standards Institute (CLSI) [11]. The MIC of colistin was determined using agar dilution method, and the result was interpreted according to European Committee On Antimicrobial Susceptibility Testing (EUCAST) guidelines [12]. *E. coli* ATCC 25922 was used as a quality control.

DNA extraction

Several colonies were suspended in 50 μl of sterile distilled water for preparing genomic DNA of the isolates, and then the bacterial suspension was heated at 100 °C for 10 min as described previously [13].

MCR-1 detection

mcr-1 gene was screened in *E. coli* clinical isolates by PCR using primers as previously described [4]. All of the PCR products were sequenced and then compared with known sequences listed in the GenBank (http://www.ncbi.nlm.nih.gov/blast/).

Detection of virulence factor genes

Twenty six virulence factors (VFs) genes associated with extraintestinal virulence [14, 15] were detected using a multiplex PCR method as previously described [15]. These genes were as follows: adhesions (*pap*AH, *pap*EF, *pap*C, *pap*G allele I, *pap*G II/III, *pap*G allele II, *sfa/foc*DE, *afa/dra*BC, *fim*H, *gaf*D, *sfa*S, *foc*G and *nfa*E), toxins (*hly*A, *cnf*1 and *cdt*B), siderophores (*fyu*A and *iut*A), protections and invasions (*kps*MTII, *kps*MTIII, *tra*T, *cva*C, kpsMT and K1/K5), miscellaneous (*rfc* and PAI). The PCR products were sequenced and then compared with known sequences listed in the GenBank (http://www.ncbi.nlm.nih.gov/blast/).

Phylogenetic analysis

The phylogenetic groups (A, B1, B2, and D) of *mcr*-1 producing *E. coli* isolates were identified by a triplex PCR as previously described [16].

Multi-locus sequence typing (MLST)

Mcr-1 positive strains were analyzed by multilocus sequence typing (MLST), which was based on 7 standard housekeeping genes (*adk, fumC, gyrB, icd, mdh, purA, recA*) (http://mlst.ucc.ie/mlst/mlst/dbs/Ecoli) [17].

DNA fingerprinting

Enterobacterial Repetitive Intergenic Consensus Sequences PCR (ERIC-PCR) was applied to typing *mcr*-1 producing *E. coli* isolates with the primers ERIC-1 and ERIC-2 [18]. DNA fingerprints were compared by visual inspection, ERIC profiles were regarded as different if there were different bands on visual inspection [19].

Results and discussion

In this study, four isolates (0.6%) were confirmed to carry *mcr*-1 gene, which is lower than previous study [4]. The age of the patients ranged between 38 and 80 years. These *mcr*-1 producing strains were isolated from two different wards (Table 1). Two strains were isolated from the same patient. The clinical data of patients with *mcr*-1 positive *E. coli* infection were shown in Table 2.

Mcr-1 was usually found to be co-localized with other resistance genes on plasmids, such as ESBL genes and carbapenemase genes [20], which might increase the emergence of pan-drug resistance. In our study, the results of antimicrobial susceptibility test showed a high drug resistance in the *mcr*-1-producing isolates. All of the *mcr*-1 positive isolates were resistance to at least 3 different kinds of antibiotics (Table 1).

All four *mcr*-1 positive strains detected in our study were resistant to colistin and the MICs ranged from 4 to 16 μg/ml. It will be worrisome once *mcr*-1 coexists with other resistant genes, especially carbapenemase genes because of limited therapeutic options [20]. Previous studies revealed that *mcr-1* co-produced with carbapenem-resistant genes in *E. coli* [8, 21]. Fortunately, all of

Table 1 Main characteristics of the *mcr*-1 *E. coli*

Isolates	Data	Ward	Specimen	Phylogenetic groups	MLST	ERIC pattern	VFs	Antibiotic resistance
E321	2014.8	Colorectal surgery	Drainage-fluid	B1	ST156	1	*traT*, *iutA*	COL, CFZ, FOX, CIP, LVX, SXT, TGC
E684	2015.1	Colorectal surgery	Secretion	B1	ST156	2	*fimH*, *traT*, *iutA*	COL, CFZ, CTX, FEP, ATM, GEN, CIP, LVX, SXT
E921	2015.4	Hepatobiliary surgery	Secretion	A	ST167	3	*fyuA*, *traT*, *iutA*	COL, CFZ, CTX, ATM, GEN, CIP, LVX, SXT
E1005	2015.5	Hepatobiliary surgery	Drainage-fluid	A	ST167	3	*fyuA*, *cvaC*, *traT*, *iutA*	COL, CFZ, CTX, ATM, GEN, CIP, LVX, SXT

CFZ cefazolin, *FOX* cefoxitin, *CTX* cefotaxime, *FEP* cefepime, *TZP* piperacillin/tazobactam, *ATM* aztreonam, *IPM* imipenem, *ETP* ertapenem, *AMK* amikacin, *GEN* gentamicin, *CIP* ciprofloxacin, *LVX* levofloxacin, *SXT* trimethoprim/sulfamethoxazole, *TIG* tigecycline, *COL* colistin, *MLST* multi-locus sequence typing, *ERIC* enterobacterial repetitive intergenic consensus, *VFs* virulence factor genes

Table 2 Clinical data of patients with mcr-1 positive *E. coli* infection

Isolates	Patients	Gender	Age (years)	Underlying diseases	Length of hospital stay (days)	Treatments used	Outcomes
E321	Patient 1	Female	80	Malignancy, hypertension, pulmonary tuberculosis	51	TZP	Survived
E684	Patient 2	Female	57	Perineal infection, hypertension	37	TZP	Survived
E921	Patient 3	Male	38	Hypertension, pancreatitis, diabetes	26	MEM	Survived
E1005	Patient 3	Male	38	Hypertension, pancreatitis, diabetes	26	MEM	Survived

TZP piperacillin/tazobactam, *MEM* meropenem

them were susceptible to carbapenems (IPM and ETP), which probably indicated that no carbapenem-resistant genes coexisted with *mcr*-1. Result of ERIC-PCR (Fig. 1) showed that four *mcr*-1 positive strains were categorized into three different genotypes, one of which contained 2 strains (from the same patient). These isolates which have different patterns suggest that they were non-clonal transmission. In a previous study, two *mcr*-1 positive *E. coli* isolates from a single fowl were belonging to phylogenetic B1 and D group [22]. The *mcr*-1-producing isolates in this study were belonged to phylogenetic groups A and B1, which were mainly distributed among human commensal *E. coli* isolates [23]. The *mcr*-1 producing isolates were assigned by MLST to two different sequence types: ST156 and ST167 (Table 1), which was similar to previous reports in other studies from China [8, 22]. *E. coli* ST156 has been found that it has connection with different ESBL genes [24, 25]. ST167 was belonged to ST10 complex and regarded as prevalent ST among ESBL-producing *E. coli* from human and animal sources [26]. In addition, *E. coli* ST167 was reported to be closely related to bla_{NDM}, which needed closely concern of spreading [27]. The similar molecular characterizations illustrated that *mcr*-1 positive isolates detected from the same department in our study were clonally related.

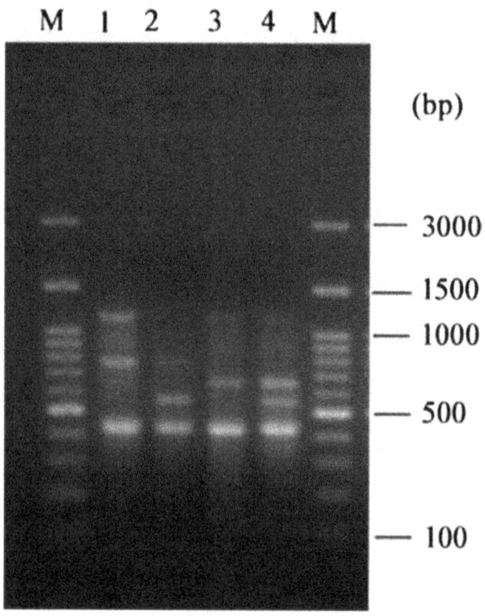

Fig. 1 ERIC-PCR products from four mcr-1 positive isolates. *M* mark, *lane 1* E321, *lane 2* E684, *lane 3* E921, *lane 4* E1005

VFs in *E. coli* were associated with colonization, bacterial fitness and virulence [28]. VFs include five main groups: (1) adhesions; (2) toxins; (3) siderophores; (4) capsule production and (5) protections and invasions.

Clinical *E. coli* strains often carry multiple VFs, and isolates belonging to groups A and B1 often have less VFs than those belonging to phylogroups B2 and D [28]. To the best of our knowledge, there is no study concerning about VFs in *mcr-1* producing *E. coli*. In our study, *mcr-1* producing isolates contained less than 4 different VFs (Table 1). Only five different kinds of VFs had been detected in our *mcr-1* positive isolates, which included *fim*H, *fyu*A, *tra*T, *iut*A and *cva*C. *fim*H is one of the most commonly VFs present in *E. coli*, which encodes the adhesion subunit of type 1 fimbriae and related to colonization [15]. Lee et al. reported that *fyu*A, *tra*T, and *iut*A were found to be independent predictors for pathogenicity. Meanwhile, *tra*T and *iut*A were thought to be closely related to ESBL genes [29]. Pitout et al. found that *cva*C was only present in non-CTX-M-producing isolates [30]. Previous reports suggested that antibiotic resistance has negative association with virulence factors [31], which could be interpreted by the loss of VFs associated with mutation to resistance [32].

It is noteworthy that two *mcr*-1 positive *E. coli* strains were isolated from the same patient but at different time (Table 1). Results of MLST and ERIC-PCR revealed that these isolates had identical genetic background. Result of antimicrobial susceptibility test showed that they had similar antibiograms. We speculate that the two isolates probably originated from a same source.

In conclusion, we have revealed a low prevalence of *mcr-1* in *E. coli* clinical isolates in a Chinese teaching hospital, and presented detailed molecular characteristics of these isolates. The presence of *mcr*-1 in *E. coli* clinical isolates suggests that it will pose a threat to public healthcare. Effective infection control measures are urgently needed to take to control the transmission of *mcr*-1 gene.

Abbreviations

MCR-1: mobile colistin resistance gene; MDR: multi-drug resistant; PCR: polymerase chain reaction; CLSI: Clinical and Laboratory Standards Institute; MLST: multi-locus sequence typing; CRE: carbapenem-resistant *Enterobacteriaceae*; ESBL: extended-spectrum β-lactamase; ERIC-PCR: Enterobacterial Repetitive Intergenic Consensus Sequences PCR; VFs: virulence factors.

Authors' contributions

QH, XX, FL, ZZ and YC conducted laboratory assays. ZW collected clinical data. QH wrote the paper. BL designed the study and reviewed the manuscript. All authors read and approved the final manuscript.

Author details

[1] Department of Clinical Laboratory, Fujian Medical University Union Hospital, 29# Xinquan Road, Fuzhou 350001, Fujian, China. [2] The Union Clinical Medical College of Fujian Medical University, Fuzhou 350004, Fujian, China. [3] Department of Pharmacy, Fujian Medical University, Union Hospital, Fuzhou 350001, Fujian, China.

Acknowledgements

We thank Prof. Jianhua Liu and Yiyun Liu of South China Agricultural University, Guangzhou, China for kindly providing us the mcr-1 positive control. We also thank Prof. Min Chen and Department of Laboratory Medicine, Medical Technology and Engineering College, Fujian Medical University for their kindly help.

Competing interests

The authors declare that they have no competing interests.

Funding

This study was supported by the National Natural Science Foundation of China (Grant No. 81201328), the Fujian Provincial Funds for Distinguished Young Scientists in Colleges and Universities, China (Grant No. JA13134), and the Medical Elite Cultivation Program of Fujian, China (Grant No. 2015-ZQN-ZD-15).

References

1. Nation RL, Li J, Cars O, Couet W, Dudley MN, Kaye KS, Mouton JW, Paterson DL, Tam VH, Theuretzbacher U, et al. Framework for optimisation of the clinical use of colistin and polymyxin B: the Prato polymyxin consensus. Lancet Infect Dis. 2015;15(2):225–34.
2. Doi Y, Paterson DL. Carbapenemase-producing Enterobacteriaceae. Semin Respir Crit Care Med. 2015;36(1):74–84.
3. Skov RL, Monnet DL. Plasmid-mediated colistin resistance (mcr-1 gene): 3 months later, the story unfolds. Euro Surveill. 2016;21:9.
4. Liu YY, Wang Y, Walsh TR, Yi L, Zhang R, Spencer J, Doi Y, Tian G, Dong B, Huang X, et al. Emergence of plasmid-mediated colistin resistance mechanism MCR-1 in animals and human beings in China: a microbiological and molecular biological study. Lancet Infect Dis. 2016;16(2):161–8.
5. Giani T, Arena F, Vaggelli G, Conte V, Chiarelli A, Henrici De Angelis L, Fornaini R, Grazzini M, Niccolini F, Pecile P, et al. Large nosocomial outbreak of colistin-resistant, carbapenemase-producing *Klebsiella pneumoniae* traced to clonal expansion of an mgrB deletion mutant. J Clin Microbiol. 2015;53(10):3341–4.
6. Olaitan AO, Morand S, Rolain JM. Mechanisms of polymyxin resistance: acquired and intrinsic resistance in bacteria. Front Microbiol. 2014;5:643.
7. Du H, Chen L, Tang Y, Kreiswirth BN. Emergence of the mcr-1 colistin resistance gene in carbapenem-resistant Enterobacteriaceae. Lancet Infect Dis. 2016;16(3):287–8.
8. Yu H, Qu F, Shan B, Huang B, Jia W, Chen C, Li A, Miao M, Zhang X, Bao C, et al. Detection of mcr-1 colistin resistance gene in carbapenem-resistant Enterobacteriaceae from different hospitals in China. Antimicrob Agents Chemother. 2016;60(8):5033–5.
9. Schwarz S, Johnson AP. Transferable resistance to colistin: a new but old threat. J Antimicrob Chemother. 2016;71(8):2066–70.
10. Haenni M, Poirel L, Kieffer N, Chatre P, Saras E, Metayer V, Dumoulin R, Nordmann P, Madec JY. Co-occurrence of extended spectrum beta lactamase and MCR-1 encoding genes on plasmids. Lancet Infect Dis. 2016;16(3):281–2.
11. CLSI. Methods for dilution antimicrobial susceptibility tests for bacteria that grow aerobically; approved standard, 10th ed. CLSI document M07-A10. Wayne: Clinical and Laboratory Standards Institute; 2015.
12. EUCAST. Breakpoints tables for interpretation of MICs and zone diameters, version 6.0; 2016.
13. He Q, Chen W, Huang L, Lin Q, Zhang J, Liu R, Li B. Performance evaluation of three automated identification systems in detecting carbapenem-resistant Enterobacteriaceae. Ann Clin Microbiol Antimicrob. 2016;15(1):40.
14. Johnson JR, Russo TA. Molecular epidemiology of extraintestinal pathogenic (uropathogenic) *Escherichia coli*. Int J Med Microbiol. 2005;295(6–7):383–404.
15. Johnson JR, Stell AL. Extended virulence genotypes of *Escherichia coli* strains from patients with urosepsis in relation to phylogeny and host compromise. J Infect Dis. 2000;181(1):261–72.

16. Clermont O, Bonacorsi S, Bingen E. Rapid and simple determination of the *Escherichia coli* phylogenetic group. Appl Environ Microbiol. 2000;66(10):4555–8.
17. Johnson JR, Clermont O, Johnston B, Clabots C, Tchesnokova V, Sokurenko E, Junka AF, Maczynska B, Denamur E. Rapid and specific detection, molecular epidemiology, and experimental virulence of the O16 subgroup within *Escherichia coli* sequence type 131. J Clin Microbiol. 2014;52(5):1358–65.
18. Smith JL, Drum DJ, Dai Y, Kim JM, Sanchez S, Maurer JJ, Hofacre CL, Lee MD. Impact of antimicrobial usage on antimicrobial resistance in commensal *Escherichia coli* strains colonizing broiler chickens. Appl Environ Microbiol. 2007;73(5):1404–14.
19. Manges AR, Johnson JR, Foxman B, O'Bryan TT, Fullerton KE, Riley LW. Widespread distribution of urinary tract infections caused by a multidrug-resistant *Escherichia coli* clonal group. N Engl J Med. 2001;345(14):1007–13.
20. Schwarz S, Johnson AP. Transferable resistance to colistin: a new but old threat. J Antimicrob Chemother. 2016;71:2066–70.
21. Li A, Yang Y, Miao M, Chavda KD, Mediavilla JR, Xie X, Tang YW. Complete sequences of mcr-1-harboring plasmids from extended-spectrum-beta-lactamase- and carbapenemase-producing Enterobacteriaceae. Antimicrob Agents Chemother. 2016;60(7):4351–4.
22. Yang RS, Feng Y, Lv XY, Duan JH, Chen J, Fang LX, Xia J, Liao XP, Sun J, Liu YH. Emergence of NDM-5 and MCR-1-producing *Escherichia coli* clone ST648 and ST156 from a single muscovy duck (*Cairina moschata*). Antimicrob Agents Chemother. 2016;60:6899–902.
23. Pitout JD. Extraintestinal pathogenic *Escherichia coli*: an update on antimicrobial resistance, laboratory diagnosis and treatment. Exp Rev Anti Infect Ther. 2012;10(10):1165–76.
24. Cortes-Cortes G, Lozano-Zarain P, Torres C, Castaneda M, Moreno Sanchez G, Alonso CA, Lopez-Pliego L, Gutierrez Mayen MG, Martinez-Laguna Y, Rocha-Gracia RD. Detection and molecular characterization of *Escherichia coli* strains producers of extended-spectrum and CMY-2 type beta-lactamases, isolated from turtles in Mexico. Vector Borne Zoonotic Dis. 2016;16:595–603.
25. Pan YS, Liu JH, Hu H, Zhao JF, Yuan L, Wu H, Wang LF, Hu GZ. Novel arrangement of the blaCTX-M-55 gene in an *Escherichia coli* isolate coproducing 16S rRNA methylase. J Basic Microbiol. 2013;53(11):928–33.
26. Schink AK, Kadlec K, Kaspar H, Mankertz J, Schwarz S. Analysis of extended-spectrum-beta-lactamase-producing *Escherichia coli isolates* collected in the GERM-Vet monitoring programme. J Antimicrob Chemother. 2013;68(8):1741–9.
27. Huang Y, Yu X, Xie M, Wang X, Liao K, Xue W, Chan EW, Zhang R, Chen S. Widespread dissemination of carbapenem-resistant *Escherichia coli* sequence type 167 strains harboring blaNDM-5 in clinical settings in China. Antimicrob Agents Chemother. 2016;60(7):4364–8.
28. Smith JL, Fratamico PM, Gunther NW. Extraintestinal pathogenic *Escherichia coli*. Foodborne Pathog Dis. 2007;4(2):134–63.
29. Lee S, Yu JK, Park K, Oh EJ, Kim SY, Park YJ. Phylogenetic groups and virulence factors in pathogenic and commensal strains of *Escherichia coli* and their association with blaCTX-M. Ann Clin Lab Sci. 2010;40(4):361–7.
30. Pitout JD, Laupland KB, Church DL, Menard ML, Johnson JR. Virulence factors of *Escherichia coli* isolates that produce CTX-M-type extended-spectrum beta-lactamases. Antimicrob Agents Chemother. 2005;49(11):4667–70.
31. Skjot Rasmussen L, Ejrnaes K, Lundgren B, Hammerum AM, Frimodt Moller N. Virulence factors and phylogenetic grouping of *Escherichia coli* isolates from patients with bacteraemia of urinary tract origin relate to sex and hospital- vs. community-acquired origin. Int J Med Microbiol. 2012;302(3):129–34.
32. Vila J, Simon K, Ruiz J, Horcajada JP, Velasco M, Barranco M, et al. Are quinolone-resistant uropathogenic *Escherichia coli* less virulent? J Infect Dis. 2002;186(7):1039–42.

10

Prevalence and characterization of extended-spectrum beta-lactamases producing *Enterobacteriaceae* in healthy children and associated risk factors

S. M. Hijazi[1*], M. A. Fawzi[2], F. M. Ali[3] and K. H. Abd El Galil[1,4]

Abstract

Background: Community acquired infections due to extended-spectrum beta-lactamase-producing *Enterobacteriaceae* (ESBL-PE) had been increased. The fecal flora of children in the community represents a huge potential reservoir for ESBLs which are located on highly transmissible plasmids. This study examined the prevalence of ESBL-PE fecal carriage, antimicrobial susceptibility pattern, possible risk factors, and characterized the genes encoding these ESBL enzymes in Lebanese children community.

Methods: A total of 125 rectal swabs were taken from healthy children aged from 1 to 5 years. Detection of ESBLs was carried out using combination-disc method test and multiplex PCR. A questionnaire concerning child's lifestyle and risk factors for ESBL carriage was illustrated.

Results: Thirty-one of 125 participants (24.8 %) carried ESBL-PE. Regular consumption of meat, and chicken were significantly associated with high carriage rate of ESBL-PE, while dairy products (milk, yogurt, cheese) association was non-significant. Intimate hygiene habits were found also affecting the carriage rate. Multiple *bla* genes were the most common, 48.4 % (15/31) of ESBL-PE carried both $bla_{CTX\text{-}M}$ and bla_{TEM}, and 22.6 % (7/31) carried $bla_{CTX\text{-}M}$, bla_{SHV}, and bla_{TEM}, 29 % (9) carried $bla_{CTX\text{-}M}$ only. Concerning CTX-M-types, CTX-M-9 was the most predominant (24/31) and mostly in combination with CTX-M-15 type.

Conclusion: High rate of colonization in healthy children with ESBL-PE was observed, regular consumption of dietary products from animal source (meat or chicken) were associated with this colonization in the community in non-hospitalized children. To our best knowledge it is the first study about regular consumption of dairy product as a risk factor for ESBL-PE community carriage, the first data about the carriage rate of ESBL-PE in community children in Lebanon and Middle East, and for the wide dissemination of CTX-M-9 type in this population.

Keywords: Extended-spectrum beta-lactamase, Children, TEM, SHV, CTX-M, CTX-9, Dairy products, Meat, Lebanon

Background

Enterobacteriaceae carrying extended-spectrum β-lactamases (ESBLs) have emerged as significant pathogens. Such strains are resistant to multiple antimicrobial agents, and can be challenging to treat, as their therapeutic options are few [1]. Resistance to β-lactams in *Enterobacteriaceae* is primarily due to β-lactamases-mediated antibiotic hydrolysis; while an altered expression of efflux pumps and/or porins play only a minor role (2). Based on substrate specificities; the β-lactamases family is divided into four functional groups: penicillinases, ESBLs, carbapenemases, and AmpC-type cephalosporinases [2]. Of these, ESBLs, which can hydrolyze virtually all penicillins and cephalosporins, including the extended-spectrum cephalosporins, like cefotaxime or ceftazidime, comprise the

*Correspondence: somayahijazi@yahoo.com
[1] Department of Pharmaceutical Sciences (Pharmaceutical Microbiology), Faculty of Pharmacy, Beirut Arab University, Beirut, Lebanon
Full list of author information is available at the end of the article

largest and most prevalent group of enzymes [3]. Many ESBL producers are multi-resistant to non-β-lactam antibiotics, including fluoroquinolones and aminoglycosides [4], trimethoprim, tetracyclines, sulfonamides, and chloramphenicol as well as aminoglycosides, and this is often encoded by the same plasmids that determine the ESBL [5]. Consequently, effective antibiotic therapy for treating these infections is limited to a small number of drugs [6] such as carbapenems and thus increasing the chance of resistance to carbapenems among the *Enterobacteriaceae.* Of major concern is the coexistence of multiple ESBL, carbapenemase genes, and other antibiotic resistance determinants on mobile elements which may lead to the emergence of organisms with resistance to all antibiotic [2].

Rapid dissemination of *Escherichia coli* and *Klebsiella pneumoniae* isolates producing ESBLs widely in the community settings, resulted in both community-onset and hospital-associated infections on a global scale [7]. More than 200 types of ESBLs have been described in various species of the *Enterobacteriaceae* family and other non-enteric organisms, including *Pseudomonas aeruginosa* and *Acinetobacter spp.* These organisms produce variants of the TEM, SHV and CTX-M β-lactamases [8]. TEM- and SHV-type β-lactamases, mainly produced by *K. pneumoniae,* have spread throughout hospital settings, and CTX-M enzymes, mainly produced by *E. coli,* have become predominant in the community [9]. CTX-M enzymes were discovered in 1989 [10] but they did not become predominant over the other ESBL enzymes until the first decade of the twenty-first century during which an extraordinary spread of these enzymes was observed [11] in both hospital and community settings [12]. The $bla_{CTX\text{-}M\text{-}15}$ gene are found mainly in *Enterobacteriaceae* and were recently named "plasmids of resistance responsible for outbreak" because of their capacity to acquire genes of resistance and to transfer among bacteria [13].

The community may thus represent a reservoir for ESBLs not detected in clinical isolates [14].

Most data on prevalence, risk factors and molecular characterization of ESBL -producing organisms are from studies in adult patients in both hospital and community settings, or from studies confined to hospitalized infants [15], only few data are available concerning the healthy pediatric populations. It is critical to better define the prevalence, risk factor, and molecular characterization of ESBLs-producing organism carried by children to adopt best-practice infection control measures and help in the appropriate choice of empirical antimicrobial coverage for infections in these populations.

The aim of this study is to investigate the prevalence and predisposing factors of intestinal carriage of ESBLs-producing *Enterobacteriaceae* (ESBL-PE) among Lebanese community children and to determine the molecular characterization of the resistance genes (bla_{TEM}, bla_{CTX}, bla_{SHV}, $bla_{CTX\text{-}M\text{-}2}$, $bla_{CTX\text{-}M\text{-}9}$, and $bla_{CTX\text{-}M\text{-}15}$).

Methods

Ethical clearance

The study protocols were approved by Institutional Review Board Committee of Beirut Arab University. Written informed consents were obtained from all patients parents (at least one parent of each child) before enrollment.

Sample population and questionnaire

The study was performed between January 2013 and May 2013 in three different pediatric clinics in Lebanon. Only 125 healthy children population aged from 1 to 5 years old coming for vaccination or general checkup were chosen for this study. However, the children who were under antibiotic treatment within 5 days before the enrollment date were excluded from this study. A questionnaire was completed for each participant regarding name, age, gender, medical history (previous antibiotic or antacid intake, previous hospital admission), dietary habits (milk, yogurt, cheese, meat, or chicken consumption), and intimate hygiene habits.

Bacterial isolation and ESBL detection and confirmation

Rectal swabs were taken by a sterile swabs moistened with sterile saline and were immediately plated onto MacConkey agar (Oxoid, UK) plates supplemented with 2 mg/l ceftazidime (used within 5 days of preparation), incubated at 37 °C for 24 h. When a sample showed positive growth on the selective medium, at least three colonies plus each distinct morphotype were selected for subsequent characterization. Bacterial identification was performed using Gram staining, biochemical testing (indole, methyl red, vogus-prauskaur, citrate, and urease), and API 20E system (bioMerieux,Marcy l'Etoile, France).

The isolates were first screened for ESBL production using ceftazidime, cefepime, cefotaxime, cefpodoxime, ceftriaxone, and aztreonam disks (Oxoid Ltd, Basingstone,UK) and then phenotypic confirmatory test was carried out by double disc synergy and the combination-disc method on Mueller–Hinton agar using ceftazidime, ceftazidime-clavulanic acid, cefotaxime, and cefotaxime-clavulanic acid. The organisms were considered to be ESBL producing when a $\geq$5-mm increase in a zone diameter for either antimicrobial agent tested in combination with clavulanic acid compared with the zone diameter of the agent when tested alone [16]. Then molecular analysis was done on all positive isolates screened.

Antimicrobial susceptibility testing

The antimicrobial susceptibility testing of all ESBL-producers were examined by agar diffusion method according to the Clinical and Laboratory Standards Institute (CLSI) guidelines [16]. Antibiotic disc (Oxoid Ltd, Basingstone, UK): cefepime 30 µg, aztreonam 30 µg, imipenem 10 µg, meropenem 10 µg, gentamicin 10 µg, amikacin 30 µg, tetracycline 30 µg, ciprofloxacin 5 µg, levofloxacin 5 µg, norfloxacin 10 µg, nalidixic acid 30 µg, trimethoprim-sulfamethoxazole 12.5/23.75 µg, and ticarcillin 75 µg were used to determine resistance patterns of the collected isolates.

Characterization of genes encoding ESBLs

Two conventional multiplex PCR was performed, the first one for the detection of TEM, SHV, CTX-M genes and the second for detection of CTX-M-2, CTX-M-9, CTX-M-15 encoding genes. Crude genomic DNA was extracted from the isolates by heat lysis. Briefly, one pure colony was suspended in 40 µl of sterile distilled water, and the cells were lysed by heating up at 95 °C for 5 min.

For the first PCR multiplex, suitable primers (Sigma-Aldrich) [17] each targeting selected region the bla_{TEM}, bla_{SHV}, and bla_{CTX-M} were used (Table 1).

Amplification reactions were performed in a 25 µl volume in which 12.5 µl of PCR master mix 2× (Thermo scientific) reaction buffer containing 0.05 *Taq* DNA polymerase, 4 mM µ/µl MgCl2, 0.4 mM of each deoxynucleoside triphosphates mix dNTP (dATP, dCTP, dGTP, and dTTP), were mixed with 12.5 µl of DNA, primers, and H_2O in the following manner; 0.5 µl TEM F, 0.5 µl TEM R, 1 µl of each remaining primers, (*SHV, CTX-M*) (10 µM/µl), 2.5 µl H_2O, and 5 µl of the template DNA. Reactions were performed in a DNA thermal cycler (BIOER) under the following conditions: denaturation at 94 °C for 5 min followed by 30 cycles at 94 °C for 20 s, 61 °C for 30 s and 72 °C for 1 min with a final extension of 72 °C for 5 min [18].

For the second multiplex PCR, suitable primers each targeting selected region the $bla_{CTX-M-2}$, $bla_{CTX-M-9}$, and $bla_{CTX-M-15}$ were used [17] (Table 2). Reactions were performed in a DNA thermal cycler under the following conditions: denaturation at 94 °C for 5 min followed by 30 cycles at 94 °C for 15 s, 56 °C for 15 s and 72 °C for 45 s with a final extension of 72 °C for 5 min.

Table 1 Primers for the bla_{TEM}, bla_{SHV}, and bla_{CTX-M} genes used in this study

Primers	Primer sequence 5′ to 3′	Size (bp)
TEM F	AGT GCT GCC ATA ACC ATG AGT G	431
TEM R	CTG ACT CCC CGT CGT GTA GAT A	
SHV F	GAT GAA CGC TTT CCC ATG ATG	214
SHV R	CGC TGT TAT CGC TCA TGG TAA	
CTX F	ATG TGC AGY ACC AGT AAR GT	593
CTX R	TGG GTR AAR TAR GTS ACC AGA	

Table 2 Primers for the $bla_{CTX-M-2}$, $bla_{CTX-M-9}$, and $bla_{CTX-M-15}$ genes used in this study

Primers	Primer sequence 5′ to 3′	Size (bp)
CTX-M-2 F	AAA CAG AGC GAG AGC GAT AAG	720
CTX-M-2 R	GGG TAA AGT AGG TCA CCA GAA C	
CTX-M-9 F	GGA TTA ACC GTA TTG GGA GTT T	164
CTX-M-9 R	GAT ACC GCA GAT AAT ACG CAG G	
CTX-M-15 F	CAC GTC AAT GGG ACG ATG T	410
CTX-M-15 R	GAA AGG CAA TAC CAC CGG T	

After PCR amplification, 2.5 µl of each reaction was separated by electrophoresis in 1.5 % agarose gel for 30 min at 100 V in 0.5× TBE buffer. DNA was stained with ethidium bromide (1 µg/ml) and the bands were detected using UV transilluminator (Cleaver Scientific Ltd).

Statistical analysis

The data were analyzed using Yates corrected χ^2 test. Chi square test was done to establish statistically difference in proportions for categorical data. Statistical significance was set as P values of <0.05 with confidence interval of 95 %. For multivariate logistic regression analysis, the two independent variables were dairy products and meat. For dairy products data were counted for consumer of any of the dairy products (milk, yogurt, or cheese). For meat variable data were counted for consumer for either animal meat or chicken collectively as meat. ESBL-PE carriage was the dependent variable. Statistical analysis was performed using Minitab program (Minitab 14 statistical software, PA, USA) and The Statistical Package for Social Sciences (SPSS, Version 20) program (IBM, Armonk, NY).

Results

Prevalence of ESBL-PE

One hundred twenty-five subjects participated in this study, 63 (50.4 %) were females and 62 (49.6 %) were males ranging in age from 1 to 5 years old. Of these participants, 31 (24.8 %) as shown in Table 3 were ESBL-PE carrier. Males had a higher colonization frequency (33.9 %) than did females (15.9 %) (P = 0.09).

Factors associated with ESBL-PE carriage

Subjects who used antibiotics or antacid in the last 8 weeks, had higher rate of ESBL-PE carriage than their counterparts (Table 3), though no significant differences between these variables, while subjects admitted to the

Table 3 Factors associated with ESBL-PE fecal carriage in healthy children in Lebanese community

Characteristic	Total N (%) 125 (100 %)	ESBL+ N (%) 31 (24.8 %)	ESBL− N (%) 94 (75.2 %)	P value
Sex				0.009
Male	62 (49.6 %)	21 (67.7 %)	41 (43.6 %)	
Female	63 (50.4 %)	10 (32.3 %)	53 (56.4 %)	
Taking antibiotic during last 8 weeks				0.072
Yes	56 (44.8 %)	18 (58.1 %)	38 (40.41 %)	
No	69 (55.2 %)	13 (41.9 %)	56 (59.6 %)	
Hospital admission in past 12 months				0.019
Yes	23 (18.4 %)	10 (32.3 %)	13 (13.8 %)	
No	102 (81.6 %)	21(67.7 %)	81 (86.2 %)	
Taking antacid drug during last 8 weeks				0.072
Yes	11 (8.8 %)	5 (16.1 %)	6 (6.4 %)	
No	114 (91.2 %)	26 (83.9 %)	88 (93.6 %)	
Drinking milk				0.011
Regularly*	75 (60 %)	25 (80.6 %)	50 (53.2 %)	
Rare^ or never	50 (40 %)	6 (19.4 %)	44 (46.8 %)	
Drinking or eating yogurt				0.039
Regularly	77 (61.6 %)	23 (74.2 %)	54 (57.4 %)	
Rare or never	48 (38.4 %)	8 (25.8 %)	40 (42.6 %)	
Eating cheese				0.019
Regularly	74 (59.2 %)	23 (74.2 %)	51 (54.3 %)	
Rare or never	51 (40.8 %)	8 (25.8 %)	43 (45.7 %)	
Eating meat				0.02
Regularly	56 (44.8 %)	19 (61.3 %)	37 (39.4 %)	
Rare or never	69 (55.2 %)	12 (38.7 %)	57 (60.6 %)	
Eating chicken				0.03
Regularly	58 (46.6 %)	19 (61.3 %)	39 (41.5 %)	
Rare or never	67 (53.6 %)	12 (38.7 %)	55 (58.5 %)	
Intimate hygiene habit				0.07
Dry tissue or wipes	51 (40.8 %)	16 (51.6 %)	35 (37.2 %)	
Water + soap or water + tissue	74 (59.2 %)	15 (48.4 %)	59 (62.8 %)	
Sharing toilet				0.12
No	87 (69.6 %)	24 (77.4 %)	63(67 %)	
Yes	38 (30.4 %)	7 (22.6 %)	31(33 %)	

P value was calculated using Chi square test

* Regularly: was considered as 3 times or more per week

^ Rare: was considered as 2 times or less per week

hospital in the last 12 months, were significantly associated with high carriage rate 43.5 % (10/23) than their counterparts 20.6 % (21/102) with P = 0.019 (Table 3).

A univariate and multivariate logistic regression analysis were performed to test for regular consumption (3 times per week or more) of milk, yogurt, cheese, chicken, or meat and ESBL-PE carriage. As seen in Table 3 the univariate analysis for each predictor revealed significant impact ($P < 0.05$) for regular consumption of milk, yogurt, cheese, meat, or chicken. However the multivariate logistic regression analysis (Table 4) failed to reveal any of these dietary products consumed as a predictor of ESBL-PE carriage. To delineate the food type as dairy products or meat (meat or chicken) as a predictor, the analysis revealed the meat and chicken as significant ($P < 0.02$) predictor for ESBL-PE carriage while dairy products impact was non-significant ($P > 0.2$) (Table 5).

For intimate hygiene habits, participant who wash with water or with soap and water then dry with tissue have lower ESBL-PE carriage rate 20.3 % (15/74) compared

Table 4 Parameter estimates for multivariate logistic regression of different types of food as predictors for ESBL-PE carriage

Food type	P value	OR	95 % confidence interval for OR	
			Lower bound	Upper bound
Milk	0.130	3.276	0.705	15.215
Yogurt	0.994	0.995	0.243	4.078
Cheese	0.884	0.893	0.197	4.062
Meat	0.402	1.700	0.492	5.877
Chicken	0.905	1.080	0.307	3.792

OR, odds ratio of regular consumer of food versus rare or non-consumer for ESBL-PE positive compared to negative

Table 5 Parameter estimates for multivariate logistic regression of dairy products or meat and chicken as predictors for ESBL-PE carriage

	P value	OR	95 % CI for OR	
			Lower	Upper
Dairy	0.217	2.006	0.664	6.063
Meat/chicken	0.019	3.077	1.200	7.889

OR, odds ratio of regular consumer of food versus rare or non-consumer for ESBL-PE positive compared to negative

to 31.4 % (16/51) for those using only dry tissue or wipes with P = 0.07, OR 1.8, 95 % CI for OR 0.94–3.42 (Table 3). Participant who used to share toilets (used public toilet) were found to have 18.4 % (7/38) carriage rate compared to 27.6 % (24/87) for those don't share toilets and this was statistically insignificant.

Antibiotic susceptibility data

All isolates were resistant to azetreonam, cefepime, cefpodoxime, and ticarcillin. One hundred percent were susceptible to imipenem and meropenem, whereas 93.5 and 54.8 % were susceptible to amikacin and gentamicin respectively. Susceptibility to the quinolones tested (levofloxacin, ciprofloxacin) were 61.3 %. Furthermore, 41.9, 32.3, and 35.5 % of the isolates were susceptible to tetracycline, trimethoprim-sulfamethoxazole and nalidixic acid, respectively (Fig. 1).

bla gene composition of ESBL-PE

Molecular characterization of 31 ESBL-PE among the pediatric isolates revealed that multiple gene producers were the most predominant 71 % (22/31), where CTX-M-type was produced by all isolates (31/31). Of the 31 CTX-M-producers isolates, 48.4 % (15/31) co-produced TEM, 22.6 % (7/31) co-produced SHV and TEM, and 29 % (9/31) produced CTX-M genes only (Fig. 2).

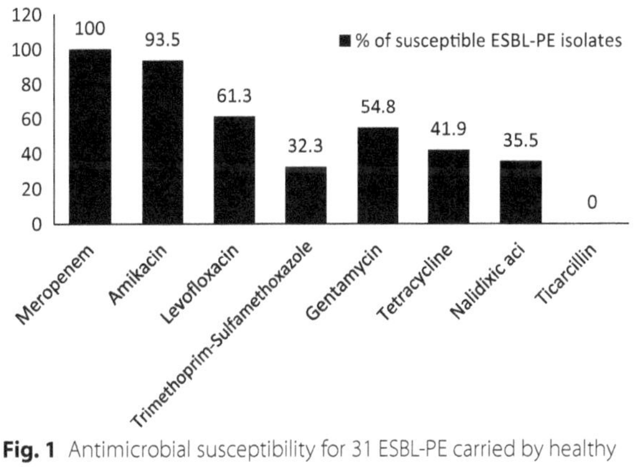

Fig. 1 Antimicrobial susceptibility for 31 ESBL-PE carried by healthy Lebanese children

The majority of ESBL-PE isolates recovered during the study were *E. coli* (n = 25), *K. pneumoniae* (n = 3), *Klebsiella* oxytoca (n = 1), and *Enterobacter cloacae* (n = 2) (Fig. 3). Fifty-six percent of isolated *E. coli* harbored $bla_{CTX\text{-}M}$ and bla_{TEM} genes, 28 % harbored $bla_{CTX\text{-}M}$ gene only, and 16 % harbored $bla_{CTX\text{-}M}$, bla_{TEM}, and bla_{SHV} genes. All *K. pneumonia* isolates harbored $bla_{CTX\text{-}M}$, bla_{TEM}, and bla_{SHV} *genes*, where one isolated *E. cloacae* harbored $bla_{CTX\text{-}M}$ gene and the other isolated one harbored $bla_{CTX\text{-}M}$ and bla_{TEM} genes.

Molecular characterization of the 31ESBL-PE isolates carrying $bla_{CTX\text{-}M}$ using specific primers for CTX-M-2, CTX-M-9, and CTX-M-15, revealed that CTX-M-9-type was the most common 77.4 % (24/31), and followed by CTX-M-15 [61.3 % (19/31)] and CTX-M-2 [29 % (9/31)] types (Fig. 4). Of these 24 CTX-M-9-producers, only 33.3 % (8/24) isolates produced CTX-M-9-type alone and the other isolates were co-producer of other types; 41.7 % (10/24) were CTX-M-15 co-producer, 25 % (6/24) were CTX-M-15 and CTX-M-2 co-producer. Two isolates produced CTX-M-15-type only, and one isolate produced both CTX-M-15-type and CTX-M-2-type (Table 6). The remaining four isolates (4/31) didn't show any of these three CTX-M-types.

Discussion

ESBL-producing organisms are increasingly common worldwide, they are recognized as important nosocomial pathogens in children, and are often associated with outbreaks [19]. Screening for intestinal carriage is crucial to predict the risk of ESBL infection, as the colon serves as a reservoir for extra-intestinal pathogenic *E. coli* [20].

This study was the first survey conducted in Lebanon on the intestinal carriage of ESBL-PE in the children community, and very rare studies were reported from

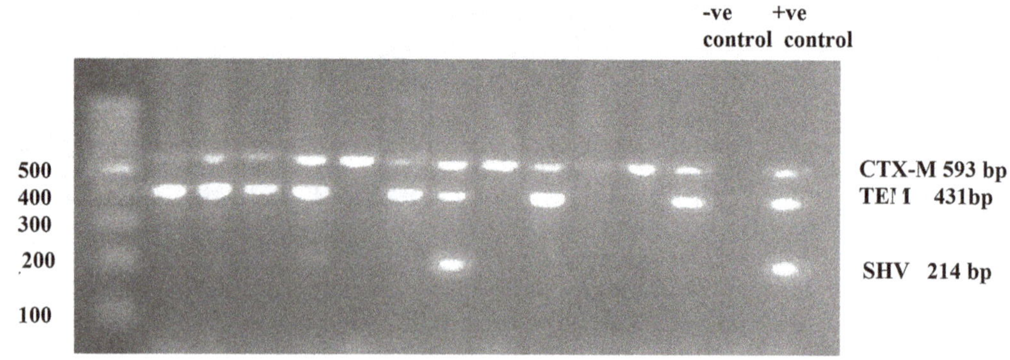

Fig. 2 Agarose gel electrophoresis for PCR products obtained from ESBL-PE isolates with TEM, SHV, and CTX-M primers

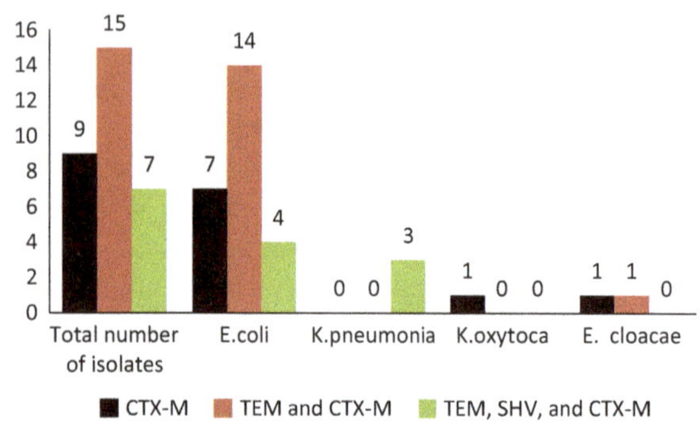

Fig. 3 *bla* gene composition of the 31 ESBL-PE isolated from 125 rectal swabs obtained from healthy Lebanese children

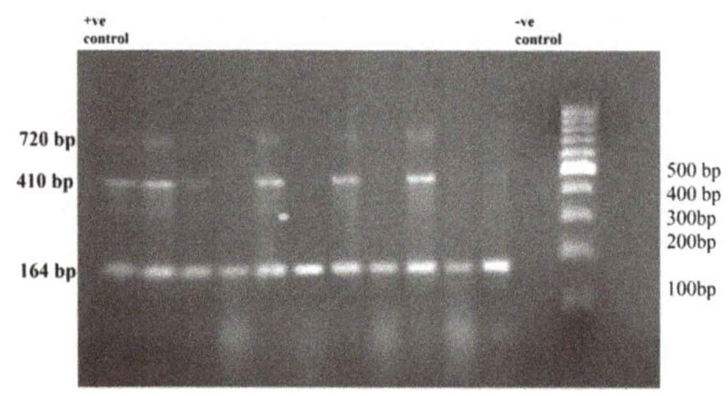

Fig. 4 Agarose gel electrophoresis for PCR products obtained from ESBL-PE isolates with CTX-M-2, CTX-M-9, and CTX-M-15 primers

Middle East. The prevalence was found to be 24.8 % which is high compared to 13.4, 2.7, and 2.9 % carriage rate in healthy pediatric in Libya, Portugal, and Sweden respectively [21–23]. Comparing this rate with fecal carriage in adult community in Saudi Arabia 12.7 % [24], in health care worker (HCW) in Egypt 21 % [25], and in adult community in 2005 in Lebanon 2.4 % [26], alarming high carriage rate was detected in this population that may serve as reservoir for dissemination of extra-intestinal ESBL-producing *E. coli* and *K. pneumoniae* and thus a source of infection in the community setting.

Males appear to have higher colonization rate than females. This observation is difficult to explain and needs to be further explored.

High carriage rate was in those individuals that used antibiotics or antacid in the last 8 weeks, or hospitalized in the last 12 months. Risk factors mentioned in the literature were prolonged hospital stays, living in nursing homes or long-term care facilities, underlying medical conditions, recent surgery, haemodialysis, and also prior use of antibiotics, particularly quinolones and third-generation cephalosporins, but also co-trimoxazole, aminoglycoside, and metronidazole [9].

Regarding antibiotic intake, although the selected children were healthy and not taking antibiotics (5 days before enrollment), it is noticed that 44.8 % of them have been taken antibiotics within last 8 weeks prior to being screened, this rate considered very high and reflects the high exposure of children to antibiotics and might explain the comparably high colonization rate. As known one of the main risk factors for the development of bacterial resistances is the increase of the consumption of several antibiotics [27]. In Lebanon there is no control measure and guidelines for antibiotic use in this age group. In addition, antibiotics are taken without medical prescription particularly in lower socioeconomic areas [28].

To the best of our knowledge, it is the first time to study regular consumption of dairy products (milk, yogurt, and cheese) and ESBL-PE carriage. In the present study, univariate analysis revealed significant association between regular consumption of dairy products, chicken, or meat with high ESBL-PE carriage rate. However analysis using multivariate logistic regression to test for the confounding factors, failed to show significant impact of any of these dietary products tested. This could be explained in part by the consumption of more than one type by most

Table 6 Molecular characterization of 31 ESBL-PE isolates producing CTX-M-type obtained from rectal swabs of 125 healthy children in Lebanese community

CTX-M type	Total number of isolates N = 31	*E. coli* N = 25 (80.6 %)	*K. pneumonia* N = 3 (9.7 %)	*K. oxytoca* N = 1 (3.2 %)	*E. cloacae* N = 2 (6.5 %)
CTX-M-9	8 (25.8 %)	7 (28 %)	1 (33.3 %)	0 (0 %)	0 (0 %)
CTX-M-9 and CTX-M-15	10 (32.3 %)	9 (36 %)	0 (0 %)	1 (100 %)	0 (0 %)
CTX-M-9, CTX-M-15, and CTX-M-2	6 (19.3 %)	5 (20 %)	1 (33.3 %)	0 (0 %)	0 (0 %)
CTX-M-15	2 (6.5 %)	1 (4 %)	1 (33.3 %)	0 (0 %)	0 (0 %)
CTX-M-15 and CTX-M-2	1 (3.2 %)	1 (4 %)	0 (0 %)	0 (0 %)	0 (0 %)
CTX-M-2	0 (0 %)	0 (0 %)	0 (0 %)	0 (0 %)	0 (0 %)
CTX-M type other than 2, 9, 15	4 (12.9 %)	2 (8 %)	0 (0 %)	0 (0 %)	2 (100 %)

of the participants. Also the number of cases that consumed one type only is few to show the power of the test. This was obvious as gathering milk, yogurt and cheese as dairy products and meat and chicken together as meat showed significant association between meat and ESBL-PE colonization. A conclusion that meat is a predictor for ESBL-PE carriage compared to dairy products was also apparent by the insignificant impact of dairy products on ESBL-PE carriage, although both had higher incidence of ESBL positive isolates compared to control rare or never users. The odd ratio was 3 and 2 for meat and dairy products respectively. These dietary products are from animal source, and as known antibiotics are used for various purposes in agriculture and livestock production, for instance to boost growth or as therapeutic treatment and disease prophylaxis. *E. coli* and some other *Enterobacteriaceae* colonize the intestinal tract of both animals and humans, and recently the number of studies describing the prevalence of ESBL-PE in meat and raw milk has increased [29, 30]. Many studies had shown significant genetic similarities among ESBL-positive *E. coli* isolates from chicken meat and human according to mobile resistance elements, virulence genes and genomic back ground [31–33]. However other fewer contrasting observations showed that considerable differences in ESBL types between poultry and humans in Europe exist [34], and meat consumption is not related to ESBL transmission suggesting environmental sources such as water for drinking and food preparation [35]. There is no direct study between consuming dairy products and ESBL-PE carriage. A recent study in Tunisia isolated *E. coli* from cattle milk harbored the $bla_{CTX\text{-}M\text{-}15}$ gene on an F2: A-:B-plasmid, a combination frequently found in humans [36]. Although the dissemination of resistance genes in *E. coli* may occur through multiple routes, our study show a potential threat posed by animal food products as sources for human ESBL-positive isolates [33]. Studies concerning ESBL-PE in dairy products and meat in the Lebanese market should be assessed to determine the impact of food products as reservoirs and disseminators of such strains through the food production chain to human.

Washing with water, or soap and water, the intimate area after urination, fecal evacuation, or diaper change might have tendency towards protective effect against ESBL-PE carriage compared to using only dry tissue or wipes, although $P = 0.07$, this might be further studied and explained.

Apart from a high rate of susceptibility to imipenem and amikacin, most isolates were resistant to other antimicrobials tested. ESBL-producing isolates were found highly resistant to nalidixic acid, tetracycline, gentamycin and to trimethoprim-sulfamethoxazole, and this result confirm carriage of multidrug-resistant ESBL-PE in this selected population of asymptomatic healthy children in Lebanon. This high carriage rate of ESBL-PE and associated resistance to aminoglycosides and trimethoprim-sulfamethoxazole, as well as high frequency of coexistance of fluoroquinolone resistance, increases the risk of infection with multi-resistant bacteria, and thus the need for usage of last resort antibiotics, such as carbapenems and colistin, in the treatment of common infections [6]. Majority of ESBL-PE carry multiple *bla* genes, where CTX-M-type was the most predominant. CTX-M ESBLs has been increased worldwide among *E. coli* and *Klebsiella spp.*, this is the first study in the Lebanon that specifically determined the high prevalence of CTX-M-type ESBLs isolated from a healthy asymptomatic children, where CTX-M type beta-lactamases enzyme were produced by all isolates, and the majority of the isolates were found to be co-producers of the TEM gene, hence, TEM type was considered also a frequent disseminated beta-lactamases type. This was in contrast to a study in Egypt HCW where SHV was the predominant [25].This massive dissemination of CTX-M-type ESBLs in our result and its rapid and global spread almost reported everywhere could be referred as 'CTX-M pandemic' [37, 38], as the CTX-M-encoding plasmids are often transmissible by conjugation in vitro; this property explains the easy dissemination of *bla* $_{CTX-M}$-harboring plasmids [39]. This dissemination of the CTX-M-type ESBLs is not restricted to the nosocomial setting but also involves the community. This phenomenon is acting to modify the epidemiology of ESBLs, whereas those enzymes were, previously, mostly restricted to the nosocomial setting [40], this may be correlated with food processing channel especially those from animal origin.

Molecular characterization of CTX-M-type ESBL revealed that the majority was CTX-M-9, followed by CTX-M-15 type. The greater number of isolates was co-producer of either 2 or 3 genes ($bla_{CTX-M-9}$, $bla_{CTX-M-15}$, $bla_{CTX-M-2}$) together. CTX-M-9 was first reported from *E. coli* obtained from urine specimen from Spain and Brazil in1996 [41, 42], and recently one report from India [43]. Where CTX-M-type was predominant in *E. coli* obtained from Libyan children with diverse groups of CTX-M-1, CTX-M-15, and CTX-M-3 [21], major type was CTX-M-15 and no CTX-M-2 and CTX-M-9-types in *E. coli* isolate obtained from stool of Tehran children suffering from diarrhea [44], and CTX-M-1, CTX-M-15, and CTX-M-14 were predominant types of ESBL-PE obtained from French children rectal swabs [45].

This is the first study from Lebanon that demonstrates such a high prevalence of CTX-M-9 enzymes among *Enterobacteriaceae* strains isolated from community children. The *bla* $_{CTX-M-9}$ was the predominant ESBL gene in this setting. Although CTX-M-15 are the most frequent CTX-M enzymes isolated in humans, animals, as well as in the environment, worldwide [46], and associated with the global CTX-M pandemic, but in our study CTX-M-9-type ESBL appears the most predominant. This is an indication that new mechanisms of resistance might be emerging in Lebanon.

Conclusion

The carriage of ESBL-PE in young children in the Lebanese community is very high compared to the other countries. A significant correlation was found between this colonization rate and regular consumption of meat or chicken. Alarming multidrug resistance ESBL-PE is of great concern especially in this age group. Furthermore ESBL-PE multiple gene carriage of TEM, SHV, and CTX-M was the predominant, where CTX-M-9 and CTX-M-15 were the mostly spreader ESBL type.

Author details

[1] Department of Pharmaceutical Sciences (Pharmaceutical Microbiology), Faculty of Pharmacy, Beirut Arab University, Beirut, Lebanon. [2] Department of Pharmaceutical Microbiology, Faculty of Pharmacy, Alexandria University, Alexandria, Egypt. [3] Department of Microbiology and Immunology, Infection Control, Faculty of Medicine, Ain Shams University, Cairo, Egypt. [4] Department of Pharmaceutical Microbiology, Faculty of Pharmacy, Mansoura University, Mansoura, Egypt.

Acknowledgements

We thank the pediatricians Maha Abou Alfa, Khalil Osta, and Nussaiba Sheik Ammar who agreed to participate in this study; Mr. Hassan Abou Zaid for his great cooperation; Nurse Ola Saad for her help in sample collection and questionnaire; Professor Ahmad EL Mallah for his help in the statistical part.

Competing interests

The authors declare that they have no competing interests.

Recommendation

Further investigation is needed to evaluate correlation between certain food consumption and ESBL-PE carriage. Dairy products and meat in the Lebanese market must be screened for ESBL-PE. Rational use of antibiotics especially in children is required. Unexpected relationship between intimate hygiene habits and ESBL-PE carriage rate warrants further investigation.

References

1. Bradford PA. Extended-spectrum beta-lactamases in the 21st century: characterization, epidemiology, and detection of this important resistance threat. Clin Microbiol Rev. 2001;14:933–51.
2. Bush K. Alarming beta-lactamase-mediated resistance in multidrug-resistant *Enterobacteriaceae*. Curr Opin Microbiol. 2010;13:558–64.
3. Livermore DM. Current epidemiology and growing resistance of Gram-negative pathogens. Korean J Intern Med. 2012;27:128–42.
4. Livermore DM, Canton R, Gniadkowski M, Nordman P, Rossolini GM, Arlet G, et al. CTX-M: changing the face of ESBLs in Europe. J Antimicrob Chemother. 2007;59:165–74.
5. Karisik E, Ellington MJ, Pike R, Warren RE, Livermore DM, Woodford N. Molecular characterization of plasmids encoding CTX-M-15 beta-lactamases from *Escherichia coli* strains in the United Kingdom. J Antimicrob Chemother. 2006;58:665–8.
6. Pitout JD. Infections with extended-spectrum beta-lactamase producing *Enterobacteriaceae*: changing epidemiology and drug treatment choices. Drugs. 2010;70:313–33.
7. Lewis JS, Herrera M, Wickes B, Patterson JE, Jorgensen JH. First report of the emergence of CTX-M-type extended-spectrum beta-lactamases (ESBLs) as the predominant ESBL isolated in a US health care system. Antimicrob Agents Chemother. 2007;51:4015–21.
8. Paterson DL, Bonomo RA. Extended-spectrum beta-lactamases: a clinical update. Clin Microbiol Rev. 2005;18:657–86.
9. Pitout JDD, Laupland KB. Extended-spectrum beta-lactamase-producing *Enterobacteriaceae*: an emerging public-health concern. Lancet Infect Dis. 2008;8:159–66.
10. Bauernfeind A, Casellas JM, Goldberg M, Holley M, Jungwirth R, Mangold P, et al. A new plasmidic cefotaximase from patients infected with *Salmonella typhimurium*. Infection. 1992;20:158–63.
11. Cantón R. Epidemiology and evolution of β-lactamases. In: Baquero F, Nombela C, Casslel GH, Gutierrez-Fuentes JA, editors. Evolutionary biology of bacterial and fungal pathogens. Washington: ASM Press; 2008. p. 249–70.
12. Cantón R, Coque TM. The CTX-M β-lactamase pandemic. Curr Opin Microbiol. 2006;9:466–75.
13. Coque TM, Novais A, Carattoli A, Poirel L, Pitout J, Peixe L, et al. Dissemination of clonally related *Escherichia coli* strains expressing extended-spectrum beta-lactamase CTX-M-15. Emerg Infect Dis. 2008;14:195–200.
14. Valverde A, Coque TM, Sánchez-Moreno MP, Rollán A, Baquero F, Cantón R. Dramatic increase in prevalence of fecal carriage of extended-spectrum beta-lactamase-producing *Enterobacteriaceae* during nonoutbreak situations in Spain. J Clin Microbiol. 2004;42:4769–75.
15. Chandramohan L, Revell PA. Prevalence and molecular characterization of extended-spectrum β-lactamase producing Enterobacteriaceae in a pediatric patient population. Antimicrob Agents Chemother. 2012;56:4765.
16. Clinical and Laboratory Standards Institute. Performance standard for antimicrobial disk susceptibility testing: approved standards. 23rd ed. Wayne, PA: CLSI; 2013 (**document M100-S20**).

17. Integrated DNA Technologies. http://eu.idtdna.com/site. Accessed 21 Sept 2013.
18. Kim J, Jeon S, Lee B, Park M, Lee H, Lee J, et al. Rapid detection of extended spectrum β-lactamase (ESBL) for *Enterobacteriaceae* by use of a multiplex PCR-based method. Infect Chemother. 2009;41:181–4.
19. Moissenet D, Salauze B, Clermont O, Bingen E, Arlet G, Denamur E, et al. Meningitis caused by *Escherichia coli* producing TEM-52 extended-spectrum beta-lactamase within an extensive outbreak in a neonatal ward: epidemiological investigation and characterization of the strain. J Clin Microbiol. 2010;48:2459–63.
20. Emori TG, Gaynes RP. An overview of nosocomial infections, including the role of the microbiology laboratory. Clin Microbiol Rev. 1993;6:428–42.
21. Ahmed SF, Ali MM, Mohamed ZK, Moussa TA, Klena JD. Fecal carriage of extended-spectrum β-lactamases and AmpC-producing *Escherichia coli* in a Libyan community. Ann Clin Microbiol Antimicrob. 2014;13:22.
22. Guimarães B, Barreto A, Radhouani H, Figueiredo N, Gaspar E, Rodrigues J, et al. Genetic detection of extended-spectrum beta-lactamasecontaining *Escherichia coli* isolates and vancomycin-resistant enterococci in fecal samples of healthy children. Microb Drug Resist. 2009;15:211–6.
23. Kaarme J, Molin Y, Olsen B, Melhus A. Prevalence of extended-spectrum beta-lactamase-producing *Enterobacteriaceae* in healthy Swedish preschool children. Acta Paediatr. 2013;102:655–60.
24. Kader AA, Kamath KA. Faecal carriage of extended-spectrum beta-lactamase-producing bacteria in the community. East Mediterr Health J. 2009;15:1365–70.
25. Bassyouni RH, Gaber SN, Wegdan AA. Fecal carriage of extended-spectrum β-lactamase- and AmpC-producing *Escherichia coli* among healthcare workers. J Infect Dev Ctries. 2015;9:304–8.
26. Moubareck C, Daoud Z, Hakime NI, Hamze M, Mangeney N, Matta H, et al. Countrywide spread of community- and hospital-acquired extended-spectrum betalactamase (CTX-M-15)-producing *Enterobacteriaceae* in Lebanon. J Clin Microbiol. 2005;43:3309–13.
27. Gómez J, García Vázquez E, Ruiz Gómez J. Clinical relevance of bacterial resistance: a historical approach (1982–2007). Rev Esp Quimioter. 2008;21:115–22.
28. Farah R, Lahoud N, Salameh P, Saleh N. Antibiotic dispensation by Lebanese pharmacists: a comparison of higher and lower socio-economic levels. J Infect Public Health. 2015;8:37–46.
29. Geser Nadine, Stephan Roger, Hächler Herbert. Occurrence and characteristics of extended-spectrum β-lactamase (ESBL) producing *Enterobacteriaceae* in food producing animals, minced meat and raw milk. BMC Vet Res. 2012;8:21–30.
30. Casella T, Rodríguez MM, Takahashi JT, Ghiglione B, Dropa M, Assunção E, et al. Detection of blaCTX-M-type genes in complex class 1 integrons carried by *Enterobacteriaceae* isolated from retail chicken meat in Brazil. Int J Food Microbiol. 2015;16:88–91.
31. Overdevest I, Willemsen I, Rijnsburger M, Eustace A, Xu L, Hawkey P, et al. Extended-spectrum β-lactamase genes of *Escherichia coli* in chicken meat and humans, The Netherlands. Emerg Infect Dis. 2011;17:1216–22.
32. Kluytmans JA, Overdevest IT, Willemsen I, Kluytmans-van den Bergh MF, van der Zwaluw K, Heck M, et al. Extended-spectrum β-lactamase producing *Escherichia coli* from retail chicken meat and humans: comparison of strains, plasmids, resistance genes, and virulence factors. Clin Infect Dis. 2013;56:478–87.
33. Leverstein-van Hall MA, Dierikx CM, Cohen Stuart J, Voets GM, van den Munckhof MP, van Essen-Zandbergen A, et al. Dutch patients, retail chicken meat and poultry share the same ESBL genes, plasmids and strains. Clin Microbiol Infect. 2011;17:873–80.
34. Wu G, Day MJ, Mafura MT, Nunez-Garcia J, Fenner JJ, Sharma M, et al. Comparative analysis of ESBL-positive *Escherichia coli* isolates from animals and humans from the UK, The Netherlands and Germany. PLoS One. 2013;8:e75392.
35. Königer D, Gastmeier P, Kola A, Schwab F, Meyer E. Vegetarians are not less colonized with extended-spectrum-b-lactamase producing bacteria than meat eaters. J Antimicrob Chemother. 2014. doi:10.1093/jac/dkt335.
36. Grami R, Dahmen S, Mansour W, Mehri W, Haenni M, Aouni M, Madec JY. BlaCTX-M-15-carrying F2: A-: B-plasmid in *Escherichia coli* from cattle milk in Tunisia. Microb Drug Resist. 2014;20:344–9.
37. Pournaras S, Ikonomidis A, Kristo I, Tsakris A, Maniatis AN. CTX-M enzymes are the most common extended-spectrum β-lactamases among *Escherichia coli* in a tertiary Greek hospital. J Antimicrob Chemother. 2004;54:574–5.
38. Yan JJ, Hsueh PR, Lu JJ, Chang FY, Shyr JM, Wan JH, et al. Extended-spectrum beta-lactamases and plasmid-mediated AmpC enzymes among clinical isolates of *Escherichia coli* and *Klebsiella pneumoniae* from seven medical centers in Taiwan. Antimicrob Agents Chemother. 2006;50:1861–4.
39. Baraniak A, Fiett J, Sulikowska A, Hryniewicz W, Gniadkowski M. Countrywide spread of CTX-M-3 extended-spectrum beta-lactamase-producing microorganisms of the family *Enterobacteriaceae* in Poland. Antimicrob Agents Chemother. 2002;46:151–9.
40. Rossolini GM, D'Andrea MM, Mugnaioli C. The spread of CTX-M-type extended-spectrum β-lactamases. Clin Microbiol Infect Rev. 2008;14(Suppl. 1):33–41.
41. Cantón R, Novais A, Valverde A, Machado E, Peixe L, Baquero F, et al. Prevalence and spread of extended-spectrum beta-lactamase-producing *Enterobacteriaceae* in Europe. Clin Microbiol Infect. 2008;14(Suppl. 1):144–53.
42. Bonnet R. Growing group of extended-spectrum beta-lactamases: the CTX-M enzymes. Antimicrob Agents Chemother. 2004;48:1–14.
43. Roy S, Krishnan R, Mukherjee S, Schneiders T, Niyogi SK, Basu S. Prevalence of ST131 virulence-associated strains among CTX-M-producing *Escherichia coli* in the gut of hospitalized neonates in India. Diagn Microbiol Infect Dis. 2013;77:158.
44. Memariani M, Najar Peerayeh S, Zahraei Salehi T, Shokouhi Mostafavi SK. Occurrence of SHV, TEM and CTX-M β-lactamase genes among enteropathogenic *Escherichia coli* strains isolated from children with diarrhea. Jundishapur J Microbiol. 2015;8(4):e15620.
45. Birgy André, Cohen Robert, Levy Corinne, Bidet Philippe, Courroux Céline, Benani Mohamed, et al. Community faecal carriage of extended-spectrum beta-lactamase-producing *Enterobacteriaceae* in French children. BMC Infect Dis. 2012;12:315.
46. Lahlaoui H, Ben Haj Khalifa A, Ben Moussa M. Epidemiology of *Enterobacteriaceae* producing CTX-M type extended spectrum β-lactamase (ESBL). Méd Mal Infect Rev. 2014;44:400–4.

11

Clinical characteristics and antimicrobial susceptibility of *Bacillus cereus* blood stream infections

Mahoko Ikeda[1], Yuka Yagihara[1], Keita Tatsuno[1], Mitsuhiro Okazaki[2], Shu Okugawa[1*] and Kyoji Moriya[1]

Abstract

Background: *Bacillus cereus* is one of the pathogens causing nosocomial bloodstream infections (BSIs). However, few reports have documented the antimicrobial susceptibility and clinical characteristics of *Bacillus cereus* BSI and the importance of empirical therapy. The aim of this study was to investigate the clinical characteristics and antimicrobial susceptibility of *B. cereus* isolates from patients with BSI and to analyze the impact of appropriate empirical therapy on the outcome of patients with *B. cereus* BSI.

Methods: All adult cases of bacteremia between April 2003 and March 2012 in a teaching hospital in Tokyo, Japan were reviewed retrospectively. Clinical data were collected from the patients' medical records and charts. Antimicrobial susceptibility testing was performed by broth microdilution method. The patients with *B. cereus* BSI were divided into an appropriate empirical therapy group and an inappropriate empirical therapy group. The primary outcome was all-cause mortality at 4 weeks after the start of BSI. The secondary outcome was early defervescence within 2 days after starting empirical therapy.

Results: There were 29 *B. cereus* bloodstream infection cases. No vancomycin, gentamicin, and imipenem-resistant isolates were found. However, 65.5 % were resistant to clindamycin and 10.3 % were resistant to levofloxacin. The main etiology was venous catheter-related (69 %). All-cause mortality at 4 weeks was not significantly different between the appropriate empirical therapy group (9 cases) and the inappropriate group (20 cases) in this study. However, early defervescence within 2 days after starting empirical therapy was significantly different ($p = 0.032$).

Conclusions: The BSI of *B. cereus* is mostly caused by venous catheter-related infections. Appropriate empirical therapy is important to achieve early clinical resolution in *B. cereus* BSI. Vancomycin is one of the appropriate selections of empirical therapy for *B. cereus* BSI.

Keywords: *Bacillus cereus*, Blood stream infection, Empirical therapy, Susceptibility

Background

The *Bacillus cereus* group contains six species, *B. cereus*, *B. thuringiensis*, *B. weihenstephanensis*, *B. mycoides*, *B. pseudomycoides*, and *B. anthracis* [1]. The most prevalent human pathogen in the *B. cereus* group is *B. cereus* [1]. The automated identification system in diagnostic laboratories cannot distinguish between *B. cereus* and *B. thuringiensis*, because they are genetically similar species. However, *B. thuringiensis* is an extremely rare human pathogen and is basically an insect pathogen [2].

B. cereus is a spore-forming Gram-positive bacillus that exists ubiquitously in soil, marine environments, vegetables, the intestinal tracts of invertebrates, and human skin [3]. The organism is a common pathogen in food poisoning [3]. Invasive *B. cereus* infections such as bacteremia, pneumonia [4], eye infection [5], central nervous system (CNS) infections [6, 7], and soft tissue infections [8, 9] have been reported in hospital settings. More information about the clinical characteristics of

*Correspondence: okugawa-tky@umin.ac.jp
[1] Department of Infection Control and Prevention, Faculty of Medicine, The University of Tokyo, 7-3-1 Hongo, Bunkyo, Tokyo 113-8655, Japan

B. cereus bloodstream infection (BSI) is urgently needed to improve the treatment of patients with *B. cereus* infection.

BSIs are important causes of morbidity and mortality. Appropriate empirical therapy should be started immediately after BSI is identified [10]. Recent reports have analyzed risk factors for *B. cereus* BSI, such as prior antimicrobial treatment [11, 12], reuse of contaminated towels [13, 14], central venous catheter insertions [12, 15], and hematological malignancy [16]. Fatal outcomes have been related to neutropenia [6], delays in treatment [17], and CNS symptoms [15, 17].

Inappropriate antibiotic therapy has been shown to be predictive of higher mortality rates in patients with bacteremia compared to appropriate therapy [10]. The antimicrobial agents for the empirical therapy should be selected according to the antimicrobial susceptibility of the pathogen. However, few studies have reported on the clinical characteristics of *B. cereus* BSI and the importance of empirical therapy [17, 18]. The aim of this study was therefore to investigate the antimicrobial susceptibility of clinical *B. cereus* isolates from patients with BSI and to analyze the impact of appropriate empirical therapy on clinical outcomes in patients with *B. cereus* BSI.

Methods

Study setting and patients

All cases of bacteremia that occurred between April 2003 and March 2012 in the microbial blood culture database of the University of Tokyo Hospital, a 1217-bed tertiary-care teaching hospital in Tokyo, Japan, were retrospectively reviewed. Patients with *B. cereus* bacteremia were divided into appropriate empirical therapy and inappropriate empirical therapy groups.

Data collection and definitions

All adult (age $\geq$18 years) patients from whose blood cultures *B. cereus* was isolated were enrolled. Bacteremia caused by *B. cereus* was defined as: (1) two or more positive blood cultures collected in one day; or (2) positive blood cultures collected on more than two consecutive days. Untreated cases and cases that received oral antimicrobial therapy were excluded, as were patients who were afebrile despite positive blood cultures for *B. cereus*.

Patients' data, clinical symptoms, laboratory results, antibiotics used, in-hospital mortality due to any cause, presence of blood cultures that became negative, and microbiological data were collected from the clinical charts and the laboratory database. Patients' data included age, sex, underlying disease (diabetes mellitus, cirrhosis, malignancy, immunosuppressants, and neutropenia), and implanted medical devices such as central venous catheters, biliary stents, and artificial joints. Clinical symptoms included fever, suspected focus of infection, and complications with BSI. Laboratory data were white blood cell counts, neutrophil counts, C-reactive protein and albumin levels. Data of antibiotics used before and after blood culture samples were obtained were also reviewed.

Fever was defined as a body temperature $\geq$37.5 °C. When a body temperature of <37.5 °C was maintained for >24 h, the patient was defined as afebrile. Body temperature was measured at least 3 times a day (at 08:00, 14:00, and 20:00). A complication was considered a focus of infection accompanied by *B. cereus* BSI.

Empirical therapy was defined as the antibiotics received on the first day of therapy for the BSI. Appropriate antimicrobial therapy was defined as systemic administration of at least one antimicrobial agent to which the *B. cereus* isolate proved susceptible in vitro.

Microbiological methods

Blood culture specimens were inoculated into BACTEC standard culture bottles in a BACTEC 9000 system (Becton, Dickinson and Company, Franklin Lakes, NJ, USA). All isolates were identified as *B. cereus*/*B. thuringiensis* using a VITEK2 system with the BCL card (SYSMEX bioMerieux, Tokyo, Japan). Antimicrobial susceptibility was determined with the Walkaway system and the standard criteria of the Clinical and Laboratory Standards Institute (CLSI) guide. The breakpoints against *B. cereus* in the CLSI guideline M45A2E [19] were used for the following agents: ampicillin, cefazolin, cefotaxime, caftazidime, imipenem, vancomycin, amikacin, gentamicin, erythromycin, levofloxacin, clindamycin, chloramphenicol and rifampin. For other antimicrobials, the breakpoints for *Staphylococcus* spp. in the CLSI guideline M 100-S22 [20] and S24 [21] were used [22].

Clinical outcomes

The primary outcome was all-cause mortality at 4 weeks after onset of bacteremia. The secondary outcome was early defervescence within 2 days after starting empirical therapy.

Statistical analysis

Fisher's exact test was used for analysis of categorical data. Non-parametric data were analyzed using the Mann–Whitney U test. Values of $P < 0.05$ were considered significant. All statistical analyses were performed using JMP Pro version 10 software (SAS Institute, Cary, NC, USA).

Results

Patients' characteristics

A total of 5894 cases with positive blood cultures was identified over the 9-year study period. Of these, *B.*

cereus was isolated in 203 cases. One hundred seventy one cases were excluded, because they had one *B. cereus*-positive blood culture. Three cases with more than two *B. cereus*-positive blood cultures were also excluded, because one case was untreated, one case was treated with oral antibiotics, and one case was afebrile. After applying the exclusion criteria, 29 cases (14.3 % of cases in which *B. cereus* was detected, 0.49 % of all culture-positive cases) were included in this study. The patients' clinical characteristics are shown in Table 1. The mean age was 65.3 years (range 18–89 years), and 55.2 % were male. The main etiology was venous catheter-related (69 %). The appropriate and inappropriate empirical therapy groups had similar baseline characteristics, sources of infection, and comorbidities that could significantly affect the clinical outcome. Complications except focuses of infection cited in Table 1 was endophthalmitis (1 case) occurred in the inappropriate empirical therapy group. In laboratory results, patients in the appropriate therapy group had a tendency to have higher white blood cell counts than patients in the inappropriate therapy group.

Antimicrobial susceptibility

All isolates showed sensitivity to vancomycin, gentamicin, and imipenem. However, 48.3–100 % of isolates were resistant to cephalosporins, 65.5 % were resistant to clindamycin, and 10.3 % were resistant to levofloxacin (Table 2).

Antibiotic treatment

In the appropriate empirical therapy group, piperacillin-tazobactam (3 cases), vancomycin (2 cases), or ampicillin–sulbactam, cefmetazole, clindamycin, amikacin, or cefoperazone–sulbactam (1 case each) was used. In the inappropriate empirical therapy group, cefepim (6 cases), ampicillin–sulbactam, cefazolin, ceftriaxone/cefotaxim (3 cases each), ceftazidime (2 cases), cefotiam, or clindamycin (1 case each) was used, and in vitro testing showed that the *B. cereus* isolated on blood culture was resistant. One patient was not treated empirically with antibiotics. The duration of antimicrobial therapy did not differ between the two groups (Table 3). All patients, but one, were changed to an appropriate antibiotic agent by 5 days.

Table 1 Characteristics of patients with *Bacillus cereus* bloodstream infection

Variable	All patients (n = 29)	Empirical therapy that was deemed		*P* value
		Appropriate (n = 9)	Inappropriate (n = 20)	
Age, years (median, range)	65.3 (18–89)	68 (18–89)	65 (47–83)	0.743
Sex (male/female)	16/13	4/5	12/8	0.688
No. of patients with comorbidity				
Diabetes mellitus	8	3	5	0.675
Malignancy	15	4	11	0.700
Liver cirrhosis	4	1	3	1.00
Immunosuppressant	5	2	3	0.633
Neutropenia	4	0	4	0.280
No. of patients with implanted device				
Central venous catheter	6	1	5	0.633
Peripheral venous catheter	22	8	14	0.382
Others	7	3	4	0.642
Source of BSI				
Total catheter-related infection	20	7	13	0.675
Peripheral blood catheter	15	6	9	0.427
Central venous catheter	5	1	4	1.00
Others[a]	5	0	5	0.153
Unknown	4	2	2	0.568
Laboratory data (average, range)				
White blood cell count (/μL)	7497 (100–22,200)	9630 (1800–22,200)	6537 (100–16,100)	0.052
C-reactive protein (g/dL)	4.19 (0.04–16.6)	3.79 (0.04–16.6)	3.34 (0.17–13.7)	0.514
Albumin (g/dL)	3.29 (2.10–4.20)	2.71 (2.10–3.90)	3.45 (2.40–4.20)	0.206

[a] Other sources of BSI in the inappropriate empirical therapy group include febrile neutropenia (2 cases), possible infective endocarditis according to modified Duke's criteria (2 cases), and peritonitis (1 case)

Table 2 Antimicrobial susceptibility of major antibiotics against *Bacillus cereus*

Antimicrobial agent	n	MIC[a] (mg/dL)			Interpretation n (%)		
		Range	50 %[b]	90 %[b]	Susceptible	Interpretive	Resistant
Vancomycin	29	≤2	≤2	≤2	29 (100)	0	0
Imipenem	29	≤0.5 to 4	≤0.5	≤0.5	29 (100)	0	0
Gentamicin	29	≤2 to 4	≤2	4	29 (100)	0	0
Amikacin	26	≤16	≤16	≤16	26 (100)	0	0
Linezolid	25	≤0.25 to 2	1	1	25 (100)		
Chloramphenicol	22	2 to 4	4	4	22 (100)	0	0
Rifampin	15	≤1	≤1	≤1	15 (100)	0	0
Levofloxacin	29	≤0.12 to >16	≤0.5	≤0.5	26 (89.7)	1 (3.4)	2 (6.9)
Clindamycin	29	<0.25 to ≥4	2	2	10 (34.5)	18 (62.1)	1 (3.4)
Erythromycin	29	≤0.25 to >16	0.5	1	18 (62.1)	6 (20.7)	2 (6.9)
Cefazolin	29	≤8 to ≥64	≤8		15 (51.7)	6 (20.7)	8 (27.6)
Daptomycin	22	≤0.12 to 4	2	4	8 (36.4)	12 (54.5)[c]	
Cefotaxime	22	4 to ≥64	16	32	2 (9.1)	18 (81.8)	2 (9.1)
Ampicillin/sulbactam	25	≤0.25 to >8	4	>8	1 (4)	–	24 (96)
Ampicillin	29	0.5 to >8	>4	>4	0	–	29 (100)
Ceftazidime	22	32 to >64	>64	>64	0	0	22 (100)

[a] Minimum inhibitory concentration

[b] MIC at which 50 or 90 % of tested isolates are inhibited

[c] This isolates were interpreted as "not susceptible" because the breakpoint was only set for susceptible

Table 3 Antibiotic empirical therapy and outcomes of *Bacillus cereus* bloodstream infection

Variable	All patients (n = 29)	Empirical therapy that was deemed		*P* value
		Appropriate (n = 9)	Inappropriate (n = 20)	
Duration of appropriate antibiotic treatment median (days, range)	15 (7–41)	13 (7–20)	16.5 (7–41)	0.050
Early defervescence (patients)	10	6	4	0.032*
Survival at 4 weeks (patients)	27[a]	8/9 (88.9 %)	19/19 (100 %)	0.321

* Statistically significant ($p < 0.05$)

[a] One patient was excluded in this analysis because of transfer to another hospital

Clinical outcome

In terms of the primary outcome, no significant difference in all-cause mortality at 4 weeks after onset of bacteremia was seen between the groups (Table 3). However, the secondary outcome of early defervescence was achieved significantly more often in the appropriate empirical therapy group. Central venous catheters were all removed in both groups. The presence of blood cultures that became negative was confirmed in 6 patients of the appropriate therapy group and 17 patients of the inappropriate therapy group. However, the intervals of taking blood cultures differed depending on the cases.

Discussion

The present data show that the BSI of *B. cereus* was mostly caused by venous catheter-related infections and that appropriate empirical therapy is important to achieve early clinical resolution in *B. cereus* bloodstream infection, although the appropriateness of therapy does not affect mortality.

In this study, cases detected *B. cereus* in more than two sets of blood cultures were enrolled as definite BSI and accounted for 14.3 % of *B. cereus*-detected cases. In our hospital, the rate of obtaining two sets of blood cultures was around 60 % at the beginning of the study period, and it increased to 75 % at the end. Although a further increase of the two-set rate may enable us to obtain more cases and uncover the detailed clinical picture of *B. cereus* BSI, the criterion used to select the definitive *B. cereus* BSI cases was more than two sets of positive blood cultures according to the BSI guideline [23]. *B. cereus* bacteremia was reported to be underestimated as contamination [24, 25], and it has recently been increasingly recognized that some cases of *B. cereus* bacteremia are definite BSIs [15, 17].

Bacteremia due to other bacteria, such as *Staphylococcus aureus* and extended-spectrum beta lactamase-producing Gram-negative bacteria, caused higher 30-day mortality in patients with various comorbidities than *B. cereus* bacteremia even when empirical therapy was inappropriate [26, 27]. In the present study, only one patient died in the appropriate therapy group, and no patient died in the inappropriate therapy group, indicating that *B. cereus* might be less virulent to humans. However, the appropriateness of therapy still has benefit for patients with *B. cereus* BSI, because early defervescence was significantly related to appropriate empirical antibiotic therapy.

Which antibiotic agents are appropriate for bacteremia due to *B. cereus*? In the present study, the *B. cereus* isolated was frequently not susceptible to empirical therapy, but an early treatment response was related to susceptible empirical therapy.

In this study, all isolates were resistant to ampicillin, and almost all were resistant to cephalosporins. All were sensitive to carbapenems. This could be explained by the fact that *B. cereus* is genetically resistant to all beta-lactams except carbapenems [3]. However, some reports showed carbapenem-resistant *B. cereus* bacteremia [28, 29], and some in vitro studies showed that *B. cereus* possesses metallo-beta lactamase genetically [30, 31]. Thus, further study is needed to determine whether carbapenems could be one of the choices for empirical treatment of *B. cereus* BSI.

Fluoroquinolones and clindamycin are also possible if a *B. cereus* isolate is susceptible. The present data showed a resistance rate of 65.5 % (19/29 cases) for clindamycin and 10.3 % (3/29) for levofloxacin. Horii et al. reported that 26 *B. cereus* isolates from blood cultures showed MIC90 of levofloxacin as 4 (CLSI's breakpoint of levofloxacin was ≤ 2 as sensitive) [11]. When empirical therapy is started with these agents, the susceptibility pattern should be considered.

All isolates showed good susceptibility to vancomycin according to CLSI's breakpoint (MIC ≤ 4 as sensitive). Other reports [11, 22] also showed no vancomycin-resistant *B. cereus* isolated from both clinical samples and environmental samples. Given that a main cause of *B. cereus* BSI is catheter-related infection, vancomycin is suitable for empirical treatment of *B. cereus* BSI, because the common causative pathogens of catheter-related infection are Gram-positive bacteria including *S. aureus* and coagulase-negative *Staphylococci*. However, BSI caused by *B. cereus* with vancomycin-reduced susceptibility (MIC 4 μg/mL) was reported in neonates [32]. We should pay attention to changes in susceptibility to vancomycin.

Other optimal choices for Gram-positive bacteria, daptomycin and linezolid, are options in *B. cereus* BSI. In the present study, the MIC90 of linezolid was 1, and all isolates were considered susceptible. In contrast, more than half of the *B. cereus* showed the MIC of daptomycin >1, although breakpoint of daptomycin was ≤ 1 as susceptible. The MIC of daptomycin was tested by microdilution assay. Luna et al. [22] reported that the MICs of daptomycin were 0.25–1 using the E test for 42 strains of *B. cereus* collected from the environment. The differences in the MICs might be due to differences in methodology or differences in whether they were clinical isolates or not. An in vitro study reported that a gene that gave daptomycin resistance was activated under swarming condition [33], and that spores were resistant to daptomycin until they germinated [34]. Thus, further study of the measurement of daptomycin MIC and the use of daptomycin for treatment is needed.

This study has some limitations. First, whether antimicrobials were susceptible was determined by antimicrobial breakpoints of *B. cereus* in CLSI's guideline M45A2E [19]. However, for some antimicrobials for which breakpoints have not been determined, breakpoints of *S. aureus* in M100 [21] were used with reference to a previous report [22]. Although breakpoints of these species were similar for various classes of antimicrobials such as cephalosporins, vancomycin was slightly different. This may be limitation of this study because undefined breakpoints of *B. cereus* may differ from those of *S. aureus* already defined in M100 [21]. We hope that various antimicrobial breakpoints of *B. cereus* would be set based on the abundant experience with the treatment of *B. cereus* infection. Second, *B. cereus and B. thuringiensis* were not distinguished in this study, because the automated identification system was used. Although *B. thuringiensis* is basically a harmless pathogen to humans, the extremely rare case with *B. thuringiensis* infection might have been missed. Third, the study was performed retrospectively based on clinical records, and the number of cases was small. To determine the most effective therapy for *B. cereus* BSI, more large-scale and prospective studies should be performed.

Conclusions

The definite BSI of *B. cereus* accounted for 14.3 % of *B. cereus*-detected cases, and they were mostly caused by venous catheter-related infections. Early clinical resolution was related to appropriate empirical antibiotic therapy. Vancomycin is optimal for empirical therapy of *B. cereus* BSI, but further clinical data are needed.

Authors' contributions

MI and SO conceived and designed the study, analysed the data, and drafted the manuscript. YY and MO performed microbiological works. MK and KT helped design the study and draft the manuscript. All authors read and approved the final manuscript.

Author details

[1] Department of Infection Control and Prevention, Faculty of Medicine, The University of Tokyo, 7-3-1 Hongo, Bunkyo, Tokyo 113-8655, Japan. [2] Department of Medical Technology, School of Health Sciences, Tokyo University of Technology, 5-23-22 Nishikamata, Ota, Tokyo 144-8535, Japan.

Acknowledgements

The authors wish to thank Dr. Takatoshi Kitazawa and Dr. Yasuo Ota for the discussion on study design.

Competing interests

The authors declare that they have no competing interests.

References

1. Kolstø AB, Tourasse NJ, Økstad OA. What sets Bacillus anthracis apart from other Bacillus species? Annu Rev Microbiol. 2009;63:451–76.
2. Ghelardi E, Celandroni F, Salvetti S, Fiscarelli E, Senesi S. Bacillus thuringiensis pulmonary infection: critical role for bacterial membrane-damaging toxins and host neutrophils. Microbes Infect. 2007;9(5):591–8.
3. Bottone EJ. *Bacillus cereus*, a volatile human pathogen. Clin Microbiol Rev. 2010;23(2):382–98.
4. Avashia SB, Riggins WS, Lindley C, Hoffmaster A, Drumgoole R, Nekomoto T, et al. Fatal pneumonia among metalworkers due to inhalation exposure to *Bacillus cereus* containing *Bacillus anthracis* toxin genes. Clin Infect Dis. 2007;44(3):414–6.
5. Rishi E, Rishi P, Sengupta S, Jambulingam M, Madhavan HN, Gopal L, et al. Acute postoperative *Bacillus cereus* endophthalmitis mimicking toxic anterior segment syndrome. Ophthalmology. 2013;120(1):181–5.
6. Gaur A, Patrick C, McCullers J, Flynn P, Pearson T, Razzouk B, et al. *Bacillus cereus* bacteremia and meningitis in immunocompromised children. Clin Infect Dis. 2001;32(10):1456–62.
7. Hansford JR, Phillips M, Cole C, Francis J, Blyth CC, Gottardo NG. *Bacillus cereus* bacteremia and multiple brain abscesses during acute lymphoblastic leukemia induction therapy. J Pediatr Hematol Oncol. 2014;36(3):e197–201.
8. Meredith FT, Fowler VG, Gautier M, Corey GR, Reller LB. *Bacillus cereus* necrotizing cellulitis mimicking clostridial myonecrosis: case report and review of the literature. Scand J Infect Dis. 1997;29(5):528–9.
9. Lee YL, Shih SD, Weng YJ, Chen C, Liu CE. Fatal spontaneous bacterial peritonitis and necrotizing fasciitis with bacteraemia caused by *Bacillus cereus* in a patient with cirrhosis. J Med Microbiol. 2010;59(Pt 2):242–4.
10. Dellinger RP, Levy MM, Rhodes A, Annane D, Gerlach H, Opal SM, et al. Surviving sepsis campaign: international guidelines for management of severe sepsis and septic shock: 2012. Crit Care Med. 2013;41(2):580–637.
11. Horii T, Notake S, Tamai K, Yanagisawa H. *Bacillus cereus* from blood cultures: virulence genes, antimicrobial susceptibility and risk factors for blood stream infection. FEMS Immunol Med Microbiol. 2011;63(2):202–9.
12. Ko JH, Kang CI, Lee WJ, Huh K, Yoo JR, Kim K, et al. Clinical features and risk factors for development of Bacillus bacteremia among adult patients with cancer: a case–control study. Support Care Cancer. 2015;23(2):377–84.
13. Dohmae S, Okubo T, Higuchi W, Takano T, Isobe H, Baranovich T, et al. *Bacillus cereus* nosocomial infection from reused towels in Japan. J Hosp Infect. 2008;69(4):361–7.
14. Sasahara T, Hayashi S, Morisawa Y, Sakihama T, Yoshimura A, Hirai Y. *Bacillus cereus* bacteremia outbreak due to contaminated hospital linens. Eur J Clin Microbiol Infect Dis. 2011;30(2):219–26.
15. Inoue D, Nagai Y, Mori M, Nagano S, Takiuchi Y, Arima H, et al. Fulminant sepsis caused by *Bacillus cereus* in patients with hematologic malignancies: analysis of its prognosis and risk factors. Leuk Lymphoma. 2010;51(5):860–9.
16. Kassar R, Hachem R, Jiang Y, Chaftari A, Raad I. Management of *Bacillus bacteremia*: the need for catheter removal. Medicine (Baltimore). 2009;88(5):279–83.
17. Uchino Y, Iriyama N, Matsumoto K, Hirabayashi Y, Miura K, Kurita D, et al. A case series of *Bacillus cereus* septicemia in patients with hematological disease. Intern Med. 2012;51(19):2733–8.
18. Kato K, Matsumura Y, Yamamoto M, Nagao M, Ito Y, Takakura S, et al. Seasonal trend and clinical presentation of *Bacillus cereus* bloodstream infection: association with summer and indwelling catheter. Eur J Clin Microbiol Infect Dis. 2014;33(8):1371–9.
19. Clinical and Laboratory Standards Institute (CLSI). Methods for antimicrobial dilution and disk susceptibility testing of infrequently isolated or fastidious bacteria; approved guideline, 2nd edn. M45A2E. Wayne: CLSI; 2010.
20. Clinical and Laboratory Standards Institute (CLSI). Performance standards for antimicrobial susceptibility testing; twenty-second informational supplement M100-S22. Wayne: CLSI; 2012.
21. Clinical and Laboratory Standards Institute (CLSI). Performance standards for antimicrobial susceptibility testing; twenty-fourth informational supplement M100-S24. Wayne: CLSI; 2014.
22. Luna VA, King DS, Gulledge J, Cannons AC, Amuso PT, Cattani J. Susceptibility of *Bacillus anthracis*, *Bacillus cereus*, *Bacillus mycoides*, *Bacillus pseudomycoides* and *Bacillus thuringiensis* to 24 antimicrobials using Sensititre automated microbroth dilution and Etest agar gradient diffusion methods. J Antimicrob Chemother. 2007;60(3):555–67.
23. Mermel LA, Allon M, Bouza E, Craven DE, Flynn P, O'Grady NP, et al. Clinical practice guidelines for the diagnosis and management of intravascular catheter-related infection: 2009 Update by the Infectious Diseases Society of America. Clin Infect Dis. 2009;49(1):1–45.
24. Hsueh PR, Teng LJ, Yang PC, Pan HL, Ho SW, Luh KT. Nosocomial pseudoepidemic caused by *Bacillus cereus* traced to contaminated ethyl alcohol from a liquor factory. J Clin Microbiol. 1999;37(7):2280–4.
25. Loeb M, Wilcox L, Thornley D, Gun-Munro J, Richardson H. Bacillus species pseudobacteremia following hospital construction. Can J Infect Control. 1995;10(2):37–40.
26. López-Cortés LE, Del Toro MD, Gálvez-Acebal J, Bereciartua-Bastarrica E, Fariñas MC, Sanz-Franco M, et al. Impact of an evidence-based bundle intervention in the quality-of-care management and outcome of *Staphylococcus aureus* bacteremia. Clin Infect Dis. 2013;57(9):1225–33.
27. Kang CI, Kim SH, Park WB, Lee KD, Kim HB, Kim EC, et al. Bloodstream infections due to extended-spectrum beta-lactamase-producing *Escherichia coli* and *Klebsiella pneumoniae*: risk factors for mortality and treatment outcome, with special emphasis on antimicrobial therapy. Antimicrob Agents Chemother. 2004;48(12):4574–81.
28. Kiyomizu K, Yagi T, Yoshida H, Minami R, Tanimura A, Karasuno T, et al. Fulminant septicemia of *Bacillus cereus* resistant to carbapenem in a patient with biphenotypic acute leukemia. J Infect Chemother. 2008;14(5):361–7.
29. Katsuya H, Takata T, Ishikawa T, Sasaki H, Ishitsuka K, Takamatsu Y, et al. A patient with acute myeloid leukemia who developed fatal pneumonia caused by carbapenem-resistant *Bacillus cereus*. J Infect Chemother. 2009;15(1):39–41.
30. Sabath LD, Abraham EP. Zinc as a cofactor for cephalosporinase from *Bacillus cereus* 569. Biochem J. 1966;98(1):11C–3C.

12

Antimicrobial resistance and virulence characterization of *Staphylococcus aureus* and coagulase-negative staphylococci from imported beef meat

Kamelia Osman[1], Avelino Alvarez-Ordóñez[2], Lorena Ruiz[3], Jihan Badr[4], Fatma ElHofy[5], Khalid S. Al-Maary[6], Ihab M. I. Moussa[6], Ashgan M. Hessain[7], Ahmed Orabi[1], Alaa Saad[4] and Mohamed Elhadidy[8,9]*

Abstract

Background: The objectives of this study were to characterize the diversity and magnitude of antimicrobial resistance among *Staphylococcus* species recovered from imported beef meat sold in the Egyptian market and the potential mechanisms underlying the antimicrobial resistance phenotypes including harboring of resistance genes (*mecA*, *cfr*, *gyrA*, *gyrB*, and *grlA*) and biofilm formation.

Results: The resistance gene *mecA* was detected in 50% of methicillin-resistant non-*Staphylococcus aureus* isolates (4/8). Interestingly, our results showed that: (i) resistance genes *mecA*, *gyrA*, *gyrB*, *grlA*, and *cfr* were absent in *Staphylococcus hominis* and *Staphylococcus hemolyticus* isolates, although *S. hominis* was phenotypically resistant to methicillin (MR-non-*S. aureus*) while *S. hemolyticus* was resistant to vancomycin only; (ii) *S. aureus* isolates did not carry the *mecA* gene (100%) and were phenotypically characterized as methicillin- susceptible *S. aureus* (MSS); and (iii) the resistance gene *mecA* was present in one isolate (1/3) of *Staphylococcus lugdunensis* that was phenotypically characterized as methicillin-susceptible non-*S. aureus* (MSNSA).

Conclusions: Our findings highlight the potential risk for consumers, in the absence of actionable risk management information systems, of imported foods and advice a strict implementation of international standards by different venues such as CODEX to avoid the increase in prevalence of coagulase positive and coagulase negative *Staphylococcus* isolates and their antibiotic resistance genes in imported beef meat at the Egyptian market.

Keywords: Coagulase-positive staphylococci, Coagulase-negative staphylococci, Antibiotic resistance genes, Imported beef meat

Background

Contamination of meat with foodborne pathogens represents a major public health threat. The increasing volume of trade and travel is considered as a potential risk factor facilitating the global transport and dissemination of pathogenic bacteria in food. Imported animal products are considered as a clear example, and risk analyses have been previously applied to characterize these products [1]. This risk analyses strategy have been implemented following the World Trade Organization (WTO) creation. The application of sanitary and phytosanitary measures in response to the sanitary and phytosanitary measures agreement (SPS Agreement) [2] requires the WTO members to remove barriers on the trade of agricultural products, except in situations where such trade can potentially create risk to the animal, human or plant health in the importing country.

Staphylococcus aureus is one of the most common foodborne pathogens causing food poisoning outbreaks worldwide [3]. Other than *S. aureus*, the clinical and

*Correspondence: mm_elhadidy@mans.edu.eg
[8] Department of Bacteriology, Mycology and Immunology, Faculty of Veterinary Medicine, Mansoura University, Mansoura 35516, Egypt
Full list of author information is available at the end of the article

veterinary importance of coagulase-positive staphylococci (CPS) and coagulase-negative staphylococci (CNS) have often been neglected. In recent years, the risk of CPS and CNS has been highlighted by recent reports [4–6] with special reference to the CNS that have been commonly found in food [7, 8]. CNS have been recorded as conveying vector for virulence genes and have been implicated in some cases of food poisoning [9]. Furthermore, food-related staphylococci could act as dissemination vectors for antibiotic resistance genes to other potentially pathogenic microorganisms causing immediate threat to the public health. The *mecA*-harboring CNS (MRCNS) have been reported to have a reservoir in animal farm facilities and in meat products, with the ability to be conveyed to *S. aureus* [10–12].

The remarkable global concern of antibiotic- resistant pathogens in the food chain and the potential for these resistant pathogens to spread through the food chain prompted the Codex Alimentarius Commission to establish an *ad hoc* Intergovernmental Task Force on antimicrobial resistance. The main task of this commission is to apply a complete risk assessment strategy on the use of antimicrobials belonging to both clinical and veterinary classes. While domestic control over antimicrobial usage policies and monitoring is achievable, negligible information is available for imported food [13], with special reference to beef meat that has been incriminated to contribute to the emergence of multidrug resistance among humans through the dispersion of resistance genes carried by resistant pathogens transmitted by contaminated meat [14, 15].

Livestock-associated methicillin-resistant *S. aureus* (LA-MRSA) have acquired a number of novel and unusual antimicrobial resistance genes including multiresistance genes such as the *cfr* gene, that confers resistance to phenicols, lincosamides, oxazolidinones, pleuromutilins, and streptogramin A [16]. Oxazolidinones are last resort antimicrobial agents for the control of serious infections caused by MRSA and vancomycin-resistant enterococci in humans. MRSA is also notoriously difficult to treat due to resistance to β-lactams (including penicillin, oxacillin, and methicillin) represent a class of antibiotics generally prescribed as the first line of defense against clinical infections caused by staphylococci, which include drugs like penicillin, oxacillin, and methicillin. This resistance was attributed to the carriage of *mecA*. The *mecA* gene encodes a different form of penicillin-binding protein, PBP2a, which β-lactam drugs cannot inactivate.

Therefore, the objectives of this study were to characterize the diversity of *Staphylococcus* strains recovered from imported meat sold in the Egyptian market and to assess recovered isolates as potential dispersion vectors for the spread of antimicrobial resistance. To achieve that aim, *Staphylococcus* isolates were tested for the presence of antimicrobial resistance phenotypes and genetic determinants (*mecA*, *cfr*, *gyrA*, *gyrB*, and *grlA*) and for their biofilm formation.

Methods

Imported beef meat samples

A total of 100 imported frozen meat samples were delivered to the Department of Poultry Diseases, Animal Health Research, Institute, Dokki, Egypt, as a routine microbiological analysis check for foodborne pathogens. Samples were collected by the food hygiene officials in ice-boxes from different supermarket chains as well as butcher shops located in the Great Cairo Zone. The meat samples (25 g) were suspended in 225 ml sterile phosphate buffered saline (PBS, pH 7.4) and homogenized in a stomacher (Lab-Blender 400, PBI, Milan, Italy) for 10 min. A total of 25 ml of the homogenate were added to 10 ml of Giolitti-Cantoni broth (BD Diagnostics, Franklin Lakes, NJ, USA). The tubes were incubated at 37 °C for 18–24 h with shaking at 200 rpm. Ten microliter aliquots of the enriched cultures were seeded on Baird Parker agar (BD Diagnostics, Franklin Lakes, NJ, USA), supplemented with egg yolk tellurite emulsion. The plates were incubated at 37 °C for 18–24 h and recovered single colonies were streaked onto blood agar plates (TSA with 5% sheep blood), and further incubated at 37 °C for 12–18 h. Characteristic staphylococci colonies (black, with or without a halo) were further identified based on Gram stain, catalase assay, tube coagulase test and further biochemical identification tests referred in standard diagnostic tables [17].

Determination of virulence factors

Production of hemolysins

Production of α-, β- and γ-hemolysins was detected by streaking each staphylococcal isolate on blood agar plates containing 5% sheep red blood cells following the protocol previously developed [18].

Vero cell cytotoxicity assay

The ability of the isolated staphylococci to initiate degeneration of Vero cells was microscopically evaluated following the validated methodology described elsewhere [19] with minor modifications. The cytotoxicity assay was carried out using Vero (African green monkey kidney) cells in 96-well microtiter trays. Suspensions of each tested strain in distilled water were adjusted to 0.5 McFarland standard. Then, 20 μl of bacterial suspensions were added to 3.5 ml of brain heart infusion broth (BBL, Becton–Dickinson Microbiology Systems). The tubes were incubated 2 days at 35 °C, and thereafter for

2 days at room temperature. After centrifugation of bacterial broth cultures, 20 µl of supernatants were added in triplicate to 180 µl of cell culture medium. After incubation at 37 °C, in a humid atmosphere and 5% CO_2, the cytotoxic effect of each staphylococcal strain on the Vero monolayer morphology was microscopically perceived up to 5 days.

Phenotypic determination of the antibiotic resistance profile

The disk diffusion method was used to investigate the antibiotic resistance phenotype of the 23 *Staphylococcus* spp. recovered from the imported beef meat on Mueller–Hinton agar plates as previously described [20]. *Escherichia coli* NCIMB 50034 and *S. aureus* ATCC 25923 were included as controls. The antibiotics tested were selected from two categories, as follows [21]: (i) Critically important antibiotics: ampicillin-sulbactam (20 µg), methicillin (5 µg), oxacillin (1 µg), penicillin (10 µg), ciprofloxacin (5 µg), erythromycin (15 µg), gentamicin (10 µg), vancomycin (30 µg) and (ii) Highly important antibiotics: chloramphenicol (30 µg), clindamycin (2 µg), tetracycline (30 µg), and sulfamethoxazole/trimethoprim (25 µg).

Molecular characterization

Overnight cultures of all *Staphylococcus* isolates were subjected to the boiling method for the preparation of cell lysates to be used for DNA templates. Genus-specific confirmation was carried out through PCR using the 16S rRNA gene *Staphylococcus*-genus-specific primers and cycling conditions previously described [22]. *S. aureus* ATCC 43300 and *E. coli* NCIMB 50034 were used as positive and negative controls, respectively. All confirmed staphylococci were submitted to further molecular analyses for the detection of the *mecA* gene, that is considered as the gold-standard for MRSA confirmation [23]. Four additional antimicrobial resistance markers frequently reported in *S. aureus* were screened by PCR, including the *gyrA*, *gyrB*, and *grlA* genes that are responsible for quinolone resistance and the *cfr* gene (chloramphenicol-florfenicol resistance gene), conferring resistance to several classes of antibiotics (phenicols, lincosamides, oxazolidinones, pleuromutilins, and streptogramin A; known as the PhLOPSA phenotype). PCR amplifications were carried out with a GeneAmp PCR System 2400 (Perkin-Elmer, Weiterstadt, Germany) using the primers and the cycling conditions previously described [8]. Two microliters of template DNA were added to 23 µl of master mix containing 1 µM of each primer and 3U of Taq polymerase. The amplicons were screened by gel-electrophoresis on 1.5% (w/v) agarose gels in TBE buffer and visualized following ethidium bromide staining. *S. aureus* reference strains EMRSA-15 and ATCC 25923 were used was used as a positive controls for the *mecA* and the *cfr* genes, respectively.

Biofilm formation

The tube method (TM) and Congo red agar (CRA) method previously described [24] were followed to assess the ability for biofilm and slime formation by the 23 *Staphylococcus* isolates using the following international reference strains as controls: the non-biofilm producers *Staphylococcus epidermidis* ATCC 12228 and *Staphylococcus warneri* ATCC 10209 (negative controls), and the biofilm producers *S. epidermidis* ATCC 35983, *Staphylococcus simulans* ATCC 27851 and *Staphylococcus xylosus* ATCC 29979 (positive controls). For the TM, adherence was observed as a ring formation on the inside walls of the test tube when stained with crystal violet. Regarding the interpretation of the TM results, strains were classified as strongly adherent (+) or negative (−). Results of the CRA method were interpreted as follows: very black, black and almost black colonies were considered to be strong biofilm formers, while very red, red and bordeaux colonies were classified as negative strains for biofilm formation.

Correlation analyses

Pearson's correlation was used to analyze the association between all studied phenotypic and genotypic features. Univariate analyses (Chi square test, $p < 0.05$) were performed to identify variables significantly associated. The p values < 0.05 were considered statistically significant. Statistical analysis and data representation were done using R software (3.3.2).

Results

Isolation and characterization of *Staphylococcus* spp. from imported beef meat samples

In this study, a total of 23 staphylococcal isolates were recovered from 100 imported meat samples (23%), including CPS strains (12/23) and CNS strains (11/23) (Table 2). The 23 *Staphylococcus* spp. (*S. aureus*, n = 3; *S. hyicus*, n = 6; *S. intermedius*, n = 3; *S. epidermidis*, n = 1; *S. hemolyticus*, n = 1; *S. hominis*, n = 1; *S. lugdunensis*, n = 3; *S. simulans*, n = 1; and *S. scuri*, n = 4) isolates were cytotoxic to Vero cells. The three types of hemolysis were manifested as α-, β- and γ-hemolysins at a percentage of 17.4, 47.8, and 34.8%, respectively (Table 1).

Biofilm formation phenotype

Using the tube method (TM), a total of 18 isolates (78.3%) were classified as positive for biofilm formation ability, while 5 isolates (21.7%) were considered negative. Using CRA method, 7 of the 23 *Staphylococcus* spp.

Table 1 Phenotypic (antibiotic resistance, haemolytic activity and biofilm formation ability) and genotypic (antibiotic resistance genes) profile of all *Staphylococcus* spp. strains isolated from imported meat

Isolate	Species	Antibiotic resistance genes					Antibiotic resistance profile												Biofilm formation		Haemolysis			Virulence
		mecA	*gyrA*	*grlA*	*gyrB*	*Cfr*	Ampicillin-sulbactam	Chloramphenicol	Ciprofloxacin	Clindamycin	Erythromycin	Gentamycin	Methicillin	Oxacillin	Penicillin	Sulfamethoxazole/ trimethoprim	Tetracycline	Vancomycin	Congo Red Agar	Tube method	α	β	δ	Vero cell
1	*S. aureus*	–	+	–	–	–	R	S	R	R	R	S	S	R	R	R	S	S	–	+	–	+	–	+
2	*S. aureus*	–	+	–	–	–	S	S	S	S	S	S	S	S	R	R	S	S	–	+	–	–	+	+
3	*S. aureus*	–	–	–	+	–	S	S	S	S	S	S	S	S	R	R	S	S	–	+	–	–	+	+
4	*S. hyicus*	+	–	+	–	–	S	S	S	R	S	R	R	R	R	R	S	R	+	+	–	+	–	+
5	*S. hyicus*	–	+	–	–	–	S	S	S	S	S	S	S	S	R	R	S	S	–	+	–	+	–	+
6	*S. hyicus*	–	–	+	–	–	S	S	S	S	S	S	S	S	R	R	S	S	–	+	–	+	–	+
7	*S. hyicus*	+	+	+	+	–	S	S	R	R	S	R	R	R	R	R	R	R	+	+	+	–	–	+
8	*S. hyicus*	+	–	–	–	–	S	S	R	R	S	R	R	R	R	R	S	R	+	+	–	–	+	+
9	*S. hyicus*	–	+	+	–	–	S	S	S	R	S	R	S	S	R	R	S	S	–	–	–	–	+	+
10	*S. intermedius*	–	+	–	–	–	S	S	S	R	R	R	S	S	R	R	S	S	–	–	–	+	–	+
11	*S. intermedius*	–	+	+	+	–	S	S	S	R	R	R	R	R	R	R	S	R	+	+	–	–	+	+
12	*S. intermedius*	+	–	+	+	–	S	S	R	R	R	R	R	R	R	R	R	R	+	+	–	–	+	+
13	*S. epidermidis*	–	+	+	–	–	S	R	R	R	R	R	S	R	R	R	S	S	–	+	–	+	–	+
14	*S. hemolyticus*	–	–	–	–	–	S	S	S	S	S	S	S	S	S	S	S	R	+	+	–	+	–	+
15	*S. hominus*	–	–	–	–	–	R	S	S	R	R	R	R	R	R	R	R	R	–	–	–	+	–	+
16	*S. lugdunensis*	+	–	–	–	–	S	S	R	R	S	R	R	R	R	R	R	R	+	–	–	+	–	+
17	*S. lugdunensis*	–	–	–	–	–	S	S	S	S	S	S	S	S	R	R	S	S	+	+	–	+	–	+
18	*S. lugdunensis*	–	+	+	+	–	S	S	S	S	S	S	S	S	R	R	S	R	–	+	–	+	–	+
19	*S. simulans*	–	+	+	–	–	S	S	R	R	S	R	S	R	R	R	R	S	–	+	–	+	–	+
20	*S. scuri*	–	+	+	+	–	R	S	R	R	S	R	R	R	R	R	R	S	+	+	–	+	–	+
21	*S. scuri*	–	+	–	–	–	R	S	S	R	S	R	S	S	R	R	S	S	–	+	–	–	–	+
22	*S. scuri*	–	–	–	–	–	R	S	S	R	S	R	S	R	R	R	S	S	–	+	–	–	–	+
23	*S. scuri*	–	–	–	–	–	R	S	S	S	S	S	S	R	R	R	S	S	–	+	–	–	–	+

isolates (30.4%) showed black colonies with shriveled lucent texture whereas 16 (69.6%) isolates showed pink colored colonies with mucoid appearance on the CRA plates that were interpreted as negative for biofilm formation (Table 1).

Antibiotic resistance phenotypic profile

The diversity in occurrence of antibiotic resistance among the tested *Staphylococcus* spp. isolates is outlined in Tables 1 and 2 . The 23 isolates were resistant to at least one antibiotic. Less than 50% of the isolates exhibited resistance to the β-lactams ampicillin (6/23) and methicillin (8/23), erythromycin (6/23), chloramphenicol (1/23), ciprofloxacin (7/23), vancomycin (9/23), and tetracycline (6/23) (Table 2). Ninety six percent of the isolates (22/23) were resistant to penicillin and sulfamethoxazole/trimethoprim, while only one isolate was resistant to chloramphenicol (Table 1). MDR, defined as resistance to ≥ 3 antimicrobial classes, was observed in 16 *Staphylococcus* isolates. Fifteen multidrug resistance (MDR) combination patterns were observed (Table 2). The penicillin/sulfamethoxazole/trimethoprim (P/SXT) resistance phenotype was evident in 14/15 of these combinations.

Antimicrobial resistance genes

From the 23 screened isolates, five isolates (3/6 *S. hyicus*; 1/3 *S. intermedius*; 1/3 *S. lugdunensis*) were identified as positive for *mecA* (5/23). Four of the 13 oxacillin-resistant isolates harbored the *mecA* gene, while 4 of the 8 methicillin resistant isolates carried the *mecA* gene (Table 3).

Table 2 Antimicrobial resistance patterns among *Staphylococcus* spp. strains isolated from imported beef meat

Antibiotics	Number of antibiotics	Total number of isolates	%
VA	1	1/23	4
P, SXT	2	6/23	26
P, TE, VA, SXT	4	1/23	4
P, CN, E, DA, SXT	5	2/23	9
P, OX, CN, DA, SXT			
P, OX, SAM, CN, DA, SXT	6	3/23	13
P, OX, MET, CN, DA, SXT			
P, OX, E, DA, C, SXT, CIP	7	5/23	22
P, CN, DA, TE, VA, SXT, CIP			
P, OX, CN, DA, TE, SXT, CIP			
P, OX, MET, CN, DA, VA, SXT			
P, OX, MET, CN, DA, VA, SXT, CIP	8	2/23	9
P, OX, MET, CN, E, DA, TE, VA, SXT	9	3/23	13
P, OX, MET, CN, E, DA, VA, SXT, CIP			
P, OX, MET, SAM, E, DA, TE, VA, SXT			

C chloramphenicol, *CIP* ciprofloxacin, *CN* gentamycin, *DA* clindamycin, *E* erythromycin, *MET* methicillin, *OX* oxacillin, *P* penicilin, *SAM* ampicillin-sulbactam, *SXT* sulfamethoxazole/trimethoprim, *TE* tetracycline, *VA* vancomycin

Interestingly, the following three observations were recorded: (i) although *S. hominis* and *S. hemolyticus* isolates were resistant to methicillin and vancomycin, respectively, the resistance genes *mecA*, *gyrA*, *gyrB*, *grlA* and *cfr* were absent. (ii) three *S. aureus* isolates did not carry the *mecA* gene (100%) and were phenotypically characterized as MSS; and (iii) one *S. lugdunensis* isolate was observed to harbor the *mecA* resistance gene but was phenotypically characterized as methicillin-susceptible non-*S. aureus* (MSNSA). The resistance gene *mecA* was detected in 4/8 (50%) methicillin-resistant non-*S. aureus* (MRNSA) isolates (Table 3). Of the three MSSA isolates, two carried the *gyrA* gene (66.66%) and one carried the *gyrB* gene (33.33%) (Table 1). The *cfr* gene was absent in all *Staphylococcus* isolates. The non-*cfr*-conveying CNS showed extensive resistance to several antimicrobials irrespective of those incorporated in the *cfr*-transmitted PhLOPSA phenotype (conferring resistance to several classes of antibiotics (phenicols, lincosamides, oxazolidinones, pleuromutilins, and streptogramin A; PhLOPSA phenotype) (Table 1). Phenotypically, 40% (8/20) of NSA (non *Staphylococcus aureus*) isolates were methicillin resistant, while the *mecA* gene was detected in only 25% (5/20) of isolates.

Correlation analyses

Correlation analyses showed that presence of *mecA* was directly correlated with resistance to ciprofloxacin, gentamicin, methicillin, oxacillin, and vancomycin (Pearson's correlation coefficients of 0.50, 0.42, 0.72, 0.46 and 0.66, respectively) (Fig. 1). There were several instances of co-occurrence of resistance to various antibiotics. Indeed, resistance to various antibiotics was directly correlated. For instance, resistance to methicillin was significantly associated with resistance to ciprofloxacin (Pearson's correlation coefficient of 0.43), clindamycin (Pearson's correlation coefficient of 0.53), gentamicin (Pearson's correlation coefficient of 0.59), oxacillin (Pearson's correlation coefficient of 0.64), tetracycline (Pearson's correlation coefficient of 0.61) and vancomycin (Pearson's correlation coefficient of 0.72). Similarly, a high correlation between resistances to several other antibiotics was found (Fig. 1). In addition, biofilm formation, as assessed by the CRA tests, was directly correlated with *mecA* presence (Pearson's correlation coefficient of 0.66), methicillin resistance (Pearson's correlation coefficient of 0.72) and vancomycin resistance (Pearson's correlation coefficient of 0.63).

Discussion

Globally, an increasing recognizable concern exists on the status of antimicrobial resistant microbial contaminants in the food chain and their capacity to be widely

Table 3 Prevalence of the *mecA* gene in imported beef samples

Staphylococcus spp. (n = number of isolates)	n = of MRS	Presence of *mecA*gene		n = of MSS	Precence of *mecA* gene	
		n=	%		n=	%
S. aureus (n = 3)	0	0	0	3	0	0
S. hyicus (n = 6)	3	3	100	3	0	0
S. intermedius (n = 3)	2	1	50	1	0	0
S. epidermidis (n = 1)	0	0	0	1	0	0
S. hemolyticus (n = 1)	0	0	0	1	0	0
S. hominus (n = 1)	1	0	0	0	0	0
S. lugdunensis (n = 3)	1	0	0	2	1	50
S. simulans (n = 1)	0	0	0	1	0	0
S. scuri (n = 4)	1	0	0	3	0	0
Total	8	4	50	15	1	6.7

MRS methicillin resistant *Staphylococcus*, *MSS* methicillin susceptible *Staphylococcus*

dispersed through the international trade of food. This prompted the Codex Alimentarius Commission to establish an ad hoc Intergovernmental Task Force on Antimicrobial Resistance in 2007, bearing in mind the occurrence of national and regional diversity in antimicrobial misuse, human subjection to resistant microorganisms and determinants and their prevalence in foodborne pathogens. Egypt imports different meat types to fill the gaps in animal protein supply. According to the U.S. Meat Export Federation (USMEF) that examines key statistics and trends in beef and pork trade from 2008 to 2017, Egypt's projection for beef-importing in 2017 would reach about 332,000 metric tons of meat imports and this is supposed to grow to 2025 by 52.28% [25]. While the importation of beef meat in Egypt is crucial to close the gap in animal protein requirements, monitoring the frequency of antimicrobial resistance in imported meat must assure that quality and safety standards are met.

The spread of MRSA is a serious public health concern for both human and veterinary medicine. Due to the occurrence of MRSA, methicillin and other β-lactamic antibiotics have become useless for clinical therapy, leaving the term MRSA to be used to describe *S. aureus* strains resistant to effectively all β-lactamase-resistant penicillins and harboring the *mecA* gene [23]. Although the development and spread of multiple antibiotic-resistant MRSA have gained much attention over the past years, yet the role of imported meat has not been given much attention. In a Danish study, Agersø et al. reported that MRSA was found in 18% of the imported broiler meat and 7.5% of the imported pork [26]. MRSA are often resistant to other antimicrobials different to methicillin, highlighting the necessity for new and effective antimicrobials. Attributed to their extended antimicrobial spectra, fluoroquinolone compounds such as ciprofloxacin and norfloxacin were recommended as useful candidates for eradicating MRSA [27]. Nonetheless, due to the misuse of these compounds in the clinical practice, resistance of MRSA to these compounds has been observed [28]. For this reason ciprofloxacin is not recommended to be used in empirical therapy against MRSA infections. Furthermore, the use of other fluoroquinolones is only allowed following accurate antimicrobial susceptibility testing. Nonetheless, vancomycin remains the drug of choice to treat MRSA infections [29].

Identification of methicillin resistant staphylococci in the laboratory is often problematic due to difficulty in detecting heterogeneous methicillin-oxacillin resistance in staphylococci [30, 31]. Moreover, Standard interpretive breakpoints for oxacillin susceptibility reporting published by the CLSI (formerly the National Committee for Clinical and Laboratory Standards) were changed in 2004, and NSA isolates of veterinary origin are now more likely than in previous years to be deemed resistant by testing laboratories that use those guidelines [32].

In this study, the susceptibility of 23 *Staphylococcus* spp. strains isolated from imported meat to 12 antibiotics from different classes was evaluated. An extreme resistance was found against penicillin and sulfamethoxazole/trimethoprim as compared to other tested antibiotics, which could be attributed to the extensive use of these antibiotics in treating mastitis cases and/or as growth promoters in animal feed in the countries from which the beef meat was imported. Resistance to other clinically important antibiotics, including β-lactamic antibiotics (such as ampicillin-sulbactam, methicillin, oxacillin), fluoroquinolones (ciprofloxacin), macrolides (erythromycin), aminoglycosides (gentamicin), glycopeptides

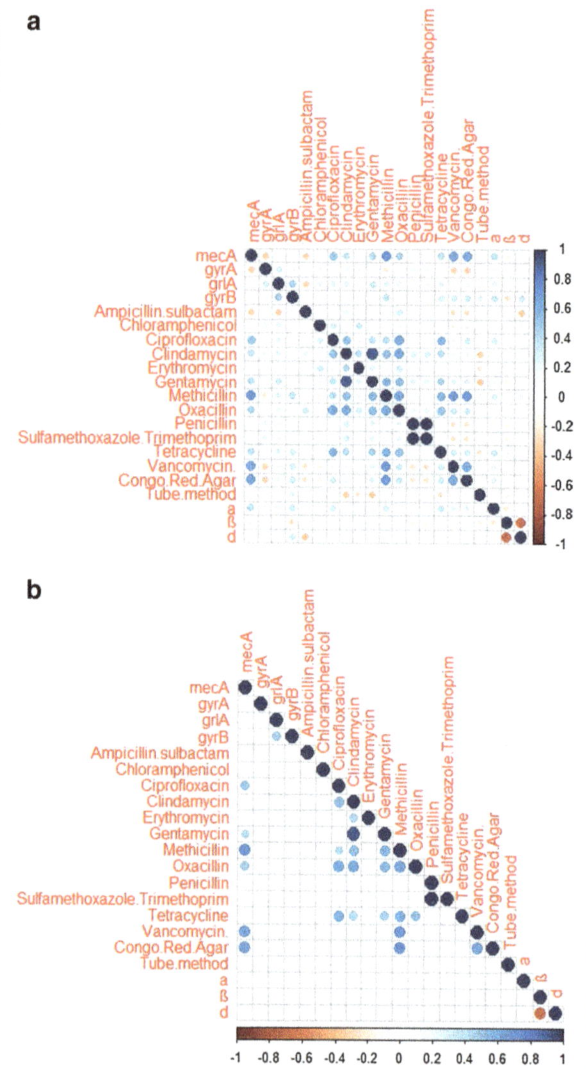

Fig. 1 **a** Correlation matrix of phenotypic (antibiotic resistance, haemolytic activity and biofilm formation ability) and genotypic (antibiotic resistance genes) features. **b** Correlation matrix showing only significant ($p < 0.05$) associations, as assessed by the Chi square test

(vancomycin), lincosamides (clindamycin) and tetracycline also occurred and, in some cases, multidrug resistance phenotypes were identified. Indeed, correlation analyses showed co-occurrence of resistance to series of antibiotics. Extended-spectrum beta-lactamases (ESBL) -producing pathogens are often resistant to fluoroquinolones and aminoglycosides since resistance mechanisms for these classes of antibiotics are often carried on the same large plasmids that contain the genetic elements for ESBL production [33]. Our results corroborate this observation. Thus, for instance, resistance to methicillin was significantly associated with resistance to ciprofloxacin and gentamycin, among others (clindamycin, oxacillin, tetracycline and vancomycin). The colonization ability in conjunction with the occurrence of MDR highlights the hazardous nature of the *Staphylococcus* spp. isolated from imported beef meat.

The antimicrobial resistance determinants *mecA*, *gyrA*, *gyrB*, *grlA* and *cfr*, frequently reported in *S. aureus* strains were also screened in recovered isolates. The emergence of the multiple drug resistance gene *cfr* in staphylococci is of global clinical and veterinary importance that has been previously investigated in staphylococci [34] and has been identified as a phenicol and lincosamide resistance gene [35]. In this study, the absence of the *cfr* gene among imported beef meat isolates suggests a decreased potential risk as an outcome of harboring the gene in the food chain through imported meat. Furthermore, the absence of the gene *cfr* poses a significant and interdisciplinary public health positive factor to the Egyptian consumers. One isolate showed chloramphenicol resistance but was negative for the *cfr* gene. This observation might be attributed to a possible heterogeneous expression of the *cfr* gene [36] or to different potential chloramphenicol resistance mechanisms.

The *mecA* gene confers methicillin resistance. It encodes the penicillin binding protein 2a, an enzyme that has low affinity for beta-lactams, and has been reported to lead to resistance to ciprofloxacin, gentamycin, methicillin, oxacillin and vancomycin [37]. In our study, the *mecA* gene was carried by 5 out of 23 *Staphylococcus* spp. isolates, and, as expected, presence of *mecA* was directly correlated with resistance to ciprofloxacin, gentamycin, methicillin, oxacillin, and vancomycin. Nevertheless, not all methicillin or oxacillin resistant isolates were *mecA* positive. It was previously indicated that some isolates missing the *mecA* gene could be identified as phenotypically resistant to oxacillin (MRSA) [38]. These results suggests that other potential resistance mechanisms might exist. Molecular investigations of a *S. aureus* isolate, which was found to be phenotypically resistant to methicillin but negative for the *mecA* gene, were able to identify the presence of a novel *mecA* homologue, which was found to be associated with cattle [39], suggesting the existence of a zoonotic MRSA reservoir [40]. In 2012, the International Working Group on the Classification of Staphylococcal Cassette Chromosome elements (IWCC) renamed the *mecA* variant, *mecC* [41]. Methicillin-resistant *S. aureus* strains carrying the *mecC* gene have been shown to cause a range of infections in humans and appear to be predominantly community associated [40]. The prevalence of *mecC* in CNS has been recently reported for 13 European countries, where it has been isolated from 14 different host species (Holmes et al. 42), and an allotype of the *mecC* gene has been detected in a *S. xylosus* strain [42]. It is also worth mentioning the fact that one *S. lugdunensis* isolate was observed to harbor the *mecA* resistance gene but was phenotypically characterized as MSNSA. The phenotypic susceptibility to oxacillin, methicillin, penicillin and ampicillin (β-lactam antibiotic of the penicillin class) regardless of the *mecA* presence may be attributed to the heterogeneous expression of *mecA* [43], which is more common in CNS than that in *S. aureus* [44]. Nevertheless, it should be noted that in 2014, Bhargava and Zhang emphasized the importance of MRCNSs as important reservoirs of *mecA* that could act as precursors of MRSA [11]. In addition, temperature abuse during storage and transportation to the importing country may result in multiplication of MRS [45]. An additional important finding was introduced by the identification and characterization of another gene on the SCC element called *mecR2* that regulates and increases *mecA* expression when MRSA bacteria encounter β-lactam drugs [46].

Besides resistance genes, mutation-mediated resistance is especially common among resistances to synthetic antibacterial agents, such as fluoroquinolones and oxazolidinones in *S. aureus* and other bacterial species [47]. The primers used in this study amplified only the copies of *gyrA*, *gyrB*, and *grlA* that contained mutations in the quinolone resistance-determining regions (QRDRs). In this study, the amplification of a *grlA* and *gyrA* product represented the presence of a mutation conferring resistance. Mutations in the *gyrB* gene does not play an important role in quinolone resistance [48]. Although the presence of resistance genes are a primary reason for antibiotic resistance, the resistance phenotype and gene presence are not exclusively linked in this study. Similarly, this inconsistency was common in other classes of antibiotics, demonstrating that the presence of a certain resistance gene was not necessary an indicator of antibiotic resistance [49]. A potential explanation for this inconsistency could be the lack of expression of some of the resistance genes and the presence of other genes encoding resistance. In addition, chromosomally encoded multidrug resistance pumps have been shown to have other primary functional or structural roles [50].

The connection between microbial biofilms and antibiotic resistance is of considerable interest to biomedical researchers. Previous reports have suggested that a correlation between antibiotic resistance and biofilm formation ability exists, a phenomenon that may be responsible for a decrease in the efficaciousness of antimicrobial agents against *S. aureus* infections [51]. As a consequence of biofilm development, the capability of horizontal gene transfer is increased and may facilitate the dispersion of antibiotic resistance [52]. In the present study, MRS and MDR isolates showed a good potential to form biofilms. In fact, correlation analyses showed that biofilm formation, as assessed by the CRA tests, was directly correlated with *mecA* presence, methicillin resistance and vancomycin resistance, and biofilm producing MRNSA showed high resistance to almost all antibiotic classes compared to non-producers, which corroborates previous observations [53].

Conclusions

Despite the alert generated by the outbreaks of foot and mouth disease and swine fever, which have been attributed to international trade of meat, little information or actionable risk management information is available yet on the dissemination of microbial hazards through retail imported meat. This study reveals that imported meat can act as a transmission vector for MRSA or MRNSA harboring the *mecA* gene, which may represent a risk for both human and veterinary medicine. The data obtained on the resistance of *Staphylococcus* spp. to antimicrobials, may be used for implementing an antimicrobial resistance spread monitoring and prevention program.

Abbreviations

ESBL: extended-spectrum beta-lactamases; CNS: coagulase-negative staphylococci; CPS: coagulase-positive staphylococci (CPS); LA-MRSA: livestock-associated methicillin-resistant *Staphylococcus aureus*; MDR: multiple drug resistance; MRNSA: methicillin-resistant non-*Staphylococcus aureus*; MRSA: methicillin-resistant *Staphylococcus aureus*; MSNSA: methicillin-susceptible non-*Staphylococcus aureus*; NSA: non *Staphylococcus aureus*; QRDRs: quinolone resistance-determining regions.

Authors' contributions

KO conceived, designed the experiments, analyzed the data and wrote the paper; AAO, LR and ME conducted the data analysis and contributed to the writing of the manuscript. FE, KAM, IM and AH contributed with their scientific advice during the work and revision of the manuscript; AO and AS contributed with reagents/materials/analysis tools and performed the experiments. All authors read and approved the final manuscript.

Author details

[1] Department of Microbiology, Faculty of Veterinary Medicine, Cairo University, Giza, Egypt. [2] Department of Food Hygiene and Technology and Institute of Food Science and Technology, University of León, León, Spain. [3] Department of Nutrition, Bromatology and Food Technology, Universidad Complutense de Madrid, Madrid, Spain. [4] Department of Poultry Diseases, Animal Health Research, Institute, Giza, Egypt. [5] Department of Bacteriology, Immunology and Mycology, Faculty of Veterinary Medicine, Benha University, Moushtohor, Egypt. [6] Department of Botany and Microbiology, College of Science, King Saud University, Riyadh, Kingdom of Saudi Arabia. [7] Department of Health Science, College of Applied Studies and Community Service, King Saud University, Riyadh, Kingdom of Saudi Arabia. [8] Department of Bacteriology, Mycology and Immunology, Faculty of Veterinary Medicine, Mansoura University, Mansoura 35516, Egypt. [9] Foodborne Pathogens, Scientific Institute of Public Health, Juliette Wytsmanstraat 14, 1050 Brussels, Belgium.

Acknowledgements

The authors extend their appreciation to the Deanship of Scientific Research at King Saud University for funding the work through the research group Project No.: RGP-162.

Competing interests

The authors declare that they have no competing interests.

References

1. MacDiarmid SC. Risk analysis and the importation of animals and animal products. Rev Sci Tech. 1993;12:1093–107.
2. WTO 2016. World Trade Organization. Sanitary and phytosanitary measures: text of the agreement. The WTO Agreement on the Application of Sanitary and Phytosanitary Measures (SPS Agreement). Centre William Rappard, 154 rue de Lausanne, Geneva, Switzerland.
3. Hennekinne JA, De Buyser ML, Dragacci S. *Staphylococcus aureus* and its food poisoning toxins: characterization and outbreak investigation. FEMS Microbiol Rev. 2012;36:815–36.
4. Bhumbra S, Mahboubi M, Blackwood RA. *Staphylococcus lugdunensis*: novel organism causing cochlear implant infection. Infect Dis Rep. 2014;6:5406.
5. Giormezis N, Kolonitsiou F, Foka A, Drougka E, Liakopoulos A, Makri A, Papanastasiou AD, Vogiatzi A, Dimitriou G, Marangos M, Christofidou M, Anastassiou ED, Petinaki E, Spiliopoulou I. Coagulase-negative staphylococcal bloodstream and prosthetic-device-associated infections: the role of biofilm formation and distribution of adhesin and toxin genes. J Med Microbiol. 2014;63:1500–8.
6. Pinheiro L, Brito CI, de Oliveira A, Martins PY, Pereira VC, da Cunha Mde L. *Staphylococcus epidermidis* and *Staphylococcus haemolyticus*: molecular detection of cytotoxin and enterotoxin genes. Toxins. 2015;7:3688–99.
7. Osman KM, Abd EL-Razik KA, Marie HSH, Arafa A. Coagulase-negative staphylococci collected from bovine milk: species and antimicrobial gene diversity. J Food Saf. 2016;36:89–99.
8. Osman KM, Amer AM, Badr JM, Helmy NM, Elhelw RA, Orabi A, Bakry M, Saad AS. Antimicrobial resistance, biofilm formation and *mecA* characterization of methicillin-susceptible *S. aureus* and non-*S. aureus* of beef meat origin in Egypt. Front Microbiol. 2016;7:222.
9. Veras JF, Carmo LS, Tong LC, Shupp JW, Cummings C, Dos Santos DA, Cerqueira MM, Cantini A, Nicoli JR, Jett M. A study of the enterotoxigenicity of coagulase-negative and coagulase-positive staphylococcal isolates from food poisoning outbreaks in Minas Gerais, Brazil. Int J Infect Dis. 2008;12:410–5.
10. Chajęcka-Wierzchowska W, Zadernowska A, Nalepa B, Sierpińska M, Łaniewska-Trokenheim Ł. Coagulase-negative staphylococci (CoNS) isolated from ready-to-eat food of animal origin–phenotypic and genotypic antibiotic resistance. Food Microbiol. 2015;46:222–6.
11. Bhargava K, Zhang Y. Characterization of methicillin-resistant coagulase-negative staphylococci (MRCoNS) in retail meat. Food Microbiol. 2014;42:56–60.
12. Tulinski P, Fluit AC, Wagenaar JA, Mevius D, van de Vijver L, Duim B. Methicillin-resistant coagulase-negative staphylococci on pig farms as a reservoir of heterogeneous staphylococcal cassette chromosome *mec* elements. Appl Environ Microbiol. 2012;78:299–304.
13. Doyle MP, Loneragan GH, Scott HM, Singer RS. Antimicrobial resistance: challenges and perspectives. Comp Rev Food Sci Food Saf. 2013;12:234–48.
14. Alabi SA, Frielinghaus L, Grobusch MP, Köck R, Becker K, Issifou S, Kremsner PG, Peters G, Mellmann A. The risk to import ESBL-producing *Enterobacteriaceae* and *Staphylococcus aureus* through chicken meat trade in Gabon. BMC Microbiol. 2014;14:286.
15. Card R, Vaughan K, Bagnall M, Spiropoulos J, Cooley W, Strickland T, Davies R, Anjum MF. Virulence characterization of *Salmonella enterica* isolates of differing antimicrobial resistance recovered from UK livestock and imported meat samples. Front Microbiol. 2016;7:640.
16. Long KS, Poehlsgaard J, Kehrenberg C, Schwarz S, Vester B. The Cfr rRNA methyltransferase confers resistance to phenicols, lincosamides, oxazolidinones, pleuromutilins, and streptogramin A antibiotics. Antimicrob Agents Chemother. 2006;50:2500–5.
17. Bannerman T. *Staphylococcus*, *Micrococcus*, and other catalase positive cocci that grow aerobically. In: Murray PR, Baron EJ, Jorgensen JH, et al., editors. Manual of clinical microbiology. Washington, DC: ASM Press; 2003. p. 384–404.
18. Futagawa-Saito K, Ba-Thein W, Sakurai N, Fukuyasu T. Prevalence of virulence factors in *Staphylococcus intermedius* isolates from dogs and pigeons. BMC Vet Res. 2006;2:4.
19. Tao M, Yamashita H, Watanabe K, Nagatake T. Possible virulence factors of *Staphylococcus aureus* in a mouse septic model. FEMS Immunol Med Microbiol. 1999;23:135–46.
20. CLSI. Performance standards for antimicrobial susceptibility testing. Clinical and Laboratory Standards Institute 2007, CLSI M100-S17, Wayne, PA, USA.
21. WHO World Health Organization. Critically important antimicrobials for human medicine—3rd rev. WHO Press, World Health Organization, 20 Avenue Appia, 1211 Geneva 27, Switzerland; 2012.
22. Zhang K, Sparling J, Chow BL, Elsayed S, Hussain Z, Church DL, Gregson DB, Louie T, Conly JM. New quadriplex PCR assay for detection of methicillin and mupirocin resistance and simultaneous discrimination of *Staphylococcus aureus* from coagulase-negative staphylococci. J Clin Microbiol. 2004;42:4947–55.
23. Paterson GK, Harrison EM, Holmes MA. The emergence of *mecC* methicillin-resistant *Staphylococcus aureus*. Trends Microbiol. 2014;22:42–7.
24. Mathur T, Singhal S, Khan S, Upadhyay DJ, Fatma T, Rattan A. Detection of biofilm formation among the clinical isolates of staphylococci: an evaluation of three different screening methods. Indian J Med Microbiol. 2006;24:25–9.
25. USDA 2016 United States Department of Agriculture Foreign Agricultural Service Foreign Ag ServiceVerified account @USDAForeignAg.
26. Agersø Y, Hasman H, Cavaco LM, Pedersen K, Aarestrup FM. Study of methicillin resistant *Staphylococcus aureus* (MRSA) in Danish pigs at slaughter and in imported retail meat reveals a novel MRSA type in slaughter pigs. Vet Microbiol. 2012;157:246–50.
27. Gilbert MJ, Boscia A, Kobasa WD, Kaye D. Enoxacin compared with vancomycin for the treatment of experimental methicillin-resistant *Staphylococcus aureus* endocarditis. Antimicrob Agents Chemother. 1986;29:461–3.
28. Pai V, Rao VI, Rao SP. Prevalence and antimicrobial susceptibility pattern of methicillin-resistant *Staphylococcus aureus* [MRSA] isolates at a tertiary care hospital in Mangalore, South India. J Lab Phys. 2010;2:82–4.
29. Gade ND, Qazi MS. Fluoroquinolone therapy in *Staphylococcus aureus* infections: where do we stand? J Lab Phys. 2013;5:109–12.
30. Tenover FC, Goering RV. Methicillin-resistant *Staphylococcus aureus* strain USA300: origin and epidemiology. J Antimicrob Chemother. 2009;64:441–6.
31. Brown DFJ. Detection of methicillin/oxacillin resistance in staphylococci. J Antimicrob Chemother. 2002;48(S1):65–70.
32. NCCLS National Committee for Clinical Laboratory Standards. Performance standards for antimicrobial disk and dilution susceptibility tests for bacteria isolated from animals; informational supplement. 2004, Document *M31-S1*. Wayne, Pa: NCCLS; 2004.
33. Karam G, Chastre J, Wilcox MH, Vincent J. Antibiotic strategies in the era of multidrug resistance. Crit Care. 2016;20:136.
34. Wang Y, He T, Schwarz S, Zhao Q, Shen Z, Wu C, Shen J. Multidrug resistance gene *cfr* in methicillin-resistant coagulase-negative staphylococci from chickens, ducks, and pigs in China. Int J Med Microbiol. 2013;303:84–7.
35. Witte W, Cuny C. Emergence and spread of *cfr*-mediated multiresistance in staphylococci: an interdisciplinary challenge. Future Microbiol. 2011;6:925–31.
36. Terlizzi V, Carnovale V, Castaldo G, Castellani C, Cirilli N, Colombo C, Corti F, Cresta F, D'Adda A, Lucarelli M, Lucidi V, Macchiaroli A, Madarena E, Padoan R, Quattrucci S, Salvatore D, Zarrilli F, Raia V. Clinical expression of patients with the D1152H CFTR mutation. J Cyst Fibros. 2015;14:447–52.
37. Lee JH. Methicillin (oxacillin)-resistant *Staphylococcus aureus* strains isolated from major food animals and their potential transmission to humans. Appl Environ Microbiol. 2003;69:6489–94.
38. Lee JH, Jeong JM, Park YH, Choi SS, Kim YH, Chae JS, Moon JS, Park H, Kim S, Eo SK. Evaluation of the methicillin-resistant *Staphylococcus aureus* (MRSA)-screen latex agglutination test for detection of MRSA of animal origin. J Clin Microbiol. 2004;42:2780–2.
39. García-Álvarez L, Holden MT, Lindsay H, Webb CR, Brown DF, Curran MD, Walpole E, Brooks K, Pickard DJ, Teale C, Parkhill J, Bentley SD, Edwards GF, Girvan EK, Kearns AM, Pichon B, Hill RL, Larsen AR, Skov RL, Peacock SJ, Maskell DJ, Holmes MA. Methicillin-resistant *Staphylococcus aureus* with a novel *mecA* homologue in human and bovine populations in the UK and Denmark: a descriptive study. Lancet Infect Dis. 2011;11:595–603.
40. Petersen A, Stegger M, Heltberg O, Christensen J, Zeuthen A, Knudsen LK, Urth T, Sorum M, Schouls L, Larsen J, Skov R, Larsen AR. Epidemiology of methicillin-resistant *Staphylococcus aureus* carrying the novel mecC gene in Denmark corroborates a zoonotic reservoir with transmission to humans. Clin Microbiol Infect. 2013;19:E16–22.

41. Ito T, Hiramatsu K, Tomasz A, de Lencastre H, Perreten V, Holden MT, Coleman DC, Goering R, Giffard PM, Skov RL, Zhang K, Westh H, O'Brien F, Tenover FC, Oliveira DC, Boyle-Vavra S, Laurent F, Kearns AM, Kreiswirth B, Ko KS, Grundmann H, Sollid JE Jr, John JF, Daum R, Soderquist B, Buist G, and International Working Group on the Classification of Staphylococcal Cassette Chromosome Elements (IWG-SCC). Guidelines for reporting novel *mec*A gene homologues. Antimicrob Agents Chemother. 2012;56:4997–9.
42. Holmes M, Zadoks R. Methicillin resistant *S. aureus* in human and bovine mastitis. Mammary Gland Biol Neoplasia. 2011;16:373–82.
43. Stegger M. Rapid detection, differentiation and typing of methicillin-resistant *Staphylococcus aureus* harbouring either *mec*A or the new *mec*A homologue *mec*A (LGA251). Clin Microbiol Infect. 2012;18:395–400.
44. Stepanovic S, Hauschild T, Dakic I, Al-Doori Z, Svabic-Vlahovic M, Ranin L, Morrison D. Evaluation of phenotypic and molecular methods for detection of oxacillin resistance in members of the *Staphylococcus sciuri* group. J Clin Microbiol. 2006;44:934–7.
45. de Boer E, Zwartkruis-Nahuis JT, Wit B, Huijsdens XW, de Neeling AJ, Bosch T, van Oosterom RA, Vila A, Heuvelink AE. Prevalence of methicillin-resistant *Staphylococcus aureus* in meat. Int J Food Microbiol. 2009;134:52–6.
46. Arêde P, Milheiriço C, de Lencastre H, Oliveira DC. The anti-repressor *MecR2* promotes the proteolysis of the *mecA* repressor and enables optimal expression of β-lactam resistance in MRSA. PLoS Pathog. 2012;8:e1002816.
47. Aldred KJ, Kerns RJ, Osheroff N. Mechanism of quinolone action and resistance. Biochemistry. 2014;53:1565–74.
48. Sierra JM, Marco F, Ruiz J, Jime´nez de Anta MT, Vila J. Correlation between the activity of different fluoroquinolones and the presence of mechanisms of quinolone resistance in epidemiologically related and unrelated strains of methicillin-susceptible and –resistant *Staphylococcus aureus*. Clin Microbiol Infect. 2002;8:781–90.
49. Xu J, Shi C, Song M, Xu X, Yang P, Paoli G, Shi X. Phenotypic and genotypic antimicrobial resistance traits of foodborne *Staphylococcus aureus* isolates from Shanghai. J Food Sci. 2014;79:M635–42.
50. Kosmidis C, Schindler BD, Jacinto PL, Patel D, Bains K, Seo SM, Kaatz GW. Expression of multidrug resistance efflux pump genes in clinical and environmental isolates of *Staphylococcus aureus*. Intl J Antimicrob Agents. 2012;40:204–9.
51. Gu¨ndog˘an N, Citak S, Turan E. Slime production, DNAse activity and antibiotic resistance of *Staphylococcus aureus* isolated from raw milk, pasteurized milk and ice cream samples. Food Control. 2006;17:389–92.
52. Lee HW, Koh YM, Kim J, Lee JC, Lee YC, Seol SY, Cho DT, Kim J. Capacity of multidrug-resistant clinical isolates of *Acinetobacter baumannii* to form biofilm and adhere to epithelial cell surfaces. Clin Microbiol Infect. 2008;14:49–54.
53. Donlan RM, Costerton W. Biofilms: survival mechanisms of clinically relevant microorganisms. Clin Microbiol Rev. 2002;15:167–93.

13

Antimicrobial activity of mul-1867, a novel antimicrobial compound, against multidrug-resistant *Pseudomonas aeruginosa*

George Tetz[1*], Daria Vikina[2] and Victor Tetz[2]

Abstract

Background: There is an urgent need for new antimicrobial compounds to treat various lung infections caused by multidrug-resistant *Pseudomonas aeruginosa* (MDR-PA).

Methods: We studied the potency of Mul-1867 against MDR-PA isolates from patients with cystic fibrosis, chronic obstructive pulmonary disease, and ventilator-associated pneumonia. The minimal inhibitory concentrations (MICs) and minimum biofilm eliminating concentrations (MBECs), defined as the concentrations of drug that kill 50 % ($MBEC_{50}$), 90 % ($MBEC_{90}$), and 100 % ($MBEC_{100}$) of the bacteria in preformed biofilms, were determined by using the broth macrodilution method.

Results: Mul-1867 exhibited significant activity against MDR-PA and susceptible control strains, with MICs ranging from 1.0 to 8.0 μg/mL. Mul-1867 also possesses anti-biofilm activity against mucoid and non-mucoid 24-h-old MDR-PA biofilms. The $MBEC_{50}$ value was equal to onefold the MIC. The $MBEC_{90}$ value ranged from two to fourfold the MIC. Moreover, Mul-1867 completely eradicated mature biofilms at the concentrations tested, with $MBEC_{100}$ values ranging between 16- and 32-fold the MIC. Mul-1867 was non-toxic to Madin-Darby canine kidney (MDCK) cells at concentrations up to 256 μg/mL.

Conclusion: Overall, these data indicate that Mul-1867 is a promising locally acting antimicrobial for the treatment and prevention of *P. aeruginosa* infections.

Keywords: Biofilms, Mucoid, Non-mucoid, Multidrug-resistant, *P. aeruginosa*, Cystic fibrosis

Background

Pseudomonas aeruginosa is an important pathogen contributing to lung infections in patients with pulmonary diseases such as cystic fibrosis (CF), chronic obstructive pulmonary disease (COPD), and ventilator-associated pneumonia (VAP) [1–3]. By 21 years of age, most CF patients are chronically infected with *P. aeruginosa* that, once established, is difficult to eradicate and is associated with major morbidity [4–6]. *P. aeruginosa* is also an important contributor to acute exacerbations in COPD and VAP [7]. Some *P. aeruginosa* strains are mucoid due to overexpression of alginate, and are less susceptible to the host immune system [8]. Overproduction of alginate, and conversion of *P. aeruginosa* to a mucoid phenotype, are considered markers of chronic lung infections and indicate a decreased life expectancy and a more rapid decline in pulmonary function [9].

Both mucoid and non-mucoid strains of *P. aeruginosa* form biofilms that are associated with persistence in chronic infections, and also contribute to bacterial colonization in acute infections [10]. Established biofilms display high resistance to antimicrobials, and finding ways to disrupt these films is a critical goal in combatting these infections [11, 12]. *P. aeruginosa* survival in

*Correspondence: georgetets@gmail.com
[1] TGV-Laboratories LLC, 303 5th avenue, # 2012, New York, NY 10016, USA
Full list of author information is available at the end of the article

biofilms may be determined by multiple factors including the surface film and the presence of extracellular polymeric substances [13, 14]. Moreover, clinical isolates of multidrug resistant *P. aeruginosa* (MDR-PA) are being observed with increasing frequency [15]. Thus, biofilms formed by MDR-PA are a serious and often fatal problem for patients with lung infections, and many antibiotics are ineffective against bacteria in biofilm communities at concentrations of 10–1000 times the expected minimum inhibitory concentration (MIC) [16].

During the last decade, it became evident that existing antibiotics were unable to treat respiratory infections caused by *P. aeruginosa* effectively [17]. Lung infections caused by MDR-PA were poorly responsive even to nebulized therapy when the aerosolized antibiotics achieved high concentrations directly at the pathological site [18]. It was also shown that many antibiotics, even when able to decrease the number of live bacteria within the biofilm, could not completely eradicate preformed biofilms [19].

The poor therapeutic results with existing antibiotics revealed a critical need for the development of new antimicrobials active against MDR-PA that can be used to treat lung infections. The goal of this study was to examine in vitro MICs and minimal biofilm eradication concentrations (MBECs) of the novel antimicrobial compound, Mul-1867 (poly-N,N'-hexamethyleneguanidine-poly-N1,N4-hexamethyleneaminoguanidine; Fig. 1). The mechanism of action of Mul-1867 involves a nonspecific attack on the cell walls of MDR-PA isolated from patients with respiratory tract infections [20]. Furthermore, the anti-biofilm efficacy of Mul-1867 against preformed mucoid and non-mucoid 24-h-old biofilms of MDR-PA was assessed.

Methods

Test substance and antibiotics

Mul-1867 (Fig. 1) was synthesized by TGV-Therapeutics (New York, NY, USA).

The antibiotics used for these studies included amikacin, aztreonam, ceftazidime, meropenem, piperacillin, and tobramycin, which are currently administered to treat lung infections in patients with CF, COPD, or VAP. These antibiotics were purchased from Sigma-Aldrich (St. Louis, MO, USA).

Bacterial strains and growth conditions

MDR-PA isolates from CF patients including the AGR14, MR45, and VT-CF-234 strains, as well as one susceptible isolate, SEV 7; were obtained from the CF Foundation Therapeutics Development Network Resource Center for Microbiology at Seattle Children's Hospital (Seattle, WA, USA) and from the Institute of Human Microbiology, LLC (DE, USA). MDR-PA isolates from COPD and VAP patients, VT-COPD-274 and VT-VAP-72, respectively, were supplied by the Institute of Human Microbiology. The three strains classified phenotypically as mucoid were SEV 7, VT-CF-234, and VT-COPD-274. The strain used for quality control of the antibiotic panels was *P. aeruginosa* ATCC 27853 from the American Type Culture Collection (Manassas, VA, USA).

All bacterial strains were subcultured from freezer stocks onto Mueller–Hinton agar plates (Oxoid Ltd., London, England) and incubated at 37 °C overnight. All subsequent liquid subcultures were derived from colonies isolated from these plates and were grown in Mueller–Hinton broth (MHB) (Oxoid). The isolates were categorized as susceptible, intermediate, or resistant according to the Clinical and Laboratory Standards Institute (CLSI) breakpoints guidelines (Table 1) [21].

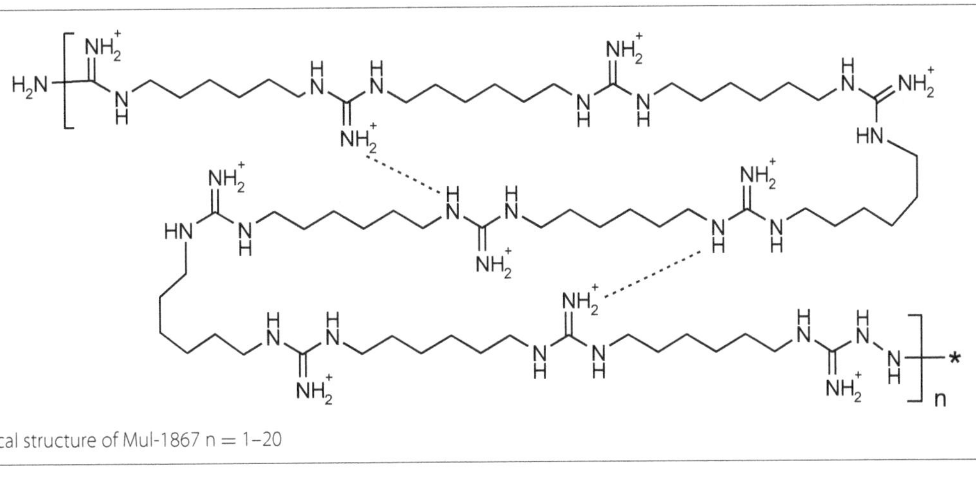

Fig. 1 Chemical structure of Mul-1867 n = 1–20

Table 1 Bactericidal activities of Mul-1867 and other antibacterials against non-mucoid *P. aeruginosa* isolates

Antibacterials	Susceptibility breakpoint (μg/mL)	*P. aeruginosa* strain minimal inhibitory concentration (μg/mL)			
		AGR14	MR 45	VT-VAP-72	ATCC 27853
Mul-1867	ND[a]	8	8	4	1
Amikacin	≤16	128	256	128	4
Aztreonam	≤8	32	128	64	2
Ceftazidime	≤8	32	32	16	2
Meropenem	≤2	32	64	32	1
Piperacillin	≤16	>256	256	128	4
Tobramycin	≤4	32	32	32	1

[a] *ND* no data

In vitro antimicrobial susceptibility testing

The MICs for antimicrobials were determined by the broth macrodilution method according to CLSI guideline [22, 23]. A standard bacterial inoculum of 5 × 10^5 colony forming units (CFU)/mL was used. Serial twofold dilutions of the antimicrobials were prepared in cation-adjusted MHB. The MIC was defined as the lowest concentration of antibiotic that completely inhibited visible growth. Experiments were conducted in triplicate.

Effect of Mul-1867 against *P. aeruginosa* biofilms

In each well of a 96-well flat-bottom polystyrene tissue culture microtiter plate (Sarstedt, Numbrecht, Germany), 200 μL of a standardized *P. aeruginosa* inoculum (5 × 10^5 CFU/mL) in cation-adjusted MHB were added. Following a 24 h incubation period at 37 °C, biofilm samples were washed twice with phosphate-buffered saline to remove non-adherent bacteria and then exposed for 24 h to 200 μL of MHB containing Mul-1867 at 1-, 2-, 4-, 8-, 16-, 32-, and 64-fold the MIC. Untreated biofilms were used as the negative controls. After the exposure, well contents were aspirated to prevent antimicrobial carryover and each well was washed three times with sterile deionized water.

To estimate the CFU number, biofilms were scraped thoroughly, with particular attention paid to the well edges [11]. The well contents were aspirated, placed in 1 mL of isotonic phosphate buffer (0.15 M, pH 7.2), and the total CFU number was determined by serial dilution and plating on Mueller-Hinton agar.

The MBECs were determined as the concentrations of drug that killed 50 % ($MBEC_{50}$), 90 % ($MBEC_{90}$), and 100 % ($MBEC_{100}$) of the bacteria in preformed biofilms compared to the untreated control (100 % viability). MBEC sensitivities were determined using the 2012 Clinical and Laboratory Standards Institute guidelines for interpretation [23]. Tests were performed in triplicate on three separate occasions, and the results were averaged.

Cytotoxicity assay

Cytotoxicity of Mul-1867 on Madin-Darby canine kidney (MDCK) cells was determined by the microculture tetrazolium (MTT) assay. Briefly, cells (1 × 10^5/well) were plated in 100 μL of minimal essential media in 96-well plates and incubated overnight in a 5 % CO_2 atmosphere. Serial dilutions of Mul-1867, with final concentrations corresponding to a range of 8–256 μg/mL, were added to the cells that were then incubated at 37 °C for a further 24 h. Control wells were treated with sterile water. MTT analysis was then performed based on the standard method [24].

After incubation, an aliquot of [3-(4,5-Dimethylthiazol-2-yl)-2,5-diphenyltetrazolium bromide] solution (Sigma-Aldrich, St. Louis, MO, USA) at 0.5 mg/mL was added to each well, and following a further 30 min incubation at 37 °C, the medium was discarded and the formazan blue formed in the cells was dissolved with 100 μL of dimethyl sulfoxide. Absorbance at 570 nm was determined with a microplate reader (Stat-Fax-2100, Awareness Technology Inc, USA). The absorbance of the formazan formed in non-treated cells was considered 100 % viability.

Statistical analyses

Results of the cytotoxicity assay are presented as mean ± standard deviation of three independent experiments. All statistical analyses were performed using the statistics package Statistica for Windows (version 5.0). Results are reported as the mean ± standard error for each group. Non-parametric paired Wilcoxon signed rank test was applied to analyse pre- and post-challenge differences. $P < 0.05$ was considered significant.

Results

In vitro antimicrobial susceptibility testing of *P. aeruginosa* isolates

The MICs of Mul-1867 and other antibiotics against non-mucoid *P. aeruginosa* isolates are shown in Table 1.

Mul-1867 exhibited significant activity against all isolates that were resistant to amikacin, aztreonam, ceftazidime, meropenem, piperacillin, and tobramycin according to CLSI criteria, as well as against susceptible and control strains.

Of the seven MDR-PA isolates, three had the mucoid phenotype that is widespread among CF patients and is associated with reduced success of treatment. Mul-1867 exhibited a high level of antimicrobial activity against mucoid MDR-PA strains irrespective of their resistance to other antibiotics (Table 2) [25, 26].

There was no statistically significant difference between the activity of Mul-1867 against the mucoid vs. non-mucoid *P. aeruginosa* strains. The MIC values ranged from 1 to 8 μg/mL for the non-mucoid strains, and from 2 to 4 μg/mL for the mucoid strains.

Effect of Mul-1867 against preformed *P. aeruginosa* biofilms

The anti-biofilm activity of Mul-1867 against 24-h-old *P. aeruginosa* biofilms was analyzed to reveal possible differences in susceptibility patterns between non-mucoid and mucoid *P. aeruginosa* strains. The activity of Mul-1867 on mature biofilms, tested at concentrations equal to a multiple of the MIC, is summarized in Table 3. After 24 h of growth, the CFUs of *P. aeruginosa* AGR14 and *P. aeruginosa* VT-CF-234 biofilms were 1.8×10^8 CFU/mL and 3.5×10^8 CFU/mL, respectively.

A comparison between the MIC and MBEC values indicated that Mul-1867 was a highly active antimicrobial exhibiting dose-dependent effects against the *P. aeruginosa* strains tested. Mul-1867 showed $MBEC_{50}$ and $MBEC_{90}$ values of 1- and 4-fold the MIC, respectively, against a non-mucoid strain. Mul-1867 displayed comparable activity against a mucoid strain with $MBEC_{50}$ and $MBEC_{90}$ values of 1- and twofold the MIC, respectively.

Table 2 Minimal inhibitory concentrations of Mul-1867 and other antibacterials against mucoid *P. aeruginosa* isolates

Antibacterials	Susceptibility breakpoint (μg/mL)	*P. aeruginosa* strain minimal inhibitory concentration (μg/ml)		
		SEV 7	VT-CF-234	VT-COPD-274
Mul-1867	ND[a]	2	2	4
Amikacin	≤16	128	64	256
Aztreonam	≤8	64	64	128
Ceftazidime	≤8	2	32	32
Piperacillin	≤16	2	64	128
Meropenem	≤2	32	8	16
Tobramycin	≤4	16	128	64

[a] *ND* No data

Table 3 Susceptibility results of Mul-1867 against *P. aeruginosa* strains

Isolate	Mucoid	$MBEC_{50}$ (μg/mL)	$MBEC_{90}$ (μg/mL)	$MBEC_{100}$ (μg/mL)
P. aeruginosa AGR14	No	8	32	256
P. aeruginosa VT-CF-234	Yes	2	4	32

MBEC minimum biofilm eliminating concentrations

Reduction in cell numbers by 90 % suggested that Mul-1867 has the potential for biofilm eradication, which is an important goal in antimicrobial treatment. Thus, we determined the $MBEC_{100}$ after treatment of *P. aeruginosa* biofilms with Mul-1867 for 24 h.

In this assay, Mul-1867 completely eradicated mature *P. aeruginosa* biofilms at the concentrations tested, with $MBEC_{100}$ values of 32- and 16-fold the MIC for the AGR14 and VT-CF-234 strains, respectively. The ability to eradicate a biofilm at a concentration eightfold higher than that required to reduce biofilm bacteria by 90 % suggested that Mul-1867 possesses significant anti-biofilm activity.

Cell cytotoxicity of Mul-1867

The compound did not exhibit any statistically significant cytotoxicity against MDCK cells at concentrations ranging from 8 to 256 μg/mL, as tested by the MTT assay 24 h after challenging with Mul-1867 (Fig. 2).

Discussion

P. aeruginosa presents substantial problems for patients with CF, and is a major predictor of morbidity [27]. For the last decade, the emergence of MDR-PA strains has posed treatment challenges in patients with COPD and VAP [28]. In the current study, we found that a novel

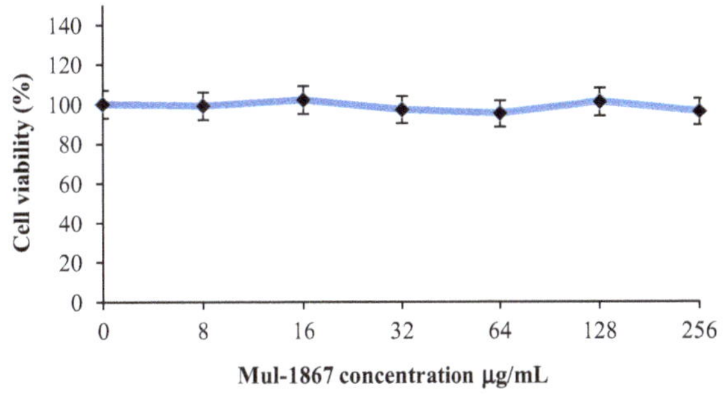

Fig. 2 Cytotoxic effect of Mul-1867 on Madin-Darby canine kidney cell lines as determined by the microculture tetrazolium assay

drug candidate, Mul-1867, exhibits a high level of antimicrobial activity against both MDR and susceptible clinical isolates of *P. aeruginosa* from patients with life-threatening lung infections.

We showed previously that Mul-1867 is a fast-acting antimicrobial whose mechanism of action involves a nonspecific attack on the bacterial cell wall that causes leakage of cell contents [20]. Mucoid strains lead to the persistence of *P. aeruginosa* infections. The data available in the literature concerning the effect of mucoidity on antimicrobial susceptibility show some differences depending on the type of antibiotic being tested [29]. Our data indicate that there is no cross-resistance between amikacin, aztreonam, ceftazidime, meropenem, piperacillin, and tobramycin vs. Mul-1867 against susceptible and MDR-PA strains tested in this study.

P. aeruginosa biofilms respond poorly to treatment with existing medicines due to the presence of additional barriers including a surface film or extracellular polymeric substances that reduce antibiotic penetration [30]. Biofilms formed by MDR-PA are almost completely insensitive to treatment with antibiotics that have high MBEC values that cannot be achieved at the site of infection using currently recommended dosages, or even with local administration directly to the site of infection [31]. There are also reports that biofilms formed by some strains of *P. aeruginosa* cannot be eradicated at any concentration of antibiotics that are commonly used for therapy. Importantly, however, Mul-1867 was equally effective against mucoid and non-mucoid *P. aeruginosa* strains.

The $MBEC_{90}$/MIC ratio is an important parameter for choosing the best antibacterial to treat *P. aeruginosa* biofilm-associated infections (lower is better). Our studies revealed that Mul-1867 possessed low $MBEC_{90}$/MIC ratios (between two and four). Moreover, biofilms formed by both non-mucoid and mucoid *P. aeruginosa* strains were totally eradicated with Mul-1867 at concentrations of 32- and 16-fold the MIC, respectively.

Positively charged antibiotics bind to extracellular polymeric substance and extracellular DNA, which decreases their bioavailability [30]. Mul-1867 is a positively charged molecule, and its antimicrobial activity was also reduced by the biofilm's components. However, its activity level remained high enough to achieve total eradication of biofilms.

Cell viability assessed by the MTT assay revealed that Mul-1867 did not display cytotoxic effects at the tested concentrations (between 8 to 256 μg/mL). The absence of apparent toxicity to MDCK cells at the highest concentration of Mul-1867 that was used against the least sensitive *P. aeruginosa* strain tested in this study (AGR14) is a notable attribute of this topical antimicrobial compound.

The high levels of Mul-1867 activity against the clinical isolates tested in this study are consistent with those found in our previous work [20]. This demonstrates the broad antimicrobial activity of this molecule against planktonic and sessile gram-positive and gram-negative bacteria. The efficacy of Mul-1867 against both non-mucoid and mucoid strains of *P. aeruginosa* raises the possibility that it may serve as a locally acting antimicrobial compound and may be able to successfully eradicate biofilm infections caused by *P. aeruginosa*.

Abbreviations

CF: cystic fibrosis; CFU: colony forming units; CLSI: Clinical and Laboratory Standards Institute; COPD: chronic obstructive pulmonary disease; MBEC: minimum biofilm eliminating concentrations; MDCK: madin-Darby canine kidney; MDR-PA: multidrug-resistant *Pseudomonas aeruginosa*; MHB: Mueller–Hinton broth; MIC: minimal inhibitory concentration; VAP: ventilator-associated pneumonia.

Authors' contributions

Conceived and designed the experiments VT GT. Performed the experiments: VT DV GT. Analyzed the data: VT GT. Contributed reagents/materials/analysis tools: VT DV GT. Contributed to the writing of the manuscript: GT. All authors read and approved the final manuscript.

Author details

[1] TGV-Laboratories LLC, 303 5th avenue, # 2012, New York, NY 10016, USA.
[2] Institute of Human Microbiology, New York, NY 10016, USA.

Acknowledgements

The authors thank Jane Burns and Adam Griffith from Seattle Children's Research Institute for generously supplying the clinical isolates.

Competing interests

The authors declare that they have no competing interests.

References

1. Garcia-Vidal C, Almagro P, Romaní V, Rodríguez-Carballeira M, Cuchi E, Canales L, Garau J, et al. *Pseudomonas aeruginosa* in patients hospitalised for COPD exacerbation: a prospective study. Eur Respir J. 2009;34:1072–8.
2. Folkesson A, Jelsbak L, Yang L, Johansen HK, Ciofu O, Hoiby N, et al. Adaptation of *Pseudomonas aeruginosa* to the cystic fibrosis airway: an evolutionary perspective. Nat Rev Microbiol. 2012;10:841–51.
3. Peña C, Gómez-Zorrilla S, Oriol I, Tubau F, Dominguez MA, Pujol M, et al. Impact of multidrug resistance on *Pseudomonas aeruginosa* ventilator-associated pneumonia outcome: predictors of early and crude mortality. Eur J Clin Microbiol Infect Dis. 2013;32:413–20.
4. Saiman L, Marshall BC, Mayer-Hamblett N, Burns JL, Quittner AL, Cibene DA, et al. Azithromycin in patients with cystic fibrosis chronically infected with *Pseudomonas aeruginosa*: a randomized controlled trial. JAMA. 2003;290:1749–56.
5. Mowat E, Paterson S, Fothergill JL, Wright EA, Ledson MJ, Walshaw MJ, et al. *Pseudomonas aeruginosa* population diversity and turnover in cystic fibrosis chronic infections. Am J Respir Crit Care Med. 2011;183:1674–9.
6. Schelstraete P, Haerynck F, Van daele S, Deseyne S, De Baets F. Eradication therapy for *Pseudomonas aeruginosa* colonization episodes in cystic fibrosis patients not chronically colonized by *P. aeruginosa*. J Cyst Fibros. 2013;12:1–8.

7. Domenech A, Puig C, Martí S, Santos S, Fernández A, Calatayud L, et al. Infectious etiology of acute exacerbations in severe COPD patients. J Infect. 2013;67:516–23.
8. Owlia P, Nosrati R, Alaghehbandan R, Lari AR. Antimicrobial susceptibility differences among mucoid and non-mucoid *Pseudomonas aeruginosa* isolates. GMS Hyg Infect Control. 2014;9:13.
9. Govan JR, Deretic V. Microbial pathogenesis in cystic fibrosis: mucoid *Pseudomonas aeruginosa* and *Burkholderia cepacia*. Microbiol Rev. 1996;60:539–74.
10. Costerton JW, Stewart PS, Greenberg EP. Bacterial biofilms: a common cause of persistent infections. Science. 1999;284:1318–22.
11. Tetz GV, Artemenko NK, Tetz VV. Effect of DNase and antibiotics on biofilm characteristics. Antimicrob Agents Chemother. 2009;53:1204–9.
12. Lopes SP, Ceri H, Azevedo NF, Pereira MO. Antibiotic resistance of mixed biofilms in cystic fibrosis: impact of emerging microorganisms on treatment of infection. Int J Antimicrob Agents. 2012;40:260–3.
13. Tetz VV, Korobov VP, Artemenko NK, Lemkina LM, Panjkova NV, Tetz GV. Extracellular phospholipids of isolated bacterial communities. Biofilms. 2004;1:149–55.
14. Hall-Stoodley L, Costerton JW, Stoodley P. Bacterial biofilms: from the natural environment to infectious diseases. Nat Rev Microbiol. 2004;2:95–108.
15. Breidenstein EB, de la Fuente-Núñez C, Hancock RE. *Pseudomonas aeruginosa*: all roads lead to resistance. Trends Microbiol. 2011;19:419–26.
16. Rodríguez-Martínez JM, Pascual A. Antimicrobial resistance in bacterial biofilms. Rev Med Microbiol. 2006;17:65–75.
17. Döring G, Flume P, Heijerman H, Elborn JS. Consensus Study Group. Treatment of lung infection in patients with cystic fibrosis: current and future strategies. J Cyst Fibros. 2012;11:461–79.
18. Morosini MI, García-Castillo M, Loza E, Pérez-Vázquez M, Baquero F, Cantón R. Breakpoints for predicting *Pseudomonas aeruginosa* susceptibility to inhaled tobramycin in cystic fibrosis patients: use of high-range Etest strips. J Clin Microbiol. 2005;43:4480–5.
19. Reiter KC, Sambrano GE, Villa B, Paim T, Oliveira C, d'Azevedo PA. Rifampicin fails to eradicate mature biofilm formed by methicillin-resistant *Staphylococcus aureus*. Rev Soc Bras Med Trop. 2012;45:471–4.
20. Tetz G, Tetz V. *In vitro* antimicrobial activity of a novel compound, Mul-1867, against clinically important bacteria. Antimicrob Resist Infect Control. 2015;4:45.
21. Clinical and Laboratory Standards Institute. Performance standards for antimicrobial susceptibility testing. Twenty-first informational supplement (M100-S21). Clinical and Laboratory Standards Institute, Wayne; 2011.
22. Clinical and Laboratory Standards Institute. Methods for determining bactericidal activity of antimicrobial agents; approved guideline (M26-A). Wayne: Clinical and Laboratory Standards Institute; 1999.
23. Clinical and Laboratory Standards Institute. Methods for dilution antimicrobial susceptibility tests for bacteria that grow aerobically; approved standard, ninth edition (M07-A9). Wayne: Clinical and Laboratory Standards Institute; 2012.
24. Sieuwerts AM, Klijn JG, Peters HA, Foekens JA. The MTT tetrazolium salt assay scrutinized: how to use this assay reliably to measure metabolic activity of cell cultures in vitro for the assessment of growth characteristics, IC50-values and cell survival. Eur J Clin Chem Clin Biochem. 1995;33:813–23.
25. Mayer-Hamblett N, Rosenfeld M, Gibson RL, Ramsey BW, Kulasekara HD, Retsch-Bogart GZ, et al. *Pseudomonas aeruginosa* in vitro phenotypes distinguish cystic fibrosis infection stages and outcomes. Am J Respir Crit Care Med. 2014;190:289–97.
26. Lam JC, Somayaji R, Surette MG, Rabin HR, Parkins MD. Reduction in *Pseudomonas aeruginosa* sputum density during a cystic fibrosis pulmonary exacerbation does not predict clinical response. BMC Infect Dis. 2015;15:145.
27. Flume PA, VanDevanter DR. Clinical applications of pulmonary delivery of antibiotics. Adv Drug Deliv Rev. 2015;85:1–6.
28. Fricks-Lima J, Hendrickson CM, Allgaier M, Zhuo H, Wiener-Kronish JP, Lynch SV, et al. Differences in biofilm formation and antimicrobial resistance of *Pseudomonas aeruginosa* isolated from airways of mechanically ventilated patients and cystic fibrosis patients. Int J Antimicrob Agents. 2011;37:309–15.
29. Schülin T. In vitro activity of the aerosolized agents colistin and tobramycin and five intravenous agents against *Pseudomonas aeruginosa* isolated from cystic fibrosis patients in southwestern Germany. J Antimicrob Chemother. 2002;49:403–6.
30. Messiaen AS, Nelis H, Coenye T. Investigating the role of matrix components in protection of *Burkholderia cepacia* complex biofilms against tobramycin. J Cyst Fibros. 2014;13:56–62.
31. Hengzhuang W, Ciofu O, Yang L, Wu H, Song Z, Oliver A, et al. High β-lactamase levels change the pharmacodynamics of β-lactam antibiotics in *Pseudomonas aeruginosa* biofilms. Antimicrob Agents Chemother. 2013;57:196–204.

The spread of bla_{OXA-48} and $bla_{OXA-244}$ carbapenemase genes among *Klebsiella pneumoniae*, *Proteus mirabilis* and *Enterobacter* spp. isolated in Moscow, Russia

Nadezhda K. Fursova[1*], Eugeny I. Astashkin[1], Anastasia I. Knyazeva[1], Nikolay N. Kartsev[1], Ekaterina S. Leonova[1], Olga N. Ershova[2], Irina A. Alexandrova[2], Natalia V. Kurdyumova[2], Svetlana Yu. Sazikina[2], Nikolay V. Volozhantsev[1], Edward A. Svetoch[1] and Ivan A. Dyatlov[1]

Abstract

Background: The spread of carbapenemase-producing *Enterobacteriaceae* (CPE) is a great problem of healthcare worldwide. Study of the spread for $bla_{OXA-48-like}$ genes coding epidemically significant carbapenemases among hospital pathogens is important for the regional and global epidemiology of antimicrobial resistance.

Methods: Antibacterial resistant isolates of *Klebsiella pneumoniae* (n = 95) from 54 patients, *P. mirabilis* (n = 32) from 20 patients, *Enterobacter aerogenes* (n = 6) from four patients, and *Enterobacter cloacae* (n = 4) from four patients were collected from January, 2013 to October, 2014 in neurosurgical intensive care unit (ICU) of the Burdenko Neurosurgery Institute, Moscow. Characteristics of the isolates were done using susceptibility tests, PCR detection of the resistance genes, genotyping, conjugation, DNA sequencing, and bioinformatic analysis.

Results: Major strains under study were multi drug resistant (MDR), resistant to three or more functional classes of drugs simultaneously—98.9 % *K. pneumoniae*, 100 % *P. mirabilis*, one *E. aerogenes* isolate, and one *E. cloacae* isolate. Molecular-genetic mechanism of MDR in *K. pneumoniae* and *P. mirabilis* isolates were based on carrying of epidemic extended-spectrum beta-lactamase $bla_{CTX-M-15}$ gene (87.2 and 90.6 % accordingly), carbapenemase $bla_{OXA-48-like}$ gene (55.3 and 23.3 % accordingly), and class 1 (54.8 and 31.3 % accordingly) and class 2 (90.6 % *P. mirabilis*) integrons. The $bla_{OXA-48-like}$-positive *K. pneumoniae* were collected during whole two-year surveillance period, while *P. mirabilis* and *Enterobacter* spp. carrying $bla_{OXA-48-like}$ genes were detected only after four and 18 months after the research start, respectively. The $bla_{OXA-48-like}$ gene acquisition was shown for *P. mirabilis* isolates collected from five patients and for *E. cloacae* isolate collected from one patient during their stay in the ICU, presumably from $bla_{OXA-48-like}$-positive *K. pneumoniae*. The source of the $bla_{OXA-244}$ gene acquired by *E. aerogenes* isolates and the time of this event were not recognized.

Conclusions: The expanding of CPE in the surveyed ICU was associated with the spread of bla_{OXA-48} and $bla_{OXA-244}$ carbapenemase genes documented not only among *K. pneumoniae*, well-known bacterial host for such genes, but among *P. mirabilis*, *E. aerogenes*, and *E. cloacae*.

Keywords: *Enterobacteriaceae*, *Klebsiella pneumoniae*, *Proteus mirabilis*, *Enterobacter aerogenes*, *Enterobacter cloacae*, OXA-48-like carbapenemase, Hospital pathogens, Antibacterial resistance, Horizontal gene transfer

*Correspondence: n-fursova@yandex.ru
[1] State Research Center for Applied Microbiology and Biotechnology, Obolensk, 142279 Moscow Region, Russia
Full list of author information is available at the end of the article

Background

One of the main problems of healthcare worldwide is hospital-acquired infections (HAI) caused by multi drug resistant (MDR) pathogens [1, 2] including carbapenemase-producing *Enterobacteriaceae* (CPE) [3]. The spread of CPE over the last decades is a great danger because carbapenems are the last treatment options for infections caused by MDR bacteria. Recently carbapenemases belonged to three Ambler-classes of beta-lactamases [4] were reported from CPE isolated in Russia: the KPC-type (class A), the NDM-type (class B), and the OXA-48-type (class D) [5]. The OXA-48 carbapenamase is enzyme that was first identified in *Klebsiella pneumoniae* clinical strains isolated in Turkey, 2003 [6]. Currently OXA-48-producers are described among many species of enterobacteria: *K. pneumoniae, Escherichia coli, Enterobacter cloacae, Citrobacter freundii, Serratia marcescens, Morganella morganii* and *Proteus mirabilis* [7–9]. The endemic areas of OXA-48-producers are Turkey, the North Africa and India. Nosocomial outbreaks caused by OXA-48-producers are registered in many European countries including France, Germany, Switzerland, Spain, Holland, and Great Britain. Sporadic cases of such infections are observed in North and South America, China, Australia, and in the Middle East countries [10]. Wide spread of $bla_{\text{OXA-48}}$-like genes among enterobacteria is explained by their localization on the 62 kb conjugative plasmid belonged to IncL/M incompatibility group. Such plasmids are characterized by a high rate of transfer and a wide range of hosts. Their high conjugative potential is due to inactivation of *tir* gene coding the repressor of conjugative plasmid transfer, by the inserting of the composite transposon Tn1991/Tn1991.2 carrying the $bla_{\text{OXA-48-like}}$ gene [11]. In several studies is shown that $bla_{\text{OXA-48}}$-carrying plasmids provide the ability of both clonal and horizontal transfer [7]. There are several variants of $bla_{\text{OXA-48-like}}$ genes coding enzymes differ from each other on some amino acid substitutions [12]. For instance, the $bla_{\text{OXA-244}}$ gene discovered in Spain in 2013 differs from the $bla_{\text{OXA-48}}$ gene in a single nucleotide substitution A640G that result in a single amino acid substitution Arg214Gly [13]. It should be noted that carbapenemase activity of all OXA-48-like enzymes are low, so they cannot provide the high levels of carbapenem resistance without additional contribution of other factors such as porin mutations resulting in decrease of cell wall permeability [14].

In this paper we present phenotypic and genotypic characterization of antibacterial resistant *K. pneumoniae, Proteus mirabilis, Enterobacter aerogenes*, and *E. cloacae* isolates carrying $bla_{\text{OXA-48}}$ and $bla_{\text{OXA-244}}$ carbapenemase genes, and discuss *K. pneumoniae* as possibly source for $bla_{\text{OXA-48-like}}$ genes spreading in the ICU.

Methods

Bioethical requirements

The materials used in the work do not contain personal data of patients, because of clinical isolates were marked without name, date of birth, address, number of the disease history, personal documents and other personal materials. At the same time, in accordance with the Requirements of the Russian Federation Bioethical Committee, each patient signed a contract with hospital at admission to the clinic. The contract contained consent to treatment and laboratory examination, including a detailed investigation using instrumental methods.

Bacterial isolates

Antibacterial resistant hospital isolates of *Klebsiella pneumoniae* (n = 95) from 54 patients, *Proteus mirabilis* (n = 32) from 20 patients, *Enterobacter aerogenes* (n = 6) from 4 patients, and *Enterobacter cloacae* (n = 4) from 4 patients with mechanical ventilation in neurosurgical intensive care unit (ICU) of the Burdenko Neurosurgery Institute, Moscow, were collected from January, 2013 to October, 2014. Bacterial cultures were grown on the Nutrient Medium No. 1 (SRCAMB, Obolensk, Russia), Luria–Bertani (LB) broth (Difco, USA) and Muller-Hinton broth (Himedia, India) at 37 °C. Bacterial isolates were stored in 10 % glycerol at minus 70 °C.

Bacterial identification

Bacterial identification was done by Vitek-2 Compact (BioMerieux, France) and MALDI-TOF Biotyper (Bruker Daltonik, Germany).

Susceptibility to antibacterial agents

Minimal inhibitory concentrations (MICs) of antibacterials were determined by Vitek-2 device (BioMerieux, France) using VITEK-2 AST N-101 and AST N-102 cards: amoxicillin/clavulanic acid (AMC), ampicillin/sulbactam (SAM), cefuroxime (CXM), cefoxitin (FOX), cefotaxime (CTX), ceftriaxone (CRO), ceftazidime (CAZ), cefoperazone/sulbactam (CFS), cefepime (FEP), ertapenem (ETP), imipenem (IPM), meropenem (MEM), tetracycline (TET), tigecycline (TGC), ciprofloxacin (CIP), chloramphenicol (CHL), gentamicin (GEN), tobramycin (TOB), amikacin (AMK), trimethoprim (TMP), trimethoprim/sulfamethoxazole (SXT), nitrofurantoin (NIT), and colistin (CST). Results were interpreted according to the 2014 European Committee on Antimicrobial Susceptibility Testing Recommendations (http://www.eucast.org/clinical_breakpoints/). *E. coli* strains ATCC 25922 and ATCC 35218 were used for quality control.

Conjugation experiment

Conjugation was performed using previously described method [15]. Donor and recipient overnight cultures were grown under aeration conditions at 120 rpm/min during 18 h at 37 °C on LB broth containing 100 mg/L cefotaxime (Sigma, USA) for donor strain, and 200 mg/L rifampicin (Sigma, USA) for recipient strain. Five milliliters of fresh LB broth without antibiotic were inoculated by 0.05 ml overnight cultures and incubated with aeration to $OD_{600} = 0.6$. Then 1 ml each donor and recipient cultures were combined into one tube and incubated at 37 °C for 3 h without shaking. After that the conjugating mixture was diluted with tenfold steps and 0.1 ml was plated in triplicate on LB agar containing 100 mg/L cefotaxime and 200 mg/L rifampicin. Bacteria were incubated at 37 °C for 48 h. To determine the efficiency of conjugation the conjugation mixture was inoculated in parallel on cefotaxime + rifampicin and rifampicin. Frequency of plasmid transfer was calculated as the number of transconjugant cells per number of recipient cells.

PCR detection of the resistance genes

PCR was performed using previously described oligonucleotide primers to detect $bla_{CTX\text{-}M}$, bla_{TEM}, bla_{SHV}, $bla_{OXA\text{-}48\text{-}like}$, bla_{NDM}, bla_{KPC} beta-lactamase genes and class 1 and 2 integrons [16–21], *repA* and *traU* genes which are the genetic markers of the IncL/M plasmid [22], and the *ompK36* gene [23]. The PCR was carried using GradientPalmCycler (Corbert Research, Australia) and Thercyc cycler (DNA-Technology, Russia). PCR products were analysed by electrophoresis in 1.5 % agarose gel in a Sub-Cell GT apparatus (BioRad, USA).

Strain genotyping

Intra-species genotyping of *K. pneumoniae*, *P. mirabilis*, and *Enterobacter* spp. strains was done by Random Amplified Polymorphic DNA (RAPD-PCR) using «random» primers OPA11 and Wil 2 accordingly previously described method [24].

DNA sequencing

Cycle sequencing reactions were performed using the ABI PRISM BigDye Terminator v.3.1 kit. Purified products were analysed on an ABI PRISM 3100-Avant automated DNA Sequencer in the SINTOL Center for collective use (Moscow, Russia).

Bioinformatic analysis

A computer analysis of DNA sequences was performed using Vector NTI9 software (Invitrogen, USA) and BLAST web resource (http://blast.ncbi.nlm.nih.gov/Blast.cgi). Class 1 and 2 integrons were analysed using INTEGRAL database (http://integrall.bio.ua.pt/?).

GenBank accession numbers

The accession numbers of *K. pneumoniae* DNA sequences are follows: 27 $bla_{CTX\text{-}M\text{-}15}$ genes [GenBank: KJ187476, KJ187477, KM058748, KM058751, KM058752, KJ469366, KC817480, KJ363319, KJ363321, KJ481796, KM085432, KM871847, KP205559, KP205560, KP205561, KP205562, KP205563, KP214528, KP214529, KP214530, KP214531, KP214532, KP214533, KP214534, KP214535, KP214536, KP214537]; one $bla_{CTX\text{-}M\text{-}3}$ gene [GenBank: KP214538]; 16 $bla_{OXA\text{-}48}$ genes [GenBank: KJ481797, KJ481798, KM085437, KP100448, KP100449, KP198287, KP198288, KP198289, KP198290, KP198291, KP198292, KP198293, KP198294, KP205554, KP205555, KP205556]; four $bla_{OXA\text{-}244}$ genes [GenBank: KJ187475, KJ481795, KJ481799, KM058746]; six class 1 integron gene cassettes arrays [GenBank: KJ363320, KM009101, KF952266, KM009102, KC862254, KF971879]; three *ompC* genes [GenBank: KJ469369,KJ579290, KJ579291]; one *ompK36* gene [GenBank: KJ579289].

The accession numbers of *P. mirabilis* nucleotide sequences are follows: 10 $bla_{CTX\text{-}M\text{-}15}$ genes [GenBank: KM009108, KM058749, KM058750, KC822920, KJ633803, KM085431, KM085433, KM085435, KM085436, KP271997]; one $bla_{CTX\text{-}M\text{-}3}$ gene [GenBank: KM871848]; six $bla_{OXA\text{-}48}$ genes [GenBank: KJ579286, KJ696733, KM058747, KP205551, KP205552, KP205553]; one $bla_{OXA\text{-}244}$ gene [GenBank: KJ579285]; one class 1 integron gene cassettes array [GenBank: KM085438]; four class 2 integron gene cassettes arrays [GenBank: KJ579284, KM085439, KM085440, KP271998].

The accession numbers of *E. aerogenes* nucleotide sequences are follows: three $bla_{OXA\text{-}244}$ genes [GenBank: KM357271, KP056309, KP205557]; the accession number of *E. cloacae* nucleotide sequence is one $bla_{OXA\text{-}48}$ gene [GenBank: KP056311].

Results and discussion

Isolate sources and resistance phenotypes

Antibacterial resistant enterobacterial hospital isolates collected on the period of January, 2013 to October, 2014 from the patients with mechanical ventilation in neurosurgical intensive care unit (ICU) of the Burdenko Neurosurgery Institute, Moscow, belonged to *Klebsiella pneumoniae* (n = 95), *Proteus mirabilis* (n = 32), *Enterobacter aerogenes* (n = 6), *Enterobacter cloacae* (n = 4), *Escherichia coli* (n = 4), *Serratia marcescens* (n = 3), and *Morganella morganii* (n = 2). Carriers of OXA-48-like genes have been identified among them: 52 *K. pneumoniae*, 7 *P. mirabilis*, 3 *E. aerogenes*, and 1 *E. cloacae* isolates.

K. pneumoniae isolates were predominantly collected from respiratory system—endotracheal aspirate, bronchial lavage, and maxillary sinus (46.3 %), fewer isolates were obtained from the urine (40.0 %), wounds (6.3 %), lumbar and ventricular liquor (4.2 %), blood (2.1 %) and rectal swab (1.1 %). The major *P. mirabilis* isolates were isolated from urine (65.6 %), fewer isolates were obtained from the respiratory system (25.0 %), wounds (6.3 %) and blood (3.1 %). *E. aerogenes* isolates were collected from liquor (n = 5) and endotracheal aspirate (n = 1). *E. cloacae* isolates were collected from endotracheal aspirate (n = 3) and urine (n = 1). Major antibacterial resistant bacteria were collected from the respiratory system and from the urine and were associated with invasive equipment and instruments, namely mechanical ventilation and urinary catheters.

The most *K. pneumoniae* and *P. mirabilis* isolates in this study were resistant to the majority of used antibacterial agents: AMC, SAM, CXM, CTX, CRO, CIP, CHL, GEN, TOB, TMP, SXT and NIT. Additionally, the *K. pneumoniae* isolates were resistant to FOX, CAZ, CFS, FEP, ETP, MEM and TET, and the *P. mirabilis* isolates were resistant to IPM, TET, TGC and CST (Fig. 1). It is noteworthy the high proportion of the pathogens were resistant to TGC (32.4 % *K. pneumoniae* and 50.0 % *P. mirabilis* isolates) and to CST (87.5 % *P. mirabilis* isolates), that are the drugs using for the treatment of severe hospital infections. So, only one antibiotic, CST remains good activity against *K. pneumoniae* (89.5 % isolates), and only three drugs, CFS (100 % isolates), ETP (100 % isolates) and CAZ (87.1 % isolates) were effective against *P. mirabilis* (Fig. 1). The antibacterials used in this study belong to the eight functional classes: beta-lactams (penicillins, cephalosporins, and carbapenems), tetracyclines, fluoroquinolones, phenicoles, aminoglycosides, polymyxins, sulfonamides, and nitrofurans. According to Magiorakos et al. [25] many strains under study were categorized as multi drug resistant (MDR) pathogens because of 98.9 % *K. pneumoniae* and 100 % *P. mirabilis* isolates were resistant to three or more functional classes of drugs simultaneously (Fig. 2). It should be noted that a large part of both *K. pneumoniae* (35.9 %) and *P. mirabilis* (54.8 %) strains were resistant to seven functional antibacterial classes. One *E. aerogenes* isolate was estimated as an extremely drug resistant because of resistance to all used antibiotics except TGC; three isolates were resistant to cefalosporins, carbapenems and NIT; two isolates were resistant to NIT only. Among *E. cloacae* isolates one isolate was MDR with sensitivity to IPM and AMK only; other isolates were resistant only to penicillins and cephalosporins.

Resistance genotypes

Detection of the $bla_{CTX\text{-}M}$, bla_{TEM}, bla_{SHV}, $bla_{OXA\text{-}48\text{-}like}$, bla_{NDM}, and bla_{KPC} beta-lactamase genes as well as class 1 and class 2 integrons in the genomes of the strains has been done for study of the resistance molecular genetic mechanisms (Fig. 3). The $bla_{CTX\text{-}M}$ genes were detected in 87.2 % *K. pneumoniae* and 90.6 % *P. mirabilis* isolates. Among 38 $bla_{CTX\text{-}M}$ genes major (n = 36) were

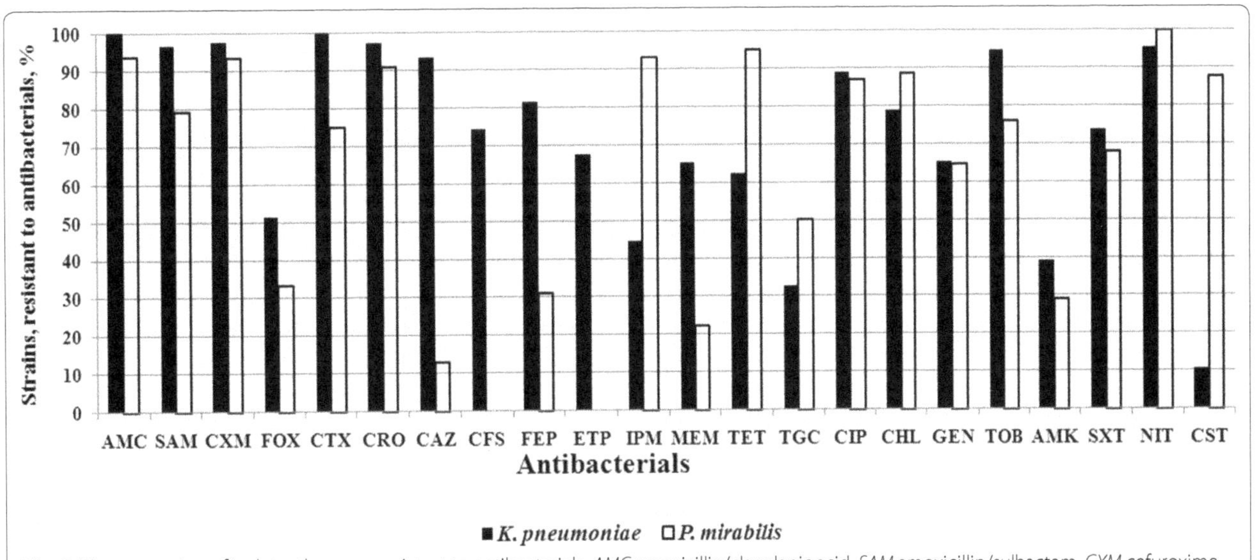

Fig. 1 The proportion of isolates those are resistant to antibacterials: *AMC* amoxicillin/clavulanic acid, *SAM* amoxicillin/sulbactam, *CXM* cefuroxime, *FOX* cefoxitin, *CTX* cefotaxime, *CRO* ceftriaxone, *CAZ* ceftazidime, *CFS* cefoperazone/sulbactam, *FEP* cefepime, *ETP* ertapenem, *IPM* imipenem, *MEM* meropenem, *TET* tetracycline, *TGC* tigecycline, *CIP* ciprofloxacin, *CHL* chloramphenicol, *GEN* gentamicin, *TOB* tobramycin, *AMK* amikacin, *TMP* trimethoprim, *SXT* trimethoprim/sulfamethoxazole, *NIT* nitrofurantoin, *CST* colistin

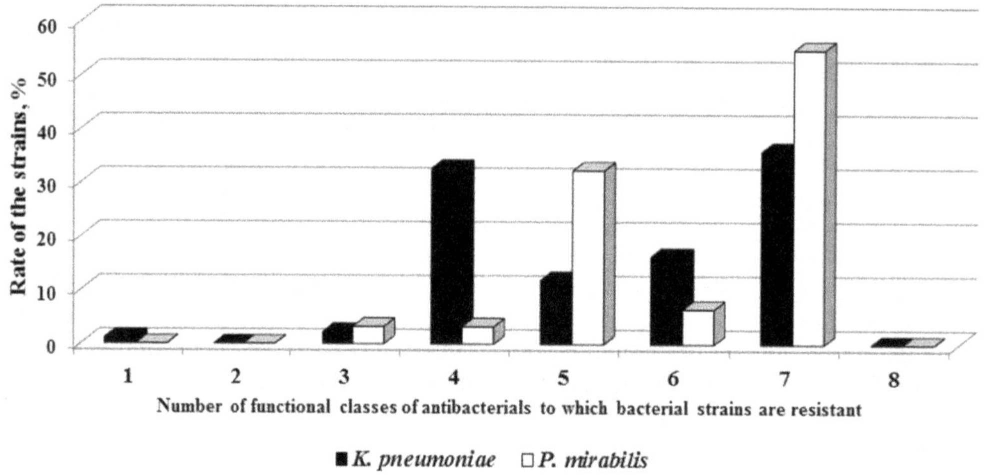

Fig. 2 The proportion of bacterial isolates those are resistant to 1–8 functional classes of antibacterials simultaneously: beta-lactams (penicillins, cephalosporins, and carbapenems) tetracyclines, quinolones, fenicoles, aminoglycosides, polymyxins, sulfonamides, nitrofuranam

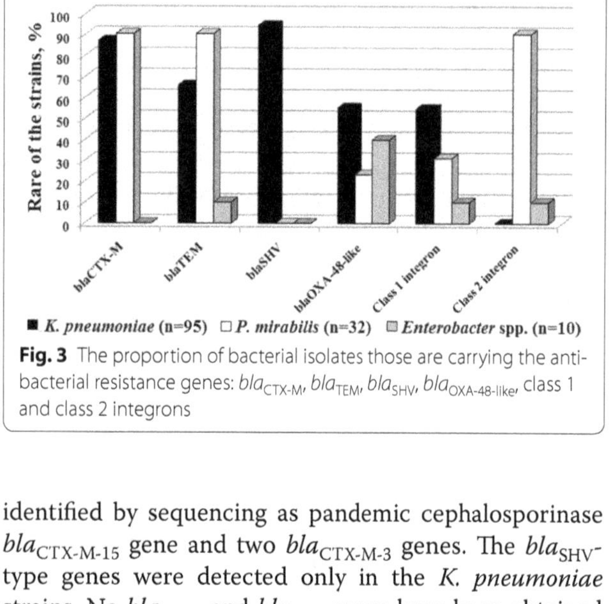

Fig. 3 The proportion of bacterial isolates those are carrying the antibacterial resistance genes: bla_{CTX-M}, bla_{TEM}, bla_{SHV}, $bla_{OXA-48-like}$, class 1 and class 2 integrons

identified by sequencing as pandemic cephalosporinase $bla_{CTX-M-15}$ gene and two $bla_{CTX-M-3}$ genes. The bla_{SHV}-type genes were detected only in the *K. pneumoniae* strains. No bla_{NDM} and bla_{KPC} genes have been obtained in our study. The $bla_{OXA-48-like}$ carbapenemase genes were detected in 55.3 % of *K. pneumoniae*, in 23.3 % of *P. mirabilis*, and in 20.0 % of *Enterobacter* spp. isolates. DNA sequencing of 28 $bla_{OXA-48-like}$ genes revealed two alleles: the bla_{OXA-48} gene was detected in *K. pneumoniae* (n = 17), *P. mirabilis* (n = 6) and *E. cloacae* (n = 1); the $bla_{OXA-244}$ gene was detected in *K. pneumoniae* (n = 4), *P. mirabilis* (n = 1) and *E. aerogenes* (n = 1).

Mobile genetic elements, class 1 integrons were detected in 54.8 % *K. pneumoniae* and in 31.3 % *P. mirabilis* isolates (Fig. 3). Variable regions of class 1 integrons identified in *K. pneumoniae* carried three types of the gene cassette array: (*dfrA1-orfC*), (*dfrA17-aadA5*), and (*dfrA12-orfF-aadA2*). The class 1 integrons detected in *P. mirabilis* carried only one type of the gene cassette array (*dfrA17-aadA5*). Class 2 integrons obtained in *P. mirabilis* (90.6 %) isolates carried a gene cassette array (*dfrA12-sat2-aadA1*). However, one class 1 integron and one class 2 integron revealed in *E. cloacae* and *E. cloacae* isolates respectively did not have any gene cassette arrays, that might be considered as a reserve for future accumulating of the resistance genes. The integron identification numbers have been obtained in accordance with the nomenclature described by Moura et al. [26] using a specialized database INTEGRAL. The (*dfrA1-orfC*) gene cassette array was attributed to the In263 integron, the (*dfrA17-aadA5*) array to the In392–395 integron, the (*dfrA12-orfF-aadA2*) array to the In27 integron, and the (*dfrA12-sat2-aadA1*) array to the In2–4 integron. According to the report of Partridge et al. from the University of Sydney, Australia, the vast majority of gene cassettes submitted into the GenBank database to date are extremely rare (presented less than 10 times), while a small group of gene cassettes are extremely frequent, they were named "successful" cassettes [27]. All gene cassettes identified in clinical isolates collected from the ICU in our study belong to this group of "successful" cassettes. Thus, on the date Feb 6, 2015, the *aadA1* cassette has been presented in the GenBank database 910 times, the *aadA2* cassette 601 times, the *aadA5* cassette 248 times, the *dfrA1* cassette 348 times, the *dfrA12* cassette 245 times, the *orfF* cassette 218 times, the *dfrA17* cassette 209 times, the *orfC* cassette 135 times, and the *sat2* cassette 79 times. These data suggest the high prevalence of the gene cassettes detected in our study among bacterial pathogens.

Since the permeability of bacterial cell wall is important for multi drug resistance [23], we carried out the detection of porin gene *ompK36* and obtained this gene in 92.4 % *K. pneumoniae* isolates.

Diversity of RAPD-genotypes

Great genetic heterogeneity of the pathogen populations was shown by RAPD-PCR genotyping for *K. pneumoniae* (n = 72) and *P. mirabilis* (n = 32). It was revealed 36 *K. pneumoniae* genotypes and 8 *P. mirabilis* genotypes. Four *K. pneumoniae* genotypes were prevalent in different periods of the study. The K23 genotype (n = 14) was major in 2013, while the K26 genotype (n = 5) was major in the first half of 2014, and the K30 (n = 6) and the K31 (n = 5) genotypes were prevalent in the second half of 2014. Interestingly, *K. pneumoniae* isolates belonged to K23, K26 and K31 genotypes carried the $bla_{\text{OXA-48-like}}$ genes, whereas isolates belonged to K30 genotype did not have these genes. Among all *P. mirabilis* isolates collected in our study, the P1 RAPD-PCR-genotype (n = 23) was prevalent. It is noteworthy that all *P. mirabilis* isolates carried $bla_{\text{OXA-48-like}}$ genes belonged to this prevalent genotype (Table 1). So, great variety of *K. pneumoniae* and *P. mirabilis* genotypes indicates no single source for dissemination of these pathogens. Perhaps presence of $bla_{\text{OXA-48-like}}$ genes in bacterial genome provides some populational advantage for certain genotypes. Two RAPD-genotypes (E1 and E2) were identified for *E. aerogenes* isolates, but all three $bla_{\text{OXA-244}}$-positive isolates were attributed to one genotype E1. Only one RAPD-genotype (E3) was determined for all *E. cloacae* isolates, including $bla_{\text{OXA-48}}$-positive one.

Spread of $bla_{\text{OXA-48-like}}$ genes in ICU

The case of the $bla_{\text{OXA-48}}$ gene acquisition by *K. pneumoniae* within ICU was demonstrated for the Patient K. The first isolate belonged to K29 genotype (May 21, 2013) had no the $bla_{\text{OXA-48}}$ gene; the next two isolates of K29 genotype (Oct 31, 2013 and Dec 12, 2013) have already acquired the $bla_{\text{OXA-48}}$ gene (Table 1; Fig. 4). The first case of the $bla_{\text{OXA-48}}$ gene emergence in a new bacterial host, *P. mirabilis*, was registered in the Patient H (Apr 08, 2013). It was happened four months after the start of the study, while such genes in *K. pneumoniae* isolates were detected during the entire two year period. Two months later, Jun 13, 2013, the $bla_{\text{OXA-244}}$ gene was identified in *P. mirabilis* isolate collected from the Patient C. Unfortunately, a retrospective epidemiological analysis has not allowed concluding relatedness of occurrence the $bla_{\text{OXA-244}}$ gene in Russia and in Spain where this gene was first described in 2013 [13]. The first case of the $bla_{\text{OXA-244}}$ gene emergence in a bacterial host *E. aerogenes* was registered in the Patient F (Jun 17, 2014), i.e. 18 months after the start of the study. The first case of the $bla_{\text{OXA-48}}$ gene identification in *E. cloacae* was obtained in the Patient O (Aug 30, 2014), i.e. 20 months after the start of the study. So, two $bla_{\text{OXA-48-like}}$ alleles have disseminated in the ICU simultaneously.

Comparative analysis of two or more *P. mirabilis* isolates collected from the same patient has been done for four patients: E, H, I, and J. All of these patients had no the $bla_{\text{OXA-48-like}}$ gene in their first isolates. The second isolates (Patients H and J) and the second and the third isolates (Patients E and I) carried the $bla_{\text{OXA-48-like}}$ genes. So, the $bla_{\text{OXA-48-like}}$ genes acquisition by *P. mirabilis* occurred in the ICU, presumably from $bla_{\text{OXA-48-like}}$-positive *K. pneumoniae* which is half of all *K. pneumoniae* isolates under study. Additional proof of this hypothesis is the concurrent isolation of $bla_{\text{OXA-244}}$-positive *K. pneumoniae* and *P. mirabilis* from urine of the Patient C (Fig. 4), as well as isolation of $bla_{\text{OXA-48}}$-positive *K. pneumoniae* and *E. cloacae* from endotracheal aspirate and urine correspondently of the Patient N. Unfortunately, such clear hypothesis cannot to explain the fact of the $bla_{\text{OXA-48}}$-positive *K. pneumoniae* isolation from endotracheal aspirate and feces of the Patient F and—on the same period—the $bla_{\text{OXA-244}}$-positive *E. aerogenes* isolates from liquor of this patient (Table 1).

Plasmid localization of $bla_{\text{OXA-48-like}}$ genes

It is known that the $bla_{\text{OXA-48-like}}$ genes localized on the IncL/M conjugative plasmids [11, 22]. PCR-detection of the specific IncL/M plasmid markers—*repA* and *traU*—showed the presence of the plasmid in all $bla_{\text{OXA-48-like}}$-positive *P. mirabilis* (n = 7) and *Enterobacter* spp. (n = 4) isolates, and the absence of such plasmid in the $bla_{\text{OXA-48-like}}$-negative isolates. The same correlation between $bla_{\text{OXA-48-like}}$ gene and the markers of the IncL/M plasmid was revealed for *K. pneumoniae* strains. So the $bla_{\text{OXA-48-like}}$ genes in bacterial isolates under study were located on IncL/M conjugative plasmids.

The acquisition of the $bla_{\text{OXA-48-like}}$ gene consisting plasmid IncL/M has been demonstrated by the experimental conjugation at *intra-* and *inter*-species transfer. Two clinical *K. pneumoniae* strains, B-500 and B-757 K, resistant to cefotaxime were used as donors. The *K. pneumoniae* M-9 Rif strain was used as a recipient at intraspecies conjugation, and the *E. coli* HB101 Rif was used as a recipient at interspecies conjugation. Selection of transconjugants was done by selective markers cefotaxime and rifampicin. The efficiency of conjugation was $2.0–8.5 \times 10^{-4}$ at *intra-* and $2.0–3.0 \times 10^{-3}$—at *inter*-species conjugation. The IncL/M transfer from the donor to the recipient was detected by the plasmid markers *repA* and *traU* appearance in the transconjugants. The $bla_{\text{CTX-M}}$, bla_{TEM}, bla_{SHV}, and class 1 integrase

Table 1 The features of *K. pneumoniae*, *P. mirabilis* and *Enterobacter* spp. isolates that were collected from the patients of the ICU in 2013–2014

Microbe	Strain	Isolation date[a]	Isolation source	Patient	bla_{TEM}	bla_{SHV}	bla_{CTX-M}	$bla_{OXA-48-like}$	*int1*	*ins1*	*int2*	*ins2*	Antibacterial resistance	RAPD type
K. pneumoniae	B-38	15.01.13	U	A	+	+	+	bla_{OXA-48}	+	+	–	–	Pn Cf Cp Tc Qn Cm Su Nf	K7
K. pneumoniae	B-500	24.04.13	EA	B	+	+	+	$bla_{OXA-244}$	+	-	–	–	Pn Cf Tc Qn Cm Su Nf	K23
K. pneumoniae	B-567	21.05.13	U	C	+	+	+	$bla_{OXA-244}$	+	-	–	–	Pn Cf Cp Qn Su Nf	K23a
K. pneumoniae	B-600	21.05.13	EA	K	+	+	+	–	–	–	–	–	Pn Cf Qn Ag Su Nf	K29
K. pneumoniae	B-757 K	13.06.13	U	C	+	+	+	$bla_{OXA-244}$	+	–	–	–	Pn Cf Cp Tc Qn Cm Ag Su Nf	K23
K. pneumoniae	B-811 K	16.07.13	IS	D	+	+	+	$bla_{OXA-244}$	+	+	–	–	Pn Cf Cp Qn Su Nf	K1
K. pneumoniae	B-1667	31.10.13	U	K	+	+	+	bla_{OXA-48}	–	–	–	–	Pn Cf Qn Cm Ag Su Nf	K29
K. pneumoniae	B-1896	12.12.13	U	K	+	+	+	bla_{OXA-48}	–	–	–	–	Pn Cf Cp Tc Qn Cm Ag Su Nf	K29
K. pneumoniae	B-481/14	25.03.14	U	E	–	+	+	bla_{OXA-48}	+	–	–	–	Pn Cf Cp Qn Cm Ag Nf	K23
K. pneumoniae	B-617/14	25.04.14	U	E	–	+	+	bla_{OXA-48}	+	–	–	–	Pn Cf Cp Qn Cm Ag Nf	K23
K. pneumoniae	B-690/14 K	06.05.14	U	E	–	+	+	bla_{OXA-48}	+	–	–	–	Pn Cf Cp Qn Cm Ag Nf	K23
K. pneumoniae	B-767/14	27.05.14	EA	N	–	+	+	bla_{OXA-48}	+	+	–	–	Pn Cf Cp Tc Qn Cm Ag Su Nf	K28
K. pneumoniae	B-941/14	24.06.14	EA	F	+	+	–	bla_{OXA-48}	+	–	–	–	Pn Cf Cp Tc Qn Cm Ag Su Nf	K36
K. pneumoniae	B-R1a	10.07.14	RS	F	–	+	+	bla_{OXA-48}	+	+	–	–	Pn Cf Cp Tc Cm Ag Su	K31
K. pneumoniae	B-1699/14 K	23.10.14	EA	L	–	+	+	bla_{OXA-48}	–	–	–	–	Pn Cf Cp Qn Cm Ag Nf	K31
P. mirabilis	B-123	07.02.13	U	G	+	–	+	–	+	+	+	+	Pn Cf Cp Qn Cm Ag Su Nf Co	P3
P. mirabilis	B-239	27.02.13	EA	H	+	–	+	–	+	+	+	+	Pn Cf Cp Qn Cm Ag Su Nf Co	$P1_1$
P. mirabilis	B-371	28.03.13	U	E	+	–	+	–	–	–	+	+	Pn Cf Cp Qn Cm Nf Co	$P1_1$
P. mirabilis	B-431 M	08.04.13	EA	H	+	–	+	bla_{OXA-48}	+	+	+	+	Pn Cf Cp Qn Cm Ag Su Nf Co	$P1_1$
P. mirabilis	B-757 M	13.06.13	U	C	+	–	+	$bla_{OXA-244}$	–	–	+	+	Pn Cf Cp Tc Qn Cm Ag Nf	$P1_1$
P. mirabilis	B-1939	17.12.13	W	M	+	–	+	–	–	–	+	+	Pn Cf Cp Qn Cm Ag Su Nf	P6
P. mirabilis	B-416/14	13.02.14	U	E	+	–	+	bla_{OXA-48}	–	–	+	–	Pn Cf Cp Tc Qn Cm Nf	$P1_1$
P. mirabilis	B-690/14 M	06.05.14	U	E	+	–	+	bla_{OXA-48}	–	–	+	+	Pn Cf Cp Tc Qn Cm Nf	$P1_1$
P. mirabilis	B-712/14 M	12.05.14	U	E	+	–	+	–	–	–	+	+	Pn Cf Tc Qn Cm Nf	$P1_2$
P. mirabilis	B-682/14	06.05.14	EA	I	+	–	+	–	+	+	+	+	Pn Cf Cp Tc Qn Cm Ag Su Nf	$P1_2$
P. mirabilis	B-799/14	26.05.14	EA	I	+	–	+	bla_{OXA-48}	+	+	+	+	Pn Cf Cp Tc Qn Cm Ag Su Nf	$P1_2$
P. mirabilis	B-828/14	02.06.14	EA	I	+	–	+	bla_{OXA-48}	+	+	+	+	Pn Cf Cp Tc Qn Cm Ag Su Nf	$P1_2$
P. mirabilis	B-1578/14	01.09.14	U	J	+	–	+	–	–	–	+	–	Pn Cf Cp Tc Qn Cm Ag Su Nf	$P1_5$
P. mirabilis	B-1672/14 M	20.10.14	U	J	+	–	+	bla_{OXA-48}	–	–	+	–	Pn Cf Cp Tc Qn Cm Ag Su Nf	$P1_5$
E. aerogenes	B-2012/14	17.06.14	L	F	+	–	–	$bla_{OXA-244}$	–	–	–	–	Pn Cf Cp Nf	E1
E. aerogenes	B-2137/14E	25.06.14	L	O	–	–	–	$bla_{OXA-244}$	–	–	–	–	Pn Cf Cp Tc Qn Cm Ag Su Nf	E1
E. aerogenes	B-2212/14	30.06.14	L	F	–	–	–	$bla_{OXA-244}$	–	–	–	–	Pn Cf Cp Nf	E1
E. cloacae	B-1530/14	30.08.14	U	N	–	–	–	bla_{OXA-48}	+	–	–	–	Pn Cf Cp Tc Qn Cm Ag Su Nf	E3

EA endotracheal aspirate, *IS* intracranial sinus, *L* liquor, *RS* rectal swab, *U* urine, *W* wound, *A, B, C, D, E, F, G, H, I, J, K, L, M, N* and *O* patients, $bla_{OXA-244}$, bla_{CTX-M}, bla_{TEM}, bla_{SHV} beta-lactamase genes, *int1* class 1 integrase gene, *ins1* genetic cassette array of class 1 integron, *int2* class 2 integrase, *ins2* genetic cassette array of class 2 integron, *Pn* penicillins, *Cf* cephalosporins, *Cp* carbapenems, *Tc* tetracyclines, *Qn* fluoroquinolones, *Cm* phenicols, *Ag* aminoglycosides, *Su* sulfonamides, *Nf* nitrofurans, «+» positive, «–» negative

[a] Day, month, year

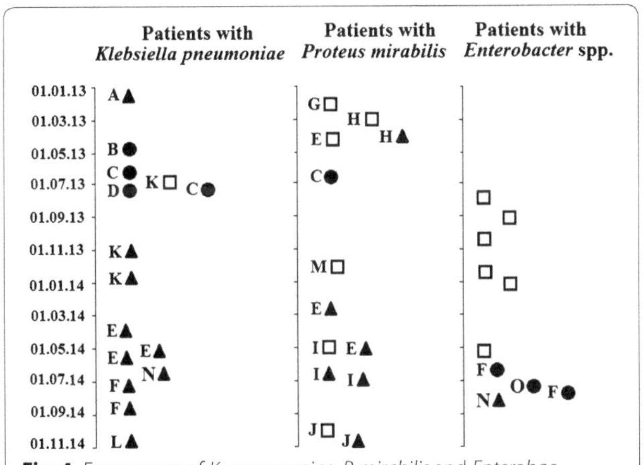

Fig. 4 Emergence of *K. pneumoniae*, *P. mirabilis* and *Enterobacter* spp. clinical isolates carrying $bla_{OXA\text{-}48\text{-}like}$ genes on the period from 01.01.2013 to 01.11.2014: *square* no gene, *filled triangle* $bla_{OXA\text{-}48}$ gene, *filled circle* $bla_{OXA\text{-}244}$ gene; *A, B, C, D, E, F, G, H, I, J, K, L, M, N* and *O* patients

genes were detected in the transconjugant cells (Table 2). The distribution of genetic markers in the transconjugants shows that both donor *K. pneumoniae* strains carried two conjugative plasmids: the IncL/M plasmid ($bla^{+}_{OXA\text{-}244}repA^{+}traU^{+}$) and the unidentified plasmid ($bla^{+}_{CTX\text{-}M}$ bla^{+}_{TEM} bla^{+}_{SHV}) (Table 2).

Conclusions

The molecular genetic mechanisms for multi-drug resistance of *K. pneumoniae*, *P. mirabilis*, *E. aerogenes* and *E. cloacae* isolates collected from a Moscow neurosurgical ICU in 2013–2014 were shown associated with $bla_{CTX\text{-}M}$, bla_{TEM}, bla_{SHV} beta-lactamase genes, class 1 and class 2 integrons, as well as with $bla_{OXA\text{-}48\text{-}like}$ carbapenemase genes. Two alleles genes, the $bla_{OXA\text{-}48}$ and the $bla_{OXA\text{-}244}$, have been identified in the isolates under study. Moreover, *P. mirabilis*, *E. aerogenes* and *E. cloacae* are first determined as bacterial hosts for the of $bla_{OXA\text{-}48\text{-}like}$ genes in Russia. The $bla_{OXA\text{-}48\text{-}like}$ genes were found to be integrated into the well-known conjugative plasmids of IncL/M incompatibility group that probably were transferred from *K. pneumoniae* to *P. mirabilis* and to *E. cloacae* during the period of the patient stay in the ICU. The source of the $bla_{OXA\text{-}244}$ gene acquired by *E. aerogenes* isolates and the time of this event were not recognized.

So, this study highlights ongoing expanding of CPE pathogens in Russia. Obtained knowledge is important for an adequate evaluation of the epidemiological situation, for predicting the development of the situation in the future, and for the correct choice of the optimal strategy for the antibacterial therapy.

Table 2 Donor, recipient and transconjugant *K. pneumoniae* and *E. coli* strains features at *intra*- and *inter*-species conjugation

Role at conjugation	Strain	Conjugation effectiveness	Genetic markers								Plasmids
			repA	*traU*	$bla_{OXA\text{-}244}$	$bla_{CTX\text{-}M}$	bla_{TEM}	bla_{SHV}	*int1*	*ompK36*	
Donor	*K. pneumoniae* B-500		+	+	+	+	+	+	+	+	L/M, UP
Donor	*K. pneumoniae* B-757 K		+	+	+	+	+	+	+	+	L/M, UP
Recipient	*K. pneumoniae* 9 Rif		–	–	–	–	–	+	–	+	–
Recipient	*E. coli* HB-101 Rif		–	–	–	–	–	–	–	–	–
Transconjugant	*K. pneumoniae* 9/500-1	2.0×10^{-4}	+	+	+	+	+	+	+	+	L/M, UP
Transconjugant	*K. pneumoniae* 9/500-2	2.0×10^{-4}	–	–	–	+	+	+	+	+	UP
Transconjugant	*E. coli* HB/500-1	2.0×10^{-3}	+	+	+	–	–	–	–	–	L/M
Transconjugant	*K. pneumoniae* 9/757-1	8.5×10^{-4}	+	+	+	+	+	+	+	+	L/M, UP
Transconjugant	*K. pneumoniae* 9/757-2	8.5×10^{-4}	–	–	–	+	+	+	+	+	UP
Transconjugant	*E. coli* HB/757-1	3.0×10^{-3}	+	+	+	–	–	–	–	–	L/M

repA, *traU* genetic markers of the IncL/M plasmid, $bla_{OXA\text{-}244}$, $bla_{CTX\text{-}M}$, bla_{TEM}, bla_{SHV} beta-lactamase genes, *int1* class 1 integrase gene, *ompK36 K. pneumoniae* porin protein gene, «+» positive, «–» negative, *L/M* conjugative plasmid IncL/M, *UP* unidentified conjugative plasmid

Authors' contributions

NKF, EIA and ONE planned this study. ONE and NVK analyzed information about the patients and obtained the clinical samples. IAA, SYS, AIK and NNK collected bacterial isolates, performed bacterial identification and susceptibility to antibacterial agents. EIA, AIK, NNK and ESL performed the conjugation experiment, PCR detection of the resistance genes, strain genotyping and DNA sequencing—under the supervision of NVV. NKF carried bioinformatic analysis. NKF, EIA and ONE wrote the manuscript while EAS and IAD made significant contributions to the manuscript preparation. All authors read and approved the final manuscript.

Author details

[1] State Research Center for Applied Microbiology and Biotechnology, Obolensk, 142279 Moscow Region, Russia. [2] The Burdenko Neurosurgery Institute, Moscow 125047, Russia.

Acknowledgements

The study was financially supported by the State Research Center for Applied Microbiology and Biotechnology, Obolensk, and The Burdenko Neurosurgery Institute, Moscow. The work of NKF, AIK, EAS, and NVV consisting in genotyping *Klebsiella pneumoniae* was also supported by the Russian Science Foundation (Grant No. 15-15-00058).

Competing interests

The authors declare that they have no competing interests.

References

1. Rosenthal VD, Bijie H, Maki DG, et al. International nosocomial infection control consortium (INICC) report, data summary of 36 countries, for 2004–2009. Am J Infect Control. 2012;40(5):396–407.
2. Glasner C, Albiger B, Buist G, et al. Carbapenemase-producing *Enterobacteriaceae* in Europe: a survey among national experts from 39 countries, February 2013. Euro Surveill. 2013;18(28):20525.
3. Birgand G, Armand-Lefevre L, Lepainteur M, et al. Introduction of highly resistant bacteria into a hospital via patients repatriated or recently hospitalized in a foreign country. Clin Microbiol Infect. 2014;20(11):O887–90.
4. Ambler RP. The structure of-lactamases. Philos Trans R Soc Lond B Biol Sci. 1036;1980(289):321–31.
5. Ageevets VA, Partina IV, Lisitsyna ES, et al. Emergence of carbapenemase-producing Gram-negative bacteria in Saint Petersburg, Russia. Int J Antimicrob Agents. 2014;44(2):152–5.
6. Poirel L, Heritier C, Tolun V, et al. Emergence of oxacillinase-mediated resistance to imipenem in *Klebsiella pneumoniae*. Antimicrob Agents Chemother. 2004;48(1):15–22.
7. Arana DM, Saez D, García-Hierro P, et al. Concurrent interspecies and clonal dissemination of OXA-48 carbapenemase. Clin Microbiol Infect. 2015;21(2):148.e1–4.
8. Hammoudi D, Moubareck CA, Aires J, et al. Countrywide spread of OXA-48 carbapenemase in Lebanon: surveillance and genetic characterization of carbapenem-non-susceptible *Enterobacteriaceae* in 10 hospitals over a one-year period. Int J Infect Dis. 2014;29:139–44.
9. Chen L, Al Laham N, Chavda KD, et al. First report of an OXA-48-producing multidrug-resistant *Proteus mirabilis* strain from Gaza, Palestine. Antimicrob Agents Chemother. 2015;59(7):4305–7.
10. Nordmann P, Poirel L. The difficult-to-control spread of carbapenemase producers among *Enterobacteriaceae* worldwide. Clin Microbiol Infect. 2014;20(9):821–30.
11. Potron A, Poirel L, Nordmann P. Derepressed transfer properties leading to the efficient spread of the plasmid encoding carbapenemase OXA-48. Antimicrob Agents Chemother. 2014;58(1):467–71.
12. Martínez-Martínez L, González-López JJ. Carbapenemases in *Enterobacteriaceae*: types and molecular epidemiology. Enferm Infecc Microbiol Clin. 2014;32(Suppl 4):4–9.
13. Oteo J, Hernández JM, Espasa M, et al. Emergence of OXA-48-producing *Klebsiella pneumoniae* and the novel carbapenemases OXA-244 and OXA-245 in Spain. J Antimicrob Chemother. 2013;68(2):317–21.
14. Poirel L, Naas T, Nordmann P. Diversity, epidemiology, and genetics of class D beta-lactamases. Antimicrob Agents Chemother. 2010;54(1):24–38.
15. Fursova NK, Pryamchuk SD, Abaev IV, et al. Genetic environments of bla(CTX-M) genes located on conjugative plasmids of *Enterobacteriaceae* nosocomial isolates collected in Russia within 2003–2007. Antibiot Khimioter. 2010;55(11-12):3–10 **(Russian)**.
16. Eckert C, Gautier V, Arlet G. DNA sequence analysis of the genetic environment of various *bla*CTX-M genes. J Antimicrob Chemother. 2006;57(1):14–23.
17. Edelstein M, Pimkin M, Palagin I, et al. Prevalence and molecular epidemiology of CTX-M extended-spectrum beta-lactamase-producing *Escherichia coli* and *Klebsiella pneumoniae* in Russian hospitals. Antimicrob Agents Chemother. 2003;47(12):3724–32.
18. Priamchuk SD, Fursova NK, Abaev IV, et al. Genetic determinants of antibacterial resistance among nosocomial Escherichia coli, *Klebsiella* spp., and *Enterobacter* spp. isolates collected in Russia within 2003–2007. Antibiot Khimioter. 2010;55(9-10):3–10 **(Russian)**.
19. Hujer KM, Hujer AM, Hulten EA, et al. Analysis of antibiotic resistance genes in multidrug-resistant *Acinetobacter* sp. isolates from military and civilian patients treated at the Walter Reed Army Medical Center. Antimicrob Agents Chemother. 2006;50(12):4114–23.
20. Yang J, Chen Y, Jia X, et al. Dissemination and characterization of NDM-1-producing *Acinetobacter pittii* in an intensive care unit in China. Clin Microbiol Infect. 2012;18(12):E506–13.
21. Rasheed JK, Biddle JW, Anderson KF, et al. Detection of the *Klebsiella pneumoniae* carbapenemase type 2 carbapenem-hydrolyzing enzyme in clinical isolates of *Citrobacter freundii* and *K. oxytoca* carrying a common plasmid. J Clin Microbiol. 2008;46(6):2066–9.
22. Poirel L, Bonnin RA, Nordmann P. Genetic features of the widespread plasmid coding for the carbapenemase OXA-48. Antimicrob Agents Chemother. 2012;56(1):559–62.
23. Chen J-H, Siu LK, Fung C-P, et al. Contribution of outer membrane protein K36 to antimicrobial resistance and virulence in *Klebsiella pneumoniae*. J Antimicrob Chemother. 2010;65:986–90.
24. Zimmer M, Barnhart H, Idris U, et al. Detection of *Campylobacter jejuni* strains in the water lines of a commercial broiler house and their relationship to the strains that colonized the chickens. Avian Dis. 2003;47(1):101–7.
25. Magiorakos AP, Srinivasan A, Carey RB, et al. Multidrug-resistant, extensively drug-resistant and pandrug-resistant bacteria: an international expert proposal for interim standard definitions for acquired resistance. Clin Microbiol Infect. 2012;18(3):268–81.
26. Moura A, Soares M, Pereira C, et al. INTEGRALL: a database and search engine for integrons, integrases and gene cassettes. Bioinformatics. 2009;25(8):1096–8.
27. Partridge SR, Tsafnat G, Coiera E, et al. Gene cassettes and cassette arrays in mobile resistance integrons. FEMS Microbiol Rev. 2009;33(4):757–84.

15

Antimicrobial resistance in coagulase-negative staphylococci from Nigerian traditional fermented foods

P. T. Fowoyo[1*] and S. T. Ogunbanwo[2]

Abstract

Background: Coagulase-negative staphylococci have become increasingly recognized as the etiological agent of some infections. A significant characteristic of coagulase-negative staphylococci especially strains isolated from animals and clinical samples is their resistance to routinely used antibiotics although, resistant strains isolated from fermented foods have not been fully reported.

Methods: A total of two hundred and fifty-five CoNS isolates were subjected to antimicrobial susceptibility test using the disc diffusion technique. The minimum inhibitory concentration of the isolates to the tested antibiotics was determined using the microbroth dilution method. Methicillin resistant strains were confirmed by detection of methicillin resistant genes (*mecA*) and also employing cefoxitin screening test.

Results: The isolates were confirmed to be methicillin resistant by the detection of *mecA* genes and the cefoxitin screening test. The isolates demonstrated appreciable resistance to ampicillin (86.7%), sulfomethoxazole–trimethoprim (74.9%), amoxicillin–clavulanic acid (52.5%) and oxacillin (35.7%). Methicillin resistance was exhibited by 13 out of the 255 isolates although no *mecA* gene was detected. It was also observed that the methicillin resistant isolates were prevalent in these traditional foods; *iru*, *kindirmo*, *nono* and *wara*.

Conclusion: This study has ameliorated the incidence of multiple antibiotic resistant coagulase-negative staphylococci in Nigerian fermented foods and if not tackled adequately might lead to horizontal transfer of antibiotic resistance from food to man.

Keywords: Antibiotic resistance, Coagulase-negative staphylococci, Fermented foods, Methicillin resistance, *mecA* gene

Background

Coagulase-negative staphylococci were previously dismissed as contaminants and were found to occur mostly in hospitalized patients, individuals suffering from nosocomial infections and infections arising from the use of catheter or other intra-uterine devices however, it has been shown that CoNS from fermented foods also exhibit virulent traits [1]. The major challenge of CoNS-related infections has been the difficulty in therapy due to antimicrobial resistance. Antimicrobial agents used in therapy and as feed supplements to promote growth in food animals may increase the spread of drug-resistant bacteria. Such bacteria may contaminate milk or meat and are subsequently found in fermented food made of such raw material [2]. The levels of antibiotic resistant infections in the developing world have increased steadily in the last few decades as a result of combination of microbial characteristics and the selective pressure of antimicrobial use [3]. Microbial mechanisms of overcoming the activities of antimicrobial agents include the production of structure-altering or inactivating enzymes (e.g. beta-lactamase or amino glycoside-modifying enzymes), alteration of penicillin-binding proteins or other cell-wall target sites, altered DNA gyrase targets, permeability mutations,

*Correspondence: seunpt@yahoo.com
[1] Biosciences Department, Salem University, P.M.B. 1060 Lokoja, Kogi State, Nigeria
Full list of author information is available at the end of the article

active efflux and ribosomal modification [4–6]. Multidrug-resistant bacteria in both the hospital and community environment are important concern to the clinician, as it is the major cause of failure in the treatment of infectious diseases, increased morbidity, and mortality and the evolution of new pathogens [7, 8].

Penicillin was initially the drug of choice for treatment of infections caused by *Staphylococcus* however, penicillin resistance in CoNS became very high since 1968 [9]. Nowadays, resistance is around 91% in clinical strains [10]. Two mechanisms confer penicillin resistance in staphylococci; the first and the most important is the production of β-lactamase which inactivates penicillin by the hydrolysis of its β-lactam ring. The second is primarily associated with human isolates and confers resistance due to a penicillin-binding protein, PBP2a, encoded by *mecA* [2]. The *blaZ* has also been identified as the cause of penicillin resistance among coagulase-negative staphylococci (CoNS) suggesting that *blaZ* is one of the main mechanism of penicillin resistance in staphylococci [2]. Methicillin resistance in *Staphylococcus* is caused by the expression of PBP2a encoded by the *mecA* gene [11]. Resistance of staphylococci to methicillin and all β-lactam antibiotics is associated with the low affinity of a penicillin-binding protein, PBP2a, which is not present in susceptible staphylococci [12–17]. This protein is encoded by the *mecA* gene, which is located in the mec region in which the DNA is of foreign origin [18]. There is evidence of horizontal transfer of SCC cassette between staphylococcal species [19] which implies that CoNS could serve as a reservoir for the spread of resistance genes. Transfer of resistance genes between CoNS and *S. aureus* has been reported thus indicating that CoNS may act as a resistance gene reservoir for *S. aureus*. It is thus possible that the different species of staphylococci that are present in the same microenvironment, for example on the skin of dairy cows can exchange *mecA* and *blaZ*, if the appropriate bacterial factors are met [2].

In this study, the incidence of antibiotic resistance against 9 antibiotics among 255 strains of coagulase-negative staphylococci of fermented food associated CoNS were investigated using disc diffusion technique according to the CLSI guidelines. The antibiotic resistant phenotypes were confirmed molecularly by the detection of *mecA* genes and cefoxitin screening test.

Methods

CoNS strains used in this study

In total, 255 CoNS strains were used in this study. The strains were isolated from six different Nigerian fermented foods, including *kindirmo* (66), *nono* (44) *iru* (58), *wara* (32), *ogi* (28) and *kunu* (27). The isolates were identified using both conventional and molecular methods employing 16S rRNA sequencing [20].

Antibiotic susceptibility testing

In vitro susceptibility of the test isolates to the antibiotics was determined using Kirby-Bauer disc diffusion [21]. A sterile wire loop was used to pick a discrete colony of the 18 h old culture of each of the test isolate cultured on mannitol salt agar (MSA) and used to inoculate sterile brain heart infusion broth inside a test tube and incubated at 37 °C for 4 h. The inoculum was standardized using the 0.5 McFarland turbidity standard which corresponds to 1.5×10^8 cfu/ml of cells. A sterile cotton swab was dipped into the adjusted suspension and excess inoculum was removed by pressing the swab firmly on the inside wall of the tube. The dried surface of a Mueller–Hinton agar plate was inoculated by streaking the swab over the entire surface. This procedure was repeated by streaking two more times, rotating the plate approximately 60° each time to ensure an even distribution of inoculum. The antimicrobial discs were placed firmly on the surface of the inoculated agar plate using sterile forceps. The plates were left for 1 h after which they were incubated at 35 °C for 18 h. After 16–18 h of incubation, the plates were examined and the diameters of the zones of inhibition were measured. The discs used were ampicillin (30 μg), amoxicillin-clavulanic acid (30 μg), cefotaxime (30 μg), oxacillin (1 μg), ciprofloxacin (5 μg), trimethoprim–sulphomethaxazole (5 μg), erythromycin (25 μg), gentamycin (10 μg) and ofloxacin (5 μg). All the antibiotic discs were procured from Oxoid, Germany. The results were classified as susceptible, intermediate, or resistant according to the approved guidelines of the Clinical and Laboratory Standards Institute [22].

Determination of minimum inhibitory concentration (MIC) using the broth micro-dilution method

The method by [21] was employed. A 96-well microtitre plate was used. Twofold serial dilutions of the different antibiotics were prepared and dispensed into the microtitre plates. The antimicrobial solutions were prepared at twice the desired final concentration and the wells filled with 0.05 ml of the antibiotic instead of 0.1 ml. Each tray labeled had a growth control well and a sterility (uninoculated) well.

The inoculum used for the broth micro-dilution was prepared using the direct colony suspension method. An 18 h old culture of CoNS was grown on blood agar. Distinct colonies were picked and each inoculated into 5 ml of Mueller–Hinton broth in a test tube. The broth culture was incubated at 35 °C for 4 h. The turbidity of the actively growing broth culture was adjusted with sterile broth using 0.5 McFarland standard. The resulting suspension contained approximately $1–2 \times 10^8$ cfu/ml. 2 ml of the suspension was dispensed into 38 ml of water (1:20 dilution). The prong of the inoculator was used to transfer 0.01 ml (1:10 dilution) into each well. The MIC panel was inoculated carefully to avoid splashing from one well to another. The microdilution trays were incubated inside a plastic bag at 35 ± 2 °C for 16–20 h in an ambient air incubator within 15 min of adding the inoculum. The amount of growth in the wells containing the antimicrobial agent was compared with the amount of growth in the growth control wells (no antimicrobial agent) used in each set of tests when determining the growth end points. A test was considered valid when acceptable growth was ≥2 mm turbidity at the bottom of the well or when a definite turbidity was observed.

Detection of methicillin resistance genes (*mecA*)

The methicillin resistant genes present in the coagulase-negative staphylococci strains were detected by polymerase chain reaction according to the method of [23]. DNA was extracted using the QIA Amp mini kit (QIAgen). Polymerase chain reaction for detection of the gene *mecA* (513 bp) was carried out using the following primers: A22f (5′ AAA ATC GAT GGT AAA GGT TGG C 3′) and A22r (AGT TCT GCA GTA CCG GAT TTG C) as described by [11]. Amplification cycles for *mecA* was carried out according to the method of [23] Considering 40 cycles of 94 °C for 30 s, 55 °C for 30 s, 72 °C for 1 min with a final extension of 72 °C for 5 min. *Staphylococcus aureus* ATCC43300 *mecA* + was used as positive control [21]. The amplicons were evaluated by agarose gel electrophoresis followed by staining in ethidium bromide (0.5 mg/ml), visualized on UV transilluminator (UVP, Inc USA) and documented by the program QuantiOne (BioRad) using molecular weight markers of 100 bp (Fermentas ®).

Results

A total of 221 (86.7%) of the isolates were resistant to ampicillin, however majority of the resistant CoNS occurred in *wara* (93.8%), *nono* (88.6%), *kindirmo* (92.4%) and *iru* (86.2%). 74.9% of the CoNS isolates were resistant to trimethoprim-sulfamethoxazole with high incidence in *iru* (84.5%), *wara* (84.4%) and *kindirmo* (72.7%). The highest resistance of amoxicillin-clavulanic acid was noted in CoNS isolated from *ogi* (60.7%), *iru* (60.3%), *nono* and *wara* (59.4%). The highest oxacillin resistance isolates were from *ogi* (42.9%), *nono* (40.9%) and *wara* (43.8%). The resistance to the other antibiotics cefotaxime, ciprofloxacin, erythromycin, gentamycin and ofloxacin were not as high as the other antibiotics as shown in Table 1.

Table 2 shows the resistance phenotype of the CoNS species. Thirty-four (13%) of the isolates were not resistant to any of the antibiotic tested. CoNS species having resistance phenotype to only ampicillin and trimethoprim-sulfamethoxazole were only 57 in number. *Staphylococcus epidermidis* (92%) demonstrated the highest resistance to ampicillin while *S. caprae* (69%) had the

Table 2 Phenotypic antimicrobial resistance patterns of CoNS species from fermented food samples

Profile	Resistance phenotypes	Number of strains	Number of antibiotic classes
1	None	34	0
2	AMP	30	1
3	AMP, SXT	57	2
4	AMP, SXT, AMC	43	2
5	AMP, SXT, AMC, OX	30	2
6	AMP, SXT, AMC, OX, CIP	21	3
7	AMP, SXT, AMC, OX, CIP, E	11	4
8	AMP, SXT, AMC, OX, CIP, E, CN	10	5
9	AMP, SXT, AMC, OX, CIP, E, CN, OFX	10	5
10	AMP, SXT, AMC, OX, CIP, E, CN, OFX, CTX	9	5

AMP ampicillin, *SXT* sulphomethoxazole-trimethoprim, *AMC* Amoxicillin–clavulanic acid, *OX* oxacillin, *CIP* ciprofloxacin, *E* erythromycin, *CN* gentamicin, *OFX* ofloxacin, *CTX* cefotaxime

Table 1 Distribution and Percentage Antimicrobial Resistance of Coagulase-Negative Staphylococci from Fermented Food Samples

Antibiotics	% Resistance of CoNS from foods						
	Total	*Iru*	*Ogi*	*Nono*	*Kindirmo*	*Kunu zaki*	*Wara*
	(255)	n = 58	n = 28	n = 44	n = 66	n = 27	n = 32
Ampicillin	221 (86.7%)	50 (86.2%)	21 (75%)	39 (88.6%)	61 (92.4%)	20 (74.1%)	30 (93.8%)
Trimethoprim–sulfamethoxazole	191 (74.9%)	49 (84.5%)	18 (64.3%)	31 (70.5%)	48 (72.7%)	18 (66.7%)	27 (84.4%)
Amoxicillin–clavulanic acid	134 (52.5%)	35 (60.3%)	17 (60.7%)	26 (59.1%)	29 (43.9%)	8 (29.6%)	19 (59.4%)
Cefotaxime	9 (3.5%)	2 (3.4%)	0 (0%)	3 (6.8%)	2 (3.0%)	1 (3.7%)	1 (3.1%)
Oxacillin	91 (35.7%)	17 (29.3%)	12 (42.9%)	18 (40.9%)	21 (31.8%)	9 (33.3%)	14 (43.8%)
Ciprofloxacin	61 (23.9%)	12 (20.7%)	3 (10.7%)	10 (22.7%)	18 (27.3%)	5 (18.5%)	13 (40.6%)
Erythromycin	40 (15.7%)	8 (13.8%)	2 (7.1%)	10 (22.7%)	11 (16.7%)	0 (0%)	9 (28.1%)
Gentamicin	29 (11.4%)	4 (6.9%)	2 (7.1%)	9 (20.5%)	7 (16.7%)	0 (0%)	7 (21.9%)
Ofloxacin	18 (7.1%)	2 (3.4%)	1 (3.6%)	4 (9.1%)	4 (6.1%)	1 (3.7%)	6 (18.8%)

least percentage of resistance to ampicillin. For trimethoprim-sulfamethoxazole, the highest resistance of 81% was recorded in *S. xylosus* with *S. caprae* having the least resistance (53%) to the antibiotic. *Staphylococcus simulans* (68%) recorded the highest resistance to amoxicillin-clavulanic acid while the least resistance was shown in *S. epidermidis* (41%). Oxacillin resistance in *S. xylosus* was 32% which was the highest and the least was in *S. kloosii* (14%). *Staphylococcus caprae* exhibited the highest resistance to ciprofloxacin, ofloxacin, gentamycin, erythromycin and cefotaxime as shown in Fig. 1.

Table 3 shows the minimum inhibitory concentration (MIC) distribution of the CoNS species. Based on the Clinical and Laboratory Standards Institute (CLSI) guidelines for MIC reading, the percentage of CoNS species resistant to the ampicillin, trimethoprim-sulfomethoxazole, amoxicillin-clavulanic acid and oxacillin were 85.5, 67.8, 49.8 and 25.9% respectively.

Cefoxitin screening test was carried out on the isolates so as to establish their status as methicillin resistant strains. Thirteen (5.1%) of the tested isolates were positive to cefoxitin screening test and most of them were multidrug resistant with the highest occurrence of the methicillin resistant species in *nono*. The species were *S. kloosii* (KIL 4), *S. xylosus* (WAIL 3, KIL 2 and WAJ 5),

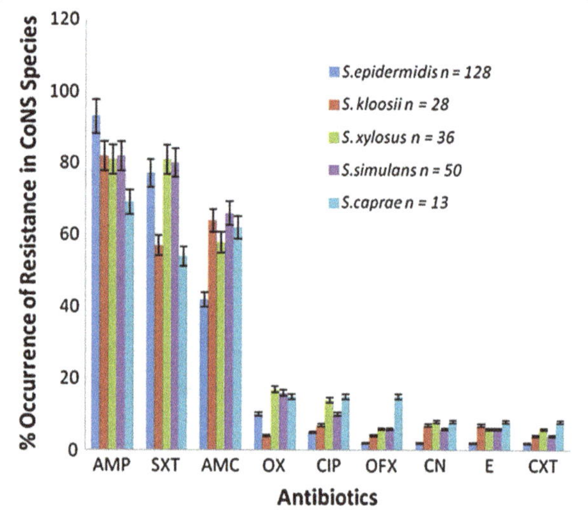

Fig. 1 Percentage occurrence of antibiotic resistance in CoNS Species. *Error bars* represent standard deviation of mean of replicate determinations

Table 4 Coagulase negative Staphylococci isolates showing methicillin resistance using cefoxitin screening

ID	Source	C–S	Resistance phenotype
S. xylosus KIL 2	*Kindirmo*	+	AMP, OX, SXT, AMC, CIP, E, CXT, CN. OFX
S. xylosus WAIL 3	*Wara*	+	AMP, OX, SXT, CIP, E, CXT, CN. OFX
S. kloosii KIL 4	*Kindirmo*	+	AMP, OX, SXT, AMC, CIP, E, CN OFX
S. epidermidis OGIL 3	*Ogi*	+	AMP, OX, AMC, CIP, E, OFX
S. epidermidis IRIL 7	*Iru*	+	AMP, OX, SXT, AMC, CIP, CN OFX
S. epidermidis NOMA 10	*Nono*	+	AMP, OX, SXT, AMC, CIP, E, CXT, CN OFX
S. simulans NOJ 6	*Nono*	+	AMP, OX, CIP, E, CXT, OFX
S. simulans KIM 5	*Kindirmo*	+	AMP, OX, SXT, AMC, CIP, E,
S. xylosus WAJ 5	*Wara*	+	AMP, OX, SXT, AMC, E, CXT
S. caprae NOMA 5	*Nono*	+	AMP, OX, SXT, AMC, CIP, E, CXT, OFX
S. caprae NOMA 6	*Nono*	+	AMP, OX, SXT, CIP, E, CN OFX
S. epidermidis NOL 3	*Nono*	+	AMP, OX, SXT, AMC, E, CXT CN OFX
S. epidermidis IRIL 5	*Iru*	+	AMP, OX, SXT, CIP, E, CN OFX

Table 3 Minimum inhibitory concentration (MIC) of antibiotics against CoNS isolated from fermented food samples

Antimicrobial agents	Numbers of CoNS with MIC[a]											Resistant isolates (%)
	≤0.12	0.25	0.5	1	2	4	8	16	32	64	128	
Ampicillin	24	13	*11*	*62*	*55*	*27*	*0*	*0*	*43*	*18*	*2*	218 (85.5%)
Trimethoprim–sulfomethoxazole	11	37	19	15	0	*0*	*0*	*0*	*0*	*70*	*103*	173 (67.8%)
Amoxicillin–clavulanic acid	101	0	27	0	0	0	*0*	*0*	*0*	*40*	*87*	127 (49.8%)
Oxacillin	53	136	0	*0*	*0*	*47*	*0*	*0*	*19*	*0*	*0*	66 (25.9%)
Ciprofloxacin	84	43	14	0	**52**	*0*	*7*	*24*	*9*	*9*	*13*	62 (24.3%)
Ofloxacin	21	12	22	69	**121**	*0*	*0*	*0*	*0*	*0*	*10*	10 (3.9%)
Gentamicin	15	151	16	**26**	**10**	**0**	*21*	*7*	*0*	*0*	*0*	37 (14.5%)
Erythromycin	98	91	15	0	0	0	*0*	6	*0*	*40*	*0*	46 (18.0%)
Cefotaxime[b]	0	181	20	0	0	49	0	0	0	3	2	–

[a] Based on the CLSI breakpoints. MICs indicative for susceptible isolates are displayed on a white background, those for intermediate on a bold and those for resistant on a italics

[b] Susceptility of staphylococci to cefotaxime may be detected from testing only penicillin and either cefoxitin or oxacillin

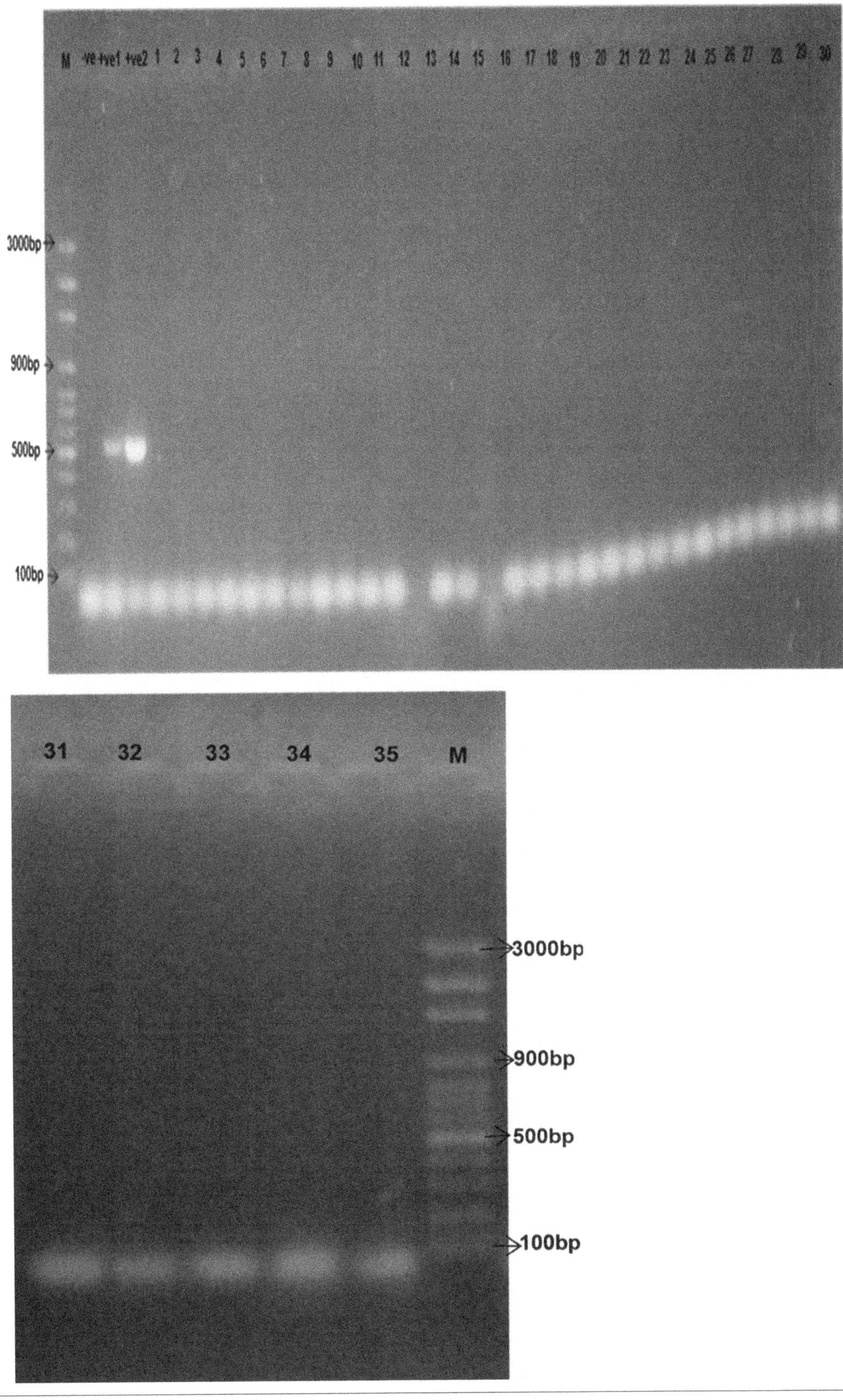
M -ve +ve1 +ve2 1 2 3 4 5 6 7 8 9 10 11 12 13 14 15 16 17 18 19 20 21 22 23 24 25 26 27 28 29 30
3000bp
900bp
500bp
100bp
31 32 33 34 35 M
3000bp
900bp
500bp
100bp

(See figure on previous page.)
Fig. 2 Gel electrophoresis micrograph of PCR product screen for *mecA* from extracted DNA (1–35) *Left* to *right*: M = O'GeneRuler 100 bp plus molecular weight marker (Thermo Scientific Fermentas™), Well 2 = Negative control for *mecA* gene, well 3 = Positive control 2, well 4 = Positive control 2 for *mecA* gene, wells 5–30 = Isolates 1–30. Weight of *mecA* gene = 513 bp. Positive isolates- none

S. epidermidis (OGIL 3, IRIL 7, NOMA 10, NOL 3 and IRIL 5), *S. simulans* (NOJ 6 and KIM 5) and *S. caprae* (NOMA 5 and NOMA 6) as indicated in Table 4. The molecular expression for *mecA* genes revealed that none of the isolates possessed the resistant genes (Fig. 2).

Discussion

Majority of the CoNS strains exhibited resistance to ampicillin, amoxicillin-clavulanic acid, sulphomethoxazole–trimethoprim, and oxacillin. A large percentage of the strains were susceptible to the antibiotics ciprofloxacin, erythromycin, gentamicin, cefotaxime and ofloxacin. *Staphylococcus epidermidis* demonstrated the highest resistance to ampicillin while *S. xylosus* exhibited the highest resistance to sulfomethoxazole–trimethoprim. The highest percentage resistance to amoxicillin-clavulanic acid was demonstrated by *S. simulans*. Oxacillin resistance was highly demonstrated by *S. xylosus*. The resistance exhibited by a large percentage of CoNS to these routinely used antibiotics in treatment of staphylococcal infections necessitates the search for newer and more effective antibiotics against this group of organisms.

There was discrepancy between the detection of methicillin resistance phenotypically using cefoxitin screening and the absence of *mecA* gene in the CoNS strains. This may be attributed to methicillin resistance being caused by other mechanisms other than expression of *mecA* gene [24]. Also the sensitivity of PCR in the detection of *mecA* may have been compromised by the presence of PCR inhibitors or other physical factors [25, 26]. The work by [27] showed that out of 15 isolates showing oxacillin resistant phenotype, only one possessed the *mecA* gene, it was noted that there were unusual methicillin resistant CoNS that have a resistance mechanism other than the production of PBP2a and they have been reported as borderline methicillin resistant strains [28]. The borderline methicillin resistant strains are resistant to oxacillin due to their plasmid borne determinants including hyper-produced penicillinases, genes conferring resistance to cadmium or other gene products [29, 30]. It is also possible that the *mecA* negative oxacillin resistant CoNS may possess *mecA* alleles which could not be detected by the primers used in this study. Many CoNS strains also show diversity in *mecA* sequences and have different impact on β-lactam resistance.

Conclusions

The high percentage of antimicrobial resistance demonstrated by the strains shows that food may serve as reservoirs for antibiotic resistance and allow for horizontal gene transfer from farm animals or their products to humans. Indigenous fermented food products may represent a critical risk for transfer of antimicrobial resistance to humans. As a consequence, transfer of antimicrobial resistance genes between bacteria after ingestion by humans may occur. Antimicrobial resistant CoNS present in food constitute a direct risk to public health as they increase the gene pool from which pathogenic bacteria can pick up resistance traits. The resistance of the organisms to routinely used antimicrobials also calls for the search for new antimicrobials and more effective management of diseases caused by CoNS in the event of an outbreak.

Abbreviations

CoNS: coagulase-negative staphylococci; *mecA*: methicillin resistant gene; PBP2a: penicillin binding protein; DNA: deoxyribonucleic acid; CLSI: Clinical and Laboratory Standards Institute; MIC: minimum inhibitory concentration.

Authors' contributions

FP carried out the laboratory analysis, OS was a major contributor in writing the manuscript. Both authors read and approved the final manuscript.

Author details

[1] Biosciences Department, Salem University, P.M.B. 1060 Lokoja, Kogi State, Nigeria. [2] Microbiology Department, University of Ibadan, Ibadan, Oyo State, Nigeria.

Acknowledgements

Not applicable.

Competing interests

The authors declare that they have no competing interests.

Funding

This research was self funded.

References

1. Fowoyo PT, Ogunbanwo ST. Occurrence and characterisation of coagulase-negative staphylococci from Nigerian traditional fermented foods. Food Sci Qual Manag. 2016;50:49–55.

2. Normanno G, Salandra GL, Dambrosio A, Quaglia NC, Corrente M, Parisi A, Olsen JE, Christensen H, Aarestrup F. Diversity and evolution of *blaZ* from *Staphylococcus aureus* and coagulase-negative staphylococci. J Antimicrob Chemother. 2006;57(3):450–60. doi:10.1093/jac/dki492.
3. Blondeau JM, Tillotson GS. Antimicrobial susceptibility patterns of respiratory pathogens-a global perspective. Semin Respir Infect. 2000;15:195–207.
4. Gold HS, Moellering RC. Antimicrobial-drug resistance. N Engl J Med. 1996;335(19):1445–53.
5. Aaterson DL. Extended-spectrum betalactamases: the European experience. Curr Opin Infect Dis. 2001;14:697–701.
6. Levy SB. Factors impacting on the problem of antibiotic resistance. J Antimicrob Chemother. 2002;49(1):25–30. doi:10.1093/jac/49.1.25.
7. Hacker J, Blum-Oehler G, Muhldorfer I, Tschape H. Pathogenicity islands of virulent bacteria: structure, function and impact on microbial evolution. Mol Microbiol. 1997;23:1089–97.
8. Jones RN, Phaller MA. Bacterial resistance; a worldwide problem. Diagn Microbiol Infect Dis. 1998;31:379–88.
9. Corse J, Williams REO. Antibiotic resistance of coagulase-negative staphylococci and micrococci. J Clin Pathol. 1968;21:722.
10. Koksal F, Yasar H, Samasti M. Antibiotic resistance patterns of coagulase negative *Staphylococcus* strains isolated from blood cultures of septicemic patients in Turkey. Microbiol Res. 2007;164(4):404–10.
11. Kumurya AS. Loss of the meca gene during storage of methicillin resistant *Staphylococcus aureus* isolates in Northwestern Nigeria. J Public Health Epidemiol. 2013;5(10):410–5. doi:10.5897/JPHE12.105.
12. Hartman BJ, Tomasz A. Low-affinity penicillin-binding protein associated with beta-lactam resistance in *Staphylococcus* aureus. J Bacteriol. 1984;158(2):513–6.
13. Pierre J, Williamson R, Bornet M, Gutmann L. Presence of an additional penicillin-binding protein in methicillin-resistant *Staphylococcus epidermidis, Staphylococcus haemolyticus, Staphylococcus hominis, and Staphylococcus simulans* with a low affinity for methicillin, cephalothin, and cefamandole. Antimicrob Agents Chemother. 1990;34:1691–4.
14. Chambers HF. Coagulase-negative staphylococci resistant to beta-lactam antibiotics in vivo produce penicillin-binding protein 2a. Antimicrob Agents Chemother. 1987;31:919–24.
15. Chambers HF. Methicillin resistance in staphylococci: molecular and biochemical basis and clinical implications. Clin Microbiol Rev. 1997;10:781–91.
16. Chambers HF. Penicillin-binding protein-mediated resistance in pneumococci andstaphylococci. J Infect Dis. 1999;179(Suppl. 2):S353–9.
17. Mohammad R, Mahmood Y, Au F. Comparison of different laboratory methods for detection of MRSA. Pak J Med Sci. 2006;22(4):442–5.
18. Matsuhashi M, Song MD, Ishino F, Wachi M, Doi M, Inoue M, Ubukata K, Yamashita N, Konno M. Molecular cloning of the gene of a penicillin-binding protein supposed to cause high resistance to P-lactam antibiotics in *Staphylococcus* aureus. J Bacteriol. 1986;167:975–80.
19. Hanssen A, Kjeldsen G, Sojlid JUE. Local variants of Staphylococcal Cassette chromosome *mec* in Sporadic methicillin-resistant *Staphylococcus aureus* and Methicillin-resistant coagulase-negative Staphylococci: evidence of horizontal gene transfer? Antimicrob Agents Chemother. 2004;48(1):285–96. doi:10.1128/AAC.48.1.285-296.2004.
20. Fowoyo PT, Ogunbanwo ST. Virulence and toxigenicity of coagulase-negative staphylococci in Nigerian traditional fermented foods. Can J Microbiol. 2016;62:1–7.
21. Bauer AW, Kirby WM, Sherris JC, Turck M. Antibiotic susceptibility testing by standardized single disc method. Am J Clin Pathol. 1996;44:493–6.
22. Clinical and Laboratory Standards Institute (CLSI). M100-S22. Performance standards for antimicrobial susceptibility testing; 22nd informational supplement. Clinical and Laboratory Standards Institute, Wayne, 2012.
23. Coelho SMO, Reinoso E, Pereira IA, Soares LC, Demo M, Bogni C, Souza MMS. Virulence factors and antimicrobial resistance of *Staphylococcus aureus* isolated from bovine mastitis in Rio de Janeiro. Pesq Vet Bras. 2009;29:369–74.
24. Gradelski E, Aleksunes L, Valera L, Bonner D, Fung- Tomc J. Correlation between genotype and phenotypic categorization of Staphylococci based on methicillin susceptibility and resistance. J Clin Microbiol. 2001;39(8):2961–3. doi:10.1128/JCM.39.8.2961-2963.2001.
25. Ingato SP, Kimangá N, Omuse G, Kariuki S, Gunturu R, Dinda V. Characteristics of archived coagulase negative staphylococci isolates at a University hospital, Nairobi, Kenya. Kenya. Open J Med Microbiol. 2014;4:236–41.
26. Procop GW, Shrestha NK, Tuohy MJ, Hall GS, Isada CM. Rapid identification of *Staphylococcus aureus* and the *mecA* Gene from BacT/ALERT blood culture bottles by using the light cycler system. J Clin Microbiol. 2002;40(7):2659–61. doi:10.1128/JCM.40.7.2659-2661.2002.
27. Han JE, Hwang SY, Kim JH, Shin SP, Jun JW, Chai JY, Park YH, Park SC. CPRMethicillin resistant coagulase-negative staphylococci isolated from South Korean ducks exhibiting tremor. Acta Vet Scand. 2013;55(1):88. doi:10.1186/1751-0147-55-88.
28. Suzuki E, Hiramatsu K, Yokota T. Survey of methicillin—resistant clinical strains of coagulase negative for *mecA* gene distribution. Antimicrob Agent Chemother. 1992;36:429–34.
29. Massida O, Montanari MP, Mingoia M, Viraldo PE. Borderline methicillin susceptible *Staphylococcus aureus* strains have more in common than reduced susceptibility to penicillase-resistant penicillins. Antimicrob Agents Chemother. 1996;40:2769–74.
30. Massida O, Mingoia M, Fadda D, Whalen MB, Montanari MP, Varaldo PE. Analysis of the beta lactamase plasmid of borderline methicillin susceptible *Staphylococcus aureus*: focus on *bla* complex genes and cadmium resistance determinants cadD and cadX. Plasmid. 2006;55:114–27.

16

Clonal dissemination of KPC-2 producing *Klebsiella pneumoniae* ST11 clone with high prevalence of *oqxAB* and *rmtB* in a tertiary hospital in China

Li Cheng†, Xiao-Li Cao†, Zhi-Feng Zhang, Ming-zhe Ning, Xue-Jing Xu, Wanqing Zhou, Jun-Hao Chen, Jin-hua Zhang, Han Shen* and Kui Zhang*

Abstract

Background: Carbapenemase-producing *Klebsiella pneumoniae* (CPKP) *strains* have emerged as a major problem for healthcare systems. The aim of this study was to determine the circulating clones and analyze the clinical and molecular characteristics of CPKP in our hospital.

Methods: A total of 74 carbapenemase producers collected from our hospital from 2012 to 2014 were analyzed for the prevalence of extended-spectrum β-lactamase (ESBLs), plasmid-mediated quinolone resistance genes (PMQRs), exogenously acquired 16S rRNA methyltransferase (16S-RMTase), and plasmid-mediated AmpC enzyme (pAmpCs) by PCR and DNA sequencing. The sequence types (STs) of the carbapenemase producers were analyzed by multi-locus sequence typing (MLST). And Pulsed-field gel electrophoresis (PFGE) was performed to investigate the genetic relationship of KPC-2 producing strains. Clinical data were retrieved from the medical records.

Results: KPC-2 (n = 72) was the predominant enzyme followed by NDM-1 (n = 2); The genes *bla*CTX-M, *bla*SHV, *bla*TEM-1, *bla*DHA-1, *rmtB*, *armA*, *oqxA*, *oqxB*, and *qnrB* were present in 29 (39.2 %), 27 (36.5 %), 46 (62.2 %), 2 (2.7 %), 25 (33.8 %), 1 (1.4 %), 60 (81.1 %) and 56 (75.7 %), 6 (8.1 %) isolates, respectively. MLST analysis revealed 10 different STs. The most dominant ST was ST11 (78.4 %, 58/74), followed by ST15 (8.1 %, 6/74). PFGE patterns of the KPC-2 producing *K. pneumoniae* isolates exhibited clonal dissemination of ST11 and ST15 clones as well as a genetic diversity of the remaining strains.

Conclusion: The intra- and inter-hospital cross-transmission of KPC-2-producing *K. pneumoniae* ST11 co-carrying *oqxAB* and *rmtB* in our hospital strongly suggested that rapid identification of colonized or infected patients and screening of carriers is quite necessary to prevent a scenario of endemicity.

Keywords: KPC-2, ST11, OqxAB, MLST, *Klebsiella pneumoniae*

*Correspondence: shenhan10366@sina.com; 13505151066@163.com
†Li Cheng and Xiao-Li Cao contributed equally to this work
Department of Laboratory Medicine, Nanjing Drum Tower Hospital, The Affiliated Hospital of Nanjing University Medical School, Zhongshan Road, 321#, Gulou District, Nanjing, Jiangsu, People's Republic of China

Background

Klebsiella pneumoniae are part of the human gut microbiota and frequently cause infections from mild urinary and gastrointestinal infections to severe bacteremia and pneumonia with a high rate of mortality and morbidity [1]. An increasing emergence of carbapenem resistance among *K. pneumoniae* isolates worldwide has limited the therapeutic options for treatment of these infections [2].

Carbapenem resistance in *K. pneumoniae* is frequently caused by the predominant production of KPC carbapenemase worldwide [3], the production of OXA-48-like carbapenemase is currently spreading most rapidly in many European countries with IMP and VIM being occasionally detected [4]. And transmission of *bla*NDM are potentially global health issues [5]. In addition, Carriage of bla_{ESBL} and/or bla_{AmpC} in combination with active efflux or porin loss has also been shown to be responsible for carbapenem-resistance in *Enterobacteriaceae* [6].

Carbapenem resistant *K. pneumoniae* (CRKP) is reported to be caused either by epidemic clones or by the horizontal dissemination of mobile elements such as plasmids and insertion sequences. In Europe and American countries, KPC-producing ST258 *K. pneumoniae* can undeniably be regarded as one of the most successful multidrug-resistant nosocomial pathogens [7]. And the international high-risk clone of *K. pneumoniae* ST11 is frequently reported as a successful pathogen at infections in Asian and European countries because of the association of important co-resistance and virulence factors [8]. And the quick expansion and evolution of this multi-resistant and virulent clone may lead to an evolving crisis of global dimensions [9].

In recent years, CRKP has been emerging with an increasing frequency worldwide [2]. All these isolates were resistant to currently available antimicrobial agents except tigecycline. Extended-spectrum β-lactamase (ESBLs), exogenously acquired 16S rRNA methyltransferase (16S-RMTase) genes, and plasmid-mediated AmpC enzyme (pAmpCs) has been frequently detected among the clinical multidrug-resistant *Enterobacteriaceae* [10]. In addition, the prevalence of PMQR genes has been reported to be associated with the increasing quinolone resistance development in *Enterobacteriaceae* which involved an increase in the diversity of the PMQR genes [11]. Nevertheless, data on the distribution of these resistant determinants among carbapenemase-producing *K. pneumoniae* (CPKP) isolates collected during a long time period is still limited, and the dissemination of the internationally predominant CPKP isolate is still unclear.

The aim of the present study was to determine the circulating clones of CPKP and our study focused on a hospital-wide screening of ESBLs, 16S-RMTase, PMQRs and pAmpCs in CPKP strains collected during a 3-year-old period.

Methods

Bacterial isolates

Nanjing Drum Tower hospital is comprehensive tertiary hospital which manages 32 clinical departments, maintains 1460 patients, and admits more than 42,000 inpatients. A total of 108 non-replicate and consecutive *K. pneumoniae* isolates including 107 CRKP and 1 strains intermediate to carbapenem were collected from our hospital from January, 2012 to December, 2014. The Vitek 2 system (bioMérieux. Firenze, Italy) was used for isolate identification and antimicrobial drug susceptibility testing. Clinical specimens consisted of sputum (n = 44), blood (n = 18), urine (n = 12), secretion (n = 11), ascites (n = 9), bile (n = 6) catheter tips (n = 6), and others (n = 2). Among them, carbapenemase producers were further analyzed in this study. Clinical data such as the clinical features, laboratory results, and treatment were retrieved from the medical records department. The study protocol was approved by the Ethics Committee of Nanjing Drum Tower Hospital and written informed consent was obtained from all patients included in the study.

Carba NP confirmatory test

For carbapenemase detection, Carba NP Confirmatory test was performed on 108 *K. pneumoniae* isolates according to the guidelines of Nordmann et al. [12] and CLSI 2015 [13]. Briefly, 2 microcentrifuge tubes for each patient isolate were labelled as "a" and "b" with 100 μL of bacterial protein extraction reagent (Tris–HCl 20 mmol/L lysis buffer) being added into each tube. A 1-μL loopful of tested bacteria from an overnight blood agar plate was emulsified in both tubes and vortexed for 5 s. Carba NP Solution A (2 mL 0.5 % phenol red solution and 180 μL 10 mM zinc sulfate solution were added into 16.6 mL clinical laboratory reagent water, pH 7.8 ± 0.1) was added into tube "a" and Carba NP Solution B (solution A + 6 mg/mL imipenem) into tube "b", respectively. After the tubes were well vortexed, An incubation at 35 ± 2 °C for up to 2 h was needed. Test results were interpreted as follows: carbapenemase producers were reported when tube "b" became into light-orange, dark yellow, or yellow before 2 h, and tube "a" kept red or red–orange.

ESBLs confirmatory testing

ESBL production was detected by using the 2015 CLSI recommendations for phenotypic confirmatory test [13]. In brief, disks containing 30 μg of cefotaxime and ceftazidime, either alone or coupled with 10 μg of clavulanate (Oxoid Ltd, Cambridge, UK), were placed at distances of 20 mm (center to center). When the inhibition zone differed by ≥5 mm, between at least 1 of the combination disks and its corresponding single antibiotic disk, the strain was identified as an ESBL producer. *E. coli* ATCC 25922 and *K. pneumoniae* ATCC 700603 were used as quality control strains.

Detection of antimicrobial resistance determinants

DNA templates were prepared by the boiling method. All the 108 strains were screened for *bla*OXA-48 and *bla*NDM genes by PCR as previously described [14]. The 74 carbapenemase-producers identified by Carba NP Confirmatory test were further analyzed for carbapenemase encoding genes (*bla*KPC, *bla*IMI, *bla*SME, *bla*GES, *bla*VIM, *bla*IMP, *bla*NDM, *bla*GIM) by PCR-based techniques with subsequent sequencing according to the protocols as previously described [15], PMQRs (*qnrA*, *qnrB*, *qnrC*, *qnrD*, *qnrS*, *aac (6′)-Ib-cr*, and *qepA*) were detected by simplex PCR, followed by sequencing [16]. Among the 74 carbapenemase-producing strains, the presence of *bla*ESBLs (*bla*CTX, *bla*TEM, *bla*SHV) were checked for 42 strains positive for the ESBLs confirmatory testing according to the previous protocol [17], The 50 strains resistant to amikacin were further analyzed for the prevalence of 16S-RMTases (*armA*, *npmA*, *rmtA*, *rmtB*, *rmtC*, *rmtD*, and *rmtE*) [18] by multiplex PCR followed by single PCR for gene confirmation. Positive products were further purified with a DNA purification kit and then sent to the Majorbio Company (Shanghai, China) for sequencing. Sequences were analyzed by using the Chromas-Pro application and BLAST (http://www.ncbi.nlm.nih.gov/BLAST), and the subtypes of β-lactamase genes were confirmed by referring to the Lahey system (http://www.lahey.org/studies/).

Multi-locus sequence typing

The sequence types of the 74 carbapenemase producers were determined by multi-locus sequence typing (MLST) analysis with 7 housekeeping genes including *gapA*, *infB*, *mdh*, *pgi*, *phoE*, *rpoB*, and *tonB* being amplified and sequenced according to Diancourt et al. [19]. Alleles and sequence types (STs) were assigned by using the MLST database (http://www.pasteur.fr/mlst/Kpneumoniae.html).

Pulsed-field gel electrophoresis

Clonal relatedness of the 72 producing KPC-2 *K. pneumoniae* strains was analyzed by pulsed-field electrophoresis (PFGE) as previously described [20]. The restriction endonuclease XbaI (Fermentas, ABI, Germany) was used to digest the prepared genomic DNA and resultant DNA fragments were separated in a PFGE CHEF-DR III system (Bio-Rad Laboratories, Hercules, CA, USA) in 0.5× Tris–borate-EDTA buffer at 120 V for 19 h, with pulse times ranging from 2.2 to 54.2 s. The banding patterns were analyzed by the BioNumerics software (Applied Math, Sint-Maten-Latem, Belgium). Cutoff lines at 80 % were used to analyze genetic relatedness.

Results

Prevalence of carbapenemase and Antimicrobial susceptibility of CPKP isolates

Carba NP Confirmatory test showed that 74 out of 108 carbapenem resistant *K. pneumoniae* isolates were confirmed to be carbapenemase producers. PCR and molecular typing identified KPC-2 among 72 out of 74 carbapenemase producers and the other 2 isolates was found to produce NDM-1. Other carbapenemase-encoding genes were not detected. All the 74 carbapenemase producers found in our study were resistant to all of the β-lactams tested with 67.6 % (50/74) exhibiting resistance to amikacin and 72.73 % (54/74) exhibiting resistance to quinolones.

Clinical characteristics of CPKP isolates

A total of 15 departments in our hospital have been involved with the clonal dissemination of KPC-2 producing *K. pneumoniae* isolates in our hospital with the intensive care units (ICU) being the commonest department (n = 21), followed by Emergency (n = 10) and Department of Neurosurgery (n = 9). Departments of Geriatrics and General Surgery, Infectious Diseases, Otolaryngology, Urology, Respiratory, Hematology, Neurology, Cardiothoracic, and Cardiology have also been included. The isolates were mainly from the respiratory tract (n = 35), blood (n = 12) and urine (n = 8). Overall, the spread of KPC-2 producing *K. pneumoniae* ST11 clones co-carrying other resistance genes in hospital wards during 2012–2014 (Table 1) showed that compared to the data in 2012, such strains rapidly increased with more hospital wards being involved, especially in ICU. And a rapid decrease of such strains was observed during 2014 resulting from the strengthening implementation of hand hygiene in our hospital at the beginning of 2014 (personal communication). In addition, the Retrieval of NDM-producing *K. pneumoniae* strains showed that one strain was isolated from the blood of a 61-year-old male diagnosed as electrolyte imbalance after colorectal cancer surgery since he was admitted into ICU, persistent fever and blood culture showed severe septicemia caused by a NDM-producing *K. pneumoniae* strain, after a combination therapy of imipenem, tigecycline, and cefepime for 20 days, the patient died; the other NDM-producing *K. pneumoniae* was recovered from the secretion of a 41-year-old male who had undergone a serious burns on his whole body. No

Table 1 The spread of KPC-2 producing *K. pneumonia* ST11 clones associated with other resistance genes in hospital wards during 2012–2014

Isolation year	KPK-ST11	Antimicrobial Resistance determinants					Ward
		ESBLs	PMQRs	16S-RMTase	Carbapenemase	AmpC	
2012	10	8	10	7	10	0	ER(3), GS(2), NL(1), GA(1), NS(1), RP(1), VS(1)
2013	36	33	32	13	36	1	ICU(11), NS(6), ER(6), GS(3) GA(2), IDS(1), OG(1), UL(1), RP(1)
2014	11	8	9	1	11	1	ICU(4), CS(3), AD(1), GA(1), NS(1)

KPK-ST11: KPC-2 producing *K. pneumonia* ST11

ER emergency room, *ICU* Intensive Care Unit, *CS* cardiothoracic surgery, *NL* neurology, *AD* andrology, *UL* urology, *VS* vascular surgery, *NS* neurosurgery, *GS* general surgery, *GA* geriatrics, *RP* respiratory, *IDS* infectious diseases, *OG* Otolaryngology

fever was observed although NDM-producing *K. pneumoniae* was isolated from the burn wounds of the patients. After a series of Rinse debridement treatment, the patient got a good wound healing and discharged.

Prevalence of antimicrobial resistant determinants

ESBLs confirmatory testing showed that 42 strains were positive for ESBLs among the 74 carbapenemase-producing strains. PCR and DNA sequencing identified CTX-M, SHV, and TEM-1 type β-lactamases in 29 (39.2 %), 27 (36.5 %), 46 (62.2 %) isolates, respectively. CTX-M variants included 24 CTX-M-14, 3 CTX-M-15, 2 CTX-M-38; one SHV-1 and multiple SHV variants including SHV-11 (n = 2), SHV-12 (n = 13), SHV-28 (n = 2), SHV-31 (n = 6), SHV-160 (n = 2), and SHV-36a (n = 1) were observed. In addition, 2 DHA-1 were identified. 16S-RMTase including RmtB (n = 25) and Arm (n = 1) were identified among 26 out of the 50 carbapenemase-producers displaying resistance to amikacin. Fifty out of 74 carbapenemase producers were found to carry *oqxAB*. And the prevalence of both *oqxA* and *oqxB* detected in *K. pneumoniae* was high: 83.3 and 77.8 %, respectively. Of them, 48 *oqxAB*, 58 *oqxA* and 56 *oqxB* were detected among 69 carbapenemase producers highly resistant to fluoroquinolones. Whereas, 2 *oqxAB*, 2 *oqxA* and 2 *oqxB* were found among the 3 carbapenemase producers susceptible to fluoroquinolones.

In addition, one novel mutants named *oqxA11* and 3 novel *oqxB* mutants named *oqxB13*, *oqxB27*, and *oqxB28* were identified. And 3 kinds of *qnrB* variants including *qnrB6* (n = 1), *qnrB10* (n = 3) and *qnrB66* (n = 2) were identified. Other PMQRs were not detected.

Of particular concern, *qnrB6*, *oqxA*, *bla*TEM-1, and *bla*CTX-M-15 were identified in one NDM-producing isolate, albeit only *oqxB*, NDM-1 was found in the other one.

MLST

MLST analysis of 74 carbapenemase producers revealed 10 different STs (Fig. 1). The most dominant ST was ST11 (78.4 %, 58/74), followed by ST15 (8.1 %, 6/74). The remaining isolates were typed as ST23, ST218, ST362, ST412, ST420, ST606, ST690, and ST709. MLST analysis of 2 NDM-1 producing *K. pneumoniae* isolates identified as ST826 and ST307, respectively.

Clonal relatedness

According to the PFGE patterns of the isolates (Fig. 1), the 57 KPC-2 producing *K. pneumoniae* ST11 isolates exhibited 7 PFGE profiles. One major clonal groups composed of 47 closely related strains was observed among all the ST11 clones according to the 80 % similarity level. The PFGE data of the other 13 KPC-2 producing *K. pneumoniae* displayed a genetic diversity (Fig. 2). Among them, 2 PFGE profiles composed of 5 ST15 clones were observed. In addition, 2 strains including 1 ST11 clone and 1 ST15 one were non-typable by PFGE.

Discussion

Clonal dissemination of CRKP in the health care settings frequently cause a potential threat to the public health with the increasing use of carbapenems in the clinical treatments worldwide. And we provided the first report on the clonal dissemination of *K. pneumoniae* ST11 with a high prevalence of OqxAB in a tertiary hospital in China.

In this study, 72 out of 74 carbapenemase producers carried KPC-2, indicating that KPC is the major CHBLs accounting for the carbapenem resistance and KPC-2 is the most prevalent enzyme which was in accordance with the previous studies both at home and abroad [3]. OqxAB, encoded by both chromosome and plasmids as a quinolone and olaquindox efflux pump, has become increasingly prevalent among members of *Enterobacteriaceae* over the past decade [21, 22]. It has been demonstrated that acquisition of the *oqxAB* encoding plasmids may facilitate the selection of CIP resistant *Salmonella typhimuriu* [23], and high expression of this pump contributes to reduced susceptibility to quinolones in clinical

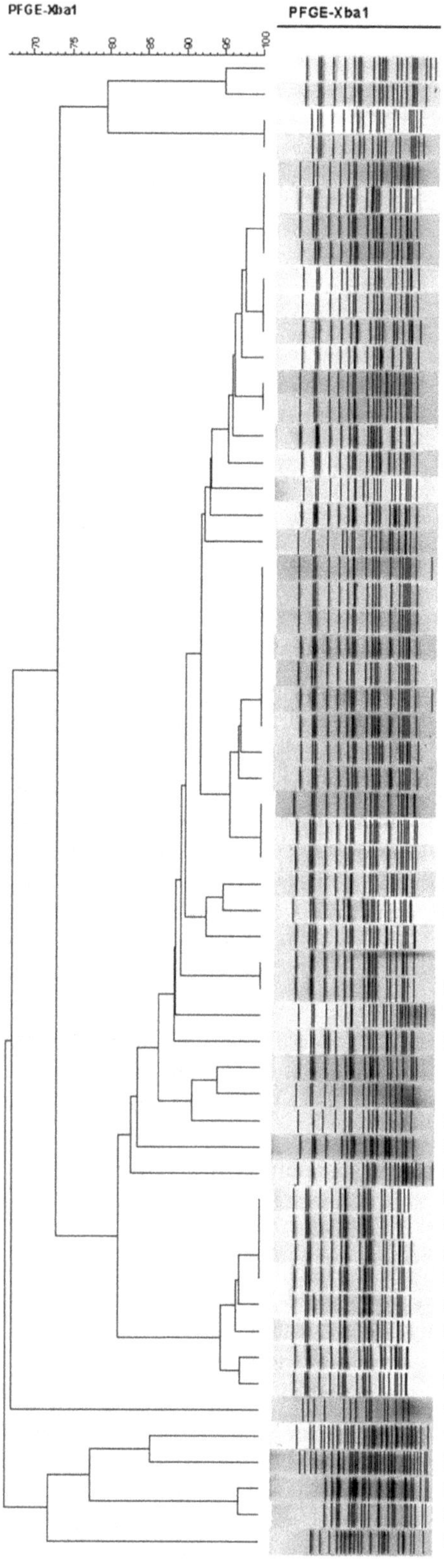

Key	ID	Ss	ward	RDs
1617	2013-05-27	secretions	ER	KPC-2,CTX-M-14,SHV-12,TEM-1,RmtB
2039	2013-09-02	sputum	ICU	KPC-2,SHV-36a,OqxAB
2711	2014-05-13	sputum	CS	KPC-2,CTX-M-14,QnrB66
2975	2014-07-19	sputum	CS	KPC-2,CTX-M-14,OqxA
1935	2013-08-14	blood	GS	KPC-2,TEM-1,OqxAB
3901	2012-09-25	sputum	NS	KPC-2,CTX-M-14,SHV-31,TEM-1,OqxAB
1943	2013-08-16	urine	NS	KPC-2,SHV-12,TEM-1,OqxAB,RmtB
2087	2013-09-20	blood	ICU	KPC-2,SHV-31,OqxAB
1638	2013-06-04	urine	GA	KPC-2,CTX-M-14,SHV-12,TEM-1,OqxA
1739	2013-07-10	sputum	NS	KPC-2,CTX-M-14,SHV-12,TEM-1,OqxAB,RmtB
2313	2013-12-15	sputum	ICU	KPC-2,SHV-11,OqxAB
1734	2013-07-10	blood	ICU	KPC-2,CTX-M-14,TEM-1,OqxAB
2025	2013-08-28	blood	ICU	KPC-2,OqxA
2104	2013-09-26	secretions	ICU	KPC-2,SHV-1,OqxAB,RmtB
1068	2012-11-11	sputum	RP	KPC-2,CTX-M-14,OqxAB,RmtB
1740	2013-07-12	catheter tip	IDs	KPC-2,CTX-M-14,TEM-1,RmtB
2159	2013-10-12	blood	GA	KPC-2,CTX-M-14,OqxAB
2660	2014-04-28	sputum	ICU	KPC-2,TEM-1,OqxAB
1848	2013-07-31	sputum	NS	KPC-2,OqxB
1153	2012-12-04	sputum	ER	KPC-2,TEM-1,OqxAB,RmtB,
1295	2013-01-03	blood	ER	KPC-2,TEM-1,OqxAB,RmtB
1325	2013-01-11	urine	ER	KPC-2,TEM-1,OqxAB,RmtB
1369	2013-01-20	sputum	ER	KPC-2,SHV-12,TEM-1,OqxAB,RmtB
1391	2013-01-29	ascites	NS	KPC-2,SHV-12,TEM-1,OqxAB,RMTB
1423	2013-02-25	sputum	ER	KPC-2,TEM-1,OqxAB,RmtB
1446	2013-03-06	sputum	NS	KPC-2,TEM-1,OqxA,RmtB
1394	2013-01-30	sputum	NS	KPC-2,TEM-1,OqxAB,RmtB
1402	2013-02-08	sputum	OG	KPC-2,SHV-12,TEM-1,OqxAB,RmtB
1183	2012-12-10	sputum	ER	KPC-2,OqxAB
1538	2013-04-16	ascites	GS	KPC-2,TEM-1,OqxAB
1549	2013-04-18	blood	ICU	KPC-2,SHV-2,TEM-1,OqxAB
2264	2013-11-20	catheter tip	ICU	KPC-2,OqxAB
2319	2013-12-16	urine	ICU	KPC-2,TEM-1,OqxB
1616	2013-05-27	catheter tip	ICU	KPC-2,SHV-2,TEM-1,OqxA,RmtB
1521	2013-04-15	blood	GA	KPC-2,SHV-12,TEM-1,OqxAB
2277	2013-11-27	sputum	ICU	KPC-2,CTX-M-14,OqxAB
1898	2013-08-07	catheter tip	ICU	KPC-2,CTX-M-14,TEM-1,OqxAB,RmtB
2505	2014-03-10	sputum	ICU	KPC-2,TEM-1,OqxAB,RmtB
1520	2013-04-14	sputum	ER	KPC-2,TEM-1,OqxAB,RmtB
1786	2013-07-22	catheter tip	ICU	KPC-2,SHV-12,OqxAB
2658	2014-04-28	sputum	NS	KPC-2,TEM-1,OqxB
2713	2014-05-12	sputum	ICU	KPC-2,CTX-M-14,OqxAB
2509	2014-03-11	sputum	GA	KPC-2,TEM-1,OqxAB
3204	2012-04-21	sputum	ER	KPC-2,SHV-160,TEM-1,CTX-M-14,RmtB
3215	2012-05-23	drainage	NL	KPC-2,SHV-31,TEM-1,CTX-M-14,OqxAB,RmtB
3618	2012-08-16	sputum	GS	KPC-2,SHV-31,CTX-M-14,TEM-1,OqxAB
3721	2102-08-31	ascites	GS	KPC-2,CTX-M-14,SHV-28,TEM-1,OqxAB
3198	2014-09-28	urine	ICU	KPC-2,CTX-M-14,TEM-1,OqxA
3409	2012-05-25	bile	GA	KPC-2,CTX-M-14,SHV-31,OqxAB
2342	2013-12-31	urine	ICU	KPC-2,TEM-1,OqxAB
2357	2014-01-07	secretions	AD	KPC-2,TEM-1,OqxAB
1975	2013-08-21	urine	UL	KPC-2,SHV-12,TEM-1
1721	2013-07-05	sputum	RP	KPC-2
2736	2014-05-17	sputum	CS	KPC-2,CTX-M-14,OqxA,QnrB10
1223	2012-12-18	blood	VS	KPC-2,TEM-1,OqxAB,RmtB
2785	2014-05-27	blood	CS	KPC-2,CTX-M-14,OqxA
1431	2013-02-28	throat	GS	KPC-2,TEM-1,OqxAB,RmtB

Fig. 1 Dendrogram based on PFGE profiles of 57 KPC-2 producing *K. pneumoniae* ST11 isolates. The dendrogram was produced by the UPGMA algorithm based on the Dice similarity coefficient included five PFGE groups as defined based on 80 % similarity of PFGE profiles. *ID* isolation date, *Ss* samples, *RDs* resistant determinants, *ER* emergency room, *ICU* Intensive Care Unit, *CS* cardiothoracic surgery, *NL* neurology, *AD* andrology, *UL* urology, *VS* vascular surgery, *NS* neurosurgery, *GS* general surgery, *GA* geriatrics, *RP* respiratory, *IDS* infectious diseases, *OG* otolaryngology

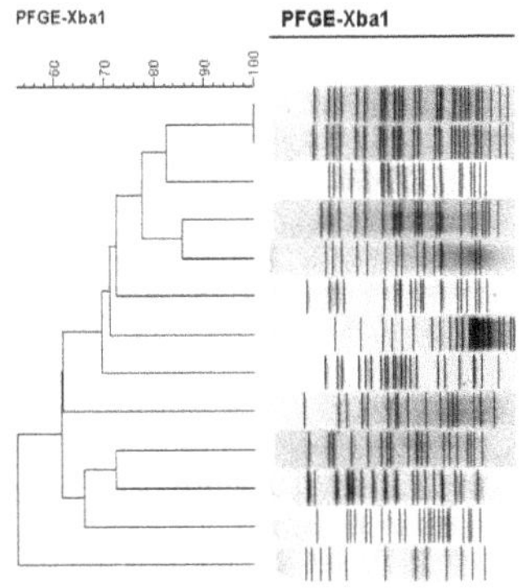

Key	ID	Ss	Ward	STs	RDs
2079	2013-9-17	blood	UL	ST15	KPC-2, OqxAB, QnrB10, DHA-1, ArmA
2094	2013-9-24	urine	UL	ST15	KPC-2, OqxAB, QnrB10, DHA-1
3213	2014-10-10	ascites	GE	ST15	KPC-2
1086	2012-11-15	sputum	NS	ST15	KPC-2, TEM-1, OqxAB
2726	2014-5-15	sputum	RP	ST15	KPC-2, CTX-M-38, OqxA
2732	2014-5-16	sputum	NL	ST420	KPC-2, CTX-M-14, OqxA, OqxB27, QnrB66
2630	2014-4-21	sputum	BS	ST412	KPC-2, CTX-M-15, TEM-1, OqxA, OqxB13
1719	2013-6-29	sputum	ER	ST709	KPC-2, CTX-M-15, TEM-1, OqxAB
3019	2014-8-1	sputum	CL	ST606	KPC-2, CTX-M-14, SHV-28, TEM-1, OqxA, OqxB28
1034	2012-11-3	sputum	GA	ST690	KPC-2, OqxA
3110	2014-8-27	blood	ICU	ST218	KPC-2, SHV-31, OqxB
2263	2013-11-21	sputum	GA	ST23	KPC-2, SHV-12, TEM-1, OqxAB
3500	2012-7-16	secrections	GS	ST362	KPC-2, SHV-160, OqxA11, OqxB

Fig. 2 Dendrogram based on PFGE profiles of 13 KPC-2 producing *K. pneumoniae* isolates. The dendrogram was produced by the UPGMA algorithm based on the Dice similarity coefficient included five PFGE groups as defined based on 80 % similarity of PFGE profiles. *ID* isolation date, *Ss* samples, *RDs* resistant determinants, *ER* emergency room, *UL* urology, *GE* gastroenterology, *NS* neurosurgery, *RP* respiratory, NL neurology, *BS* burn surgery, *ER* emergency room, *CL* cardiology, *GA* geriatrics, *ICU* Intensive Care Unit, *GS* general surgery

isolates of ESBL-producing *K. pneumoniae* [24]. A more recently published paper also described that overexpression of the *oqxAB* efflux pump in *K. pneumoniae* has been linked to an antibiotic cross-resistance phenotype [25] and OqxAB may contribute to tigecycline resistance in *K. pneumoniae* isolates [26]. Furthermore, a previous analysis of the genotypic and phenotypic characteristics of *K. pneumoniae* harboring *oqxAB*-like elements found that chromosomal *oqxAB* elements in *K. pneumoniae* strains exhibited cross resistance to olaquindox, chloramphenicol and the quinolones, whereas, transposition of the oqxAB operon from bacterial chromosome to plasmids results in more than 80-fold increase in the level of expression of the *oqxAB* pump, confirming that *oqxAB* efflux system is constitutively expressed when located in bacterial mobile elements [27]. The resistance mediated by the mutations in the quinolone-resistance determining regions in DNA gyrase and DNA topoisomerase IV of *K. pneumoniae* makes it difficult for us to speculate whether *oqxAB* in our study locates on plasmids or on the chromosome, and further study is needed to analyze the locations of these *oqxAB* operons and the role that *oqxAB*, *oqxA* and *oqxB* played in the fluoroquinolone development.

All together, the observed high prevalence of pump gene *oqxA* and *oqxB* in combination or alone in the KPC-2 producing *K. pneumoniae* ST11 represents a potential reservoir for the spread of these genes.

Of note, it's the first time that we identified a new variant *qnrB66* as well as the novel mutant named *oqxA11* and 3 novel *oqxB* mutants named *oqxB13*, *oqxB27*, and *oqxB28* in *K. pneumoniae* which indicate that these PMQRs have been rapidly evolving under the selection pressure of antimicrobial agents in the healthcare settings.

Furthermore, the high prevalence of *rmtB* among KPC-2 producing *K. pneumoniae* isolates has been reported in China [28], it has also been characterized that *rmtB* and *bla*KPC-2 were located in the same plasmid and frequently disseminated among *K. pneumoniae* isolates under the selection pressure of antimicrobial agents [29].

Up to date, ST11 strains has been frequently reported to be the carriage of multiple resistant determinants such as CTX-M, KPC-2, as well as RmtB [8]. And the co-carriage of different ESCs (extended-spectrum cephalosporinaes) and 16S-RMTases, alone or in combination, were also noted among the KPC-2 isolates in our study, indicating that the clone dissemination of ST11 strain may carry different types of plasmids or more than one plasmid. Additionally, recent reports showed that ST11 is the dominant strain associated with carbapenem resistance in *K. pneumoniae* [30] and even also the predominant clone of tigecycline-resistant *K. pneumoniae* strains [26], indicating that *K. pneumoniae* ST11 has been developing as major high-risk clone. Taken together, these data indicated rapid evolution and expansion of the KPC-2 producing ST11 isolates with acquisition and spread of transferable resistance determinants in our hospital [31].

Noticeably, there is a potential dissemination of ST15 clone secondary to the ST11 clones in our study, indicating that ST15 is another major high-risk clones. This is consistent with a recent study [32]. ST23 has been frequently reported to be the carbapenem resistant strains [33], whereas, the other clones including ST218, ST362, ST412, ST420, ST606, ST690, and ST709 has not been reported to be involved with carbapenem resistance.

Of particular concern, NDM has been frequently found in *K. pneumoniae* isolates and involved with the healthcare associated outbreaks in China [34, 35] and the emergence of NDM-producing *K. pneumoniae* isolates in our hospital showed a spread potential of these strains and infection control measures should be emergently implemented to prevent the healthcare associated outbreaks since the choice of antimicrobial agents is quite limited once the patients were infected with NDM-producing *K. pneumoniae* isolates. Additionally, to the best of our knowledge, it's the first time that we provide data on the *K. pneumoniae* ST826 and ST307 clones carrying NDM.

In recent years, the clonal dissemination of CRKP ST11 among Chinese hospitals has been frequently reported [32] and the wide distribution of the KPC-2-producing *K. pneumoniae* ST11 isolates co-carrying *oqxAB* and *rmtB* in our study indicate an intra- and inter- hospital cross-transmission of such strains in our hospital, which further strongly suggested that these isolates have a high potential to cause healthcare-associated outbreaks. Careful monitoring of carbapenem susceptibilities and rapid identification of colonized or infected patients as well as screening of carriers is quite necessary for implementation of infection control measures to prevent a scenario of endemicity.

Abbreviations

CPKP: carbapenemase-producing *Klebsiella pneumoniae*; ESBLs: extended-spectrum β-lactamase; PMQRs: plasmid-mediated quinolone resistance genes; 16S-RMTase: 16S rRNA methyltransferase; pAmpCs: plasmid-mediated AmpC enzyme; STs: sequence types; MLST: multi-locus sequence typing; PFGE: pulsed-field gel electrophoresis; ID: isolation date; Ss: samples; RDs: resistant determinants; ER: emergency room; ICU: Intensive Care Unit; CS: general surgery; NL: neurology; AD: andrology; UL: urology; VS: vascular surgery; NS: neurosurgery; GS: general surgery; GA: geriatrics; RP: respiratory; IDs: infectious diseases; OG: otolaryngology; GE: gastroenterology; BS: burn surgery; CL: cardiology.

Authors' contributions

LC and XC performed experimental work and drafted manuscript; ZZ and MN analyzed the study data; WZ, JC and JZ provided interpretation of data; KZ, HS conceived the study and provided data interpretation. All authors read and approved the final manuscript.

Acknowledgements

This study was supported by the Youth Fund of Jiangsu Province (Grant no. BK2014099) and Nanjing Medical Technology Development Fund (ZKX13028).

Competing interests

The authors declare that they have no competing interests.

References

1. Hussein K, Raz-Pasteur A, Finkelstein R, Neuberger A, Shachor-Meyouhas Y, Oren I, Kassis I. Impact of carbapenem resistance on the outcome of patients' hospital-acquired bacteraemia caused by Klebsiella pneumoniae. J Hosp Infect. 2013;83(4):307–13.
2. Hussein K, Sprecher H, Mashiach T, Oren I, Kassis I, Finkelstein R. Carbapenem resistance among Klebsiella pneumoniae isolates: risk factors, molecular characteristics, and susceptibility patterns. Infect Control Hosp Epidemiol. 2009;30(7):666–71.
3. Munoz-Price LS, Poirel L, Bonomo RA, Schwaber MJ, Daikos GL, Cormican M, Cornaglia G, Garau J, Gniadkowski M, Hayden MK, Kumarasamy K, Livermore DM, Maya JJ, Nordmann P, Patel JB, Paterson DL, Pitout J, Villegas MV, Wang H, Woodford N, Quinn JP. Clinical epidemiology of the global expansion of Klebsiella pneumoniae carbapenemases. Lancet Infect Dis. 2013;13(9):785–96.
4. Canton R, Akova M, Carmeli Y, Giske CG, Glupczynski Y, Gniadkowski M, Livermore DM, Miriagou V, Naas T, Rossolini GM, Samuelsen Ø, Seifert H, Woodford N, Nordmann P. Rapid evolution and spread of carbapenemases among Enterobacteriaceae in Europe. Clin Microbiol Infect. 2012;18(5):413–31.
5. Wei WJ, Yang HF, Ye Y, Li JB. New Delhi metallo-beta-lactamase-mediated carbapenem resistance: origin, diagnosis, treatment and public health concern. Chin Med J (Engl). 2015;128(14):1969–76.
6. Shin SY, Bae IK, Kim J, Jeong SH, Yong D, Kim JM, Lee K. Resistance to carbapenems in sequence type 11 Klebsiella pneumoniae is related to DHA-1 and loss of OmpK35 and/or OmpK36. J Med Microbiol. 2012;61(Pt 2):239–45.
7. Tzouvelekis LS, Markogiannakis A, Psichogiou M, Tassios PT, Daikos GL. Carbapenemases in Klebsiella pneumoniae and other Enterobacteriaceae: an evolving crisis of global dimensions. Clin Microbiol Rev. 2012;25(4):682–707.
8. Andrade LN, Vitali L, Gaspar GG, Bellissimo-Rodrigues F, Martinez R, Darini AL. Expansion and evolution of a virulent, extensively drug-resistant (polymyxin B-resistant), QnrS1-, CTX-M-2-, and KPC-2-producing Klebsiella pneumoniae ST11 international high-risk clone. J Clin Microbiol. 2014;52(7):2530–5.
9. Li H, Zhang J, Liu Y, Zheng R, Chen H, Wang X, Wang Z, Cao B, Wang H. Molecular characteristics of carbapenemase-producing Enterobacteriaceae in China from 2008 to 2011: predominance of KPC-2 enzyme. Diagn Microbiol Infect Dis. 2014;78(1):63–5.
10. Cao X, Xu X, Zhang Z, Shen H, Chen J, Zhang K. Molecular characterization of clinical multidrug-resistant Klebsiella pneumoniae isolates. Ann Clin Microbiol Antimicrob. 2014;13:16.
11. Carattoli A. Plasmids and the spread of resistance. Int J Med Microbiol. 2013;303(6–7):298–304.
12. Nordmann P, Poirel L, Dortet L. Rapid detection of carbapenemase-producing Enterobacteriaceae. Emerg Infect Dis. 2012;18(9):1503–7.
13. Clinical Laboratory Standards Institute. Performance standards for antimicrobial susceptibility testing; 25th informational supplement. M100-S25. CLSI, Wayne, PA. 2015.
14. Zowawi HM, Sartor AL, Balkhy HH, Walsh TR, Al Johani SM, AlJindan RY, Alfaresi M, Ibrahim E, Al-Jardani A, Al-Abri S, Al Salman J, Dashti AA, Kutbi AH, Schlebusch S, Sidjabat HE, Paterson DL. Molecular characterization of carbapenemase-producing Escherichia coli and Klebsiella pneumoniae in the countries of the Gulf cooperation council. Dominance of OXA-48 and NDM producers. Antimicrob Agents Chemother. 2014;58(6):3085–90.
15. Poirel L, Dortet L, Bernabeu S, Nordmann P. Genetic features of blaNDM-1-positive Enterobacteriaceae. Antimicrob Agents Chemother. 2011;55(11):5403–7.
16. Elgorriaga-Islas E, Guggiana-Nilo P, Dominguez-Yevenes M, González-Rocha G, Mella-Montecinos S, Labarca-Labarca J, García-Cañete P, Bello-Toledo H. Prevalence of plasmid-mediated quinolone resistance determinant aac(6')-Ib-cr among ESBL producing enterobacteria isolates from Chilean hospitals. Enferm Infecc Microbiol Clin. 2012;30(8):466–8.
17. Dallenne C, Da Costa A, Decre D, Favier C, Arlet G. Development of a set of multiplex PCR assays for the detection of genes encoding important beta-lactamases in Enterobacteriaceae. J Antimicrob Chemother. 2010;65(3):490–5.
18. Doi Y, Arakawa Y. 16S ribosomal RNA methylation: emerging resistance mechanism against aminoglycosides. Clin Infect Dis. 2007;45(1):88–94.
19. Diancourt L, Passet V, Verhoef J, Grimont PA, Brisse S. Multilocus sequence typing of Klebsiella pneumoniae nosocomial isolates. J Clin Microbiol. 2005;43(8):4178–82.
20. Carrer A, Lassel L, Fortineau N, Mansouri M, Anguel N, Richard C, Nordmann P. Outbreak of CTX-M-15-producing Klebsiella pneumoniae in the intensive care unit of a French hospital. Microb Drug Resist. 2009;15(1):47–54.

21. Yuan J, Xu X, Guo Q, Zhao X, Ye X, Guo Y, Wang M. Prevalence of the oqxAB gene complex in Klebsiella pneumoniae and Escherichia coli clinical isolates. J Antimicrob Chemother. 2012;67(7):1655–9.
22. Perez F, Rudin SD, Marshall SH, Coakley P, Chen L, Kreiswirth BN, Rather PN, Hujer AM, Toltzis P, van Duin D, Paterson DL, Bonomo RA. OqxAB, a quinolone and olaquindox efflux pump, is widely distributed among multidrug-resistant Klebsiella pneumoniae isolates of human origin. Antimicrob Agents Chemother. 2013;57(9):4602–3.
23. Wong MH, Chan EW, Liu LZ, Chen S. PMQR genes oqxAB and aac(6′)Ib-cr accelerate the development of fluoroquinolone resistance in Salmonella typhimurium. Front Microbiol. 2014;5:521.
24. Rodriguez-Martinez JM, Diaz de Alba P, Briales A, Machuca J, Lossa M, Fernández-Cuenca F, Rodríguez Baño J, Martínez-Martínez L, Pascual Á. Contribution of OqxAB efflux pumps to quinolone resistance in extended-spectrum-beta-lactamase-producing Klebsiella pneumoniae. J Antimicrob Chemother. 2013;68(1):68–73.
25. Bialek-Davenet S, Lavigne JP, Guyot K, Mayer N, Tournebize R, Brisse S, Leflon-Guibout V, Nicolas-Chanoine MH. Differential contribution of AcrAB and OqxAB efflux pumps to multidrug resistance and virulence in Klebsiella pneumoniae. J Antimicrob Chemother. 2015;70(1):81–8.
26. Zhong X, Xu H, Chen D, Zhou H, Hu X, Cheng G. First emergence of acrAB and oqxAB mediated tigecycline resistance in clinical isolates of Klebsiella pneumoniae pre-dating the use of tigecycline in a Chinese hospital. PLoS One. 2014;9(12):e115185.
27. Wong MH, Chan EW, Chen S. Evolution and dissemination of OqxAB-like efflux pumps, an emerging quinolone resistance determinant among members of Enterobacteriaceae. Antimicrob Agents Chemother. 2015;59(6):3290–7.
28. Li JJ, Sheng ZK, Deng M, Bi S, Hu FS, Miao HF, Ji ZK, Sheng JF, Li LJ. Epidemic of Klebsiella pneumoniae ST11 clone coproducing KPC-2 and 16S rRNA methylase RmtB in a Chinese University Hospital. BMC Infect Dis. 2012;12:373.
29. Sheng JF, Li JJ, Tu S, Sheng ZK, Bi S, Zhu MH, Shen XM, Li LJ. blaKPC and rmtB on a single plasmid in Enterobacter amnigenus and Klebsiella pneumoniae isolates from the same patient. Eur J Clin Microbiol Infect Dis. 2012;31(7):1585–91.
30. Sun K, Chen X, Li C, Yu Z, Zhou Q, Yan Y. Clonal dissemination of multilocus sequence type 11 Klebsiella pneumoniae carbapenemase—producing K. pneumoniae in a Chinese teaching hospital. APMIS. 2015;123(2):123–7.
31. Wang JT, Wu UI, Lauderdale TL, Chen MC, Li SY, Hsu LY, Chang SC. Carbapenem-nonsusceptible enterobacteriaceae in taiwan. PLoS ONE. 2015;10(3):e0121668.
32. Yan JJ, Wang MC, Zheng PX, Tsai LH, Wu JJ. Associations of the major international high-risk resistant clones and virulent clones with specific ompK36 allele groups in Klebsiella pneumoniae in Taiwan. New Microbes New Infect. 2015;5:1–4.
33. Qu TT, Zhou JC, Jiang Y, Shi KR, Li B, Shen P, Wei ZQ, Yu YS. Clinical and microbiological characteristics of Klebsiella pneumoniae liver abscess in East China. BMC Infect Dis. 2015;15(1):161.
34. Jin Y, Shao C, Li J, Fan H, Bai Y, Wang Y. Outbreak of multidrug resistant NDM-1-producing Klebsiella pneumoniae from a Neonatal Unit in Shandong Province, China. PLoS One. 2015;10(3):e0119571.
35. Liu Y, Wan LG, Deng Q, Cao XW, Yu Y, Xu QF. First description of NDM-1-, KPC-2-, VIM-2- and IMP-4-producing Klebsiella pneumoniae strains in a single Chinese teaching hospital. Epidemiol Infect. 2015;143(2):376–84.

17

Comparison of in-house and commercial real time-PCR based carbapenemase gene detection methods in *Enterobacteriaceae* and non-fermenting gram-negative bacterial isolates

M. Smiljanic[1], M. Kaase[2,3], P. Ahmad-Nejad[1] and B. Ghebremedhin[1*]

Abstract

Background: Carbapenemase-producing gram-negative bacteria are increasing globally and have been associated with outbreaks in hospital settings. Thus, the accurate detection of these bacteria in infections is mandatory for administering the adequate therapy and infection control measures. This study aimed to establish and evaluate a multiplex real-time PCR assay for the simultaneous detection of carbapenemase gene variants in gram-negative rods and to compare the performance with a commercial RT-PCR assay (Check-Direct CPE).

Methods: 116 carbapenem-resistant *Enterobacteriaceae*, *Pseudomonas aeruginosa* and *Acinetobacter baumannii* isolates were genotyped for carbapenemase genes by PCR and sequencing. The defined isolates were used for the validation of the in-house RT-PCR by use of designed primer pairs and probes.

Results: Among the carbapenem-resistant isolates the genes bla_{KPC}, bla_{VIM}, bla_{NDM} or bla_{OXA} were detected. Both RT-PCR assays detected all bla_{KPC}, bla_{VIM} and bla_{NDM} in the isolates. The in-house RT-PCR detected 53 of 67 (79.0%) whereas the commercial assay detected only 29 (43.3%) of the OXA genes. The in-house sufficiently distinguished the most prevalent OXA types (23-like and 48-like) in the melting curve analysis and direct detection of the genes from positive blood culture vials.

Conclusion: The Check-Direct CPE and the in-house RT-PCR assay detected the carbapenem resistance from solid culture isolates. Moreover, the in-house assay enabled the identification of carbapenemase genes directly from positive blood-culture vials. However, we observed insufficient detection of various OXA genes in both assays. Nevertheless, the in-house RT-PCR detected the majority of the OXA type genes in *Enterobacteriaceae* and *A. baumannii*.

Keywords: RT-PCR, Carbapenemases, *Acinetobacter baumannii*, MDR gram-negative bacteria

Background

An increase of infection triggered by multidrug-resistant gram-negative bacteria is a global problem because it is related to longer hospitalization, increased morbidity and mortality rates and to increased medical costs. The production of β-lactamase enzymes is the most common mechanism of bacterial resistance [1]. Carbapenemases are β-lactamases that have the ability to hydrolyse all β-lactam antibiotics, including carbapenem [2]. Rapid diagnostic tests for the identification and detection of specific resistance mechanism are necessary for therapy and prevent dissemination. Different techniques can be applied to identify carbapenem-resistant gram-negative bacteria. Phenotypic tests are used for detecting the carbapenemase activity while molecular based assays identify the resistance genes

*Correspondence: beniam.ghebremedhin@uni-wh.de
[1] Center for Clinical and Translational Research, Institute for Medical Laboratory Diagnostics, HELIOS University Clinic Wuppertal; Witten/Herdecke University, Heusnerstr. 40, 42283 Wuppertal, Germany
Full list of author information is available at the end of the article

[3]. Carbapenem-resistance can be detected by disc diffusion tests or Etest with imipenem, ertapenem or meropenem using agar plates or by automated systems (e.g. BD Phoenix, VITEK 2), selective chromogenic media for carbapenemase screening or the modified Hodge test (MHT) as additional phenotypic method [4]. The MHT is the only Clinical and Laboratory Standards Institute (CLSI)—recommended carbapenemase-screening method [4]. However, the gold standard for the detection of carbapenem-resistance are molecular based methods e.g. polymerase chain reaction (PCR)—either single- or multiplex PCR followed by a sequencing step if needed [3, 4]. However, these molecular methods are mainly implemented in reference laboratories. These diagnostic tools are necessary to administer the adequate therapeutic management for instance in septicaemia caused by carbapenemase-producing pathogens. Therefore, the distinction between carbapenem-resistance mediated by carbapenemases and those by other mechanisms is important for infection control in hospital setting. As the carbapenemase-producing gram-negative bacteria causing severe infections are generally multidrug-resistant, treatment options are compromised. Thus, the timely detection and monitoring of carbapenemases is important for therapeutic and prognostic means. Various carbapenemase genes may disseminate differently in the European countries, in the USA or the Asian countries. In the study region the predominance of the class D carbapenemase genes in *Enterobacteriaceae* and *Acinetobacter baumannii* is true [5].

In this study we established and evaluated a multiplex RT-PCR assay for the simultaneous detection of carbapenem resistance genes in gram-negative rods using the RT BD MAX™ system and compared the in-house RT-PCR with the commercial assay, the Check-Direct CPE kit.

Methods

Culture methods

Bacterial isolates

116 multidrug-resistant gram-negative isolates were collected from urine, blood-culture, wound swabs, tracheal secretions and other clinical specimens. Patient material were plated on Mac Conkey agar (BD, Becton–Dickinson and company, Heidelberg) and incubated at 37 °C over night. Species identification of these bacterial isolates was confirmed using MALDI-TOF mass-spectrometer. Carbapenem-resistance was approved using phenotypically methods (antibiotic disk diffusion and Etests on Muller–Hinton agar with imipenem, meropenem and ertapenem (BD Heidelberg, 10 µg and BD Phoenix system). All isolates have been characterized by the National Reference Centre (NRZ) at the molecular level.

For the identification of carbapenemase-producers directly from positive blood-cultures, negative Bactec™ Plus Aerobic/F blood-culture bottles containing clinical blood samples were inoculated with carbapenemase-producing isolates and incubated in a shaking incubator at 37 °C. For this purpose, a bacterial cell suspension was prepared with NaCl until a density of 0.5 McFarland turbidity standard was achieved. The blood-culture was inoculated with 500 µL of the bacterial suspension.

As negative controls we analysed 15 *Pseudomonas aeruginosa* and 20 *A. baumannii* isolates which were resistant to carbapenems but negative for the carbapenemase genes.

Molecular methods

DNA extraction

Some colonies of an overnight bacterial culture were suspended in 1.5 mL of 0.9% NaCl and centrifuged at 13,000 rpm for 10 min. The supernatant was discarded, the pellet resuspended in 500 µL NaCl and incubated for 15 min at 95 °C. Thereafter the suspension was incubated for further 10 min at room temperature and centrifuged at 13,000 rpm for 10 min. The supernatant was transferred in a new tube and the DNA concentration was measured.

For the bacterial extraction from positive blood culture vials 1.5 mL of the blood-culture was centrifuged for 5 min at 900 rpm. 500 µL of the supernatant was transferred in a new tube, mixed with 500 µL SDS (2%) and centrifuged at 13,000 rpm for 2 min. The supernatant was discarded and the DNA was extracted from the bacterial pellet as described above.

BD MAX™ diagnostic system

The BD MAX™ diagnostic system is an open RT-PCR system which allows the application of user defined protocols (UDPs). The advantage of this technology is the combined automatization of sample lysis, extraction, amplification and detection. This diagnostic system is time saving and avoids human errors. The fluorescence detection of the BD MAX™ is based on LEDs and photodiode filtering components to monitor fluorescence up to five different channels.

Primer and probes design/sets for the detection of β-lactamase genes

The primers used in this study were designed after aligning variations of the target gene using MUSCLE (http://www.ebi.ac.uk/Tools/msa/muscle/). The used sequences were downloaded from the National Center for Biotechnology Information (NCBI).

The aligned sequence was then used to design primers with the NCBI primer designing tool (http://www.ncbi.nlm.nih.gov/tools/primer-blast) and ordered at Eurofins Genomics, Ebersberg. Initially, singleplex PCR using the mastercycler (Eppendorf, Hamburg) was done to proof the primer pairs. The probes for each designed primer were ordered at TIB MOLBIOL Syntheselabor. The primers and the corresponding probes are listed in the Table 1.

In-house RT PCR on BD MAX™ system

For amplification, we used the Absolute qPCR Mix, no ROX (2×) (Thermo Fisher Scientific) and suspended the mix with 0.5 µL of the OXA-23 primer, OXA-48 Light Mix Modular, 0.75 µL of KPC, NDM and VIM primers, 0.3 µL OXA-23 probe and with 0.45 µL KPC, NDM and VIM probes. The primers primer master stock concentration was 10 pmol/µL for VIM, KPC, OXA-23 and NDM, and the probe concentration was 0.5 pmol/µL. 0.5 µL of the extracted DNA with a concentration of 80 ng/µL was added and a final volume of 12.5 µL were pipet into the microfluidic PCR cartridge (BD, Heidelberg).

The PCR was run at 95 °C for 5 min for 45 PCR cycles (95 °C, 15 s; 59 °C, 30 s; 72 °C, 11.7 s) followed by melt curve analysis for OXA-23 and OXA-48 variants with SYBR green from 40 to 100 °C in 0.2 °C steps. For the amplification and the analysis of the results the BD MAX software 4.32 A was used.

Check Direct CPE on BD MAX™ system

Bacterial isolates were directly analysed from culture media. Therefore a bacterial cell suspension to an optical density of 0.5 McFarland was diluted 1:100 and approximately 500 µL of this suspension was transferred into the DNA sample buffer tube SB-1. The rack and instrument were prepared according to the manufacturers' guidelines as well as the amplification program and the interpretation of the results.

Kappa (κ) statistics

To rather analyse the concordance between the two RT-PCR methods (in-house and commercial) for the detection of the various carbapenemase genes we performed kappa statistical analysis by use of the VassarStats platform http://vassarstats.net/index.html.

Results

Detection of the carbapenemase genes from solid culture isolates by use of the in-house method

A total of 18 KPC (*bla*$_{KPC-2}$ and *bla*$_{KPC-3}$), 19 NDM (*bla*$_{NDM-1/6, -2, -3, -5}$ and $_{-9}$) and 13 VIM (*bla*$_{VIM-1, -2, -4}$ and $_{-11}$) were detected by the in-house RT-PCR. Sixty seven (56.3%) of the 116 carbapenem-resistant gram-negative isolates harboured carbapenemase genes of oxacillinase-type carbapenemase (OTC)-variants (*bla*$_{OXA-23, -40, -48}$, and $_{-58}$-like). Within this family we observed the highest diversity of subtypes. The prevalence rate of the gene variant *bla*$_{OXA-23-like}$ was 41.8% among the different carbapenemase genes, primarily in *A. baumannii* isolates. 57 (85.1%) of the OXA types were detected by multiplex RT-PCR by use of OXA-23/-48 primer pairs. The *bla*$_{OXA-23-like}$ variants were amplified with the OXA-23 primer pair and *bla*$_{OXA-48, -162, -204}$, and *bla*$_{OXA-232}$ with the OXA-48 primer pair. Weak signals were observed during the amplification of *bla*$_{OXA-181}$ (OXA-48-like) ($n = 4$ out of 5; 80%) with the OXA-48 primer pair. The remaining *A. baumannii* isolates and other gram-negative species carrying the genes *bla*$_{OXA-40}$-like and *bla*$_{OXA-58}$-like could not be detected by the in-house RT-PCR assay.

In comparison to the in-house RT-PCR assay the isolates were analysed by use of the commercial Check-Direct CPE kit on the BD MAX™ system as well. All isolates harbouring the *bla*$_{KPC}$, *bla*$_{NDM}$ and *bla*$_{VIM}$ genes were sufficiently detected by the commercial assay. One *bla*$_{NDM}$ lost the resistance gene and has been excluded from the analysis. However, not all *bla*$_{OXA}$ gene variants were detected by use of the Check-Direct CPE assay. Only two of the 28 *bla*$_{OXA-23}$-like and all the *bla*$_{OXA-48}$-like (including 16 OXA 48, one OXA-162, five OXA-181, one OXA-204, and two OXA-232) isolates were detected

Table 1 Primer and probe sequences for the in-house RT-PCR assay

Gene	Primer pairs	Product size, bp	Probe
bla$_{KPC}$	for-GCGATACCACGTTCCGTCTG rev-CGGTCGTGTTTCCCTTTAGC	183	6FAM-AGCGGCAGCAGTTTGTTGATTG–BBQ
bla$_{NDM}$	for-TTTGGCGATCTGGTTTTCCG rev-ATCAAACCGTTGGAAGCGAC	101	LC610-AGACATTCGGTGCGAGCTGGC–BBQ
bla$_{OXA-23-like}$	for-CGCGACGTATCGGTCTTGAT rev-CGCGACGTATCGGTCTTGAT	162	HEX-ACGTATTGGTTTCGGTAATGCTGA–BBQ
bla$_{OXA-48-like}$	for-GGCACGTATGAGCAAGATGC rev-GTTTGACAATACGCTGGCTGC	182	[a]
bla$_{VIM}$	for-CCGAGTGGTGAGTATCCGAC rev-GAATGCGTGGGAATCTCGTTC	337	Cy5-CGCTGTATCAATCAAAAGCAACTCATCA–BBQ

[a] The melting-curve analysis for the OXA gene variants was performed with the OXA-48 primer. For the multiplex RT-PCR analysis a Light Mix Modular from TIB MOLBIOL Syntheselabor GmbH Berlin was used for OXA-48

in the OXA-48-like channel of the BD MAX system. Moreover, the commercial system also detected incorrectly two of the 6 $bla_{OXA\text{-}72}$ (OXA-40-like) isolates in the same channel. The two *A. baumannii* isolates harbouring $bla_{OXA\text{-}23}$-like and $bla_{NDM\text{-}1/\text{-}6}$ were only identified as NDM gene carrying isolates. Figure 1 illustrates the differences of the two assays in distinguishing the carbapenemase genes. The unweighted kappa (κ) for the KPC, NDM and VIM detection was 1—showing 100% concordance between the commercial and the in-house method—whereas for the OXA gene detection the unweighted κ was 0.4298 (95% CI 0.1251–0.7345). Noteworthy, both the in-house and the commercial RT-PCR assay did not detect any carbapenemase genes in our negative controls: 35 carbapenem non-susceptible *P. aeruginosa* and *A. baumannii* isolates. Therefore, the unweighted κ for the analysis of the non-carbapenmase isolates was 1.

Due to the high prevalence rate of $bla_{OXA\text{-}23}$ and $bla_{OXA\text{-}48}$ variants a stepwise diagnostic workflow by use of melting-curve analysis on BD MAX™ system was performed to rather differentiate these OXA subtypes. Figure 2 demonstrates the results of the in-house assay for OXA-23- and OXA-48-like with distinct melting points (T_m).

Detection of the carbapenmase genes from positive blood culture

Based on the in-house RT-PCR assay, 58 of 116 investigated carbapenemase-producing isolates were additionally analysed directly from spiked blood-culture vials and all the bla_{NDM} and bla_{VIM} isolates were sufficiently detected. One (7.1%) of the 14 bla_{KPC} carrying isolates and five (19.2%) of the 26 bla_{OXA} gene variants carrying isolates were not verified by the in-house assay. The amplification of one $bla_{OXA\text{-}232}$ (OXA-48-like) indicated weak signal and isolates carrying $bla_{OXA\text{-}181}$ (OXA-48-like) were not detected directly from positive blood-culture vials. The two *A. baumannii* isolates co-harbouring the genes $bla_{OXA\text{-}23\text{-}like}$ and $bla_{NDM\text{-}1/\text{-}6}$ were detected in both channels (Table 2).

Discussion

Multidrug resistance in gram-negative bacterial strains is increasing globally and turn out to be a very urgent challenge in health care facilities. Several phenotypic screening methods have been developed to detect or confirm carbapenemase production. These phenotypic methods are time consuming and might be difficult to interpret, e.g. occurrence of extended-spectrum betalactamases (ESBL) and porin loss or AmpC production. Therefore, the resistance gene detection by specific nucleic acid detection methods is the gold standard [3, 4, 6].

In this study we established and evaluated a multiplex RT-PCR assay in the PCR-only mode on the BD MAX™ system for the simultaneously detection of carbapenemase gene variants and the data were compared to those gained by commercial test kit. Another advantage is the combined sample lysis, extraction, amplification and detection using the fully automated BD MAX™ system. Hindiyeh et al. [7] detected bla_{KPC} genes and Naas et al. [8] $bla_{NDM\text{-}1}$ using RT-PCR. However, these assays can only detect the presence of one carbapenemase gene. Hofko et al. [9] reported the detection of carbapenemase gene variants with a multiplex SYBR green RT-PCR assay on the BD MAX™ system using two different master mixes (master mix 1: IMP-1, IMP-2, GES, VIM-2, KPC and 16S rRNA; master mix 2: OXA-23-like, OXA-48-like, VIM-1 and NDM). Nevertheless, this assay detects the carbapenemase genes in one channel (wavelength 475/520). The melting-curve analysis was performed to rather differentiate the different genes. In our RT-PCR assay we identified four different carbapenemase genes

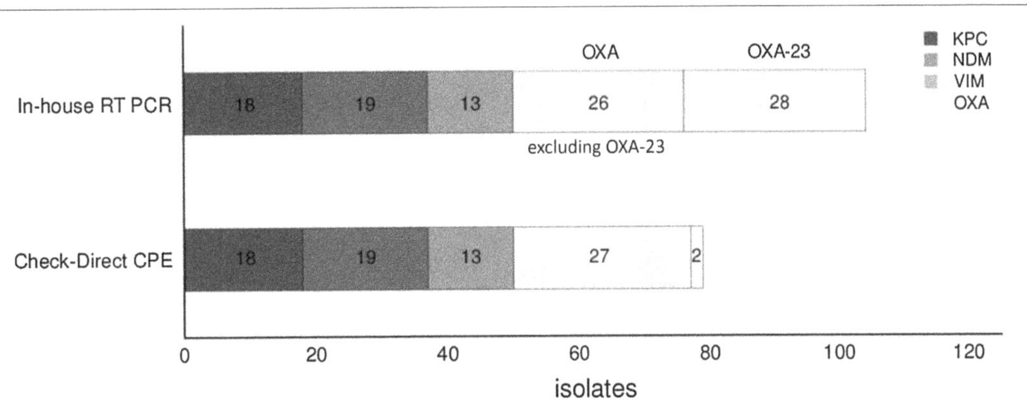

Fig. 1 Comparison of the in-house PCR assay and the Check-Direct CPE assay for the identification of carbapenemase-producing isolates ($n = 116$ isolates)

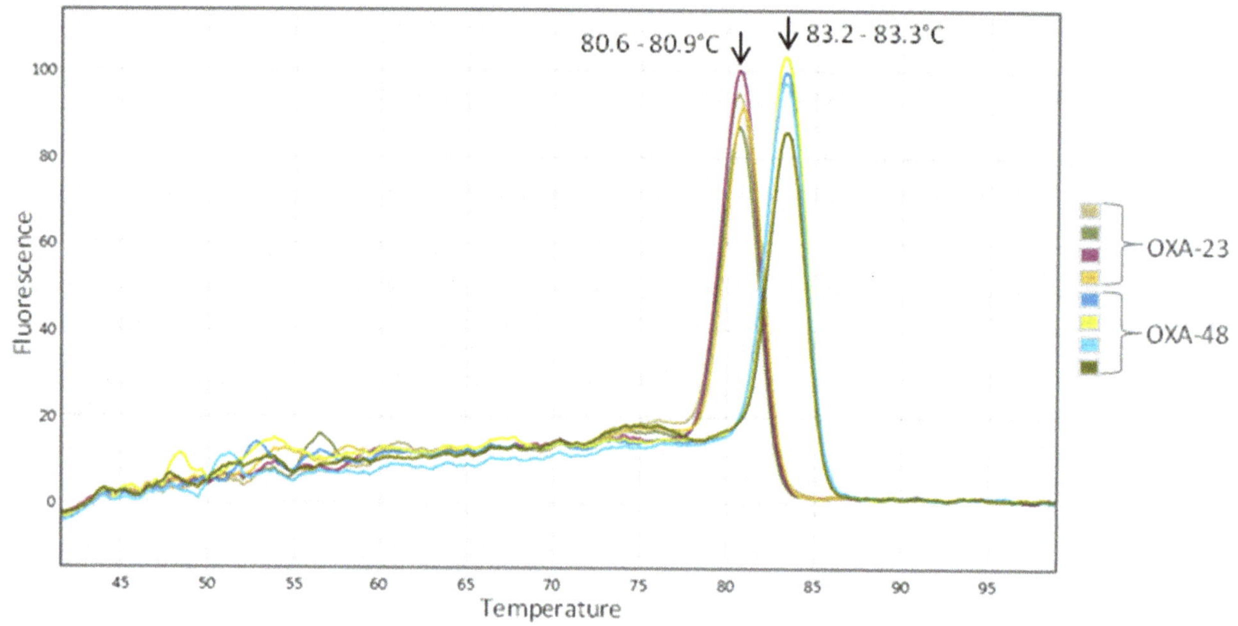

Fig. 2 Melting-curve analysis of OXA-23-like and OXA-48-like gene variants. The carbapenemase genes were amplified by SYBR green multiplex PCR mix with OXA-23-like and OXA-48-like primer followed by melt curve analysis. The melting-curve was visualised at the wavelength channel of 475/520 nm. The melting peak for OXA-23-like was observed between 80.6 and 80.9 °C and for OXA-48-like between 83.2 and 83.3 °C

Table 2 Detection of carbapenemase genes directly from positive blood culture vials by use of the in-house multiplex RT-PCR ($n = 58$)

Species	OXA23-/48-like ($n = 26$)	NDM ($n = 11$)	VIM ($n = 9$)	KPC ($n = 14$)
A. baumannii	18[a]	2[a]		
C. freundii	1		1	
E. asburiae		1		
E. cloacae			2	
E. coli	2	4		2
K. oxytoca			1	1
K. pneumoniae	5	4	1	11
P. aeruginosa			4	
Detected by in-house RT-PCR	21	11	9	13

[a] 2 isolates carrying $bla_{\text{OXA-23-like}}$ and $bla_{\text{NDM-1/-6}}$

(bla_{KPC}, bla_{NDM}, bla_{OXA} and bla_{VIM}) in four different channels using five different probes labelled with four fluorescent dyes for each primer pair. Based on the in-house PCR assay all investigated isolates carrying $bla_{\text{KPC-2, -3}}$ (18/18), $bla_{\text{NDM-1/-6, -2, -3, -5, -9}}$ (19/19) and $bla_{\text{VIM-1, -2, -4, -11}}$ (12/12) gene variants were correctly identified. In case of the two bacterial isolates carrying more than one carbapenem-resistance gene ($bla_{\text{OXA-23}}$-like and $bla_{\text{NDM-1/-6}}$) both variants were identified simultaneously.

The detection of oxacillinases seems to be more challenging. Today five main phylogenetic subgroups of the OXA-type carbapenemases (OTC) have been recognised in *A. baumannii*: OXA-23-like, OXA-40-like, OXA-51-like, OXA-58-like and OXA-143-like. The master mix containing two different OXA primer pairs (OXA-23- and OXA-48-like) detected 53 of 67 (79.0%) bla_{OXA} genes. The in-house assay was specific in a manner that it did not detect $bla_{\text{OXA-40}}$- and $bla_{\text{OXA-58}}$-like variants. However, the detection of $bla_{\text{OXA-181}}$ (4 out of $n = 5$; OXA-48-like) in *Klebsiella pneumoniae* isolate was insufficient. Further primer pairs aligned to the undetected genes could be included to rather enable the detection of more OTC variants. This was also consistent with the commercial Check-Direct CPE kit which also missed some oxacillinases positive isolates. The kit identified all five investigated $bla_{OXA-181}$. Unfortunately, this kit was not specific by detecting two of the six bla_{OXA-40}-like isolates. The primers should not cover this enzyme sub-group. However, the identification of bla_{OXA-23}-like variant remains as one of the challenging issues that yet to be improved. Only two (7.1%) of the 28 *A. baumannii* isolates carrying this gene variant were identified with the Check-Direct CPE kit. Lau et al., Antonelli et al., and Nijhuis et al. [10–12] reported 100% sensitivity for the detection of carbapenemase-producing bacteria comprising of bla_{NDM}, bla_{KPC}, bla_{VIM} and bla_{OXA-48}-like performed by the Check-Direct CPE kit which is consistent with our results. The comparison of the simultaneous detection of bla_{OXA-23}-like gene variants and the other carbapenemase genes with previous studies was not possible due to the fact that no corresponding data exist yet. However, in comparison to the Rotor-Gene instrument Monteiro et al. [13] reported the detection of bla_{IMP}, bla_{OXA-48}-like, bla_{NDM-1}, bla_{GES}, bla_{VIM} and bla_{KPC} in 21 *Enterobacteriaceae*, 1 *A. baumannii* and 8 *P. aeruginosa* isolates ($n = 30$) using the Rotor-Gene 6000 instrument with 100% sensitivity. Compared to the BD MAX™ where the genes were differentiated in five separate channels by use of the Rotor gene instrument, the genes were distinguished via melting curve analysis. Ellington et al. [14] reported in 2016 100% sensitivity for the detection of bla_{KPC}, bla_{NDM}, bla_{OXA-48}-like and bla_{VIM} carbapenemase genes using a multiplex real-time PCR assay on the Rotor-Gene Q as well as on the ABI 7500 instrument. The ABI Prism 7500 Fast instrument was also used by another research group to simultaneously detect bla_{NDM} and bla_{KPC} genes [15]. Yang and Rui [16] reported the simultaneous detection of bla_{NDM}, bla_{OXA-23}-like, bla_{OXA-40}-like, and bla_{OXA-58}-like genes in *A. baumannii* and other *Acinetobacter* spp. by performing two multiplex RT-PCR assays on the ABI Prism 7500 FAST apparatus. However, their assays did not include the identification of different carbapenemase gene variants from other species, so that the comparison of the simultaneous detection of bla_{OXA-23}-like gene variants with bla_{KPC} and bla_{VIM} with our data was not possible.

Another insufficiency of the Check Direct CPE kit is that it was not able to detect bla_{OXA-40}-like and bla_{OXA-58} due to the fact that the assay was designed for the detection of OXA-48-like. In outbreak situations this may increasingly become a problem, especially in outbreaks with *A. baumannii* isolates, the detection for such emerging subtypes in clinical specimens is mandatory for preventive and control measures in hospital setting. Fournier [17] reviewed a large number of numerous outbreaks caused by *A. baumannii* occurred in France and in the United States. Many of the outbreak strains have been found at intensive care units. Kohlenberg et al. [18] reported an outbreak of carbapenem-resistant *A. baumannii* carrying the carbapenemase gene OXA-23-like in a German university medical centre and Rolain et al. [19] reported this for Qatar during the period of 2011–2012.

In brief, the simultaneous identification of bla_{OXA}-like gene variants needs to be improved. However, our in-house assay displays a sensitivity rate of 100% for the detection of bla_{OXA-23}-like. With our in-house RT-PCR assay we were not able to differentiate the subtypes of the individual gene variants. Considering the high number of the analysed isolates positive for bla_{OXA-23}-like and bla_{OXA-48}-like variants a stepwise diagnostic workflow with melting-curve analysis was performed to rather differentiate the most prevalent OXA subtypes in this study. The peak between 80.6 and 80.9 °C was observed for OXA-23-like and between 83.2 and 83.3 °C for OXA-48-like. This assay is advantageous for the epidemiological surveillance for outbreaks with isolates carrying carbapenemase bla_{OXA} gene variants and might be extended for other carbapenemase gene variants. Roth et al. [6] reported the differentiation and identification of bla_{KPC-2} and bla_{KPC-3} genes with high-resolution melting analysis with 100% specificity and sensitivity for the detection of bla_{KPC}.

Regarding the importance of identification and antimicrobial susceptibility testing from positive blood-cultures due to septicaemia and septic shock [20] carbapenemase-producers were additionally identified directly from positive blood-culture isolates using the in-house assay. In brief, all investigated bla_{VIM} and bla_{NDM} isolates were identified by the in-house assay. In case of isolates carrying bla_{KPC} genes one (7.1%) out of 14 could not be detected. The bacterial pellet of this isolate was bloody after the second centrifugation step and not whitish as was observed for the other bacterial pellets, which might be the cause for the unsuccessful detection. For isolates containing bla_{OXA} gene variants the identification directly from positive blood vials could be observed for bla_{OXA-23}-like and bla_{OXA-48}-like (OXA-48 and -162). One $bla_{OXA-181}$ (bla_{OXA-48}-like) isolate could not be detected which is consistent with the PCR results from solid culture media. The amplification of one $bla_{OXA-232}$ showed weaker PCR product. It should be emphasized that we used negative blood-culture bottles spiked with bacterial isolates to investigate the performance of the in-house RT-PCR. Noteworthy, whereas the phenotypic assays, e.g. MHT, are eligible to detect the carbapenemase activity irrespective of the carbapenemase encoding gene sequence the RT-PCR based assay can only detect known carbapenemase encoding genes and the number of carbapenemase encoding genes and allelic variants thereof is expanding rapidly.

We would like to address a few limitations of our study, e.g. the low number and diversity of the gram-negative bacterial isolates producing VIM subtypes and OXA-48-like enzymes—in contrast to OXA-23-like—and thus representing only one or few isolates of particular subtype. Based on our findings, we plan to conduct a longitudinal surveillance study to further elucidate the epidemiology of carbapenem non-susceptible gram-negative bacteria in our region.

In conclusion, we have demonstrated that the in-house multiplex RT-PCR was a successful tool for the identification of carbapenemase gene variants directly from different solid culture isolates as well as from positive blood-culture vials. The assay is easy to perform, interpret and allows distinction between $bla_{\text{OXA-23}}$ and $bla_{\text{OXA-48}}$ variants, e.g. for outbreak analysis. Our in-house RT-PCR assay is an easy and rapid method for the detection of carbapenem resistance genes as compared to the routine microbiological diagnostic methods which need 2–3 days. Such same day analysis is crucial in hospital setting to rather implement the infection control and prevention measures, and moreover to administer the appropriate antimicrobial therapy in severe infections.

Authors' contributions

BG and MS proposed, designed, carried out the study, MS and BG analyzed the generated data and drafted the manuscript and performed the data analysis. MK provided with some of the strains from NRZ. MK and PAN participated in proofreading of the manuscript and in critical revision. All authors read and approved the final manuscript.

Author details

[1] Center for Clinical and Translational Research, Institute for Medical Laboratory Diagnostics, HELIOS University Clinic Wuppertal; Witten/Herdecke University, Heusnerstr. 40, 42283 Wuppertal, Germany. [2] Department of Medical Microbiology, Ruhr-University Bochum, Bochum, Germany. [3] Department of Infection Control, University Medical Center Göttingen, Göttingen, Germany.

Competing interests

The authors declare that they have no competing interests.

References

1. Saini A. Insights on the structural characteristics of NDM-1: the journey so far. Adv Biol Chem. 2012;02:323–34.
2. Cantón R, Akóva M, Carmeli Y, Giske CG, Glupczynski Y, Gniadkowski M, Livermore DM, Miriagou V, Naas T, Rossolini GM, Samuelsen Ø, Seifert H, Woodford N, Nordmann P. Rapid evolution and spread of carbapenemases among *Enterobacteriaceae* in Europe. Clin Microbiol Infect. 2012;18:413–31.
3. Nordmann P, Poirel L. Strategies for identification of carbapenemase-producing E*nterobacteriaceae*. J Antimicrob Chemother. 2013;68:487–9.
4. Birgy A, Bidet P, Genel N, Doit C, Decré D, Arlet G, Bingen E. Phenotypic screening of carbapenemases and associated β-lactamases in carbapenem-resistant *Enterobacteriaceae*. J Clin Microbiol. 2012;50:1295–302.
5. Ghebremedhin B, Halstenbach A, Smiljanic M, Kaase M, Ahmad-Nejad P. MALDI-TOF MS based carbapenemase detection from culture isolates and from positive blood culture vials. Ann Clin Microbiol Antimicrob. 2016;15:5.
6. Roth AL, Hanson ND. Rapid detection and statistical differentiation of KPC gene variants in gram-negative pathogens by use of high-resolution melting and ScreenClust analyses. J Clin Microbiol. 2013;51:61–5.
7. Hindiyeh M, Smollen G, Grossman Z, Ram D, Davidson Y, Mileguir F, Vax M, David DB, Tal I, Rahav G, Shamiss A, Mendelson E, Keller N. Rapid detection of bla_{KPC} carbapenemase genes by real-time PCR. J Clin Microbiol. 2008;46:2879–83.
8. Naas T, Ergani A, Carrer̈ A, Nordmann P. Real-time PCR for detection of NDM-1 carbapenemase genes from spiked stool samples. Antimicrob Agents Chemother. 2011;55:4038–43.
9. Hofko M, Mischnik A, Kaase M, Zimmermann S, Dalpke AH. Detection of carbapenemases by real-time PCR and melt curve analysis on the BD Max system. J Clin Microbiol. 2014;52:1701–4.
10. Lau AF, Fahle GA, Kemp MA, Jassem AN, Dekker JP, Frank KM. Clinical performance of Check-Direct CPE, a multiplex PCR for direct detection of bla_{KPC}, bla_{NDM} and/or bla_{VIM} and $bla_{\text{OXA-48}}$ from perirectal swabs. J Clin Microbiol. 2015;53:3729–37.
11. Nijhuis R, Samuelsen Ø, Savelkoul P, van Zwet A. Evaluation of a new real-time PCR assay (Check-Direct CPE) for rapid detection of KPC, OXA-48, VIM, and NDM carbapenemases using spiked rectal swabs. Diagn Microbiol Infect Dis. 2013;77:316–20.
12. Antonelli A, Arena F, Giani T, Colavecchio OL, Valeva SV, Paule S, Boleij P, Rossolini GM. Performance of the BD MAX™ instrument with Check-Direct CPE real-time PCR for the detection of carbapenemase genes from rectal swabs, in a setting with endemic dissemination of carbapenemase-producing *Enterobacteriaceae*. Diagn Microbiol Infect Dis. 2016;86(1):30–4.
13. Monteiro J, Widen RH, Pignatari ACC, Kubasek C, Silbert S. Rapid detection of carbapenemase genes by multiplex real-time PCR. J Antimicrob Chemother. 2012;67:906–9.
14. Ellington MJ, Findlay J, Hopkins KL, Meunier D, Alvarez-Buylla A, Horner C, McEwane A, Guivere M, McCraec LX, Woodforda N, Hawkey P. Multicentre evaluation of a real-time PCR assay to detect genes encoding clinically relevant carbapenemases in cultured bacteria. Int J Antimicrob Agents. 2016;47:151–4.
15. Zheng F, Sun J, Cheng C, Rui Y. The establishment of a duplex real-time PCR assay for rapid and simultaneous detection of bla_{NDM} and bla_{KPC} genes in bacteria. Ann Clin Microbiol Antimicrob. 2013;12:1.
16. Yang Q, Rui Y. Two multiplex real-time pcr assays to detect and differentiate *Acinetobacter baumannii* and *Non-baumannii* $bla_{\text{OXA-58-Like}}$ genes. PLoS ONE. 2016;11(7):e0158958.
17. Fournier PE. The epidemiology and control of *Acinetobacter baumannii* in health care facilities. Clin Infect Dis. 2006;42:692–9.
18. Kohlenberg A, Brümmer S, Higgins PG, Sohr D, Piening BC, De Grahl C, Halle E, Rüden H, Seifert H. Outbreak of carbapenem-resistant *Acinetobacter baumannii* carrying the carbapenemase OXA-23 in a German university medical centre. J Med Microbiol. 2009;58:1499–507.
19. Rolain J, Loucif L, Elmagboul E, Shaukat A, Ahmedullah H. Emergence of multidrug-resistant *Acinetobacter baumannii* producing OXA-23 Carbapenemase in Qatar. New Microbes New Infect. 2016;11:47–51.
20. Moore DF, Hamada SS, Marso E, Martin WJ. Rapid identification and antimicrobial susceptibility testing of gram-negative bacilli from blood cultures by the rapid identification and antimicrobial susceptibility testing of gram-negative bacilli from blood cultures by the automicrobic system. J Clin Microbiol. 1981;13:934–9.

18

Raoultella planticola bacteremia-induced fatal septic shock following burn injury

Tetsuya Yumoto[1*], Hiromichi Naito[1], Hiromi Ihoriya[1], Kohei Tsukahara[1], Tomoyuki Ota[2], Toshiyuki Watanabe[2] and Atsunori Nakao[1]

Abstract

Background: *Raoultella planticola*, a Gram-negative, aerobic bacillus commonly isolated from soil and water, rarely causes invasive infections in humans. Septic shock from *R. planticola* after burn injury has not been previously reported.

Case presentation: A 79-year-old male was admitted to the emergency intensive care unit after extensive flame burn injury. He accidently caught fire while burning trash and plunged into a nearby tank filled with contaminated rainwater to extinguish the fire. The patient developed septic shock on day 10. The blood culture detected *R. planticola*, which was identified using the VITEK-2 biochemical identification system. Although appropriate antibiotic treatment was continued, the patient died on day 12.

Conclusions: Clinicians should be aware of fatal infections in patients with burn injury complicated by exposure to contaminated water.

Keywords: Burn, Sepsis, *Raoultella planticola*

Background

Raoultella planticola is a Gram-negative, aerobic bacillus commonly found in soil and aquatic environments [1]. *R. planticola* infection is a relatively uncommon clinical entity, but sometimes causes fatal infection in immunocompromised patients [2]. Contaminated water used to extinguish a fire can lead to severe wound infections caused by waterborne microorganisms [3]. To our knowledge, *R. planticola* bacteremia has not been previously described in a burn patient. Herein, we report a case of fatal septic shock due to *R. planticola* bacteremia following flame burn injury complicated by exposure to contaminated water to extinguish the fire.

Case presentation

A 79-year-old male was referred to our tertiary hospital after extensive flame burn injury. He accidently caught fire while burning trash in a steel drum. The fire was extinguished when he plunged into a nearby water storage tank filled with dirty rainwater. His medical history was unremarkable except for hemiparesis of the right side as sequelae of ischemic stroke.

Upon arrival in the emergency department, he was alert and oriented, but he appeared distressed, complaining of dyspnea. His vital signs were as follows: Glasgow Coma Scale score: 15 (E4V5M6); respiratory rate: 20 breaths/min; pulse rate: 86 beats/min, blood pressure: 194/64 mmHg; and oxygen saturation: 99% via 10 L/min through a reservoir mask. Burn wounds were distributed on his face, neck, anterior trunk, and both upper extremities. Total body surface area (TBSA) affected was 35, 30% with third-degree burns and 5% with deep dermal burns (Fig. 1). As the patient had extensive burns, including on his face and neck, he was immediately intubated and fluid resuscitation was initiated. The burned areas were gently scrubbed with soapy water and covered with non-adherent dressing. The patient was admitted to the emergency intensive care unit.

Silver-coated dressings were applied 2 days after the injury to prevent wound infection. As *Aeromonas*

*Correspondence: tyumoto@cc.okayama-u.ac.jp
[1] Advanced Emergency and Critical Care Medical Center, Okayama University Hospital, 2-5-1 Shikata-cho, Kita-ku, Okayama-shi, Okayama 700-8558, Japan
Full list of author information is available at the end of the article

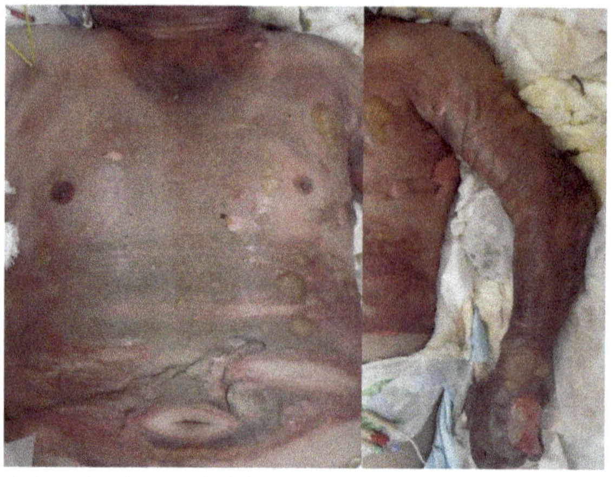

Fig. 1 The patient at admission. Burn wounds were distributed on the face, neck, anterior trunk, and both upper extremities. The total body surface area affected was 35, 30% with third-degree burns and 5% with eventual deep dermal burns

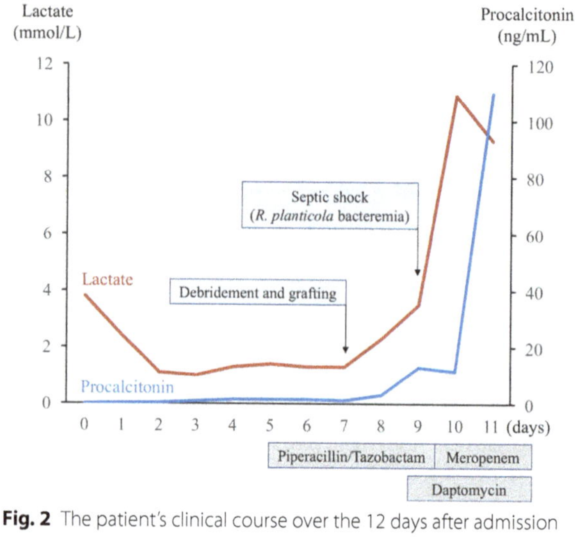

Fig. 2 The patient's clinical course over the 12 days after admission

hydrophila was isolated in the wound culture on day 5, 4.5 g doses of piperacillin/tazobactam three times daily were initiated. The medications were continued to treat *Pseudomonas aeruginosa,* which was isolated in the wound on day 7. Tangential debridement and skin grafting were performed for 30% of his TBSA on day 7. The procedure was successfully completed in 3 h.

Two days after surgery, the patient developed septic shock. White blood cell counts showed 33,470/μL with 97.7% neutrophils. His lactate and procalcitonin levels were found to be increased (Fig. 2). Noradrenaline infusion was initiated to support blood pressure following adequate fluid resuscitation. Empirical antibiotic therapy with daptomycin was administered and two sets of blood cultures were obtained. His abdomen was soft and not distended, without any evidence of intra-abdominal infections including cholecystitis or bowel necrosis based on laboratory data and radiological findings. The patient developed refractory septic shock despite the addition of vasopressin. Piperacillin/tazobactam was replaced by 1 g doses of meropenem three times daily for concerning antibiotic resistance on day 10; however, the patient's condition continued to deteriorate. His blood culture was positive for *R. planticola,* which was identified using the VITEK-2 biochemical identification system. The strain was susceptible to both piperacillin/tazobactam and meropenem. The results of antimicrobial susceptibility testing are summarized in Table 1. Cultures of the patient's urine and sputum at the onset of septic shock were revealed to be negative. Repetitive burn wound cultures yielded *P. aeruginosa,* which was sensitive to both piperacillin/tazobactam and meropenem with minimum inhibitory concentration (MIC) of ≦2 μg/mL and MIC≦0.5 μg/mL, respectively, and methicillin-sensitive *Staphylococcus aureus* (MSSA). The patient ultimately expired due to refractory septic shock and subsequent multiple organ failure on day 12. Figure 2 shows the patient's clinical course over the 12 days after admission.

Table 1 Results of antimicrobial susceptibility testing (μg/mL)

Antimicrobial agent	MIC
Cefazolin	>16
Ampicillin/sulbactam	8
Ceftriaxone	≦0.5
Cefepime	≦0.5
Gentamicin	≦1
Levofloxacin	≦0.25
Imipenem	≦0.5
Meropenem	≦0.5
Piperacillin/tazobactam	≦2
Trimethoprim/sulfamethoxazole	≦5

Discussion

This is the first report of fatal septic shock due to *R. planticola* bacteremia after flame burn injury. Extinguishing a fire with contaminated water can cause infection, and an impaired immune response after extensive burn injury may be responsible for the development of fatal septic shock.

Raoultella planticola is a Gram-negative, non-motile, encapsulated bacillus previously classified in the genus *Klebsiella,* including the species *K. planticola* and *K. trevisanii* [4]. In 1986, both microorganisms were combined as *K. planticola* because of deoxyribonucleic acid similarities [5]. The new genus *Raoultella* was established in 2001 on the basis of 16S rRNA and *rpoB* sequences [4]. *R. planticola* is considered an environmental organism commonly isolated from water and soil and does not typically cause human infections [6]. In recent years, infections due to *R. planticola* have been reported, including necrotizing fasciitis, bacteremia, severe pancreatitis, cholecystitis, cholangitis, urinary tract infection, and pneumonia [1, 6–11]. These infections mainly occur in immunocompromised patients with conditions such as cancer and hematological malignancies, and those post-transplant and/or with comorbidities including diabetes and alcoholic cirrhosis [1, 2, 8].

Several infection routes are possible in our case. Although the burn wound culture had been negative for *R. planticola*, the burn wound may have been a possible infection route, considering that *A. hydrophila*, the most common cause of wound infection related to a history of body immersion in untreated water [3], had been identified initially. In addition, both *R. planticola* and *A. hydrophila* are deemed uncommon organisms isolated from outbreaks in burn patients [12]. O'Connell et al. [13] described a case of soft tissue infection caused by *R. planticola* in a healthy individual 1 week after injury to the thumb in a soiled environment. Otherwise, since the patient had plunged into a tank of contaminated water to extinguish the fire on his body, including his face, it was speculated that the oral or gastrointestinal routes might also have contributed to the infection. Lam et al. [6] reported a case of *R. planticola* infection 4 days after a patient with metastatic cancer consumed seafood. Furthermore, extensive burn injury is well-known to lead to host immune system impairment, rendering the patient susceptible to opportunistic infections [14]. Also, escharotomy and skin grafting may be predisposed to bacteremia, as previous reports have suggested the potential risk factors of *R. planticola* bacteremia in invasive medical procedures [9].

Clinical outcomes of *R. planticola* infections have been fair unless polymicrobial bacteremia was present [2, 15]. Chun et al. summarized 20 cases of *R. planticola* bacteremia, six of which were polymicrobial infections; half of those failed to recover [2]. Even though *R. planticola* as a sole pathogen had been isolated from blood cultures in the present case, *P. aeruginosa* and MSSA burn wound infections may accelerate the patient's development of refractory septic shock. In the past few years, carbapenem-resistant *R. planticola* cases have been reported sporadically, resulting in unfavorable outcomes [15, 16]. In the present case, empiric administration of piperacillin/tazobactam had been initiated prior to the development of septic shock and isolated organisms were susceptible to piperacillin/tazobactam and meropenem. As limited data is available regarding this pathogen and its virulence, the mechanisms of its pathogenesis in the present case with poor outcomes remained unclear. We cannot assert whether the clinical course was associated with *R. planticola* bacteremia; however, it may have played a critical role in the development of fatal septic shock. Further research regarding its virulence is necessary.

The effects of prophylactic antibiotics use for patients with severe burns remains controversial, as a small volume and low-quality data is available [17]. However, a recent systematic review suggests that prophylactic antibiotics may be beneficial for patients requiring mechanical ventilation [18]. Although a history of exposure to soil or water is not always essential for *Aeromonas* spp. infection in burn patients [19], a history of extinguishing the fire with dirty water should alert the physician to consider the possibility of infection from *A. hydrophila* and other microorganisms, including *P. aeruginosa* and *Bacillus cereus* [3]. Hence, initial therapeutic antibiotics may contribute to favorable outcomes in such a specific situation.

To the best of our knowledge, this is the first report of fatal septic shock due to *R. planticola* bacteremia, which was an extremely unusual pathogen in a burn patient. Exposure to contaminated water to extinguish a fire may contribute to *R. planticola* infection. In addition, an impaired immune system due to an extensive third degree burn may further progress to refractory septic shock. Initial empirical antibiotics may be beneficial for burn patients with aquatic exposure.

Conclusions

We reported a rare case of fatal septic shock due to *R. planticola* bacteremia following flame burn injury. Clinicians should be aware of such fatal infections when a patient is exposed to contaminated water.

Abbreviations

TBSA: total body surface area; MIC: minimum inhibitory concentration; MSSA: methicillin-sensitive *Staphylococcus aureus*.

Authors' contributions

TY, HN, HI, TO and TW cared for the patient. TY and HI drafted the manuscript. TY, TO, and TW collected and analyzed the data. HN, KT, and AN evaluated the draft and suggested revisions. All authors read and approved the final manuscript.

Author details

[1] Advanced Emergency and Critical Care Medical Center, Okayama University Hospital, 2-5-1 Shikata-cho, Kita-ku, Okayama-shi, Okayama 700-8558, Japan.
[2] Department of Plastic and Reconstructive Surgery, Okayama University Graduate School of Medicine, Dentistry and Pharmaceutical Sciences, 2-5-1 Shikata-cho, Kita-ku, Okayama-shi, Okayama 700-8558, Japan.

Acknowledgements
Not applicable.

Competing interests
The authors declare that they have no competing interests.

Funding
No funding was obtained for this report.

References

1. Kim SH, Roh KH, Yoon YK, Kang DO, Lee DW, Kim MJ, et al. Necrotizing fasciitis involving the chest and abdominal wall caused by *Raoultella planticola*. BMC Infect Dis. 2012;12:59.
2. Chun S, Yun JW, Huh HJ, Lee NY. Low virulence? Clinical characteristics of *Raoultella planticola* bacteremia. Infection. 2014;42:899–904.
3. Ribeiro NF, Heath CH, Kierath J, Rea S, Duncan-Smith M, Wood FM. Burn wounds infected by contaminated water: case reports, review of the literature and recommendations for treatment. Burns. 2010;36:9–22.
4. Drancourt M, Bollet C, Carta A, Rousselier P. Phylogenetic analyses of *Klebsiella* species delineate *Klebsiella* and *Raoultella* gen. nov., with description of *Raoultella ornithinolytica* comb. nov., *Raoultella terrigena* comb. nov. and *Raoultella planticola* comb. nov. Int J Syst Evol Microbiol. 2001;51:925–32.
5. Gavini F, Izard D, Grimont PAD, Beji A, Ageron E, Leclerc H. Priority of *Klebsiella planticol* Bagley, Seidler, and Brenner 1982 over *Klebsiella trevisani* Ferragut, Izard, Gavini, Kersters, DeLey, and Leclerc 1983. Int J Syst Bacteriol. 1986;36:486.
6. Lam PW, Salit IE. *Raoultella planticola* bacteremia following consumption of seafood. Can J Infect Dis Med Microbiol. 2014;25:e83–4.
7. Alves MS, Riley LW, Moreira BM. A case of severe pancreatitis complicated by *Raoultella planticola* infection. J Med Microbiol. 2007;56:696–8.
8. Ershadi A, Weiss E, Verduzco E, Chia D, Sadigh M. Emerging pathogen: a case and review of *Raoultella planticola*. Infection. 2014;42:1043–6.
9. Yokota K, Gomi H, Miura Y, Sugano K, Morisawa Y. Cholangitis with septic shock caused by *Raoultella planticola*. J Med Microbiol. 2012;61:446–9.
10. Skelton WP 4th, Taylor Z, Hsu J. A rare case of *Raoultella planticola* urinary tract infection in an immunocompromised patient with multiple myeloma. IDCases. 2017;8:9–11.
11. Westerveld D, Hussain J, Aljaafareh A, Ataya A. A rare case of *Raoultella planticola* pneumonia: an emerging pathogen. Respir Med Case Rep. 2017;21:69–70.
12. Yun HC, Tully CC, Mende K, Castillo M, Murray CK. A single-center, six-year evaluation of the role of pulsed-field gel electrophoresis in suspected burn center outbreaks. Burns. 2016;42:1323–30.
13. O'Connell K, Kelly J, Niriain U. A rare case of soft-tissue infection caused by *Raoultella planticola*. Case Rep Med. 2010;2010:134086.
14. Bohr S, Patel SJ, Vasko R, Shen K, Golberg A, Berthiaume F, et al. The role of CHI3L1 (Chitinase-3-Like-1) in the pathogenesis of infections in burns in a mouse model. PLoS ONE. 2015;10:e0140440.
15. Demiray T, Koroglu M, Ozbek A, Altindis M. A rare cause of infection, *Raoultella planticola*: emerging threat and new reservoir for carbapenem resistance. Infection. 2016;44:713–7.
16. Castanheira M, Deshpande LM, DiPersio JR, Kang J, Weinstein MP, Jones RN. First descriptions of blaKPC in *Raoultella* spp. (*R. planticola* and *R. ornithinolytica*): report from the SENTRY Antimicrobial Surveillance Program. J Clin Microbiol. 2009;47:4129–30.
17. Avni T, Levcovich A, Ad-El DD, Leibovici L, Paul M. Prophylactic antibiotics for burns patients: systematic review and meta-analysis. BMJ. 2010;340:c241.
18. Ramos G, Cornistein W, Cerino GT, Nacif G. Systemic antimicrobial prophylaxis in burn patients: systematic review. J Hosp Infect. 2017;97:105–14.
19. Chim H, Song C. Aeromonas infection in critically ill burn patients. Burns. 2007;33:756–9.

19

Transmission and characterization of bla_{NDM-1} in *Enterobacter cloacae* at a teaching hospital in Yunnan, China

Na Du, Shumin Liu, Min Niu, Yong Duan, Shuangmeng Zhang, Jing Yao, Jian Mao, Ran Chen and Yan Du*

Abstract

Background: In recent years, New Delhi metallo-beta-lactamases 1 (bla_{NDM-1}) has been reported with increasing frequency and become prevalent. The present study was undertaken to investigate the epidemiological dissemination of the bla_{NDM-1} gene in *Enterobacter cloacae* isolates at a teaching hospital in Yunnan, China.

Methods: Antimicrobial susceptibility testing was performed using VITEK 2 system and E test gradient strips. The presence of integrons and insertion sequence common region 1 were examined by PCR and sequencing. Clonal relatedness was assessed by pulsed-field gel electrophoresis (PFGE) and multilocus sequence typing. Conjugation experiments and Southern blot hybridization were performed to determine the transferability of plasmids.

Results: Ten *E. cloacae* isolates and their *Escherichia coli* transconjugants were exhibited similar resistant patterns to carbapenems, cephalosporins and penicillins. 8 (80%) of *E. cloacae* isolates carried class 1 integron and 1 (12.5%) carried class 2 integron. Integron variable regions harbored the genes which encoded resistance to aminoglycosides (*aadA1, aadA2, aadA5, aadB, aac(6′)-Ib-cr*), sulfamethoxazole/trimethoprim (*dfrA17, dfrA12, dfrA15*) and Streptozotocin (*sat2*). Six *E. cloacae* isolates belonged to ST74 and exhibited highly similar PFGE patterns. Each isolate shared an identical plasmid with ~33.3 kb size that carried the bla_{NDM-1} gene, except T3 strain, of which the bla_{NDM-1} gene was located on a ~50 kb plasmid.

Conclusions: Our findings suggested that plasmid was able to contribute to the dissemination of bla_{NDM-1}. Hence, more attention should be devoted to monitor the dissemination of the bla_{NDM-1} gene due to its horizontal transfer via plasmid. In addition, nosocomial surveillance system should actively monitor the potential endemic clone of ST74 to prevent their further spread.

Keywords: *Enterobacter cloacae*, NDM-1, ST74, Integron, ISCR1

Background

Enterobacter cloacae is an important nosocomial pathogen, which can cause various infections including urinary tract, skin and soft tissue, respiratory tract, surgical site, biliary tract, sepsis, intravenous catheters, central nervous system and outbreaks at neonatal units [1, 2]. New Delhi metallo-beta-lactamases 1 (bla_{NDM-1}) are Ambler class B Metallo-β-lactamases(MBLs)with carbapenemase activity that confers resistance to all β-lactams except aztreonam, was first identified in a carbapenem-resistant *Klebsiella pneumoniae* strain recovered from a Swedish patient who was hospitalized in India in 2008 [3], and mainly detected in carbapenem-resistant *Acinetobacter* spp. in mainland China. However, NDM-1-mediated carbapenem resistance in *E. cloacae* has been rarely reported in China.

The widespread dissemination of bla_{NDM-1} is mainly due to plasmids, integrons, insertion sequence common region (ISCR) and clonal outbreaks [4]. Plasmids are extrachromosomal DNA molecules capable of autonomous replication, and can confer resistance

*Correspondence: 329663495@qq.com
Department of Clinical Laboratory, the First Affiliated Hospital of Kunming Medical University, Yunnan Institute of Laboratory Diagnosis, Yunnan Key Laboratory of Laboratory Medicine, No. 295, Xichang Road, Wuhua, Kunming Yunnan, China

to the major antimicrobials [5]. Integrons are bacterial genetic elements able to capture and express genes contained within mobile gene cassettes. Typically, integrons are composed of two conserved regions, a 3′ conserved segment (3′CS) and a 5′ conserved segment (5′CS), as well as an internal variable region containing gene cassettes that encode antimicrobial resistance determinants [6]. ISCR elements can transpose adjacent DNA sequences by a process called rolling-circle replication, now it is recognized as powerful antibiotic resistance gene capture systems and playing a major role in spread of antibiotic resistance genes. However, whether these mobile elements mediate the dissemination of $bla_{\text{NDM-1}}$ gene is still an unsolved mystery in the region. Therefore, the aim of this study is to explore the epidemiological dissemination of the $bla_{\text{NDM-1}}$ gene in *E. cloacae* isolates at a teaching hospital in Yunnan, China.

Methods

Bacterial strains

In total, ten NDM-1-producing *E. cloacae* isolates were collected from hospitalized patients in the First Affiliated Hospital of Kunming Medical University between June 2012 and January 2016. All isolates were identified by VITEK2 automated identification system (bioMerieux, France). Carbapenemase activity was assessed by the modified Hodge test, MBL production was examined by imipenem-ethylenediaminetetraacetic acid (EDTA) disk method and the $bla_{\text{NDM-1}}$ gene was determined by PCR in the early stage of the study. All patients were of Yunnan descent and none had a recent history of travelling epidemic area (Table 1).

Antimicrobial susceptibility testing

Antimicrobial susceptibilities for the NDM-1-producing isolates and transconjugants were initially tested using the VITEK2 system. MICs of imipenem, meropenem and ertapenem were re-evaluated using E test gradient strips (bioMerieux, France) on Mueller–Hinton agar plates and the results interpreted according to the CLSI guidelines [7]. *Escherichia coli* ATCC 25922 was used as quality control strain.

PCR amplification and sequencing

Isolates were grown overnight in M–H Agar plates at 37 °C and genomic DNA was extracted using boiling method. Class 1, 2, 3 integrons and ISCR1 were, respectively, amplified using the primers intI1/intI1, intI2/intI2, intI3/intI3, hep58/hep59, hep74/hep51, orf513F/orf513R and orf513F/sul1R (Table 2). The amplified PCR products were analyzed by electrophoresis in 2% agarose gels and finally visualized in gel documentation system. PCR amplification products were sequenced. The resulting DNA sequences were analyzed by the BLAST program (http://www.ncbi.nlm.nih.gov/BLAST/).

Pulsed-field gel electrophoresis (PFGE) and multilocus sequence typing (MLST)

Bacterial genomic DNA was prepared in agarose plugs and digested with the restriction enzymes XbaI (Promega, USA). The DNA fragments were separated by use of a CHEF Mappar XA PFGE system (Bio-Rad, USA), with running time of 22 h and pulse times ranging from 5 to 40 s. The running buffer was 0.5 × Tris-boric acid-EDTA (TBE). *Salmonella ser. Braenderup H9812* was used as a standard for comparison. PFGE patterns were compared visually following previously described criteria [12]. Multilocus sequence typing (MLST) was performed

Table 1 Clinical characteristics of the cases

Isolates	Age (years)	Gender	Specimen	Ward	Average hospital stay (days)	History of travel epidemic area	Outcome
T1	58	Male	Secreta	Orthopedics Department	66	No	Discharge
T2	96	Male	Sputum	General Practice	33	No	Discharge
T3	87	Female	Urine	EICU	117	No	Death
T4	36	Female	Urine	Transplantation Center	20	No	Discharge
T5	32	Male	Urine	Transplantation Center	39	No	Discharge
T6	65	Female	Pleural effusion	EICU	1	No	Death
T7	32	Male	Urine	Transplantation Center	23	No	Discharge
T8	22	Female	Urine	Transplantation Center	35	No	Discharge
T9	11	Female	Blood	NICU	18	No	Discharge
T10	34	Male	Urine	Transplantation Center	32	No	Discharge

EICU emergency intensive care unit, *NICU* neonatal intensive care unit

Table 2 Primers used in PCR and DNA sequencing

Gene	Nucleotide sequence (5′ to 3′)	Expected size of amplicon (bp)	Reference or source
intI1/intI1	F1: GCATCCTCGGTTTTCTGG R1: GGTGTGGCGGGCTTCGTG	457	[8]
intI2/intI2	F2: CACGGATATGCGACA AAA AGGT R2: GTAGCA AACGAGTGACGA AATG	789	[8]
intI3/intI3	F3: ATCTGCCAA ACCTGACTG R3: CGA ATGCCCCAACAACTC	922	[8]
hep58/hep59	F4: TCATGGCTTGTTATGACTGT R4: GTAGGGCTTATTATGCACGC	Unknown	[9]
hep74/hep51	F5: CGGGATCCCGGACGGCATGCACGATTTGTA R5: GATGCCATCGCAAGTACGAG	Unknown	[10]
orf513F/orf513R	F6: ATGGTTTCATGCGGGTT R6: CTGAGGGTGTGAGCGAG	475	[11]
orf513F/sul1R	F7: ATGGTTTCATGCGGGTT R7: TTTGAAGGTTCGACAGC	Unknown	[11]

on representative isolates. Internal fragments of the seven housekeeping genes were amplified using the primers given at the Institute Pasteur MLST Databases web site (http://pubmlst.org/ecloacae/). The PCR products were sequenced. Sequence types (STs) were assigned using online database tools.

Conjugation experiments and Plasmid analysis

The transfer of carbapenem resistance was tested using a conjugation test, *E. coli* 600 (rifampicin-resistant) was used as the recipient strain, NDM-1-producing *E. cloacae* clinical isolates were used as the donor strains. Donor and recipient cells from M–H broth cultures were mixed in a ratio of 2:1 and transconjugant clones were screened on M–H agar plates containing rifampicin (256 mg/L) and Imipenem (1 mg/L). Conjugation events occurred at 37 °C. The presence of the $bla_{\text{NDM-1}}$ gene in transconjugants was determined by PCR and sequencing. Genomic DNA was digested with S1 nuclease (Promega, USA). The linearized plasmids and partially digested genomic DNA were separated through the CHEF-Mapper XA PFGE system with a switch time from 2.16 to 63.8 s for 18 h at 6 V/cm at 14 °C. Linear plasmids generated by S1-PFGE were transferred to nvlon membrane (Millipore, USA) and hybridized with a digoxigenin-labeled probe specific to $bla_{\text{NMD-1}}$. Probe labeling and signal detection were carried out with DIG high primer DNA labeling and detection starter kit according to the manufacturer's instructions (Roche Applied Sciences, Germany).

Results

Antimicrobial susceptibility testing

The antibiotic susceptibility results showed that all the NDM-1-producing *E. cloacae* isolates exhibited resistance to carbapenems, cephalosporins and penicillins. Only one isolates remained susceptible to aztreonam, which was not hydrolysed by metallo-carbapenemases, thus suggesting the presence of additional β-lactamases in the remaining isolates. Ten isolates exhibited different level resistance to tetracycline, amikacin, ciprofloxacin and tigecycline, seven isolates were resistance to tetracycline, one to amikacin, nine to ciprofloxacin and one to tigecycline. These results are summarized in Table 3.

Detection of integrons and ISCR1

Class 1 integrase gene was detected in 80% (8/10), while the variable region of class 1 integron was detected in 70% (7/10) NDM-1-producing *E. cloacae* isolates. Among them, six different gene cassette arrays were found, which included: *dfrA12+aadA2, dfrA15+dfrA17, aadA2+aadA5+dfrA17, dfrA15+aadB+aadA2, dfrA15* and *dfrA15+aac (6′)-Ib-cr*. Those genes encoded resistance to aminoglycosides and sulfamethoxazole/trimethoprim. 10% (1/10) strains possessed class 2 integron, and the variable region of class 2 integron harbored *sat2+aadA1* genes, which mediated antibiotic resistance to streptothricin and streptomycin. None of the isolates harbored class 3 integron. 50% (5/10) isolates carried ISCR1 elements. However, in the five ISCR1 positive isolates, the cassette arrays could not be detected.

PFGE and MLST typing

According to Tenover's criteria [12], Six *E. cloacae* isolates, of which four obtained from transplantation center, one from general practice and one from emergency intensive care unit, belonged to ST74 and shared the same PFGE fingerprint pattern (Fig. 1), suggesting they were clonally related, the remaining strains were

Table 3 Antimicrobial drug susceptibility profiles (MICs in mg/L) for clinical isolates and transconjugants

Isolate no.	VITEK2										E test		
	PIP	TCY	ATM	CAZ	CIP	AMK	MEM	IMP	ETP	TGC	MEM	IMP	ETP
T1	≥128	≥16	≥64	≥64	≥4	16	8	8	≥8	1	>32	32	>32
T2	≥128	4	≥64	≥64	≥4	≤2	≥16	≥16	≥8	1	>32	>32	>32
T3	≥128	≥16	≥64	≥64	≥4	≥64	8	≥16	≥8	≥8	>32	>32	>32
T4	≥128	8	≥64	≥64	≥4	4	≥16	≥16	≥8	1	>32	24	>32
T5	≥128	≥16	16	≥64	≥4	4	≥16	≥16	≥8	2	>32	>32	>32
T6	≥128	≥16	≥64	≥64	≥4	16	≥16	≥16	≥8	1	32	>32	>32
T7	≥128	≥16	16	≥64	≥4	16	≥16	≥16	≥8	2	>32	>32	>32
T8	≥128	≥16	≥64	≥64	≥4	16	≥16	≥16	≥8	1	>32	>32	>32
T9	≥128	≥16	≤1	≥64	0.5	≤2	≥16	≥16	≥8	1	>32	>32	>32
T10	≥128	4	≥64	≥64	≥4	≤2	4	4	≥8	2	6	8	8
T1-EC600	≥128	≤1	≤1	≥64	0.5	≤2	8	≥16	≥8	1	8	8	8
T2-EC600	≥128	≤1	32	≥64	0.5	≤2	≥16	≥16	≥8	1	8	16	>32
T3-EC600	≥128	≤1	≤1	≥64	0.5	≤2	8	≥16	≥8	2	16	16	>32
T4-EC600	≥128	≥16	32	≥64	0.5	≤2	8	≥16	≥8	1	>32	6	8
T5-EC600	≥128	≤1	≤1	≥64	0.5	≤2	8	≥16	≥8	2	>32	>32	>32
T6-EC600	≥128	≤1	≤1	≥64	0.5	≤2	≥16	≥16	≥8	1	>32	>32	>32
T7-EC600	≥128	≤1	≤1	≥64	0.5	≤2	≥16	≥16	≥8	1	24	8	8
T8-EC600	≥128	≤1	≤1	≥64	0.5	≤2	8	≥16	≥8	1	>32	>32	>32
T9-EC600	≥128	≤1	≤1	≥64	0.5	≤2	≥16	≥16	≥8	1	24	>32	24
T10-EC600	≥128	≤1	≤1	≥64	0.5	≤2	≥16	≥16	≥8	1	>32	>32	16
EC600	≤4	≤1	≤1	≤1	≤0.25	≤2	≤0.25	≤1	≤0.5	≤0.5	0.032	0.019	0.008
ATCC25922	≤4	≤1	≤1	≤1	≤0.25	≤2	≤0.25	≤1	≤0.5	≤0.5	0.032	0.019	0.008

EC600 Escherichia coli 600, *T1-EC600* the transconjugants of T1 strain, *PIP* piperacillin, *TCY* tetracycline, *ATM* aztreonam, *CAZ* ceftazidime, *CIP* ciprofloxacin, *AMK* amikacin, *MEM* meropenem, *IPM* imipenem, *ETP* ertapenem, *TGC* tigecycline

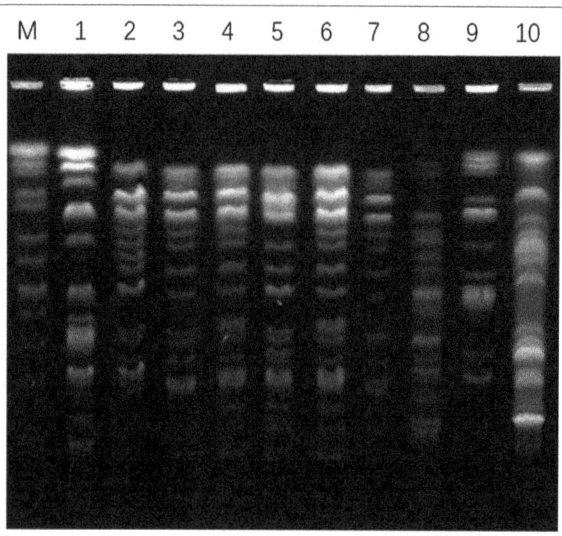

Fig. 1 Pulsed-field gel electrophoresis (PFGE) of XbaI-digested DNA of *E. cloacae* isolates. *Lane M* PFGE marker, *Salmonella ser. Braenderup* H9812; *lanes 1–10* representative NDM-1-producing *E. cloacae*

characterized by unique genotypes. MLST of representative isolates assigned the *E. cloacae* to four sequence type (ST), ST74, ST182, ST754 and ST175, respectively.

Plasmid analysis

Conjugation experiments revealed that plasmids harboring bla_{NDM-1} were transformed into *E. coli* 600. All transconjugants conferred resistance to carbapenems, cephalosporins and penicillins while all of them remained susceptible to ciprofloxacin and amikacin (Table 1). Isolates harbored three to five plasmids according to S1-PFGE electrophoresis. Southern hybridization analysis with a bla_{NDM-1}-specific probe revealed that bla_{NDM-1} was located on a ~33.3 kb plasmid in nine isolates and on a ~50 kb plasmid in one isolates (Fig. 2).

Discussion

The bla_{NDM-1} was first identified in a clinical isolate of *K. pneumoniae* in New Delhi, India, and suddenly got disseminated around the world. The bla_{NDM-1}-carrying

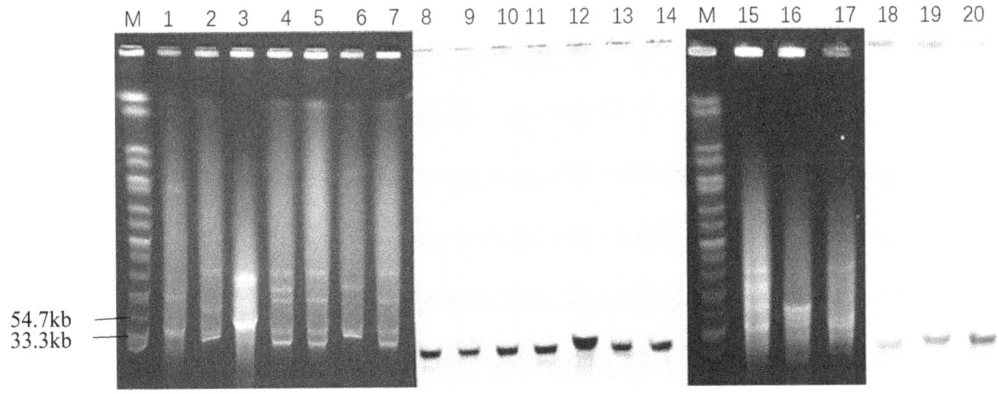

Fig. 2 Results of S1 nuclease PFGE and Southern blot hybridization. *Lane M* PFGE marker, *Salmonella ser. Braenderup* H9812; *lanes 1–7* Strains (T1–T7) digested with S1 nuclease; *lanes 8–14* hybridized plasmids of strains (T7–T1) with the bla_{NDM-1} probe; *lanes 15–17* strains (T8–T10) digested with S1 nuclease; *lanes 18–20* hybridized plasmids of strains (T8–T10) with the bla_{NDM-1} probe

bacteria conferred resistance to all most β-lactam antibiotics. Thus, treatment of infections with NDM-producing bacteria was a major challenge, leaving few options for clinical treatment beside tigecycline or colistin. The bla_{NDM-1} gene have been identified in a variety of gram-negative bacilli, including *Acinetobacter* spp. [13], *Enterobacteriaceae* [14] and *Pseudomonas aeruginosa* [15]. Lack of uncontaminated potable water and abuse of over-the-counter antibiotic administration offered the ideal setting for the development of a latent endemic situation, and international "medical tourism" played an important role in the spread of bla_{NDM-1} gene [16]. Yunnan Kunming is a famous tourist city in the world, and large numbers of domestic and foreign tourists come here every year, thus "medical tourism" may play an important role in the spread of bla_{NDM-1} among carbapenem-resistant bacteria in this region.

In China, plasmid-carrying bla_{NDM-1} have been identified in *Enterobacteriaceae* isolates in several regions including Beijing, Shanghai, Hong Kong, Shandong Henan and Yunnan province, the size of plasmids harboring bla_{NDM-1} were vary from ~50 to 360 kb [17, 18]. Our research shows that bla_{NDM-1} gene was mainly located on a plasmid with ~33.3 kb size, were different from previously reported in China before. The bla_{NDM-1} gene was not detected in integrons and ISCR1 mobile elements. Integrons only carried these genes encoding resistance to aminoglycosides [*aadA1, aadA2, aadA5, aadB, aac(6')-Ib-cr*], sulfamethoxazole/trimethoprim (*dfrA17, dfrA12, dfrA15*) and Streptozotocin (*sat2*). Those results suggested that plasmid was the most important mobile element that mediated the dissemination of bla_{NDM-1} and integrons were the basis for the formation of multiple drug-resistant bacteria in the region. In addition, it was worth noting that there had been some evidences which demonstrated that integrons and ISCR mobile elements were located on plasmids [4], thus, the resistance gene through the plasmids spreading was not a single element, but by 1 + 1 or 1 + 2 mode. This mode of dissemination should arouse high concern of the relevant departments.

Clonal spread was an important factor involved in the prevalence of NDM-1-producing *Enterobacteriaceae*. Outbreak of NDM-1-producing *K. pneumoniae* ST105 and ST147 have been reported in Yunnan [17] and Xi'an [19], and NDM-1-producing *E. cloacae* ST120 have been reported in Henan [18], China, respectively. Our study showed that 5 clusters for 10 strains, 1 cluster from 6 closely related isolates was found to exhibit similarities which is more than 90%. The result suggested that 6 NDM-1-producing *E. cloacae* isolates were clonally related. However, there was no significant epidemiological relatedness among them. Hence, we could not trace their origin. MLST analysis revealed four ST types including ST74, ST754, ST175 and ST182, among them, ST74 was the major type in NDM-1-producing *E. cloacae* isolates, which was different from previous types reported before such as ST66, ST78, ST108, ST114 and ST120 [18]. ST74 has been identified among non-susceptible to ertapenem of *E. cloacae* isolates in North-Eastern France, and was associated with OXA-48-producing *E. cloacae* isolates in Spain [20, 21]. The present study is the first to report on an outbreak of NDM-1-producing *E. cloacae* ST74.

Infection control measures were strengthened to prevent the further transmission of bla_{NDM-1}. They included hand hygiene, contact isolation, active screening, environmental surface disinfection, standard aseptic manipulation techniques, among them, hand hygiene was the most effective and economical strategy for reducing cross infection [16].

To conclude, our study demonstrated that plasmids were the most important elements that mediate horizontal transfer of the bla_{NDM-1} gene. Furthermore, we identified a potential endemic clone of ST74. The emergence of NDM-1-producing *E. cloacae* ST74 isolates is worrying, nosocomial surveillance system should pay more attention to prevent their further spread.

Abbreviations

NDM-1: New Delhi metallo-beta-lactamase 1; ISCR1: insertion sequence common region 1; PCR: polymerase chain reaction; PFGE: pulse field gel electrophoresis; MLST: multilocus sequence typing; MBLs: metallo-β-lactamases; 5CS & 3CS: 5′ & 3′-conserved segments; CLSI: Clinical and Laboratory Standards Institute; M–H: Mueller–Hinton; MIC: minimum inhibitory concentration.

Authors' contributions

YD designed the study; ND drafted the first version of this manuscript; SL and MN collected the isolates and clinical informations; ND performed the PFGE; ND and JM preformed the antimicrobial susceptibility test and conjugation experiment; RC, JY, MZ, SL, MN and ND carried out the molecular biology experiments. YD and YD participated in manuscript correction. All authors read and approved the final manuscript.

Acknowledgements

Escherchia coli 600 and *Salmonella ser. Braenderup* H9812 was a kind gift from Prof. Yunsong Yu, the First Affiliated Hospital of Zhejiang University. This study was supported by grants from the Health and Family Planning Commission of Yunnan Province (Grant No. 2016NS030).

Competing interests

The authors declare that they have no competing interests.

References

1. Miyoshi-Akiyama T, Hayakawa K, Ohmagari N, Shimojima M, Kirikae T. Multilocus sequence typing (MLST) for characterization of *Enterobacter cloacae*. PLoS ONE. 2013;8(6):e66358. doi:10.1371/journal.pone.0066358.
2. Yang FC, Yan JJ, Hung KH, Wu JJ. Characterization of ertapenem-resistant *Enterobacter cloacae* in a Taiwanese University Hospital. J Clin Microbiol. 2012;50(2):223–6. doi:10.1128/JCM.01263-11.
3. Yong D, Toleman MA, Giske CG, Cho HS, Sundman K, Lee K, Walsh TR. Characterization of a new metallo-beta-lactamase gene, bla(NDM-1), and a novel erythromycin esterase gene carried on a unique genetic structure in *Klebsiella pneumoniae* sequence type 14 from India. Antimicrobial Agents Chemother. 2009;53(12):5046–54.
4. Zhao WH, Hu ZQ. Acquired metallo-β-lactamases and their genetic association with class 1 integrons and ISCR elements in Gram-negative bacteria. Futur Microbiol. 2015;10(5):873–87. doi:10.2217/fmb.15.18.
5. Carattoli A. Resistance plasmid families in *Enterobacteriaceae*. Antimicrob Agents Chemother. 2009;53(6):2227–38. doi:10.1128/AAC.01707-08
6. Lima AM, de Melo ME, Alves LC, Brayner FA, Lopes AC. Investigation of class 1 integrons in *Klebsiella pneumoniae* clinical and microbiota isolates belonging to different phylogenetic groups in Recife, State of Pernambuco. Rev Soc Bras Med Trop. 2014;47(2):165–9.
7. Clinical and Laboratory Standards Institute. Performance standards for antimicrobial susceptibility testing: twenty-fourth informational supplement update document M100-S24. Wayne: CLSI; 2014.
8. Shibata N, Doi Y, Yamane K, Yagi T, Kurokawa H, Shibayama K, Kato H, Kai K, Arakawa Y. PCR typing of genetic determinants for metallo-beta-lactamases and integrases carried by gram-negative bacteria isolated in Japan, with focus on the class 3 integron. J Clin Microbiol. 2003;41(12):5407–13.
9. White PA, McIver CJ, Deng Y, Rawlinson WD. Characterisation of two new gene cassettes, aadA5 and dfrA17. FEMS Microbiol Lett. 2000;182(2):265–9.
10. White PA, McIver CJ, Rawlinson WD. Integrons and gene cassettes in the *Enterobacteriaceae*. Antimicrob Agents Chemother. 2001;45(9):2658–61.
11. Quiroga MP, Andres P, Petroni A, Soler Bistué AJ, Guerriero L, Vargas LJ, Zorreguieta A, Tokumoto M, Quiroga C, Tolmasky ME, Galas M, Centrón D. Complex class 1 integrons with diverse variable regions, including aac(6′)-Ib-cr, and a novel allele, qnrB10, associated with ISCR1 in clinical enterobacterial isolates from Argentina. Antimicrob Agents Chemother. 2007;51(12):4466–70.
12. Tenover FC, Arbeit RD, Goering RV, Mickelsen PA, Murray BE, Persing DH, Swaminathan B. Interpreting chromosomal DNA restriction patterns produced by pulsed-field gel electrophoresis: criteria for bacterial strain typing. J Clin Microbiol. 1995;33(9):2233–9.
13. Huang TW, Lauderdale TL, Liao TL, Hsu MC, Chang FY, Chang SC, Khong WX, Ng OT, Chen YT, Kuo SC, Chen TL, Mu JJ, Tsai SF. Effective transfer of a 47 kb NDM-1-positive plasmid among *Acinetobacter* species. J Antimicrob Chemother. 2015;70(10):2734–8. doi:10.1093/jac/dkv191.
14. Qu H, Wang X, Ni Y, Liu J, Tan R, Huang J, Li L, Sun J. NDM-1-producing *Enterobacteriaceae* in a teaching hospital in Shanghai, China: IncX3-type plasmids may contribute to the dissemination of bla_{NDM-1}. Int J Infect Dis. 2015;34:8–13. doi:10.1016/j.ijid.2015.02.020.
15. Zafer MM, Amin M, El Mahallawy H, Ashour MS, Al Agamy M. First report of NDM-1-producing *Pseudomonas aeruginosa* in Egypt. Int J Infect Dis. 2014;29:80–1. doi:10.1016/j.ijid.2014.07.008.
16. Voulgari E, Gartzonika C, Vrioni G, Politi L, Priavali E, Levidiotou-Stefanou S, Tsakris A. The Balkan region: NDM-1-producing *Klebsiella pneumoniae* ST11 clonal strain causing outbreaks in Greece. J Antimicrob Chemother. 2014;69(8):2091–7. doi:10.1093/jac/dku105.
17. Zheng R, Zhang Q, Guo Y, Feng Y, Liu L, Zhang A, Zhao Y, Yang X, Xia X. Outbreak of plasmid-mediated NDM-1-producing *Klebsiella pneumoniae* ST105 among neonatal patients in Yunnan. China. Ann Clin Microbiol Antimicrob. 2016;15:10. doi:10.1186/s12941-016-0124-6.
18. Liu C, Qin S, Xu H, Xu L, Zhao D, Liu X, Lang S, Feng X, Liu HM. New Delhi metallo-β-lactamase 1(NDM-1), the dominant carbapenemase detected in carbapenem-resistant *Enterobacter cloacae* from Henan province, China. PLoS ONE. 2015;10(8):e0135044. doi:10.1371/journal.Pone.
19. Wang X, Xu X, Li Z, Chen H, Wang Q, Yang P, Zhao C, Ni M, Wang H. An outbreak of a nosocomial NDM-1-producing *Klebsiella pneumoniae* ST147 at a teaching hospital in mainland China. Microb Drug Resist. 2014;20(2):144–9. doi:10.1089/mdr.2013.0100.
20. Fernández J, Montero I, Martínez Ó, Fleites A, Poirel L, Nordmann P, Rodicio MR. Dissemination of multiresistant *Enterobacter cloacae* isolates producing OXA-48 and CTX-M-15 in a Spanish hospital. Int J Antimicrob Agents. 2015;46(4):469–74. doi:10.1016/j.ijantimicag.2015.07.003.
21. Guillard T, Cholley P, Limelette A, Hocquet D, Matton L, Guyeux C, Lebreil AL, Bajolet O, Brasme L, Madoux J, Vernet-Garnier V, Barbe C, Bertrand X, de Champs On Behalf of CarbaFrEst Group C. Fluoroquinolone Resistance Mechanisms and population structure of *Enterobacter cloacae* non-susceptible to Ertapenem in North-Eastern France. Front Microbiol. 2015; 6:1186. doi:10.3389/fmicb.2015.01186.

20

An evaluation of *E. coli* in urinary tract infection in emergency department at KAMC in Riyadh, Saudi Arabia

Menyfah Q. Alanazi[1*], Fulwah Y. Alqahtani[2] and Fadilah S. Aleanizy[2]

Abstract

Background: Urinary tract infection (UTIS) is a common infectious disease in which level of antimicrobial resistance are alarming worldwide. Therefore, this study aims to describe the prevalence and the resistance pattern of the main bacteria responsible for UTIS *Escherichia coli* (*E. coli*).

Methods: Retrospective chart review for patients admitted to emergency department and diagnosed with UTIS at KAMC, in Riyadh, Saudi Arabia between January to March 2008 was performed. Antimicrobial susceptibility to ampicillin, augmentin (amoxicillin/clavulanate), cefazolin, co-trimoxazole (sulfamethoxazole/trimethoprim), ciprofloxacin, and nitrofurantoin, and cefpodoxime was determined for 101 *E. coli* urinary isolates.

Results: *Escherichia coli* was the most prevalent pathogen contributing to UTIS representing 93.55, 60.24, and 45.83% of all pathogen isolated from urine culture of pediatric, adult, and elderly, respectively. High rates of resistance to ampicillin (82.76, 58, and 63.64%) and co-trimoxazole (51.72, 42, and 59.09%), among *E. coli* isolated from pediatric, adult and elderly respectively. Nitrofurantoin was the most active agent, followed by ciprofloxacin, augmentin and cefazolin. 22.77% of *E. coli* isolates exhibited multiple drug resistance (MDR). Among 66 and 49 isolates resistant to ampicillin and co-trimoxazole, respectively, 34.84 and 42.85% were MDR. In contrast, all isolates resistant to augmentin and nitrofurantoin were MRD, while 72.7 and 82.4% of isolates resistant to ciprofloxacin and cefazolin were MDR.

Conclusions: High resistance was observed to ampicillin and co-trimoxazole which commonly used as empirical treatments for UTIS, limiting their clinical use. This necessitates continuous surveillance for resistance pattern of uropathogens against antibiotics.

Keywords: Antibiotics resistance, *E. coli*, Empirical therapy, UTIS

Background

Urinary tract infections (UTIs) are among the most common types of bacterial infections occurring both in the community and hospital settings [1, 2]. There are two types of UTIs: hospital associated urinary tract infection (HAUTIs), and community-associated urinary tract infection (CAUTIs) [3]. Women are the predominant group of patients with CAUTIs [1, 2]. UTIs was estimated to represent 100,000 hospitalizations, 7 million visits and 1 million admissions to emergency services in USA [4, 5]. The economic and public health burdens of UTIs is substantial and markedly affect the quality of life of infected patients [6]. In Saudi Arabia, UTIs were reported to be the second leading cause of infections predominately in women at ED [7].

The majority of UTIs are caused by *E. coli* bacteria, followed by *Proteus* spp., *Staphylococcus saprophyticus*, *Klebsiella* spp. and other *Enterobacteriaceae* [8, 9]. However, among bacteria causing UTIS, *E. coli* is considered as the most predominant cause of both community and nosocomial UTIs. Antibiotics commonly recommended for treatment of UTIs include co-trimoxazole (trimethoprim/sulfamethoxazole), nitrofurantoin, ciprofloxacin

*Correspondence: anizim1@ngha.med.sa; Dr.Monifah@gmail.com
[1] Clinical Pharmacy Practice, Drug Policy and Economics Center, King Abdulaziz Medical City, Ministry of National Guard, Health Affairs, Riyadh 22490, Saudi Arabia
Full list of author information is available at the end of the article

and ampicillin [3, 10]. However, there is global increase in antibiotic resistance among urinary tract pathogens, including resistance pattern observed in Saudi Arabia [11–14], which limit treatment options.

Evidence suggest significant relationship between extensive use of antimicrobial and antimicrobial resistance [10, 11]. Therefore, appropriate antibiotic prescription and usage will reduce the disease burden of UTIs and hence lower its complications and costs [10, 15]. For this reason, surveillance of antibiotics resistance is crucial to determine the pattern of antimicrobial resistance and consequently guide the selection of empirical therapy. Therefore, this study aims to determine the current prevalence and susceptibility to ampicillin, augmentin (amoxicillin/clavulanate), co-trimoxazole (trimethoprim/sulfamethoxazole), nitrofurantoin, cefazolin, and ciprofloxacin amongst all *E. coli* isolated from patients with UTIs. Associations between patient's demographic parameters and multidrug resistance *E. coli* isolates were also investigated.

Methods

Study setting

This study was conducted in the emergency department (ED) of King Abdulaziz Medical City (KAMC), which is a tertiary care hospital in Riyadh, the capital of Saudi Arabia. The ED at KAMC is composed of Urgi Center, Pediatric Emergency Units, Adult Emergency unit, Observation Unit, and Critical Care unit.

Study design

Retrospective cohort study of physician medication prescription over a period of 3 months from January to March 2008 in ED at KAMC, Riyadh, Saudi Arabia.

Study population

Charts of 101 patients diagnosed with UTIs due to *E. coli* were reviewed. Samples of those patients showed significant growth, bacteria growing > 10^5 colony-forming units (CFU/mL) with a single type of bacteria from a properly collected midstream "clean catch" urine sample, were considered as UTIs and processed further for identification and susceptibility testing.

Antibiotic sensitivity testing

The sensitivity and resistance of *E. coli* isolates against six antimicrobial agents including ampicillin, augmentin, co-trimoxazole (trimethoprim/sulphamethoxazole), ciprofloxacin, nitrofurantoin, and cefazolin were determined using VITEK test method which measure minimum inhibitory concentration (MIC). Susceptibility results are interpreted according to the Clinical Laboratory Standards Institute (CLSI) guidelines. Then association between resistance of *E. coli* to one or more of three antibiotics (ampicillin, co-trimoxazole and ciprofloxacin) were studied and classified to SSR (sensitive to ampicillin, sensitive co-trimoxazole, and resistance ciprofloxacin); RRR (resistance ampicillin, resistance co-trimoxazole and resistance ciprofloxacin); SSS (sensitive ampicillin, sensitive co-trimoxazole and Sensitive ciprofloxacin); RRS (resistance ampicillin, resistance co-trimoxazole and sensitive ciprofloxacin); SRS (sensitive ampicillin, resistance co-trimoxazole and sensitive ciprofloxacin), and SRR (sensitive ampicillin, resistance co-trimoxazole and resistance ciprofloxacin). Multiple resistance which defined as multidrug resistance (MDR) was defined as resistance to three or more antimicrobials. The population was classified as pediatric, adolescent and adult, and elderly. Pediatric stratified into three groups: less than 2 years, from 2 years to 6 years and between 7 and 12 years. The age category between 13–17 and 18–64 years were defined as adults, while those age 65 years or over were defined as elderly.

Measurement

Data for the period of January 1, 2008, through March 30, were obtained from the prescription and Quadra Med system. All prescriptions with UTIs diagnosis were collected and reviewed for the demographic characteristic, the name of antibiotics and microbiology data. Microbiology data include name of the uropathogen which isolated from urine culture and cause UTIs, sensitivity, and resistance of *E. coli* for six antimicrobials agents as prescribed above.

Statistical analysis

Antimicrobial susceptibility or resistant rates were calculated as the number of susceptible or resistant organisms divided by the total number of tested organisms, for a given antibiotic, and a given organism. Statistical analyses were performed using the Statistical Package for the Social Sciences (SPSS version 16.0).

Ethical approval

This study approved by the research committee at King Abdullah International Medical Research Center, Riyadh, Saudi Arabia.

Results

During the study period from January to March 2008, a total 565 urinary cultures were collected. Of a total isolate, positive cultures were representing 28.67% of all cultures collected. Gram-negative organisms totaled 149 (91.98%), Gram-positive organisms constituted 11 (6.79%) and fungal 2 (1.23%) of all isolates. There are 56.14% of all pediatric visits requested culture. 35.67%

of all adult visits and 39.75% of all elderly. In pediatric, 32.29% of culture was positive, 62.50% was negative, and 5.21% of the result was mixed of normal flora, while in the adult the result of urine culture showed 68.62% negative, 24.34% positive and 7.05% was mixed. In elderly, the result of culture was 57.81% negative, 37.50% positive and 5.21% mixed of normal flora.

The most common uropathogen isolated from urine culture was *E. coli*, which represent 93.55% of all pathogen that isolated from pediatric urine culture, 60.24% of all pathogen which isolated from adult urine culture and 45.83% of all pathogen that isolated from elderly urine culture (Table 1). Extended Spectrum Beta-Lactamases enzymes (ESBL) producing *E. coli* detected in 8.33, 4.82 and 3.23% of uropathogens isolated from elderly, adult and pediatric respectively. Other organisms, in elderly, were *Enterobacter* species (10.42%), *Klebsiella* species (10.42%), and *Acinetobacter* species (6.25%), and *Pseudomonas aeruginosa* (4.14%). Other organisms were caused UTIs in adult were *Klebsiella* species (10.42%) *Pseudomonas aeruginosa* (8.43%), and *Streptococcus* species (8.43%) (Table 1).

The overall rate of resistance for 101 *E. coli* isolates analyzed was provided in Table 2. Of the agents tested nitrofurantoin, ciprofloxacin and augmentin were the lowest rates of resistance in three age categories. Nitrofurantoin was the lowest rate of resistance among three age categories representing (0, 2, 9%) followed by ciprofloxacin representing (6.90, 8, 27.27%), and augmentin representing (10.34, 10, 27.27%) in pediatric, adult and elderly

Table 1 Distribution of uropathogens that cause urinary tract infection according age category in period from January to March 2008

Uropathogens	Frequency among patients					
	Elderly (n = 48)		Adult (n = 83)		Pediatric (n = 31)	
	n	%	n	%	n	%
Escherichia coli	22	45.83	50	60.24	29	93.55
Enterobacter species	5	10.42	4	4.82	0	0
Klebsiella species	5	10.42	7	8.43	0	0
Extended spectrum B lactamase (ESBL)	4	8.33	4	4.82	1	3.23
Acinetobacter species	3	6.25	1	1.20	0	0
Group B sterptococcus	2	4.17	7	8.43	0	0
Pseudomonas aeruginosa	2	4.17	7	8.43	0	0
Candida species	1	2.08	1	1.20	0	0
Morganella morganii	1	2.08	0	0.00	0	0
Proteus merabilis	1	2.08	1	1.20	1	3.23
Serratia marcescens	1	2.08	0	0.00	0	0
Staphylococcus aureus	1	2.08	0	0.00	0	0
Methicillin resistance Staphylococcus aureus (MRSA)	0	0	1	1.20	0	0

Table 2 Antimicrobial susceptibility result for 101 *E. coli* urinary tract isolates in study period from January to March 2008

Antibiotic name	Number of isolates n (%) classified as					
	Pediatric (n = 29 isolates)		Adult (n = 50 isolates)		Elderly (n = 22 isolates)	
	Sensitive	Resistance	Sensitive	Resistance	Sensitive	Resistance
Ampicillin	5 (17.24%)	24 (82.76%)	21 (42%)	29 (58%)	8 (36.36%)	14 (63.64%)
Augmentin	26 (89.66%)	3 (10.34%)	45 (90%)	5 (10%)	16 (72.73%)	6 (27.27%)
Co-trimoxazole	14 (48.28%)	15 (51.72%)	29 (58%)	21 (42%)	9 (40.91%)	13 (59.09%)
Ciprofloxacin	27 (93.1%)	1 (3.44%)	46 (92%)	4 (8%)	16 (72.73%)	6 (27.27%)
Nitrofurantoin	29 (100%)	0 (0.00%)	49 (98%)	1 (2%)	20 (90.91%)	2 (9.09%)
Cefazolin	25 (86.21%)	4 (13.79%)	43 (86%)	7 (14%)	15 (68.18%)	7 (31.82%)

Co-trimoxazole (sulfamethoxazole/trimethoprim)

respectively. Ampicillin demonstrated the highest rate of resistance (82.76, 58, and 63.64%) in pediatric, adult and elderly respectively. The rate of co-trimoxazole resistance among the *E. coli* isolates was (51.72, 42%), and 59.09% in pediatric, adult and elderly respectively (Table 2).

Antimicrobial resistance to individual antibiotics and the percentage of isolates demonstrating MDR phenotype were stratified by patient demographic characteristic and summarized in (Table 3). Nitrofurantoin resistance was approximately three times as common among *E. coli* isolates from males (7.14%) more than females (2.3%) and was highest (9.09%) among patients > 65 years old. Augmentin resistance was approximately comparable among *E. coli* isolates from male (14.29%) and female (13.79%) and the highest (27.27, and 15.78%) among patients more than 65 years old and equal or less than 6 years old respectively. Higher rates of ciprofloxacin resistance (27.27%) among patients > 65 years was demonstrated (Table 3). There was no resistance against augmentin and cefazolin among *E. coli* isolated from patients aged between 7 years to 17 years old. The rate of resistance of *E. coli* to co-trimoxazole was high in patients < 2 years old and > 65 years old representing 85.71% and 95.09%, respectively. Trend toward higher rates of MDR *E. coli* were demonstrated among males' patients (28.57%). By age category, the prevalence of MDR was higher in elderly 50% (n = 11 of 22), followed by adult 18% (n = 9 of 50), and pediatric 10.34% (n = 3 of 29) (Table 3).

Among the 101 *E. coli* isolates that were tested against all six antimicrobials, 31.68% found to be susceptible (Table 4). The majority (68.31%) was resistant to one or more antimicrobial and 15.84% were resistant to a single agent, predominantly ampicillin, and 29.7% were resistant to two antimicrobials. MDR isolates accounted for 22.77% (n = 23) of the 101 isolates. The majority of MDR isolates (n = 13; 56.52%) were resistant to three antimicrobial, and these accounted for 12.87% of all isolates. Isolates were also identified to be resistant to four agents were (n = 8; 34, 78% of MDR isolates; 7.92% of all isolates) and all five antimicrobials were (n = 2; 8, 69% of MDR isolates; 1.98% of all isolates) (Table 4). Resistant to ampicillin represent 34.84% (n = 23 of 23) of the MDR isolates. Among 66 and 49 isolates resistant to ampicillin and co-trimoxazole, respectively, 34.84 and 42.85% were MDR (Table 4). In contrast, all isolates resistant to augmentin and nitrofurantoin were MRD, while 72.7 and 82.4% of isolates resistant to ciprofloxacin and cefazolin were MDR.

The analysis of co-resistance between ampicillin, co-trimoxazole and ciprofloxacin were summarized in Table 5. The correlation between ampicillin and co-trimoxazole were 51.72, 34 and 27.27% in pediatric, adult and elderly respectively. *E. coli* were resistant to ampicillin, ciprofloxacin, and co-trimoxazole in adult and elderly were 4 and 27.27% respectively. In adult, the correlation between resistance of ciprofloxacin and co-trimoxazole was 2% (Table 5).

Discussion

Global spread of antibiotics resistance among uropathogens causing UTIs is alarming. This study reports the etiology of UTIs and antimicrobial susceptibility of uropathogens at KAMC in Riyadh, a capital city of Saudi Arabia. Similar to previous studies that conducted in Saudi Arabia, *E. coli* remains the majority of pathogen which isolated from urine culture in pediatric, adult, and elderly [11–14, 16], and other countries [17–19].

In this study, the resistance of *E. coli* to ampicillin was the highest, followed by co-trimoxazole. The observed resistance pattern of *E. coli* to ampicillin and co-trimoxazole are in agreement with the findings of previous studies carried out at different provinces of Saudi Arabia [11–13, 16]. Other study taken place in USA showed that that MDR *E. coli* exhibited 97.8% resistance to Ampicillin, 92.8% to trimethoprim–sulfamethoxazole, and 38.8% to ciprofloxacin [20]. In UK, high rates of resistance to ampicillin (55%) and trimethoprim (40%) were observed in *E. coli* isolates [18]. These results suggest the prevalence of ampicillin and trimethoprim/sulfamethoxazole resistance among urinary tract isolates and are consistent with finding of our study. *E. coli* showed the highest sensitivity to nitrofurantoin in the current study, which are in line with those of previous studies in Saudi Arabia [12, 14], and other countries [21, 22]. These data further support recommendations made in previous studies, in which, nitrofurantoin may be more effective than co-trimoxazole or amoxicillin in the empiric treatment of UTIs [21, 23].

The current data showed a high percentage of correlation between co-trimoxazole and ampicillin resistance among *E. coli* isolates (37.62%). Previous data from Canadian study revealed limited activity of ampicillin (79.6% resistance) against co-trimoxazole-resistant *E. coli* isolates from UTIs patients [24]. In the same study, the rates of co-trimoxazole resistance for ampicillin-resistant *E. coli* was (35.7% resistance) [24], corroborating finding of our study. In addition, high ciprofloxacin resistant (100%) was found among co-trimoxazole resistance isolates [24]. This finding is contrary to current study results as there is no evidence of high prevalence in ciprofloxacin resistant among ampicillin and/or co-trimoxazole resistant *E. coli* isolates from UTIs.

The current study found that 22.77% of *E. coli* isolates were MDR, which is higher than that observed in ED of previous study [25]. MDR prevalence was higher in *E. coli* isolates resistant to augmentin, nitrofurantoin, followed

Table 3 Patients demographic characteristic for 101 *E. coli* urinary tract isolates during period from January to March 2008

	Total no isolates	Susceptibility to all antibiotic	Resistance to one or more	n (%) isolate resistance to						
				Ampicillin	Augmentin	Co-trimoxazole	Ciprofloxacin	Nitofurantoin	Cefazolin	% MDR
Gender										
Male	14 (13.86%)	4 (28.57%)	10 (71.42%)	9 (64.29%)	2 (14.29%)	6 (42.86%)	2 (14.29%)	1 (7.14%)	2 (14.29%)	4 (28.57%)
Female	87 (86.14%)	28 (32.18%)	59 (67.82%)	57 (65.52%)	12 (13.79%)	43 (49.43%)	9 (10.34%)	2 (2.3%)	15 (17.24%)	19 (21.84%)
Total	101	32 (31.68%)	69 (68.31%)	66 (65.34%)	14 (13.9%)	49 (39.60%)	11 (10.90%)	3 (3%)	17 (16.83%)	23 (22.77%)
Category of age										
< 2 years	7 (6.93%)	1 (14.29%)	6 (85.71%)	6 (85.71%)	1 (14.29%)	6 (85.71%)	0 (0)	0 (0)	1 (14.29%)	1 (14.29%)
2 to 6 years	12 (11.88%)	3 (25%)	9 (75%)	9 (75%)	2 (16.67%)	6 (50%)	0 (0)	0 (0)	2 (16.67%)	2 (16.67%)
7 to 12 years	10 (10%)	2 (20%)	8 (80%)	8 (80%)	0	3 (30%)	1 (10%)	0 (0)	0 (0)	0 (0)
13 to 17 years	2 (2%)	1 (50%)	1 (50%)	1 (50%)	0	1 (50%)	0 (0)	0 (0)	0 (0)	0 (0)
18 to 64 years	48 (47.52%)	18 (37.5%)	30 (62.50%)	28 (58.33%)	5 (10.42%)	20 (41.67%)	4 (8.33%)	1 (2.08%)	7 (14.58%)	9 (18.75%)
65 years or more	22 (21.78%)	7 (31.82%)	15 (68.18%)	14 (63.64%)	6 (27.27%)	13 (59.09%)	6 (27.27%)	2 (9.09%)	7 (31.82%)	11 (50%)
Total	101	32	69	66	14	49	11	3	17	23

Table 4 Resistance to one or more antimicrobials among 101 *E. coli* urinary tract isolates tests against all six antimicrobials in study period

No of agents which isolates were resistance	N, % of isolates	n (%) isolates resistant to					
		Ampicillin	Augmentin	Co-trimoxazole	Ciprofloxacin	Nitrofurantoin	Cefazolin
0	32 (31.68%)						
1	16 (15.84%)	14 (87.50%)	0	2 (12.50%)	0	0	1 (6.25%)
2	30 (29.70%)	29 (96.67%)	0	26 (86.67%)	3 (10%)	0	2 (6.67%)
3	13 (12.87%)	13 (100%)	5 (38.46%)	12 (92.31%)	5 (38.46%)	0	5 (38.46%)
4	8 (7.92%)	8 (100%)	7 (87.5%)	7 (87.50%)	2 (25%)	2 (25%)	7 (87.50%)
5	2 (1.98%)	2 (100%)	2 (100%)	2 (100%)	1 (50%)	1 (50%)	2 (100%)
Total	101	66	14	49	11	3	17
MDR	23	23	14	21	8	3	14
% MDR	77.22%	34.84%	100%	42.85%	72.72%	100%	82.35%

Table 5 Resistance profile to the three antibiotics (ampicillin, ciprofloxacin and co-trimoxazole) among 101 isolates of *E. coli*

Antibiotype	Ampicillin	Co-trimoxazole	Ciprofloxacin	Pediatric n (%)	Adult n (%)	Elderly n (%)	Total n (%)
A	S	S	S	6 (20.69%)	19 (38%)	7 (31.82%)	32 (31.68%)
B	R	R	S	15 (51.72%)	17 (34%)	6 (27.27%)	38 (37.62%)
C	R	R	R	0	2 (4%)	6 (27.27%)	8 (7.92%)
D	R	S	R	1 (3.45%)	1 (2%)	0	2 (1.98%)
E	R	S	S	7 (24.14%)	9 (18%)	2 (9.09%)	18 (17.82%)
F	S	R	R	0	1 (2)	0	1 (0.99%)
G	S	R	S	0	1 (2)	1 (4.55%)	2 (1.98%)
Total				29	50	22	101

S susceptible, *R* resistance

by cefazolin and ciprofloxacin, then co-trimoxazole and ampicillin.

Despite the lowest rate of nitrofurantoin resistance (3%) when compared to other antibiotics used in the current study (only 3 of 101), these isolates were MDR. Similarly, 100% of isolates resistant to augmentin were also MDR. However, in our study we described MDR phenotypes for ampicillin, co-trimoxazole, and ciprofloxacin but not for other antibiotics. Therefore, we cannot conclude the correction between MDR with specific antibiotic.

According to patient age, the prevalence of resistance to ampicillin or co-trimoxazole was higher among isolates from patients ≤ 12 years and ≤ 2 years, respectively. This pattern seemed relatively consistent with findings of previous study which revealed higher level of resistance among isolates from patients ≤ 17 years old than among older patients [22]. For augmentin, cefazolin, ciprofloxacin, and nitrofurantoin, the prevalence of resistant isolates were higher among patients aged ≥ 65 years. This match results observed in earlier studies that found ciprofloxacin resistance was highest among patients older than 65 years (7.1%) [22]. However, nitrofurantoin resistance pattern in our study is contrary to that described by Sham et al. study, in which resistance prevalence of nitrofurantoin resistance was consistent irrespective of patient age [22].

The present study has some limitations. First, the study was only conducted only in ED setting, which not representing other health care settings in KAMC. Thus, the findings cannot be generalized. Second, the study period was short (3 months) and small sample size. Third, there was no follow-up study to investigate the consequences of observed resistance. Therefore, large-scale prospective studies are recommended to determine the extent and outcomes of resistance and MDR in UTIs at KAMC in Saudi Arabia.

Conclusions

Increased resistance of urinary tract *E. coli* isolates to both ampicillin and co-trimoxazole was demonstrated, suggesting revaluation empirical therapies for the treatment of UTIs in ED setting. This continuous evolvement in antimicrobial resistance pattern necessitates national surveillance studies to monitor and ensure safe and effective empiric therapy.

Abbreviations

KAMC: King Abdulaziz Medical City; KAIMRC: King Abdullah International Medical Research Center, augmentin, (amoxicillin/clavulanate); ED: emergency department, co-trimoxazole, (sulfamethoxazole/trimethoprim); UTIs: urinary tract infections; MDR: multiple drug resistance; MRSA: methicillin resistance *S. aureus*.

Authors' contributions

All authors contributed towards the study concept, data analysis, drafting, and revising of the paper and agreed to be accountable for all aspects of the work. All authors read and approved the final manuscript.

Author details

[1] Clinical Pharmacy Practice, Drug Policy and Economics Center, King Abdulaziz Medical City, Ministry of National Guard, Health Affairs, Riyadh 22490, Saudi Arabia. [2] Department of PharmaceUTIscs, College of Pharmacy, King Saud University, Riyadh 22452, Saudi Arabia.

Acknowledgements

The authors would like to acknowledge the King Abdullah International Medical Research Center (KAIMRC) for the support. Also, authors would like to thank Prof. Amin Kashmeery, Dr. Abdullah Adlan, Prof. Abdulhaleem Sawas and Mohmmed Assiri from King Abdullah International Medical Research Center (KAIMRC). And special thank for Dr. Abdul Rahman Jazieh, Chairman Department of Oncology King Abdulaziz Medical City, Ministry of National Guard Health Affairs.

Competing interests

The authors declare that they have no competing interests.

Funding

The study was supported by the Research Centre at King Abdullah International Medical Research Center (KAIMRC).

References

1. Car J. Urinary tract infections in women: diagnosis and management in primary care. BMJ. 2006;332(7533):94–7.
2. Lee JBL, Neild GH. Urinary tract infection. Medicine. 2007;35(8):423–8.
3. Tandogdu Z, Wagenlehner FM. Global epidemiology of urinary tract infections. Curr Opin Infect Dis. 2016;29(1):73–9.
4. Taur Y, Smith MA. Adherence to the infectious diseases society of America guidelines in the treatment of uncomplicated urinary tract infection. Clin Infect Dis. 2007;44(6):769–74.
5. Schappert SM, Burt CW. Ambulatory care visits to physician offices, hospital outpatient departments, and emergency departments: United States, 2001–2002. Vital Health Stat. 2006;13(159):1–66.
6. Kostakioti M, Hultgren SJ, Hadjifrangiskou M. Molecular blueprint of uropathogenic *Escherichia coli* virulence provides clues toward the development of anti-virulence therapeUTIscs. Virulence. 2012;3(7):592–4.
7. Alanazi MQ, Al-Jeraisy MI, Salam M. Prevalence and predictors of antibiotic prescription errors in an emergency department, Central Saudi Arabia. Drug Healthc Patient Saf. 2015;7:103–11.
8. Gupta K, et al. The prevalence of antimicrobial resistance among uropathogens causing acute uncomplicated cystitis in young women. Int J Antimicrob Agents. 1999;11(3–4):305–8.
9. Kahlmeter G. The ECO.SENS Project: a prospective, multinational, multicentre epidemiological survey of the prevalence and antimicrobial susceptibility of urinary tract pathogens—interim report. J Antimicrob Chemother. 2000;46(Suppl 1):15–22 **(discussion 63–5)**.
10. Foxman B. The epidemiology of urinary tract infection. Nat Rev Urol. 2010;7(12):653–60.
11. Al Yousef SA, et al. Clinical and laboratory profile of urinary tract infections associated with extended spectrum beta-lactamase producing *Escherichia coli* and *Klebsiella pneumoniae*. Ann Clin Lab Sci. 2016;46(4):393–400.
12. Kader AA, Kumar A. Prevalence and antimicrobial susceptibility of extended-spectrum beta-lactamase-producing *Escherichia coli* and *Klebsiella pneumoniae* in a general hospital. Ann Saudi Med. 2005;25(3):239–42.
13. Al-Harthi AA, Al-Fifi SH. Antibiotic resistance pattern and empirical therapy for urinary tract infections in children. Saudi Med J. 2008;29(6):854–8.
14. Al-Tawfiq JA, Anani AA. Antimicrobial susceptibility pattern of bacterial pathogens causing urinary tract infections in a Saudi Arabian hospital. Chemotherapy. 2009;55(2):127–31.
15. Foxman B, et al. Urinary tract infection: self-reported incidence and associated costs. Ann Epidemiol. 2000;10(8):509–15.
16. Al-Otaibi FE, Bukhari EE. Clinical and laboratory profiles of urinary tract infections caused by extended-spectrum beta-lactamase-producing *Escherichia coli* in a tertiary care center in central Saudi Arabia. Saudi Med J. 2013;34(2):171–6.
17. Bours PH, et al. Increasing resistance in community-acquired urinary tract infections in Latin America, five years after the implementation of national therapeUTIsc guidelines. Int J Infect Dis. 2010;14(9):e770–4.
18. Bean DC, Krahe D, Wareham DW. Antimicrobial resistance in community and nosocomial *Escherichia coli* urinary tract isolates, London 2005–2006. Ann Clin Microbiol Antimicrob. 2008;7:13.
19. Assefa A, et al. Bacterial profile and drug susceptibility pattern of urinary tract infection in pregnant women at Tikur Anbessa Specialized Hospital Addis Ababa, Ethiopia. Ethiop Med J. 2008;46(3):227–35.
20. Karlowsky JA, et al. Trends in antimicrobial resistance among urinary tract infection isolates of *Escherichia coli* from female outpatients in the United States. Antimicrob Agents Chemother. 2002;46(8):2540–5.
21. Gupta K, Scholes D, Stamm WE. Increasing prevalence of antimicrobial resistance among uropathogens causing acute uncomplicated cystitis in women. JAMA. 1999;281(8):736–8.
22. Sahm DF, et al. Multidrug-resistant urinary tract isolates of *Escherichia coli*: prevalence and patient demographics in the United States in 2000. Antimicrob Agents Chemother. 2001;45(5):1402–6.
23. Cormican M, et al. Extended spectrum beta-lactamase production and fluorquinolone resistance in pathogens associated with community acquired urinary tract infection. Diagn Microbiol Infect Dis. 1998;32(4):317–9.
24. Zhanel GG, et al. A Canadian national surveillance study of urinary tract isolates from outpatients: comparison of the activities of trimethoprim-sulfamethoxazole, ampicillin, mecillinam, nitrofurantoin, and ciprofloxacin. The Canadian Urinary Isolate Study Group. Antimicrob Agents Chemother. 2000;44(4):1089–92.
25. Khawcharoenporn T, Vasoo S, Singh K. Urinary tract infections due to multidrug-resistant enterobacteriaceae: prevalence and risk factors in a Chicago Emergency Department. Emerg Med Int. 2013;2013:258517.

21

Quality control of malaria microscopy reveals misdiagnosed non-falciparum species and other microscopically detectable pathogens in Senegal

Mamadou Alpha Diallo[1*], Khadim Diongue[1], Mame Cheikh Seck[1], Mouhamadou Ndiaye[1], Ibrahima Diallo[2], Younouss Diedhiou[1], Tolla Ndiaye[1], Yaye Die Ndiaye[1], Aida Sadikh Badiane[1] and Daouda Ndiaye[1]

Abstract

Background: In developing countries, malaria diagnosis relies on microscopy and rapid diagnostic tests. In Senegal, national malaria control program (NMCP) regularly conducts supervisory visits in health services where malaria microscopy is performed. In this study, expert microscopists assessed the performance of laboratory technicians in malaria microscopy.

Methods: The present external quality assessment (EQA) was conducted in three different areas of malaria transmission. Participants were laboratory technicians previously trained by NMCP on malaria microscopy. Stored read slides were randomly collected for blinded re-checking by expert microscopists. At the same time a set of 8 slides (3 positive *P. falciparum* and 5 negative slides) were submitted to participants for proficiency testing. Microscopists performance were evaluated on the basis of the errors rates on slide reading—high false positive (HFP), high false negative (HFN), low false positive (LFP) and low false negative (LFN)—and the calculation of their sensitivities and specificities relative to expert microscopy. Data were entered and analysed using Microsoft Excel software.

Results: A total of 450 stored slides were collected from 17 laboratories for re-checking. Eight laboratories scored 100% of correct reading. Only one major error was recorded (HFP). Six laboratories recorded LFN results: Borrelia, *P. ovale*, and low parasite densities (95 and 155 p/µl) were missed. Two *P. falciparum* slides were misidentified as *P. malariae* and one *P. ovale* slide as *P. vivax*. The overall sensitivities and specificities for all participants against expert microscopists were 97.8 and 98.2% respectively; Sensitivities and specificities of hospital microscopists (96.7 and 98.9%) were statistically similar to those of health centre microscopists (98.5 and 97.8% respectively) ($p=0.3993$ and $p=0.9412$ respectively). Overall, a very good agreement was noted with kappa value of 0.96 ($CI_{95\%}$ 93.4–98.6%) relative to expert microscopy. Proficiency testing showed that among the 17 participants, 11 laboratories scored 100% of correct reading. Three LFN and four LFP results were recorded respectively. The *P. falciparum* slide with Maurer dots was misidentified as *P. ovale* in 1 centre and the same slide was misread as *P. vivax* in another centre; No major error (HFP or HFN) was noted.

Conclusion: EQA of malaria microscopy showed an overall good performance especially regarding *P. falciparum* detection. However, efforts need to be made addressing the ability to detect non-falciparum species and others endemic blood pathogens such as *Borrelia*. The further NMCP training sessions and evaluations should consider those aspects to expect high quality-assured capacity for malaria microscopy.

*Correspondence: mamadoualpha.diallo@ucad.edu.sn
[1] Laboratory of Parasitology and Mycology, Cheikh Anta Diop University, Avenue Cheikh Anta Diop, BP 5005 Fann, Dakar, Senegal
Full list of author information is available at the end of the article

Keywords: External quality assessment, EQA, Microscopy, Diagnosis, Malaria, Senegal

Background

Despite the development of new diagnostic tools, microscopy still remains the gold standard method for malaria diagnosis [1]. Microscopy of thick and thin smears is relatively simple and inexpensive, and particularly suitable to rapidly diagnose malaria. Moreover, microscopy allows species identification and parasite count [2], and it is also suitable to diagnose infections with other pathogens that may be detected microscopically in routinely Giemsa-stained smears, such as spirochetes of *Borrelia*, which are common in Senegal [3]. However, reliability of malaria microscopy is highly dependent on competency of laboratory staff [2]. As a result, reinforcing strategies to promote good quality of microscopy-based malaria diagnosis has been gaining an increased interest in the global malaria agenda [4, 5].

In order to evaluate laboratory performance on malaria microscopy, WHO recognize the need to establish comprehensive external quality assessment (EQA) system [5]. However, little research on the evaluation of EQA systems in malaria microscopy has been conducted in Senegal. National Malaria Control Programs (NMCP) has defined a procedure to ensure good quality of malaria microscopy. This study aimed to evaluate the performances in malaria microscopy among laboratory technicians in Senegal.

Methods

Description

In Senegal, EQA procedures have been established by NMCP and regularly supervisory visits are conducted in all levels of malaria laboratory services. Also, NMCP organize periodic training towards lab technicians in conventional methods of malaria diagnosis. During the training sessions, participant laboratories are notified to store read slides in two separate provided boxes (Negative and Positive) for further quality control re-check. During the NMCP supervisory visits, senior microscopists assess the competence of laboratory technicians in performing thick and thin smear, reading slides, microscope maintenance and reagents management.

The collected results are analysed and reported to the NMCP, which conducts corrective actions for quality improvement.

Sites and participants

A cross-sectional study was conducted in three different strata of malaria distribution: (1) Saint Louis in the north (pre-elimination stage), (2) Dakar and Thies in the west centre (low prevalence) and (3) Kedougou in the south (high prevalence). Seventeen laboratories (seven hospitals and eleven health centres) participated (Fig. 1); Participants were lab technicians previously trained during training sessions conducted by NMCP.

On-site evaluation

A supervisory checklist was submitted to participants to assess the status of infrastructure, availability of comprehensive standard operating procedure (SOP), appropriate use of reagents and equipment, maintenance of microscope, laboratory safety, training related to malaria microscopy, data and supply management, internal quality control (QC) procedure.

Also, supervisors examined that the slides are stored according to the appropriate SOPs and that the results are reported in a register with the following mentions: species identification (instead of mentioning "Positive results"), parasite stages (young trophozoites, mature trophozoites, schizonts and gametocytes), and assessment of parasite density.

Slides rechecking

Supervisors randomly selected 30 slides from each participant laboratory (15 samples of the smears from each negative and positive boxes where slides were stored). Seventeen laboratories were supervised. Two health centres were not able to store their read slides as required by NMCP so they were not included on the rechecking evaluation. Thus, a total of 450 slides (225 declared positives and 225 declared negatives) were collected from the 15 remaining laboratories. The selected smears were sent to the national reference laboratory (NRL) where they are blindly re-examined by two WHO level 1 malaria microscopists. Slides yielding discrepant results between two experts are resolved by a third expert microscopist.

Proficiency testing

Along with collecting stored slides, a set of eight reference slides was distributed to all involved participant microscopists: slide (1) *Plasmodium falciparum* moderate parasite density (28,000 p/μl) with Maurer dots (Fig. 2), slide (2) *P. falciparum* low parasite density (192 p/μl), slide (3) *P. falciparum* gametocyte and trophozoites with high parasite density and slides 4–8) five slides with no parasites.

The set of submitted slides consisted of reference slides from national malaria slide bank. The malaria slide bank is certified by WHO and is hosted in the Laboratory of

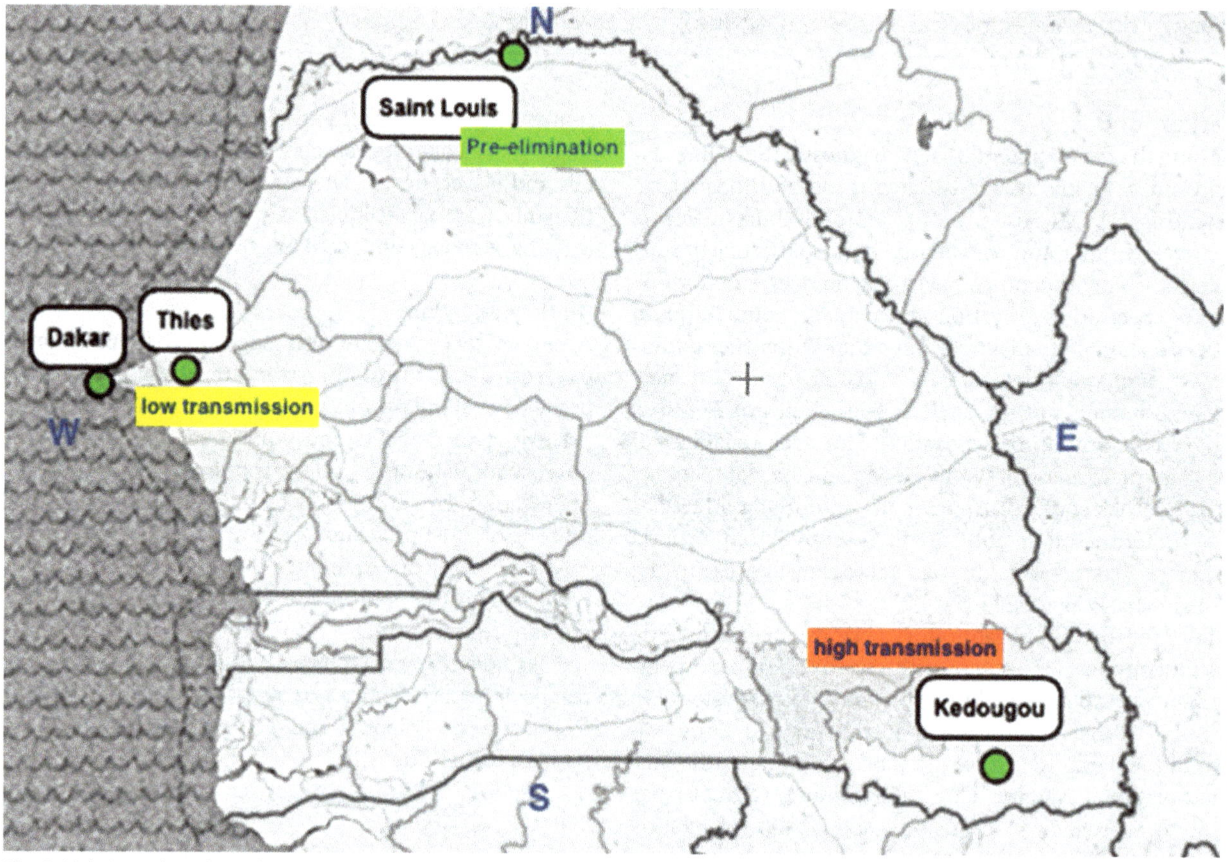

Fig. 1 Malaria epidemiological strata with sites where supervision was conducted; 7 hospital laboratories: Dakar (3), Thies (1) Saint Louis (2), Kedougou (1); 11 health centre laboratories: Dakar (2), Thies (2), Saint Louis (4), Kedougou (3)

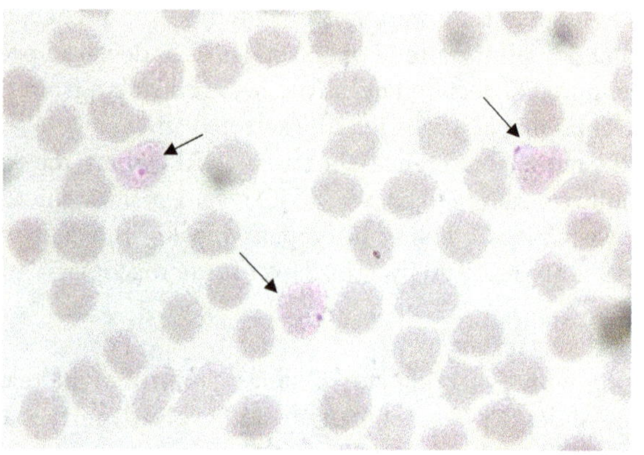

Fig. 2 Trophozoites of *P. falciparum* with specific Maurer dots inside the infected red blood cells, Giemsa stained thin smear (×1000)

Parasitology-Mycology of Aristide Le Dantec Hospital which is the national reference laboratory (NRL) for the Senegal NMCP. The NRL had six expert microscopists during past external competency assessment of malaria microscopy (ECAMM) courses.

Data analysis

The results of the EQA system were evaluated using the following indicators: major errors [high false-positive (HFP), high false-negative (HFN)], minor errors [low false-positive (LFP), low false-negative (LFN)] and misidentification; these indicators were defined depending on the modality of the evaluation:

Slides rechecking

LFP was defined as only one false positive is noted among the ten collected labelled negative by participants and HFP when there was more than one false positive. LFN was considered if the following slides were missed by participants among the ten labelled positive slides: parasite density less than 200 p/µl, spirochetes, non-falciparum species. HFN was considered when slides with parasite density more than 200 was missed.

Misidentification refers to true positive slides that were detected positive by participants but species identification was not correct.

Proficiency testing

LFP was defined when only one submitted reference negative slide is read positive by the participant and HFP when there were more than one false positive among the five negative slide. LFN was noted if only the slide with *P. falciparum* low parasite density (192 p/µl) was missed and HFN when slide with medium and high parasite density was missed by the participant.

Misidentification refers to reference positive slides that were detected positive by participants but species identification was not correct.

Sensitivity and specificity were calculated to assess the microscopy reading performance of the participants relative to the expert microscopy. Data were analysed using Excel (version 15.27). kappa statistic test was used to assess the magnitude of agreement between expert microscopists and participants. Exact Chi square analysis was used to determine the significance differences between sensitivities, specificities, negative predictive value (NPV) and positive predictive value (PPV). The p-values less than 0.05 were considered as statistical significance.

Ethical consideration

This study did not require informed consent from participants as no human subjects were involved. Ethical approval was obtained from Senegalese National Ethic Committee of Ministry of Health.

Results

On-site evaluation

Among the 17 participants, 14 laboratories have posted smear & staining procedure and parasite counting method and 15 laboratories have arranged read slides in boxes accordingly to NMCP procedure. Two laboratories were using expired Giemsa reagent. Internal quality control (QC) was followed only by 1 laboratory.

All laboratories were using standardized laboratory register provided by NMCP; however, only 5 reported their results with complete information on the different sections of the registers; concerning the positive slide reporting results, 5 laboratories mentioned "Positive" without giving any details, 7 laboratories reported the specie "*Plasmodium falciparum*" without the differentiation stage. None laboratory mentioned the presence of gametocytes nor schizonts, although those stages were seen during re-examination process. Three participants did not report the parasite counting on their registers.

All reagents related to malaria microscopy were supplied directly through NMCP. All participant facilities were suitable for standards of infrastructure, safety and waste disposal practices. Microscope maintenance was respected by all laboratories.

Proficiency testing

Among the 17 participants, 11 laboratories scored 100% as they correctly detected negative and positive reference slides. Three laboratories (one hospital and two health centres) misread negative slides as positive (LFN errors), four laboratories (one hospital and three health centres) misread low parasite density slide as negative (LFP errors); Two centres misread the *P. falciparum* slide with Maurer dots (Fig. 2) as *P. ovale* while one centre misread it as *P. vivax*; No major errors (HFP or HFN) were noted (Table 1).

Cross-checking of slides

Overall, 450 stored and collected slides from 15 participant laboratories were rechecked by WHO expert microscopists. Two health centres were excluded for this evaluation as they could not store their read slides as required by NMCP;

Eight laboratories achieved zero error. Only one major error was recorded as one health centre misread 2 negative slides as positive (HFP). Six laboratories recorded LFN results with the following positive slides misread as negative: spirochetes of Borrelia (missed by two hospital microscopists), *P. ovale* (missed by two health centres), and two slides with low parasite density of *P. falciparum* (missed by two health centres); the low parasite densities that were missed were 95 and 155 p/µl. Three laboratories detected parasites on true positive slides but species identification was incorrect: two hospitals misidentified *P. falciparum* slides as *P. malariae* and one health centre participant misidentified *P. ovale* slide as *P. vivax* (Tables 2, 3). When re-examining misidentified *P. falciparum* slides, expert microscopists observed "band-like forms" of trophozoites similar to that of *P. malariae* (Fig. 3); however, the absence of malarial pigments associated with high parasitaemia and the

Table 1 Reported errors from participants on panel testing slides

Participants	Slide 1	Slide 2	Slide 3	Slide 4–8	Total errors
Hospital 1	Negative			*P. falciparum*	2
Hospital 5		*P. ovale*			1
HC 1	Negative			*P. falciparum*	2
HC 5		*P. ovale*			1
HC 8	Negative	*P. vivax*		*P. falciparum*	3
HC 10	Negative				1
Total errors	4	3	0	3	10

Slide 1: *P. falciparum*, 192 p/µl

Slide 2: *P. falciparum*, 28,000 parasites with Maurer dots (see Fig. 1)

Slide 3: *P. falciparum*, with both trophozoites and gametocytes

Slides 4,5,6,7 and 8: No parasites

Table 2 Errors reported during cross-checking of read slides

Participants laboratories	Errors types					Total errors
	HFP	HFN	LFP	LFN[a]	Misidentification[a]	
Hospital 1	0	0	1	1	3	5
Hospital 2	0	0	0	1	0	1
Hospital 3	0	0	0	0	0	
Hospital 4	0	0	0	1	1	2
Hospital 5	0	0	0	0	0	
Hospital 6	0	0	0	0	0	
HC 1	0	0	0	0	0	
HC 2	2	0	0	0	0	2
HC 3	0	0	0	0	0	
HC 4	0	0	0	0	0	
HC 5	0	0	1	0	0	1
HC 6	0	0	0	0	1	1
HC 7	0	0	0	0	0	
HC 8	0	0	0	0	0	
HC 9	*NA*	*NA*	*NA*	*NA*	*NA*	
HC 10	*NA*	*NA*	*NA*	*NA*	*NA*	
HC 11	0	0	0	2	0	2

HC9 and HC10 were not involved as they could not store the required number of slides

[a] See details on Table 3

Table 3 Results of missed slides and misidentified slides when controlled by expert microscopists

	Results of participants	Results of controllers
	Misidentification	
Hospital 1	*P. malariae*	*P. falciparum*
Hospital 4	*P. vivax*	*P. ovale*
	LFN	
Hospital 1	Negative	Spirochetes
Hospital 2	Negative	Spirochetes
Hospital 4	Negative	*P. falciparum*, 95 p/µl
HC 4	Negative	*P. ovale*
HC 11	Negative	*P. ovale*
HC 11	Negative	*P. falciparum*, 155 p/µl

not-variegated aspect of the smear, were indicative of atypical *P. falciparum*.

The overall sensitivities and specificities for all participants against expert microscopists were 97.8 and 98.2% respectively; Sensitivities and specificities of hospital microscopists were 96.7 and 98.9% respectively while those of health centre microscopists were 98.5 and 97.8% respectively (Table 4). Overall, very good agreement was noted with kappa value of 0.96 ($CI_{95\%}$ 93.4–98.6%). No statistically significant differences of sensitivities and specificities were found between hospital and health centre microscopists (p = 0.3993 and p = 0.9412 respectively).

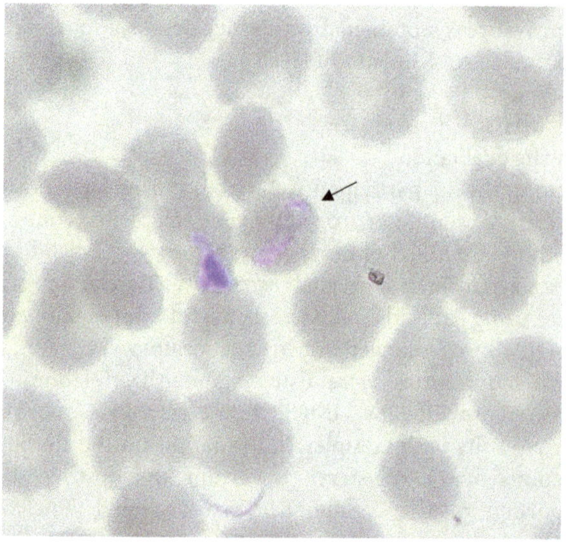

Fig. 3 *P. falciparum* trophozoite presenting an equatorial-like band in Giemsa stained thin smear (×1000)

Discussion

In Senegal, malaria transmission usually occurs during the rainy season (June–December) and the beginning of the dry season (January). This period corresponds to development of high density of vector populations. The prevalence of parasitaemia at the nation level have

Table 4 Sensitivities, specificities, PPV and NPV of participant microscopists against expert microscopists

		Controllers		Total
		Positive	Negative	
Hospital technicians	Positive	89	1	90
	Negative	3	87	90
	Total	92	88	180
Sensitivity (%)	96.7			
Specificity (%)	98.9			
PPV (%)	98.9			
NPV (%)	96.7			
Health centers technicians	Positive	132	3	135
	Negative	2	133	135
	Total	134	136	270
Sensitivity (%)	98.5			
Specificity (%)	97.8			
PPV (%)	97.8			
NPV (%)	*98.5*			

decreased from 5.9% in 2008 to 2.8% in 2013 in relationship to policies carried out by NMCP. However, high disparities of malaria prevalence exist between endemic regions. Mainly, three different epidemiological profiles have been identified [6] in which three human infecting species, *P. falciparum*, *P. malariae* and *P. ovale* are known to circulate [7]. Low values of parasitaemia prevalence are concentrated in the northern Senegal, particularly in the region of Saint-Louis, Louga and Matam. Malaria risk increases in some areas of central Senegal and reaches the highest values in the southern (Kolda, Tambacounda and Kedougou) [8, 9]. In the west centre, the parasite prevalence is about 1% in Dakar and Thies [6]. The urban malaria burden is concentrated in the cities where the anopheles vector density is very low [8].

Malaria diagnosis is one of the key strategy for effective malaria control and elimination programs. Microscopy still remains the mainstay of malaria diagnosis in endemic countries [1]. Maintaining a quality-assured microscopy service is a major challenge [10]. The quality of microscopy-based malaria diagnosis has been questioned in several studies [11–14].

This study showed that malaria microscopy in Senegal had shown an overall low total errors during this supervisory visit, particularly when addressing *P. falciparum* detection. Senegal NMCP arranged regular training system, an effective supply management and regular periodic supervisions visits with on-site corrective actions; this most probably contributed to achieve this good performance.

In Senegal, for many years the NMCP targeted especially falciparum malaria to fight against malaria. Yet, it is well known that non-falciparum species are circulating in the country [15–17]. Moreover, WHO has recommended to integrate in the EQA other local pathogens that may be detected microscopically. In Senegal, *Borrelia crocidurae*, a bacterial spirochete, is a major cause of fever (thick-borne relapsing fever). The bacteria may be observed by experienced microscopists when examining routinely malaria thick and thin smears [18]. As a result, slides positive with spirochetes were included in the NRL malaria slide bank with the aim to train and evaluate malaria microscopists on this.

In this evaluation, the *P. falciparum* slide with Maurer dots was introduced on purpose to assess the skills of microscopists to recognize such granulations. In fact, most of the time in peripheral laboratories and even in hospital laboratories, Giemsa stain is diluted with tap water; in this condition, *P. falciparum* Maurer dots do not appear and lab technicians may be unfamiliar with those findings when slides are stained appropriately using buffered solution.

In endemic African countries it has been reported misidentifications of *Plasmodium* species, particularly for the non-falciparum species [11]. Difficulties to distinguish the non-falciparum species are common, especially for those with low prevalence [12]. Moreover, the NMCP tends to neglect non-falciparum malaria due to its less severe clinical picture compared to falciparum malaria [15].

The non-identification of the stages of *P. falciparum* was a real challenge. In fact, presence of gametocytes can be an indicator of therapeutic failure and even resistance to some antimalarial drugs [19]. Moreover, in low transmission areas where malaria elimination is planned, the proportion of individuals carrying gametocytes is critical to the maintain the transmission of the disease.

In Senegal, during the previous NMCP training sessions and proficiency testing, only *P. falciparum* slides were used to train malaria microscopists and to evaluate their performance. This supervisory report led the NMCP to consider revisions on the training format for the further sessions. For the first time, the training is supported by a validated reference slide set. Currently, the NRL through the malaria slide bank is able to provide reference slides for all non-falciparum species, falciparum low parasite densities, atypical trophozoites of *P. falciparum* and spirochetes of *Borrelia*.

Also, the NMCP initiated a program for microscopists to undergo WHO external competency assessment on malaria microscopy (ECAMM) courses; the first round allowed to identify a core group of microscopists (WHO level 1 and 2). Some of those leading microscopists have been selected to undergo training-of-facilitators courses.

Thus, the next EQA should include more restringing requirements and this study could be considered as the baseline. Microscopists in the country will be assessed and certified in a national competence assessment (NCA) system. The protocol for these assessment and certification will include parasite density determination, non-falciparum species identification, falciparum low parasite density detection, atypical trophozoites of *P. falciparum* recognition and spirochetes of *Borrelia* detection. It is expected, with this program, to increase trust among clinicians so they will prescribe appropriately antimalarial drugs [20]. A preceded retraining program is planned before evaluation. In fact, refresher training as well as adequate equipment and reagents, good working conditions, motivated and qualified personnel are known to improve microscopists skills [12, 14, 21].

In Senegal, according to NMCP procedure for cross-checking slides, the number of randomly selected slides is higher than that of WHO recommendations [22]. The advantage of a large number of taken slides is to increase the power of the study to detect slide reading errors; this is particularly relevant in regions striving to eliminate malaria, such as in north Senegal.

Conclusion

In Senegal, the performance quality of malaria microscopy is relatively satisfactory especially when addressing *P. falciparum* detection. However, non-falciparum species and blood bacterial such as Borrelia are likely to be missed when performing malaria microscopy. Another approaches are recommended to be adapted by future trainings and evaluations on microscopic laboratories.

Abbreviations

ECAMM: external competency assessment of malaria microscopists; EQA: external quality assessment; HC: health centre; HFN: high false-negative; HFP: high false-positive; LFN: low false-negative; LFP: low false-positive; NCA: national competence assessment; NMCP: national malaria control program; NPV: negative predictive value; NRL: national reference laboratory; PPV: positive predictive value; QC: quality control; RDT: rapid diagnostic test; SOP: standard operating procedures; WHO: World Health Organization.

Authors' contributions

MAD, YD, MCS and KD are WHO level 1 expert microscopists; they performed the microscopy re-examinations of taken slides. MAD drafted the manuscript; MAD, BD, YD, ID and YDN were involved in the fields during supervisory visits. ASB, ID and DN critically commented on the manuscript. All authors read and approved the final manuscript.

Author details

[1] Laboratory of Parasitology and Mycology, Cheikh Anta Diop University, Avenue Cheikh Anta Diop, BP 5005 Fann, Dakar, Senegal. [2] National Malaria Control Program (NMCP), Rue Aimé Césaire, Fann Résidence, Dakar, Senegal.

Acknowledgements

We would like to thank Amy K. Bei for her help to English review this manuscript. We are thankful to the NMCP staff for their help to collect and transport slides.

Competing interests

The authors declare that they have no competing interests.

Funding

Not applicable.

References

1. Maguire JD, Lederman ER, Barcus MJ, Wendy A, Meara PO, Jordon RG, Duong S, Muth S, Sismadi P, Bangs MJ, Prescott WR, Baird JK, Wongsrichanalai C. Production and validation of durable, high quality standardized malaria microscopy slides for teaching, testing and quality assurance during an era of declining diagnostic proficiency. Malar J. 2006;5:1–8.
2. Hawkes M, Kain KC. Advances in malaria diagnosis. Expert Rev Anti Infect Ther. 2007;5:485–95.
3. Trape JF, Diatta G, Arnathau C, Bitam I, Sarih M, Belghyti D, Bouattour A, Elguero E, Vial L, Mané Y, Baldé C, Pugnolle F, Chauvancy G, Mahé G, Granjon L, Duplantier JM, Durand P, Renaud F. The epidemiology and geographic distribution of relapsing fever borreliosis in West and North Africa, with a review of the *Ornithodoros erraticus* complex (Acari: Ixodida). PLoS ONE. 2013;8:1–19.
4. Ashraf S, Kao A, Hugo C, Christophel EM, Fatunmbi B, Luchavez J, Lilley K, Bell D. Developing standards for malaria microscopy: external competency assessment for malaria microscopists in the Asia-Pacific. Malar J. 2012;11:352.
5. WHO. Malaria microscopy quality assurance manual. 2nd ed. Geneva: WHO; 2015.
6. PNLP. Cadre strategique national de lutte contre le paludisme AU Senegal 2014–2018. 2014.
7. Lucchi NW, Gaye M, Diallo MA, Goldman IF, Ljolje D, Deme AB, Badiane A, Ndiaye YD, Barnwell JW, Udhayakumar V, Ndiaye D. Evaluation of the Illumigene Malaria LAMP: a robust molecular diagnostic tool for malaria parasites. Sci Rep. 2016;6(October):36808.
8. Giardina F, Gosoniu L, Konate L, Diouf MB, Perry R, Faye O, Vounatsou P. Estimating the burden of malaria in Senegal: Bayesian zero-inflated binomial geostatistical modeling of the MIS 2008 data. PLoS ONE. 2012;7:1–10.
9. Niang M, Thiam LG, Sow A, Loucoubar C, Bob NS, Diop F, Diouf B, Niass O, Mansourou A, Varela ML, Perraut R, Sall AA, Balde AT. A molecular survey of acute febrile illnesses reveals *Plasmodium vivax* infections in Kedougou, southeastern Senegal. Malar J. 2015;14:1–8.
10. Amexo M, Tolhurst R, Barnish G, Bates I. Malaria misdiagnosis: effects on the poor and vulnerable. Lancet. 2004;364:1896–8.
11. Mukadi P, Lejon V, Barbé B, Gillet P, Nyembo C. Performance of microscopy for the diagnosis of malaria and human African trypanosomiasis by diagnostic laboratories in the Democratic Republic of the Congo: Results of a Nation-Wide external quality assessment. PLoS ONE. 2016;11:e0146450.
12. Obare P, Ogutu B, Adams M, Odera JS, Lilley K, Dosoo D, Adhiambo C, Owusu-agyei S, Binka F, Wanja E, Johnson J. Misclassification of Plasmodium infections by conventional microscopy and the impact of remedial training on the proficiency of laboratory technicians in species identification. Malar J. 2013;12:1–6.
13. Kahama-maro J, Acremont VD, Mtasiwa D, Genton B, Lengeler C. Low quality of routine microscopy for malaria at different levels of the health system in Dar es Salaam. 2011;10:332.
14. Biadglegne F, Belyhun Y, Ali J, Walle F, Gudeta N, Kassu A, Mulu A. Does the practice of blood film microscopy for detection and quantification of malaria parasites in northwest Ethiopia fit the standard ? BMC Health Serv Res. 2014;14:529.
15. Diallo MA, Badiane AS, Diongue K, Deme A, Lucchi NW, Gaye M, Ndiaye T, Ndiaye M, Sene LK, Diop A, Gaye A, Ndiaye YD, Samb D, Yade MS, Ndir O, Udhayakumar V, Ndiaye D. Non-falciparum malaria in Dakar: a confirmed case of *Plasmodium ovale* wallikeri infection. Malar J. 2016;15:429.
16. Daniels RF, Deme AB, Gomis JF, Dieye B, Durfee K, Thwing JI, Fall FB, Ba M, Ndiop M, Badiane AS, Ndiaye YD, Wirth DF, Volkman SK, Ndiaye D. Evidence of non-*Plasmodium falciparum* malaria infection in Kédougou, Sénégal. Malar J. 2017;16:9.

22

Extreme diversity and multiple SCC*mec* elements in coagulase-negative Staphylococcus found in the Clinic and Community in Beijing, China

Xiao-Ping Chen[1†], Wen-Ge Li[1†], Hao Zheng[1], Hai-Yan Du[2], Li Zhang[2], Lei Zhang[2], Jie Che[1], Yuan Wu[1], Shu-Mei Liu[2,3*] and Jin-Xing Lu[1,4*]

Abstract

Background: Coagulase-negative staphylococci (CoNS) are recognized as a large reservoir of staphylococcal cassette chromosome *mec* (SCC*mec*) harboured by *Staphylococcus aureus*. However, data of SCC*mec* in CoNS are relatively absent particularly in China.

Methods: Seventy-eight CoNS clinical and 47 community isolates were collected in Beijing. PCR was performed to classify SCC*mec* types. Under oxacillin treatment, quantitative real-time reverse transcription PCR (qRT-PCR) was performed to compare *mecA* mRNA levels and mRNA half-life between isolates with single SCC*mec* element and those with multiple one. Their growth curves were analysed. Their bacterial cell wall integrity was also compared by performing a Gram stain. All *ccr* complex segments were sequenced and obtained *ccr* segments were analysed by phylogenetic analyses.

Results: All 78 clinical isolates had *mecA* segments compared with 38% in community isolates (total 47). Only 29% clinical isolates and 33% community isolates (among *mecA* positive isolates) harboured a single previously identified SCC*mec* type; notably, 17% clinical isolates and 28% community isolates had multiple SCC*mec* types. Further studies indicated that isolates with multiple SCC*mec* elements had more stable *mecA* mRNA expression compared with isolates with single SCC*mec* elements. CoNS with multiple SCC*mec* elements demonstrated superior cell wall integrity. Interestingly, phylogenetic analyses of obtained 70 *ccr* segments indicated that horizontal gene transfer of the *ccr* complex might exist among various species of clinical CoNS, community CoNS and *S. aureus*.

Conclusions: CoNS recovered from patients carried extremely diverse but distinctive SCC*mec* elements compared with isolates from the community. More attention should be given to CoNS with multiple SCC*mec* not only because they had superior cell wall integrity, but also because CoNS and *S. aureus* might acquire *multiple SCCmec* through the *ccr* complex.

Keywords: Coagulase-negative staphylococci, Multiple SCC*mec*, Bacterial cell wall integrity

*Correspondence: lsmlucky@126.com; lujinxing6688@yahoo.com
†Xiao-Ping Chen and Wen-Ge Li contributed equally to this work
[3] FuXingMenWai Road 20, XiCheng, Beijing 100038, China
[4] Changbai Road 155, ChangPing, Beijing 102206, China
Full list of author information is available at the end of the article

Background

Coagulase-negative staphylococcus (CoNS) is a part of the commensal bacterial microflora of healthy people. However, with the development of interventional therapy and the increasing number of immunocompromised patients, these bacteria are becoming the most important causes of nosocomial infections [1, 2]. CoNS bloodstream infections have been estimated in as many as 250,000 cases annually in the US. The mortality rate of these infections is 1–25%, representing a great burden to the public health system [3]. The most common CoNS in nosocomial infection are *Staphylococcus epidermidis*, followed by *Staphylococcus haemolyticus*, *Staphylococcus hominis* and *Staphylococcus capitis* [4]. Another important reason for the increasing concern for CoNS is the fact that they also harbour SCC*mec* elements, which are found in methicillin-resistant *S. aureus* (MRSA). SCC*mec* elements harbour *mec* genes (*mecA/mecC*), providing resistance to methicillin and nearly all other beta-lactam antibiotics [5].

In general, SCC*mec* has two essential components, i.e., the *mec* gene complex and the cassette chromosome recombinase (*ccr*) gene complex. The *mec* gene complex consists of *mecA/mecC*, regulatory genes and associated insertion sequences and has been classified into five main classes, i.e., class A, class B, class C1, class C2, class D, which has been observed only in *Staphylococcus caprae*, and newly found class E [6, 7]. Encoding recombinases mediating integration and excision of SCC*mec* into and from the chromosome, *ccr* genes (*ccrC* or the pair of *ccrA* and *ccrB*) play an important role in the transfer of SCC*mec* elements [8]. The *ccr* gene(s) and surrounding genes form the *ccr* gene complex. At present, two distinct *ccr* gene complexes have been reported based on the composition of *ccr* genes, one carrying two adjacent *ccr* genes, *ccrA* and *ccrB*, and the second carrying *ccrC*. The *ccrA* and *ccrB* genes identified in *S. aureus* strains are categorized into four and five allotypes respectively, resulting in six *ccr* gene complex types, designated as type 1 (*ccrA1B1*), type 2 (*ccrA2B2*), type 3 (*ccrA3B3*), type 4 (*ccrA4B4*), type 7 (*ccrA1B6*) and type 8 (*ccrA1B3*). In contrast, all identified *ccrC* variants to date show high nucleotide similarity and are designed to only one allotype, *ccrC1*, constituting type 5 of *ccr* gene complex [7, 9]. Because of the high diversity of *ccr* gene complex and *mec* gene complex, an extensive genetic diversity of SCC*mec* elements has been revealed in *S. aureus* and a total of twelve types of SCC*mec* have been assigned for *S. aureus* based on the classes of the *mec* gene complex and *ccr* gene complex [9].

Previous studies have found that specific SCC*mec* elements, or components, exist in particular CoNS. For example, type IV was preferentially associated with *S. epidermidis* and type V was prevalently found in *S. haemolyticus* in the hospital [10, 11]. However, in recent years, more diverse SCC*mec* elements including non-*mecA*-encoding cassettes had been revealed from CoNS, and many SCC*mec* elements in methicillin-resistant CoNS (MR-CoNS) could not be typed using currently available schemes applied to MRSA. Moreover *mecA* gene has been found more widely distributed among CoNS than among *S. aureus* indicating a potential reservoir for the transfer of SCC*mec* elements to *S. aureus* [10, 12, 13]. However, only a small number of SCC*mec* elements of CoNS have been characterized in China [14]. In addition, the precise role of SCC*mec* elements of CoNS in the emergence and evolution of MRSA remains obscure, which requires characterization of additional SCC*mec* elements. Furthermore, multiple SCC*mec* have been found in CoNS recovered from patients in several studies [14, 15]. To obtain information on the SCC*mec* of local CoNS in Beijing and to reveal the function of multiple SCC*mec* in CoNS, clinical and community isolates were investigated and the features (including *mecA* mRNA quantity, mRNA half life, growth curve, bacterial cell wall integrity) of CoNS with multiple SCC*mec* elements were compared with those harbouring a single SCC*mec* element.

Methods

Sample collection and bacterial isolation

Only one isolate from each subject was collected and further analysed in the study. The demographic, hospital, and microbiological data were anonymously collected. Clinical CoNS isolates were collected from two hospitals in Beijing from July 2013 to December 2015. These CoNS strains were isolated from the blood of inpatients. The ages ranged from 34 to 98 years (mean ± SD, 50 ± 16). These patients were hospitalized for more than 48 h and were suspected of having a blood bacterial infection. Collected blood samples were inoculated into aerobic BacT/Alert FAN blood culture bottles and incubated in the BACT/Alert machine (bioMérieux, Marcy l'Etoile, France) for up to 5 days. Positive culture samples were directly inoculated onto Mueller–Hinton Broth (MH broth, Oxoid LID, Basingstoke, Hampshire, England) supplemented with 2% NaCl and incubated aerobically at 37 °C for 72 h. Species identification were determined using the Vitek II (bioMerieux, Durham, NC, USA) automated microbiology system and further confirmed by partially sequencing 16S rRNA genes amplified with primers 5F and 1194R and *rpoB* genes with primers 2491F and 3241R [13].

Community CoNS isolates were collected from healthy subjects (aged from 20 to 48) in two communities in Beijing in June 2016. Three groups of subjects, including office workers, construction workers and soldiers, were recruited. Samples were collected from the forehead and elbow with cotton swabs wetted with sterilized PBS. The swabs were placed into Mueller–Hinton Broth (MH broth, Oxoid LID, England) supplemented with 2% NaCl and incubated aerobically at 37 °C for 72 h. Ten microliters of culture suspected of bacteria growth were inoculated onto Brain Heart Infusion (BHI, Oxoid LID, England) agar and suggestive colonies with white color and smooth edge were subjected to screening tests with partial sequencing of 16S rRNA and *rpoB* genes as described above.

Detection of *mec* gene and SCC*mec* typing

The existence of the *mecA* gene was identified using primers met1/met2 and *mecC* gene with primers mecCF/mecCR [5, 16]. For *mecA* positive isolates, SCC*mec* typing was defined by the combination of *ccr* type and *mec* class, which were obtained using PCR [6, 9]. The *mec* class was assigned with five primers to identify the gene lineages of *mecA–mecI* (class A *mec* with primer mA7/mI6), *mecA*-IS1272 (class B *mec* with primer mA7/IS7), *mecA*-IS431 (class C *mec* with primer mA7/IS2) and *mecA*-IS431L (class C1 *mec* with primer mA7/IS2L). To further discriminate class C1 or C2 *mec* complexes, sequences between IS431 and *mecA* were examined using PCR with primer (IS431-F2 or IS431-R1) located in either direction of IS431 paired with primer mecA-R2 in *mecA* [14]. Five *ccr* gene complexes were identified with eight primers: four primers consisting of a common reverse primer (common to *ccrB1-3*, i.e., primer BC) and three forward primers specific for *ccrA1*, *ccrA2*, and *ccrA3* to confirm *ccr1–3* based on differences in *ccrA* genes; two primers to identify *ccr4*; and two primers to identify *ccrC* [6, 11].

For *mecA* negative isolates, *ccr* complexes were also analysed with primers as described above. The primers and lengths of amplicons used to identify the *mec* gene, *mecA* classes and *ccr* complexes are listed in Additional file 1: Table S1. PCR products of *ccr* complexes from all isolates were sent to Sangon Biotechnology Company (Sangon Biotech, Shanghai, China) for sequencing. The results were blasted with sequences in GenBank, and *ccr* genes with nucleotide identities more than 85% were designed to the same allotype [9].

Those with two *mecA* classes were designated CoNS with multiple SCC*mec* elements; those with one class of *mecA* complex and one *ccr* complex detected were classified into CoNS with a single SCC*mec* element. All strains with multiple SCC*mec* elements and those with single elements were further characterized.

Determination of minimal inhibitory concentrations (MIC) to oxacillin

For MIC determination, a broth microdilution broth susceptibility assay was performed according to CLSI guidelines [17]. The oxacillin (oxacillin sodium monohydrate, Sigma-Aldrich, St. Louis, MO, USA) concentration ranged from 256 to 0.125 μg/ml. The plates were incubated under normal atmospheric conditions for 24 h at 37 °C. The presence of a white pellet on the bottom of the tube indicated bacterial growth. The MIC value was identified by the lowest concentration of oxacillin at which no visible growth could be observed.

Growth curves of CoNS under oxacillin treatment

Samples of bacterial culture were prepared as follows: a single colony of the strain was cultured with MH broth overnight at 37 °C. Bacterial suspensions were diluted with MH broth to 0.5 McFarland standards and added to oxacillin (final concentration 2 μg/ml) and cultured at 37 °C. Two millilitres of culture was removed at the indicated time point. The growth curves were measured by plate counts on MHI agar (Oxoid LID, Basingstoke, Hampshire, England). The experiments were repeated three times, and the results were reported as an average of the replicate samples.

Quantification of *mecA* mRNA in CoNS under oxacillin treatment

Samples of bacterial culture were prepared as described above. Total RNA was extracted using the OMEGA bacterial RNA kit (OMEGA Biotech, Doraville, GA, USA) and eluted into 50 μl ddH_2O. Three microliters of RNA was reverse transcribed into cDNA using the TransScript TM Two-Step RT-PCR Super Mix (TransGene Biotech, Beijing, China) in a total volume of 20 μl. Using standard PCR and real-time PCR, 2 μl of cDNA was used to evaluate and represent the quantity of total *mecA* mRNA in each 2 ml sample because it held the same proportion of total RNA in each sample.

For standard PCR, 2 μl of cDNA was amplified via PCR with TransScript 2× PCR Super Mix (Transgene Biotech, Beijing, China) in a total volume of 30 μl. The primer pairs (mecAF/mecAR) are shown in Additional file 1: Table S1 [18].

For qRT-PCR analyses, real-time PCR amplification was performed in a total volume of 25 μl containing 12.5 μl of 2× SYBR Fast qPCR Mix (TAKARA, Dalian, China), 1.0 μl primer and 2 μl template cDNA. The specific primers (mecA-1501F, mecA-1598R) used for the detection of *mecA* gene are listed in Additional file 1: Table S1 [19]. Data were presented as the relative copies of *mecA* mRNA levels compared with that of untreated CoNS with a single SCC*mec* element.

mecA mRNA half-life identification

Samples of bacterial culture were prepared as described above except with oxacillin cultured at 37 °C for 3 h. Transcriptional arrest was induced with actinomycin D as references except that the dosage of actinomycin D was modified to 2 μg/ml according to a preliminary experiment [20]. Two millilitres of culture was removed at the indicated time point. Total RNA was extracted and subjected to *mecA* mRNA analyses as described above.

Bacterial cell wall integrity assays

Samples of bacterial culture were prepared as described above except with 8 μg/ml oxacillin treatment. Samples were collected for Gram stain at 0, 1, and 3 h to visualize the bacterial cell wall integrity under a microscope.

Phylogenetic analyses of *ccr*

The reference sequences of the ccr complex in GenBank (Additional file 1: Table S2) and those derived here (Additional file 1: Tables S3, S4) were used to construct a phylogenetic tree. Using MEGA version 5.0, neighbour-joining trees were constructed with the maximum composite likelihood model assuming rate uniformity and pattern homogeneity.

Statistical analysis

Statistical analysis and graphic presentations were performed with Microsoft Excel XP software. The results are expressed as the average of three assays. A *P* value of 0.05 (Student's t test) was considered significant.

Results

Sample collection

In this study, a total of 78 clinical CoNS isolates and 47 community CoNS isolates were recovered and identified to species.

Identification of CoNS

CoNS obtained from the clinic were classified into 4 different Staphylococcal species. These included *S. epidermidis* (n = 30), *S. hominis* (n = 20), *S. capitis* (n = 15) and *S. haemolyticus* (n = 13). However, most of the CoNS recovered from community were *S. epidermidis* (n = 40), and the other CoNS were few, including *S. hominis* (n = 5) and *S. haemolyticus* (n = 2).

Extremely diverse SCC*mec* types and multiple SCC*mec* elements

No *mecC* gene was detected in all these isolates. Not surprisingly, *mecA* was detected in 100% (78/78) clinic isolates compared to 38% (18/47) of the community isolates. The SCC*mec* typing results of these isolates are summarized in Table 1. Interestingly, only a small portion of CoNS were assigned as harbouring a single previously identified SCC*mec* type in both the clinical and community strains (23/78, 29% and 6/18, 33%, respectively). Those identified in clinical isolates included SCC*mec* type III (n = 7), type V (n = 7), type IV (n = 3), type VIII (n = 3), type II (n = 2), and type IX (n = 1). For community strains, only six strains of *S. epidermidis* were confirmed to harbour single SCC*mec* type II. Moreover, 11% (9/78) of clinical CoNS and 5% (1/18) of community isolates recovered carried a new single SCC*mec* type. Strains with an previously identified single SCC*mec* type or new single SCC*mec* type were assigned as CoNS with a single SCC*mec* element.

Interestingly, 54% (42/78) of clinical isolates and 39% (7/18) of community isolates (including new single SCC*mec* types, new types with a single *mecA* class and multiple *ccr* complexes) could not be classified into any SCC*mec* type, most of them carried more than one *ccr* complex. Surprisingly, 17% (13/78) of the clinical isolates and 28% (5/18) of the community isolates had two classes of SCC*mec* types (assigned as CoNS with multiple SCC*mec* elements), particularly some clinical isolates that harboured five *ccr* complexes (i.e., *ccrA1B1*, *ccrA2B2*, *ccrA3B3*, *ccrA4B4* and *ccrC*).

Strains (both clinical and community isolates) that did not fit into the SCC*mec* typing criteria, including those harbouring multiple SCC*mec* elements, were designated new SCC*mec* types (total n = 67), which accounted for approximately 70% of the total CoNS with *mecA* segments determined. It was unexpected that among the 29 community strains without a *mecA* or *mecC* segment detected, 24 (83%) contained a *ccr* complex. Furthermore, multiple *ccr* complexes were detected in 5 (21%) strains.

More stable *mecA* mRNA transcription in CoNS with multiple SCC*mec* elements compared to single elements

As shown in Fig. 1b, total *mecA* mRNA in CoNS with multiple SCC*mec* elements exhibited constant and stable expression during the 10 h experiment. However, total *mecA* mRNA in CoNS with single SCC*mec* element was transcribed unsteadily during this experimental course (Fig. 1a). To further assay *mecA* mRNA stability, *mecA* mRNA half-life was analysed in randomly selected *S. epidermidis* H67 and H30. As demonstrated in Fig. 1c, the *mecA* mRNA half-life was approximately 40–50 min in *S. epidermidis* H30. In contrast, *mecA* mRNA was very unstable in *S. epidermidis* H67, in which the *mecA* mRNA half-time probably was no more than 10 min.

Quantitative RT-PCR analyses of randomly selected isolates further confirmed that the total *mecA* mRNA in *S. epidermidis* H30 demonstrated continuously sustainable expression during the 10 h experiment. In contrast,

Table 1 Detection of *mecA* segments and SCC*mec* typing results of CoNS isolates

Character of SCC*mec*	Source	Species	*mecA* PCR	*mec*A class	*ccr* type	SCC*mec* type	No. of isolate	Example isolate
Previously identified single SCC*mec* type	Clinic	*S. homi*	+	A	4	VIII	3	H80, H86
			+	A	2	II	1	H59
		S. epid	+	A	3	III	4	H8
			+	B	2	IV	3	H67, H11
			+	C2	5	V	2	H81
			+	A	2	II	1	
		S. haem	+	C2	1	IX	1	
		S. capi	+	A	3	III	3	H4
			+	C2	5	V	5	H7, H26, H54, H60, H85
						Total number	*23*	
	Community	*S. epid*	+	A	2	II	6	
						Total number	*6*	
New identified single SCC*mec* type	Clinic	*S. homi*	+	A	1	New	3	H29, H34
		S. haem	+	C1	4	New	5	H2
			+	C1	2	New	1	
						Total number	*9*	
	Community	*S. haem*	+	C1	2	New	1	CJ31-1
						Total number	*1*	
New type with a single *mecA* class and multi *ccr* complexes	Clinic	*S. homi*	+	A	1, 4	New	2	H1
			+	A	1, 2	New	1	H73
			+	A	2, 4	New	2	
			+	A	3, 4	New	1	HA1
			+	A	1, 4, 5	New	2	H6
			+	A	1, 3, 4, 5	New	1	
		S. epid	+	A	1, 3	New	5	H22
			+	A	1, 3, 4	New	2	H21
			+	A	3, 4, 5	New	1	H92
			+	C2	4, 5	New	1	H76
			+	C2	1, 2, 5	New	1	
			+	B	2, 4	New	3	H24, H77
		S. haem	+	A	1, 2, 4	New	1	
			+	C2	2, 4	New	1	H28
			+	C2	4, 5	New	1	H68
			+	C2	1, 4	New	2	H15, H36
		S. capit	+	A	3, 4	New	1	H23
			+	A	1, 2, 4, 5	New	1	H37
			+	A	1, 2, 3, 5	New	1	H83
			+	A	1, 2, 3, 4, 5	New	1	H72
			+	C2	2, 4, 5	New	1	H78
			+	C2	1, 2, 4, 5	New	1	
						Total number	*33*	
New type with a single *mecA* class and multi *ccr* complexes	Community	*S. epid*	+	A	2, 4	New	1	
			+	A	2, 4, 5	New	1	
			+	B	1, 2	New	3	
			+	B	2, 4	New	1	
						Total number	*6*	

Table 1 continued

Character of SCC*mec*	Source	Species	*mecA* PCR	*mecA* class	*ccr* type	SCC*mec* type	No. of isolate	Example isolate
New type with multi SCC*mec*	Clinic	*S. homi*	+	A, C2	1, 4, 5	New	1	
			+	A, C2	1, 2, 4, 5	New	2	H33-2
			+	A, C2	1, 2, 3, 4, 5	New	1	H62
		S.epid	+	A, B	2, 4, 5	New	1	
			+	A, B	2, 3, 5	New	1	
			+	A, B	2, 3, 4, 5	New	1	H30
			+	A, B	1, 2, 3, 4, 5	New	1	
			+	A, C2	1, 5	New	1	
			+	A, C2	2, 4, 5	New	1	H87
			+	A, C2	1, 2, 3, 4, 5	New	1	H57
		S. haem	+	A, B	1, 2, 3, 4	New	1	HA11
		S.capit	+	A, C2	1, 2, 4, 5	New	1	H14
						Total number	*13*	
	Community	*S. homi*	+	A, B	2	New	1	
			+	A, B	1	New	1	CV34
			+	A, B	2, 4	New	1	C3-1
		S. epid	+	A, B	1, 2	New	1	
			+	A, C2	2, 5	New	1	
						Total number	*5*	
Isolates without *mecA* detected	Community	*S. homi*	–	–	2	N	2	C13-2
		S. epid	–	–	2	N	15	C5-1, CJ29
			–	–	1, 2	N	1	
			–	–	2, 5	N	2	
			–	–	5	N	2	CJ28-3
			–	–	2, 4	N	1	CV33-1
			–	–	–	N	5	
		S. haem	–	–	2, 4	N	1	
						Total number	*29*	

S. homi, S. hominis; S. epid, S. epidermidis; S. haem, S. haemolyticus; S.capit, S. capitis, –, *mecA* negative; N, not available

the total *mecA* mRNA in *S. epidermidis* H8 showed very unstable transcription during this experimental course. Furthermore, the number of *mecA* mRNA relative copies of *S. epidermidis* H8 at many time points was significantly less than that of *S. epidermidis* H30 (lower right panel in Fig. 2). However, no significant differences in growth curves were observed between these two isolates (upper left panel in Fig. 2). Moreover, qRT-PCR of *mecA* mRNA transcription and growth curve assays in other *S. epidermidis* isolates and CoNS species also demonstrated the same phenomenon (Additional file 2: Figure S1).

CoNS with multiple SCC*mec* elements demonstrated better bacterial cell wall integrity than those carrying a single element

Randomly selected *S. epidermidis* H30, H57 (with multiple SCC*mec* elements) and *S. epidermidis* H8, H67 (with single SCC*mec*) were recruited for analyses of bacterial cell wall integrity. As shown in Fig. 3, most cells of *S. epidermidis* H57, H30 still demonstrated Gram-positivity after 3 h treatment of oxacillin (91.6 ± 1.3, 82.6 ± 2.8%, respectively). In contrast, a smaller number of cells of *S. epidermidis* H8, H67 demonstrated Gram-positivity at 3 h under oxacillin treatment (12.3 ± 1.7, 14.2 ± 2.6%, respectively). The differences between *S. epidermidis* H30, H57 and *S. epidermidis* H8, H67 were significant ($P < 0.001$).

Phylogenetic association of *ccr* among CoNS and *S. aureus*

A total of 70 *ccr* complex segments were sequenced successfully in this study, including 60 clinical isolates and 10 community isolates (Additional file 1: Tables S3, S4). No new *ccr* allotypes or alleles were identified. The *ccrAB* alleles were assigned based on a BLAST search with sequences in GenBank, resulting in 13 *ccrA1B1*, 13 *ccrA2B2*, 9 *ccrA3B3*, 10 *ccrA4B4* and 15 *ccrC* from clinical CoNS and 1 *ccrA1B1*, 5 *ccrA2B2*, 3 *ccrA4B4*, and 1 *ccrC* from community CoNS. As shown in Fig. 4, all species of CoNS recovered from patients contained various types of *ccr* complexes

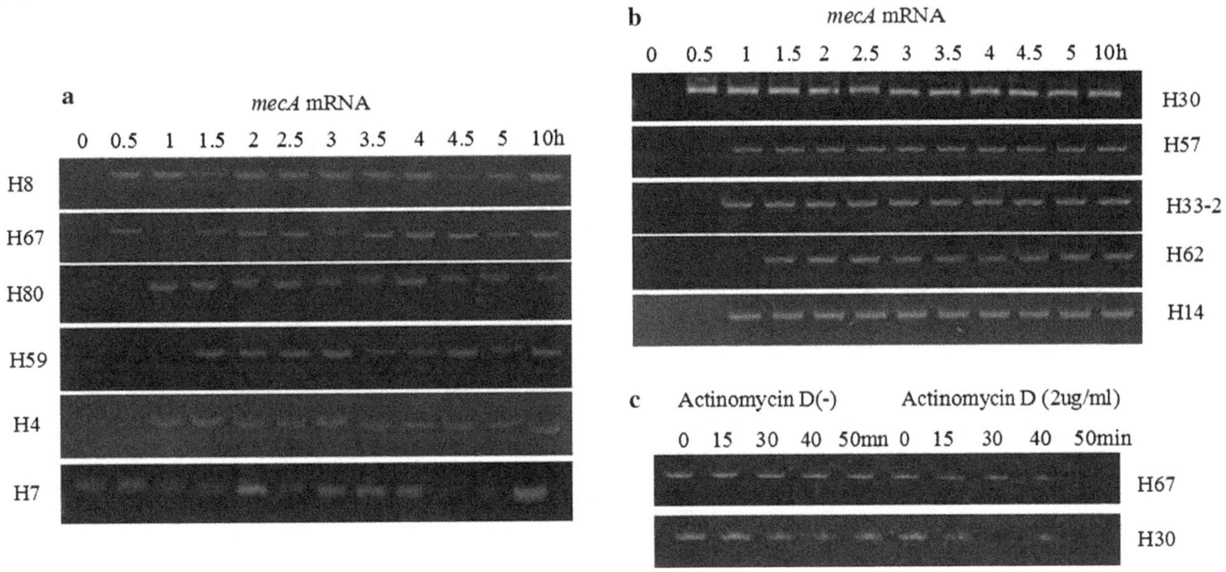

Fig. 1 mRNA expression analyses of the amplified fragments of *mecA* in CoNS with single SCC*mec* elements (**a**) and those with multiple SCC*mec* elements (**b**). Two-millilitres culture of CoNS treated with oxacillin (2 µg/ml) for 10 h were used for *mecA* mRNA transcription analyses by reverse transcription PCR (RT-PCR); after treatment with oxacillin (2 µg/ml) and actinomycin D (2 µg/ml), *mecA* mRNA half-lives were determined by RT-PCR (**c**). mRNA expression levels were described in terms of intensity using Quantity One Imager. Data are shown as the image of three independent experiments with similar results

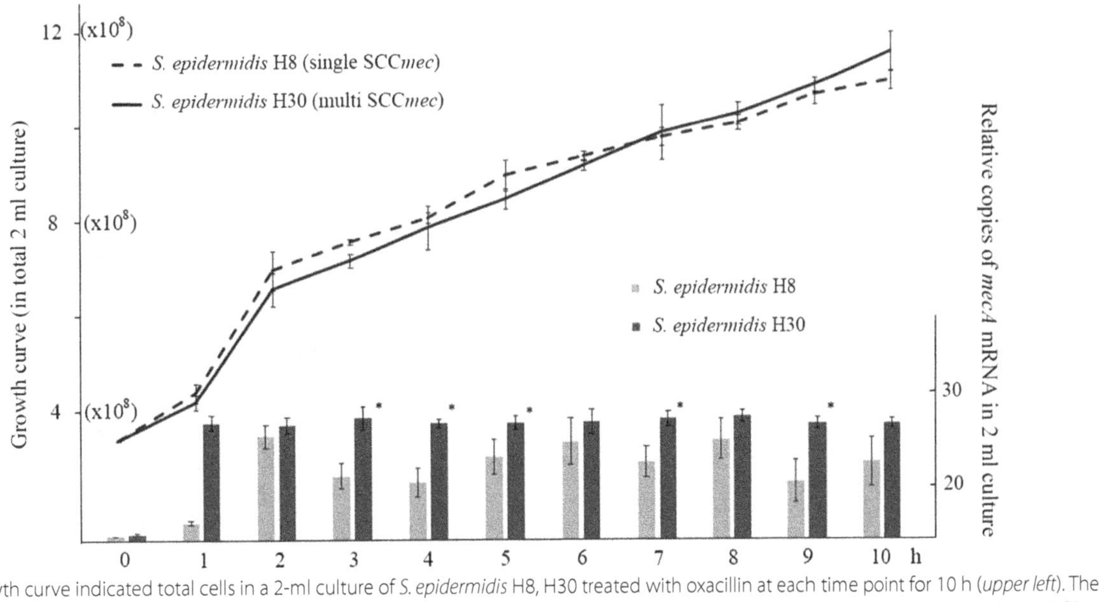

Fig. 2 Growth curve indicated total cells in a 2-ml culture of *S. epidermidis* H8, H30 treated with oxacillin at each time point for 10 h (*upper left*). The corresponding relative total *mecA* mRNA in 2-ml sample treated with oxacillin at each time point was measured by quantitative RT real-time PCR (*lower right*). Data were presented as the relative copies of *mecA* mRNA levels compared with that of *S. epidermidis* H8 (0 h). *Each bar* represents the mean ± SD of at least three independent experiments. *P < 0.05 between two strains at each time point

except *ccrA3B3*, which had not been discovered from *S. haemolyticus* in this study. For community isolates, *ccrA3B3* had not been recovered in this study. In each phylogenetic tree, *ccr* segments recovered from clinical CoNS were grouped with those from community isolates in this study and those from around the world. No specific cluster formed for either the clinical isolates or community isolates.

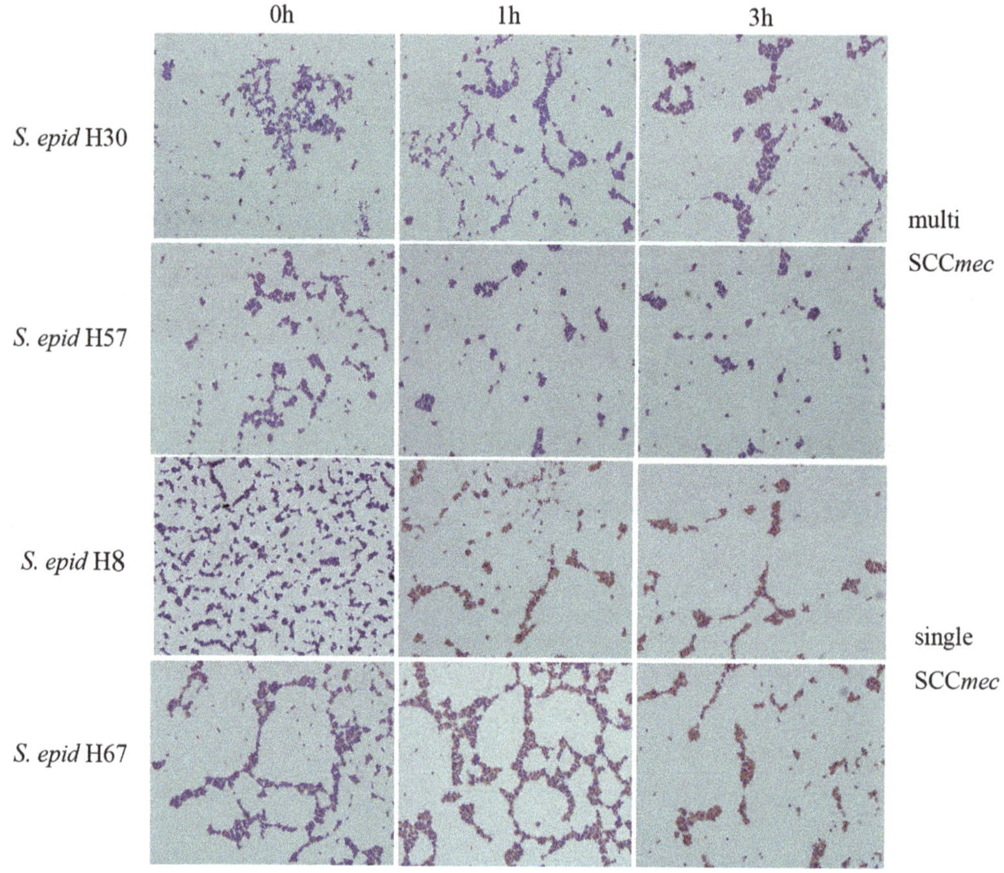

Fig. 3 Bacterial cell wall integrity under oxacillin treatment (8 μg/ml). Samples were collected for Gram staining at 0, 1, and 3 h to visualize the bacterial cell wall under a microscope. The proportion of bacteria cells demonstrated as Gram-negative among every 100 total cells, was manually calculated according to three microscope fields for each sample. The results are shown as the mean value of three microscope fields. Data are shown as the images of three independent experiments with similar results

Importantly, *ccrA3B3* segments in clinical CoNS demonstrated high similarity (nearly 100%) with those in *S. aureus* worldwide. In contrast, *ccrA1B1* segments from both the clinic and community were grouped together but separated from those found in *S. aureus*. Interestingly, *ccrA2B2*, *ccrA4B4* and *ccrC* showed an intermediate state, i.e., some clustered with those in *S. aureus* and others had separated from them.

Discussion

In general, the existence of different types of SCC*mec* in MR-CoNS is dependent on the host species and geographical locations [11]. In this study, SCC*mec* types, II, III, and V were prevalent in MR-CoNS in Beijing. Another study performed from southwest China demonstrated that SCC*mec* types III, IV and V were dominant in MR-CoNS [14]. Moreover, specific SCC*mec* types (in some instances, specific *ccr* or *mec* complex genes) were found particularly in specific CoNS species. Consistent with previous reports, type IV SCC*mec* was preferentially associated with *S. epidermidis* in our study. However, most type V SCC*mec* had been recovered in *S. capitis* in this study, unlike previous study which demonstrated type V dominates in *S. haemolyticus* [10–12]. Although in this study class C *mec* was dominantly associated with *S. haemolyticus* as previous reports [21, 22], *most S. haemolyticus* isolates (clinic or community) carried new SCC*mec* type. We also did not find type VII SCC*mec* in CoNS in this study as other researchers; however, one isolate of type IX was disclosed in *S. haemolyticus* in clinic, which had not been previously confirmed in CoNS [12, 23]. A recent study also reported SCC*mec* type IX in CoNS in the community [24]. Significantly, most CoNS strains recovered in this study (clinic and community) consisted of untypable SCC*mec* elements as many other reports [14–16, 23, 25]. Importantly, the differences between clinical CoNS and community isolates might result from sampling bias as most CoNS recovered from the community were *S. epidermidis*.

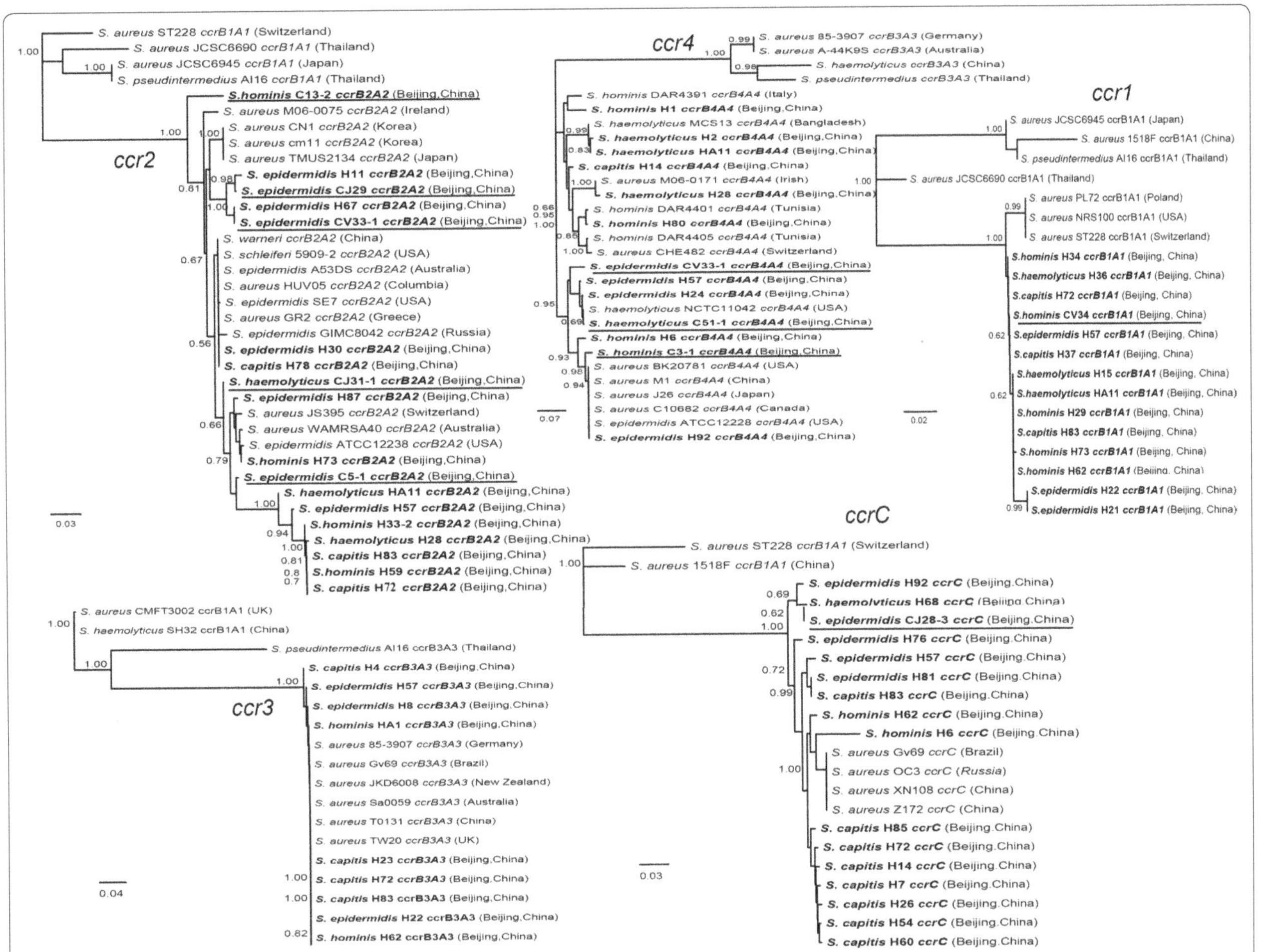

Fig. 4 Neighbour-joining tree based on *ccr* sequences determined in this study and those downloaded from GenBank. Those with *bold italic* font represent *ccr* sequences recovered in this study and those *underlined* represent isolates from the community

Intriguingly, various combinations of *ccr* types were revealed in a single CoNS strain, including clinical and community isolates in this study. Multiple copies of *ccr* complex have been reported in *S. aureus*, *S. epidermidis* and other CoNS. However, most are combinations of *ccrAB* and *ccrC* [6, 25]. To the best of our knowledge, this is the first report of a heterogeneous combination of *ccr* complex in a single CoNS strain, particularly all five types of *ccr* complexes existing in a single clinical isolate. Thus, it was not surprising that these CoNS strains contained multiple SCC*mec* elements. Multiple SCC*mec* elements have been reported in clinical MR-CoNS and the incidences were as high as that observed in our finding [6, 14]. Although it was likely that the two SCC*mec* elements actually constituted a composite rather than two independent units, multiple copies of *mecA* existed in one single CoNS strain both in the clinic and community as revealed in our study. Intriguingly, whether the existence of multiple SCC*mec* in community isolates was attributed to spill over from the hospital or to antibiotic abuse in the community requires further investigation.

It is well-known that acquisition of antibiotic resistance in bacterial cells is often accompanied by fitness cost in the absence of antibiotics, most of which demonstrated slower growth rates and finally resulted in the dilution of antibiotic resistant genes [26]. However, we did not identify any significant differences in the growth rates between CoNS strains with multiple SCC*mec* and those with a single isolate with or without oxacillin, and no correlation of multiple SCCmec with MIC in response to oxacillin was disclosed (data not shown). We speculated that MIC in response to oxacillin might also be correlated with other antibiotic genes [27]. Interestingly, we demonstrated that multiple SCC*mec* elements in CoNS strains ensure stable and continuous transcription of antibiotic-resistant genes, i.e., *mecA* gene, whose transcript, PBP2a, was capable of maintaining cell wall integrity [28]. Further analyses by Gram staining demonstrated that the cell wall in CoNS with multiple SCC*mec* demonstrated much stronger resistance and better integrity under oxacillin treatment than those CoNS with single SCC*mec* element. Interestingly, although the bacteria cell number dramatically increased, total *mecA* mRNA levels sustained constantly from 1 h to 10 h incubation with oxacillin. We suspected that the amount of *mecA* mRNA at the 1 h time point was sufficient to resist the antibiotics added into the culture.

Finally, phylogenetic analyses of *ccr* indicated potential horizontal gene transfer among different CoNS species of clinic and community isolates, even among CoNS and *S. aureus*. In particular, nearly 100% similarity of all ccr*A3B3* might result from a recent gene transfer among different CoNS species and *S. aureus*. As observed in previous studies [16], we also detected the *ccr* complex in *mec* negative strains. Specifically, some community CoNS strains had multiple *ccr* but lacked the *mec* gene. Their potential to acquire *mec* genes with these *ccr* complexes requires further attention. However, the limitation of our work is that we could not determine which *ccr* complex was linked to the specific SCC*mec*, particularly for those that had two types of *mecA* classes (multiple SCC*mec*). The presence of untypable and multiple SCC*mec* elements represent great challenges for SCC*mec* typing in MR-CoNS [11, 14, 15, 23]. Whole genome sequencing of more MR-CoNS would be helpful to construct a new typing method through understanding the relative position and precise composition of multiple SCC*mec* and to further elucidate the role of *ccr* complexes in spreading SCC*mec* elements among CoNS and *S. aureus*.

Conclusions

Overall, CoNS recovered in Beijing carried extremely diverse SCC*mec* elements including multiple SCC*mec* elements, which demonstrated superior cell wall integrity. Our data revealed potential horizontal gene transfer among different CoNS species of clinic and community isolates, even among CoNS and *S. aureus*.

Additional files

Additional file 1: Table S1. Primers used for *mec* gene detection and SCC*mec* Typing. **Table S2.** The *ccr* gene sequences obtained from GenBank for phylogenetic analyses. **Table S3.** The *ccr* gene sequences obtained in this study for phylogenetic analyses. **Table S4.** Origins of the CoNS strains whose *ccr* segments were applied to phylogenetic analyses.

Additional file 2: Figure S1. Growth curve indicating the total cells in a 2-ml culture of CoNS treated with oxacillin at each time point for 10 h (upper left in panel A, B, and C). The corresponding relative total *mecA* mRNA in the 2-ml sample treated with oxacillin at each time point was measured by quantitative RT real-time PCR (lower right in each panel). Data are presented as the relative copies of *mecA* mRNA levels compared with that of *S. epidermidis* H8 (0 h). Each bar represents the mean±SD of at least three independent experiments. $^*P<0.05$ between two strains at each time point.

Abbreviations

CoNS: coagulase-negative staphylococci; SCC*mec*: staphylococcal cassette chromosome *mec*; *ccr*: cassette chromosome recombinase; MIC: minimal inhibitory concentrations.

Authors' contributions

XPC, SML and JXL wrote the manuscript. XPC, WGL and HZ implemented PCR and sequence analyses; HYD, LZ, and LZ performed bacterial culture experiments; JC and YW did raw data analyses. All authors read and approved the final manuscript.

Author details

[1] State Key Laboratory for Infectious Disease Prevention and Control, Collaborative Innovation Center for Diagnosis and Treatment of Infectious Diseases, National Institute for Communicable Disease Control and Prevention, Chinese Center for Disease Control and Prevention, Beijing 102206, China. [2] Microbiology Laboratory, Fu Xing Hospital, Capital Medical University, Beijing 100038, China. [3] FuXingMenWai Road 20, XiCheng, Beijing 100038, China. [4] Changbai Road 155, ChangPing, Beijing 102206, China.

Acknowledgements

Not applicable.

Competing interests

The authors declare that they have no competing interests.

Funding

This work was supported by the National Key Technology Support Program (2012BAI11B05) and National Natural Science Foundation of China (Grants 81201250).

References

1. Ghazal SS, Stevens MP, Bearman GM, Edmond MB. Utility of surveillance blood cultures in patients undergoing hematopoietic stem cell transplantation. Antimicrob Resist Infect Control. 2014;3:20.
2. Widerström M. Significance of *Staphylococcus epidermidis* in health care-associated infections, from contaminant to hospital relevant pathogen: this is a wake-up call! J Clin Microbiol. 2016;54:1679–81.
3. Raad I, Hanna H, Maki D. Intravascular catheter-related infections: advances in diagnosis, prevention, and management. Lancet Infect Dis. 2007;7:645–57.
4. Dong Y, Speer CP. The role of *Staphylococcus epidermidis* in neonatal sepsis: guarding angel or pathogenic devil? Int J Med Microbiol. 2014;304:513–20.
5. García-Álvarez L, Holden MT, Lindsay H, Webb CR, Brown DF, Curran MD, et al. Meticillin-resistant *Staphylococcus aureus* with a novel mecA homologue in human and bovine populations in the UK and Denmark: a descriptive study. Lancet Infect Dis. 2011;8:595–603.
6. Kondo Y, Ito T, Ma XX, Watanabe S, Kreiswirth BN, Etienne J, et al. Combination of multiplex PCRs for staphylococcal cassette chromosome mec type assignment: rapid identification system for mec, ccr, and major differences in junkyard regions. Antimicrob Agents Chemother. 2007;51:264–74.
7. Turlej A, Hryniewicz W, Empel J. Staphylococcal cassette chromosome mec (SCCmec) classification and typing methods: an overview. Pol J Microbiol. 2011;60:95–103.
8. Misiura A, Pigli YZ, Boyle-Vavra S, Daum RS, Boocock MR, Rice PA. Roles of two large serine recombinases in mobilizing the methicillin-resistance cassette SCCmec. Mol Microbiol. 2013;88:1218–29.
9. International Working Group on the Classification of Staphylococcal. Cassette chromosome elements (IWG-SCC). Classification of staphylococcal cassette chromosome mec (SCCmec): guidelines for reporting novel SCCmec elements. Antimicrob Agents Chemother. 2009;53:4961–7.

10. Tessler AT, Billerbeck C, Kadlec K, Schwarz S. Identification and characterization of methicillin-resistant coagulase-negative staphylococci from bovine mastitis. J Antimicrob Chemother. 2010;65:1576–82.
11. Ruppé E, Barbier F, Mesli Y, Maiga A, Cojocaru R, Benkhalfat M, et al. Diversity of staphylococcal cassette chromosome mec structures in methicillin-resistant *Staphylococcus epidermidis* and *Staphylococcus haemolyticus* strains among outpatients from four countries. Antimicrob Agents Chemother. 2009;53:442–9.
12. Ibrahem S, Salmenlinna S, Virolainen A, Kerttula AM, Lyytikäinen O, Jägerroos H, et al. Carriage of methicillin-resistant Staphylococci and their SCCmec types in a long-term-care facility. J Clin Microbiol. 2009;47:32–7.
13. Petti CA, Simmon KE, Miro JM, Hoen B, Marco F, Chu VH, International Collaboration on Endocarditis-Microbiology Investigators, et al. Genotypic diversity of coagulase-negative staphylococci causing endocarditis: a global perspective. J Clin Microbiol. 2008;46:1780–4.
14. Zong Z, Peng C, Lü X. Diversity of SCCmec elements in methicillin-resistant coagulase-negative staphylococci hospital isolates. PLoS ONE. 2011;6:e20191.
15. Tulinski P, Fluit AC, Wagenaar JA, Mevius D, van de Vijver L, Duim B. Methicillin-resistant coagulase-negative staphylococci on pig farms as a reservoir of heterogeneous staphylococcal cassette chromosome mec elements. Appl Environ Microbiol. 2012;78:299–304.
16. Hanssen AM, Kjeldsen G, Sollid JU. Local variants of staphylococcal cassette chromosome mec in sporadic methicillin-resistant *Staphylococcus aureus* and methicillin-resistant coagulase-negative staphylococci: evidence of horizontal gene transfer? Antimicrob Agents Chemother. 2004;48:285–96.
17. Clinical and Laboratory Standards Institute (CLSI). Methods for dilution antimicrobial susceptibility tests for bacteria that grow aerobically. Approved Standard M07-A8. 8th ed. CLSI: Wayne; 2009.
18. Lee JW, Ji YJ, Lee SO, Lee IS. Effect of *Saliva miltiorrhiza* bunge on antimicrobial activity and resistant gene regulation against methicillin-resistant *Staphylococcus aureus* (MRSA). J Microbiol. 2007;45:350–7.
19. Wang HY, Kim S, Kim J, Park SD, Uh Y, Lee H. Multiplex real-time PCR assay for rapid detection of methicillin-resistant staphylococci directly from positive blood cultures. J Clin Microbiol. 2014;52:1911–20.
20. Chen X, Yoza BK, El Gazzar M, Hu JY, Cousart SL, McCall CE. RelB sustains IkappaBalpha expression during endotoxin tolerance. Clin Vaccine Immunol. 2009;16:104–10.
21. Berglund C, Söderquist B. The origin of a methicillin-resistant Staphylococcus aureus isolate at a neonatal ward in Sweden-possible horizontal transfer of a staphylococcal cassette chromosome mec between methicillin-resistant *Staphylococcus haemolyticus* and *Staphylococcus aureus*. Clin Microbiol Infect. 2008;14:1048–56.
22. Bouchami O, Ben Hassen A, de Lencastre H, Miragaia M. High prevalence of mec complex C and ccrC is independent of SCCmec type V in *Staphylococcus haemolyticus*. Eur J Clin Microbiol Infect Dis. 2012;31:605–14.
23. Li M, Wang X, Gao Q, Lu Y. Molecular characterization of Staphylococcus epidermidis strains isolated from a teaching hospital in Shanghai, China. J Med Microbiol. 2009;58:456–61.
24. Sinlapasorn S, Lulitanond A, Angkititrakul S, Chanawong A, Wilailuckana C, Tavichakorntrakool R, et al. SCCmec IX in meticillin-resistant *Staphylococcus aureus* and meticillin-resistant coagulase-negative staphylococci from pigs and workers at pig farms in Khon Kaen, Thailand. J Med Microbiol. 2015;64:1087–93.
25. Hanssen AM, Sollid JU. Multiple staphylococcal cassette chromosomes and allelic variants of cassette chromosome recombinases in *Staphylococcus aureus* and coagulase-negative staphylococci from Norway. Antimicrob Agents Chemother. 2007;51:1671–7.
26. Suzuki S, Horinouchi T, Furusawa C. Phenotypic changes associated with the fitness cost in antibiotic resistant *Escherichia coli* strains. Mol BioSyst. 2016;12:414–20.
27. Wassenaar TM, Ussery D, Nielsen LN, Ingmer H. Review and phylogenetic analysis of qac genes that reduce susceptibility to quaternary ammonium compounds in Staphylococcus species. Eur J Microbiol Immunol (Bp). 2015;5:44–61.
28. Niemeyer DM, Pucci MJ, Thanassi JA, Sharma VK, Archer GL. Role of mecA transcriptional regulation in the phenotypic expression of methicillin resistance in *Staphylococcus aureus*. J Bacteriol. 1996;178:5464–71.

23

Emergence of multidrug-resistant *Providencia rettgeri* isolates co-producing NDM-1 carbapenemase and PER-1 extended-spectrum β-lactamase causing a first outbreak in Korea

Saeam Shin[1], Seok Hoon Jeong[2], Hyukmin Lee[2], Jun Sung Hong[2], Min-Jeong Park[1] and Wonkeun Song[1*]

Abstract

Background: Nosocomial outbreak due to carbapenem-resistant Enterobacteriaceae has become serious challenge to patient treatment and infection control. We describe an outbreak due to a multidrug-resistant *Providencia rettgeri* from January 2016 to January 2017 at a University Hospital in Seoul, Korea.

Methods: A total of eight non-duplicate *P. rettgeri* isolates were discovered from urine samples from eight patients having a urinary catheter and admitted in a surgical intensive care unit. The β-lactamase genes were identified using polymerase chain reaction and direct sequencing, and strain typing was done with pulsed-field gel electrophoresis (PFGE).

Results: All isolates showed high-level resistance to extended-spectrum cephalosporins, aztreonam, meropenem, ertapenem, ciprofloxacin, and amikacin. They harbored the bla_{NDM-1} carbapenemase and the bla_{PER-1} type extended-spectrum β-lactamases genes. PFGE revealed that all isolates from eight patients were closely related strains.

Conclusions: The 13-month outbreak ended following reinforcement of infection control measures, including contact isolation precautions and environmental disinfection. This is the first report of an outbreak of a *P. rettgeri* clinical isolates co-producing NDM-1 and PER-1 β-lactamase.

Keywords: *Providencia rettgeri*, Outbreak, Urinary tract infection, NDM-1, PER-1

Background

The genus *Providencia* comprises part of the natural human gut flora but may also cause infections, including travelers' diarrhea, urinary tract infections, and other nosocomial infections [1]. Treatment of these infections is challenging because *Providencia rettgeri* strains are intrinsically resistant to many antimicrobials including ampicillin, first generation cephalosporins, polymyxins and tigecycline [2]. Furthermore, in recent years *P. rettgeri* has become increasingly important because of the emergence of carbapenemase-producing strains [3, 4]. Carbapenemases are enzymes known to hydrolase almost all types of β-lactams [5]. The New Delhi metallo-β-lactamase (NDM-1) has been firstly identified in 2009 in a Swedish patient who had been previously hospitalized in New Delhi, India [6]. The first occurrence of NDM-1 producers was reported in clinical isolates of *P. rettgeri* in Israel in 2013 [7]. Since then, other cases have been reported in Mexico, Brazil, Argentina, Ecuador, Canada, and Nepal [3, 4, 8–13].

PER-1 enzyme is belong to class A extended-spectrum β-lactamases (ESBLs) and firstly discovered in a plasmid of *Pseudomonas aeruginosa* in France [14]. Later, it has

*Correspondence: swonkeun@hallym.or.kr
[1] Department of Laboratory Medicine, Hallym University College of Medicine, Seoul, South Korea
Full list of author information is available at the end of the article

also found among several Gram-negative species including *Acinetobacter baumannii, Salmonella enterica* serovar Typhimurium, and also in *P. rettgeri* [15, 16]. PER-1 is widely spread in Turkey, however, high prevalence of PER-1 ESBL in *A. baumannii* has been reported in Korea [17].

Here, we report the first outbreak of multidrug-resistant *P. rettgeri* strain co-producing NDM-1 and PER-1 in Korea.

Materials and methods

Patients and bacterial isolates

From January 2016 to January 2017, a total of eight *P. rettgeri* isolates from eight patients were included in this study. Bacterial identification was done with a Vitek-MS (bioMérieux, Marcy I'Etoile, France). Medical records of the patients were retrospectively reviewed. This study protocol was approved by the hospital institutional review board.

Antimicrobial susceptibility testing

Minimum inhibitory concentrations (MICs) for cefotetan, cefotaxime, ceftazidime, cefepime, ertapenem, imipenem, meropenem, aztreonam, amikacin, ciprofloxacin, gentamicin, and tigecycline were determined using Etest strips (bioMérieux) on the Mueller–Hinton agar (Becton–Dickinson, Sparks, MD, USA). Colistin MIC was determined by broth microdilution. When available, antimicrobial susceptibility was interpreted based on the Clinical and Laboratory Standards Institute (CLSI) guideline [18]. For tigecycline and colistin, the European Committee for Antimicrobial Susceptibility Testing (EUCAST) criteria were used [19].

Detection of β-lactamase genes

The carbapenemase genes and ESBL genes were detected using specific PCR primers (Table 1) [20–27]. Amplified products were directly sequenced on the ABI 3730xl automatic sequencer (Applied Biosystems, Foster City, CA, USA) using the same primer pair. The sequences obtained were compared to those in GenBank

Table 1 Primers used in this study for identifying antimicrobial resistance genes

Classification	Primer	Target	Nucleotide sequence, 5′ to 3′	Product size, bp	References
Class A β lactamases	VEB-1F	bla_{VEB}	CGACTTCCATTTCCCGATGC	642	[20]
	VEB-1R		GGACTCTGCAACAAATACGC		
	PER-1F	bla_{PER-1}	ATGAATGTCATTATAAAAGCT	927	[20]
	PER-1R		TTAATTTGGGCTTAGGG		
	CTX-M-1F	$bla_{CTX-M-1}$	GCAGCACCAGTAAAGTGATGG	591	[21]
	CTX-M-1R		GCTGGGTGAAGTAAGTGACC		
	CTX-M-825F	$bla_{CTX-M-8}$	CGCTTTGCCATGTGCAGCACC	307	[22]
	CTX-M-825R		GCTCAGTACGATCGAGCC		
	CTX-M-914F	$bla_{CTX-M-9}$	GCTGGAGAAAAGCAGCGGAG	474	[22]
	CTX-M-914R		GTAAGCTGACGCAACGTCTG		
	SHV-OS5	bla_{SHV}	TTATCTCCCTGTTAGCCA	797	[23]
	SHV-OS6		GATTTGCTGAATTCGCTC		
	TEM-A	bla_{TEM}	TAAAATTCTTGAAGACG	1074	[23]
	TEM-B		TTACCAATGCTTAATCA		
	KPC-F	bla_{KPC}	ATGTCACTGTATCGCCGTCT	893	[24]
	KPC-R		TTTTCAGAGCCTTACTGCCC		
Class B β lactamases	VIM-F	bla_{VIM}	GATGGTGTTTGGTCGCATA	390	[25]
	VIM-R		CGAATGCGCAGCACCAG		
	IMP-F	bla_{IMP}	GGAATAGAGTGGCTTAATTC	232	[26]
	IMP-R		TCGGTTTAATAAAACAACCACC		
	NDM-1-F	bla_{NDM-1}	CAATATTATGCACCCGGTCG	726	[27]
	NDM-1-R		ATCATGCTGGCCTTGGGGAA		
Class D β lactamases	OXA-10F	bla_{OXA-10}	TATCGCGTGTCTTTCGAGTA	760	[20]
	OXA-10R		TTAGCCACCAATGATGCCC		
	OXA-F	bla_{OXA-48}	GCGTGGTTAAGGATGAACAC	438	[26]
	OXA-R		CATCAAGTTCAACCCAACCG		

(www.ncbi.nlm.nih.gov/GenBank) using the BLAST program (www.ncbi.nlm.nih.gov/BLAST/).

Pulsed-field gel electrophoresis

The bacterial genetic relatedness was evaluated by Pulsed-field gel electrophoresis (PFGE). Genomic DNA was digested with *SfiI* enzyme, and DNA fragments were separated on a CHEF-DRII System (Bio-Rad, Hercules, CA, USA). A lambda ladder (Bio-Rad) was used as a DNA size marker. The band patterns were analyzed using UVIband/Map software (UVItech Ltd., Cambridge, UK) and the dendrograms were generated based on the unweighted pair group method using arithmetic averages from the Dice coefficient. Isolates that exhibited a PFGE profile with more than 90% similarity (pulsotype) were considered as closely related strains.

Results

The characteristics of these patients and antimicrobial susceptibility patterns of *P. rettgeri* isolates were summarized in Table 2. In total, eight *P. rettgeri* isolates were recovered from urine samples of eight patients admitted in a surgical intensive care unit (SICU). All patients were admitted to a SICU from hospitalization and had a urinary catheter. The median days of the SICU stay before *P. rettgeri* isolation was 21.5 days (range, 8–38 days) (Fig. 1). All patients except one (P5) were recovered and discharged during the outbreak. A patient (P5) died following *Enterococcus faecalis* bacteremia. All *P. rettgeri* isolates showed similar antibiogram with high MIC levels to various classes of antimicrobial agents tested (cefotetan, cefotaxime, ceftazidime, cefepime, azteronam, meropenem, ertapenem, ciprofloxacin, amikacin, and tigecycline). Imipenem MICs were 0.5–4 μg/mL (6/8 susceptible isolates, 1/8 intermediate isolate, and 1/8 resistant isolate) and gentamicin MICs were 8–16 μg/mL (4/8 intermediate isolates and 4/8 resistant isolates). Molecular testing revealed that all the *P. rettgeri* isolates were positive for bla_{NDM-1} and bla_{PER-1}. No amplicons were observed for the other primer pairs for bla_{VEB}, $bla_{CTX-M-1}$, $bla_{CTX-M-8}$, $bla_{CTX-M-9}$, bla_{SHV}, bla_{TEM}, bla_{KPC}, bla_{VIM}, bla_{IMP}, bla_{OXA-10}, and bla_{OXA-48}. PFGE revealed that all isolates closely related one pulsotype with > 90% similarity (Fig. 2). The eight isolates had the three kinds of dendrogram patterns.

Discussion

In the present study we reported and characterized an outbreak of bla_{NDM-1} and bla_{PER-1} carrying *P. rettgeri*. All patients were admitted to the same SICU and had a urinary catheter. *P. rettgeri* is well known to be isolated from urine of hospitalized and catheterized patients [16]. Although periods of hospitalization of our patients were not completely overlapping, PFGE revealed that all isolates were closely related. This suggests clonal cross-transmission of this strain in the SICU, and there is a possibility of transmission between patients and medical personnel by hand colonization or by environmental contamination. Infection control measures were reinforced in the SICU to include extensive environmental disinfection, active screening for carbapenemase-producing Enterobacteriaceae, and exhaustive contact isolation precautions. The outbreak did not eradicate in a short time, but the outbreak was eventually interrupted in January 2017.

Carbapenem resistance in Enterobacteriaceae has become a major public health challenge [28]. While carbapenem is a drug of choice for treatment of Enterobacteriaceae producing ESBL and plasmid-mediated AmpC cephalosporinase, production of carbapenemase in Enterobacteriaceae can be emerged. Carbapenemase gene is important due to its potential transferability to other species, by plasmids and transposons [28]. NDM-1 encoding plasmids are diverse and can also carry other antimicrobial resistance genes, including carbapenemase genes, ESBL genes, plasmid-mediated cephalosporinase genes, and aminoglycoside resistance genes [28, 29]. Among these, most ESBLs found with NDM-1 have been reported to be as CTX-M-15 type [29, 30]. Until now, this is the first report of Enterobacteriaceae co-carrying NDM-1 and PER-1 type ESBL. Although the NDM-1 enzyme is known to inactivate all β-lactams except aztreonam [6], our *P. rettgeri* isolates showed high MIC to aztreonam, possibly due to production of PER-1 type ESBL. The range of MIC to imipenem revealed 0.5–4 μg/mL. Imipenem MICs for *Providencia* spp. tend to be higher (e.g., MICs in the intermediate or resistant range) naturally. These isolates may have elevated imipenem MICs by mechanisms other than production of carbapenemases [18].

It is known that the multidrug-resistant bacteria have superior ability to survive and spread successfully in a hospital environment. In addition, the patient's risk factor is also responsible for the nosocomial transmission of multidrug-resistant bacteria. Patient's underlying disease, exposure to antimicrobial agents, and history of having invasive procedures are known as risk factors for the acquisition of carbapenem-resistant Enterobacteriaceae [28]. This outbreak persisted for 13 months, although the prompt infection control strategy was initiated after recognition of the first few cases. Because ICU admission patients often have one or more of risk factors, so it could be very difficult to eradicate once the outbreak occurs.

In conclusion, we report an alarming outbreak of high-level of multidrug-resistant *P. rettgeri* isolates co-producing NDM-1 and PER-1 β-lactamases. Infection

Table 2 Clinical characteristics of the outbreak cases and antimicrobial susceptibility profiles of *Providencia rettgeri* isolates

Patient ID	P1	P2	P3	P4	P5	P6	P7	P8
Isolate no.	KN756	KN762	KN764	KN774	KN779	KN784	KN803	KN804
Sex/age (year)	M/63	M/50	M/52	M/66	F/75	M/81	F/40	M/53
Diagnosis	Brain hemorrhage	Deep neck infection	Central nervous system infection	Bladder cancer	Pneumonia	Pneumonia	Brain hemorrhage	Brain hemorrhage
Comorbidities	–	Diabetes mellitus	–	–	Cerebral infarction	Diabetes mellitus	–	–
Outcome	Survival	Survival	Survival	Survival	Death	Survival	Survival	Survival
Hospital admission date	18-Dec-15	05-Apr-16	28-Apr-16	01-Jul-16	28-Jul-16	14-Aug-16	16-Dec-16	19-Dec-16
P. rettgeri collection date	11-Jan-16	09-May-16	19-May-16	08-Aug-16	19-Aug-16	22-Aug-16	30-Dec-16	05-Jan-17
Antimicrobial agents used before *P. rettgeri* isolation (days)	Colistin (13), piperacillin-tazobactam (8), teicoplanin (11)	Colistin (21), metronidazole (10), piperacillin-tazobactam (10), ampicillin-sulbactam (3), teicoplanin (20), netilmicin (5), levofloxacin (9)	Colistin (13), piperacillin-tazobactam (3), vancomycin (8), teicoplanin (13), meropenem (7)	Ceftriaxone (6), tigecycline (4), doripenem (7), piperacillin-tazobactam (18), flomoxef (3), teicoplanin (5)	Metronidazole (10), moxifloxacin (6), piperacillin-tazobactam (2), teicoplanin (2)	Piperacillin-tazobactam (5), ampicillin-sulbactam (3)	Ceftriaxone (3)	Ceftriaxone (8)
MIC (μg/mL)								
Cefotetan	> 256	> 256	> 256	> 256	> 256	> 256	> 256	> 256
Cefotaxime	> 32	> 32	> 32	> 32	> 32	> 32	> 32	> 32
Ceftazidime	> 256	> 256	> 256	> 256	> 256	> 256	> 256	> 256
Cefepime	> 256	> 256	> 256	> 256	> 256	> 256	> 256	> 256
Aztreonam	> 256	> 256	> 256	> 256	> 256	> 256	> 256	> 256
Imipenem	0.5	0.5	2	4	0.5	1	0.5	0.5
Meropenem	> 32	> 32	> 32	> 32	> 32	> 32	> 32	> 32
Ertapenem	> 32	> 32	> 32	> 32	> 32	> 32	> 32	> 32
Ciprofloxacin	> 32	> 32	> 32	> 32	> 32	> 32	> 32	> 32
Amikacin	> 256	> 256	> 256	> 256	> 256	> 256	> 256	> 256
Gentamicin	8	16	16	16	8	16	8	8
Tigecycline	4	4	4	8	4	8	8	8
Colistin	2	2	8	2	2	64	4	4

MIC minimum inhibitory concentration

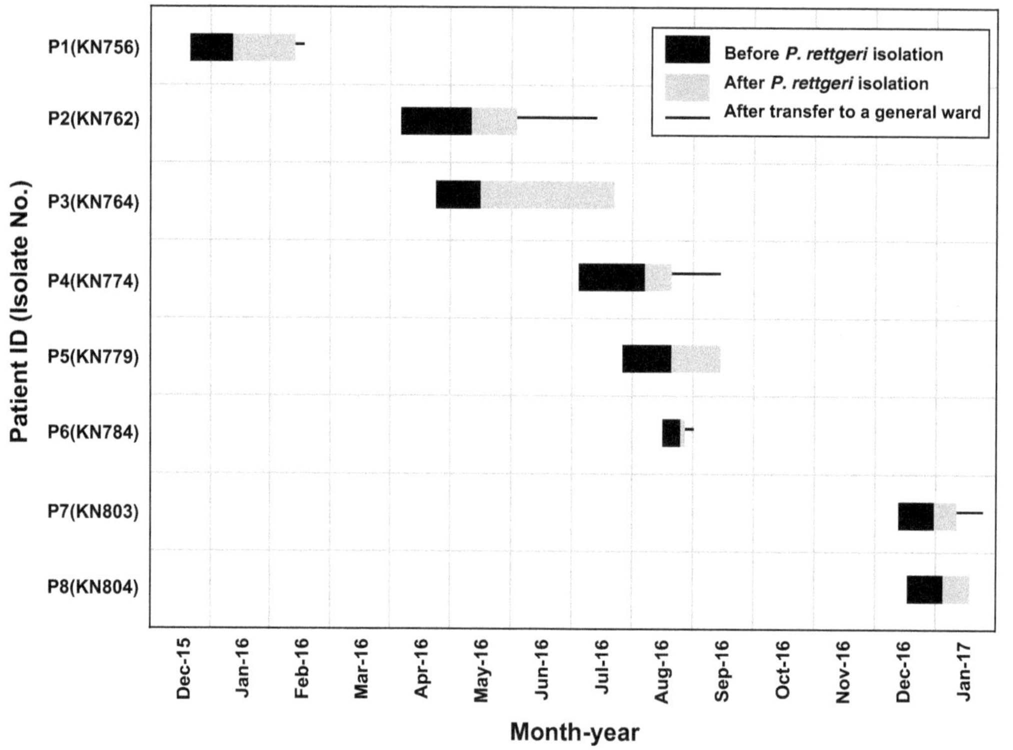

Fig. 1 Time course of the outbreak by multidrug-resistant *Providencia rettgeri*. Black bars indicate the pre-infection period and gray bars the post-infection period in the surgical intensive care unit. Solid lines indicate the period during patients was hospitalized in a general ward

prevention and control efforts should be continuously made to prevent nosocomial transmission of these threatening bacteria.

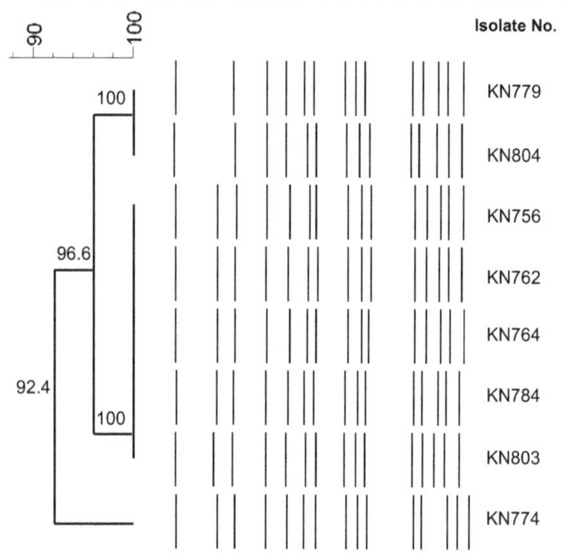

Fig. 2 Pulsed-field gel electrophoresis patterns of *Providencia rettgeri* clinical isolate co-producing NDM-1 and PER-1. All eight isolates from the outbreak were closely related strains

Author's contributions

SS performed the experiment, data analysis, and wrote the manuscript. SHJ, HL, JSH, and MJP performed the experiment and gave advice. WS designed study, data analysis, and critically reviewed and edited the manuscript. All authors read and approved the final manuscript.

Author details

[1] Department of Laboratory Medicine, Hallym University College of Medicine, Seoul, South Korea. [2] Department of Laboratory Medicine and Research Institute for Antimicrobial Resistance, Yonsei University College of Medicine, Seoul, South Korea.

Acknowledgements

Not applicable.

Competing interests

The authors declare that they have no competing interests.

Funding

This study has been funded by grant from the Korean Health Technology R&D Project, Ministry of Health & Welfare, Republic of Korea (HI12C0756).

References

1. O'Hara CM, Brenner FW, Miller JM. Classification, identification, and clinical significance of Proteus, Providencia, and Morganella. Clin Microbiol Rev. 2000;13(4):534–46.
2. Magiorakos AP, Srinivasan A, Carey RB, Carmeli Y, Falagas ME, Giske CG, Harbarth S, Hindler JF, Kahlmeter G, Olsson-Liljequist B, et al. Multidrug-

resistant, extensively drug-resistant and pandrug-resistant bacteria: an international expert proposal for interim standard definitions for acquired resistance. Clin Microbiol Infect. 2012;18(3):268–81.

3. Mataseje LF, Boyd DA, Lefebvre B, Bryce E, Embree J, Gravel D, Katz K, Kibsey P, Kuhn M, Langley J, et al. Complete sequences of a novel blaNDM-1-harbouring plasmid from *Providencia rettgeri* and an FII-type plasmid from *Klebsiella pneumoniae* identified in Canada. J Antimicrob Chemother. 2014;69(3):637–42.
4. Tada T, Miyoshi-Akiyama T, Dahal RK, Sah MK, Ohara H, Shimada K, Kirikae T, Pokhrel BM. NDM-1 Metallo-beta-Lactamase and ArmA 16S rRNA methylase producing *Providencia rettgeri* clinical isolates in Nepal. BMC Infect Dis. 2014;14:56.
5. Nordmann P, Poirel L. Emerging carbapenemases in Gram-negative aerobes. Clin Microbiol Infect. 2002;8(6):321–31.
6. Yong D, Toleman MA, Giske CG, Cho HS, Sundman K, Lee K, Walsh TR. Characterization of a new metallo-beta-lactamase gene, bla(NDM-1), and a novel erythromycin esterase gene carried on a unique genetic structure in *Klebsiella pneumoniae* sequence type 14 from India. Antimicrob Agents Chemother. 2009;53(12):5046–54.
7. Gefen-Halevi S, Hindiyeh MY, Ben-David D, Smollan G, Gal-Mor O, Azar R, Castanheira M, Belausov N, Rahav G, Tal I, et al. Isolation of genetically unrelated bla(NDM-1)-positive *Providencia rettgeri* strains in Israel. J Clin Microbiol. 2013;51(5):1642–3.
8. Barrios H, Garza-Ramos U, Reyna-Flores F, Sanchez-Perez A, Rojas-Moreno T, Garza-Gonzalez E, Llaca-Diaz JM, Camacho-Ortiz A, Guzman-Lopez S, Silva-Sanchez J. Isolation of carbapenem-resistant NDM-1-positive *Providencia rettgeri* in Mexico. J Antimicrob Chemother. 2013;68(8):1934–6.
9. Carvalho-Assef AP, Pereira PS, Albano RM, Beriao GC, Chagas TP, Timm LN, Da Silva RC, Falci DR, Asensi MD. Isolation of NDM-producing *Providencia rettgeri* in Brazil. J Antimicrob Chemother. 2013;68(12):2956–7.
10. Pasteran F, Meo A, Gomez S, Derdoy L, Albronoz E, Faccone D, Guerriero L, Archuby D, Tarzia A, Lopez M, et al. Emergence of genetically related NDM-1-producing *Providencia rettgeri* strains in Argentina. J Global Antimicrob Resist. 2014;2(4):344–5.
11. Zurita J, Parra H, Gestal MC, McDermott J, Barba P. First case of NDM-1-producing *Providencia rettgeri* in Ecuador. J Global Antimicrob Resist. 2015;3(4):302–3.
12. Carmo Junior NV, Filho HF, Gomes ECDA, Calvalcante AJ, Garcia Dde O, Furtado JJ. First report of a NDM-producing *Providencia rettgeri* strain in the state of Sao Paulo. Braz J Infect Dis. 2015;19(6):675–6.
13. Bocanegra-Ibarias P, Garza-Gonzalez E, Morfin-Otero R, Barrios H, Villarreal-Trevino L, Rodriguez-Noriega E, Garza-Ramos U, Petersen-Morfin S, Silva-Sanchez J. Molecular and microbiological report of a hospital outbreak of NDM-1-carrying Enterobacteriaceae in Mexico. PLoS ONE. 2017;12(6):e0179651.
14. Nordmann P, Ronco E, Naas T, Duport C, Michel-Briand Y, Labia R. Characterization of a novel extended-spectrum beta-lactamase from Pseudomonas aeruginosa. Antimicrob Agents Chemother. 1993;37(5):962–9.
15. Bradford PA. Extended-spectrum β-lactamases in the 21st century: characterization, epidemiology, and detection of this important resistance threat. Clin Microbiol Rev. 2001;14(4):933–51 **(table of contents)**.
16. Bahar G, Erac B, Mert A, Gulay Z. PER-1 production in a urinary isolate of *Providencia rettgeri*. J Chemother. 2004;16(4):343–6.
17. Yong D, Shin JH, Kim S, Lim Y, Yum JH, Lee K, Chong Y, Bauernfeind A. High prevalence of PER-1 extended-spectrum beta-lactamase-producing *Acinetobacter* spp. in Korea. Antimicrob Agents Chemother. 2003;47(5):1749–51.
18. CLSI. Performance standards for antimicrobial susceptibility testing; twenty-fifth informational supplement. Wayne: CLSI Document M100-S25, Clinical and Laboratory Standards Institute; 2015.
19. Testing ECoAS. Breakpoint tables for interpretation of MICs and zone diameters, version 5.0. Växjö: European Committee on Antimicrobial Susceptibility Testing; 2015.
20. Mirsalehian A, Feizabadi M, Nakhjavani FA, Jabalameli F, Goli H, Kalantari N. Detection of VEB-1, OXA-10 and PER-1 genotypes in extended-spectrum beta-lactamase-producing *Pseudomonas aeruginosa* strains isolated from burn patients. Burns. 2010;36(1):70–4.
21. Abdalhamid B, Pitout JD, Moland ES, Hanson ND. Community-onset disease caused by *Citrobacter freundii* producing a novel CTX-M beta-lactamase, CTX-M-30, in Canada. Antimicrob Agents Chemother. 2004;48(11):4435–7.
22. Pitout JD, Hossain A, Hanson ND. Phenotypic and molecular detection of CTX-M-β-lactamases produced by *Escherichia coli* and *Klebsiella* spp. J Clin Microbiol. 2004;42(12):5715–21.
23. De Champs C, Sirot D, Chanal C, Bonnet R, Sirot J. A 1998 survey of extended-spectrum beta-lactamases in Enterobacteriaceae in France. The French Study Group. Antimicrob Agents Chemother. 2000;44(11):3177–9.
24. Schechner V, Straus-Robinson K, Schwartz D, Pfeffer I, Tarabeia J, Moskovich R, Chmelnitsky I, Schwaber MJ, Carmeli Y, Navon-Venezia S. Evaluation of PCR-based testing for surveillance of KPC-producing carbapenem-resistant members of the Enterobacteriaceae family. J Clin Microbiol. 2009;47(10):3261–5.
25. Österblad M, Kirveskari J, Hakanen AJ, Tissari P, Vaara M, Jalava J. Carbapenemase-producing Enterobacteriaceae in Finland: the first years (2008–11). J Antimicrob Chemother. 2012;67(12):2860–4.
26. Poirel L, Walsh TR, Cuvillier V, Nordmann P. Multiplex PCR for detection of acquired carbapenemase genes. Diagn Microbiol Infect Dis. 2011;70(1):119–23.
27. Samuelsen O, Thilesen CM, Heggelund L, Vada AN, Kummel A, Sundsfjord A. Identification of NDM-1-producing Enterobacteriaceae in Norway. J Antimicrob Chemother. 2011;66(3):670–2.
28. Nordmann P, Naas T, Poirel L. Global spread of Carbapenemase-producing Enterobacteriaceae. Emerg Infect Dis. 2011;17(10):1791–8.
29. Kumarasamy KK, Toleman MA, Walsh TR, Bagaria J, Butt F, Balakrishnan R, Chaudhary U, Doumith M, Giske CG, Irfan S, et al. Emergence of a new antibiotic resistance mechanism in India, Pakistan, and the UK: a molecular, biological, and epidemiological study. Lancet Infect Dis. 2010;10(9):597–602.
30. Nordmann P, Poirel L, Toleman MA, Walsh TR. Does broad-spectrum β-lactam resistance due to NDM-1 herald the end of the antibiotic era for treatment of infections caused by Gram-negative bacteria? J Antimicrob Chemother. 2011;66(4):689–92.

24

Comparative and molecular analysis of MRSA isolates from infection sites and carrier colonization sites

Khaled R. Alkharsah[1,2*], Suriya Rehman[1], Fatimah Alkhamis[1], Amani Alnimr[2], Asim Diab[2] and Amein K. Al-Ali[3]

Abstract

Background: Methicillin resistant *Staphylococcus aureus* (MRSA) constitutes a major global health concern causing hospital and community acquired infections. A wide diversity of MRSA genotypes are circulating in geographically related regions. Therefore understanding the molecular epidemiology of MRSA is fundamental to design control and clearance measures.

Methods: A total of 106 MRSA isolates from infection (51) and carrier colonization sites (55) are characterized genetically based on SCCmec and MLST genotyping methods in addition to detection of PVL, TSST-1 and enterotoxins.

Results: Sccmec-IV was the most frequently detected genotype (77.3%) followed by genotype V (13.2%) and III (9.4%). SCCmec-IVa was more prevalent among the carrier group (p value 0.002). CC80 was the most commonly identified clonal complex (CC). CC6 and CC22 were significantly more prevalent among the carrier group (p value 0.02 and 0.01, respectively). PVL was highly prevalent among the isolates (58.5%). PVL was detected in 70.6% of isolates from infection sites and 47.3% of isolates from carriers. All strains were sensitive to vancomycin, however, MRSA strains isolated from infection sites had significantly higher MICs compared to strains isolated from carrier colonization sites (p value 0.021). Five new sequence types mainly from the carrier group were identified and described in the study.

Conclusions: MRSA population is genetically very diverse among carriers and infected individuals. With SCCmec type IV being most prevalent, this suggests a community origin of most MRSA strains. Therefore very well designed surveillance and clearance strategies should be prepared to prevent emergence and control spread of MRSA in the community.

Keywords: MRSA, SCCmec, MLST, Carrier, Infection, Saudi Arabia, CA-MRSA, HA-MRSA

Background

Methicillin-resistant *Staphylococcus aureus* (MRSA) causes a wide variety of infections including life threatening infections. Consequently, MRSA is a global concern and it is one of the biggest threats in a health care facility [1]. The emergence of *S. aureus* strains resistant to methicillin and other categories of β-lactam antimicrobials was reported as early as 1960s and was later attributed to the expression of a protein that binds penicillin with low affinity (PBP2a) [2]. PBP2a is encoded by *mecA* gene (a small 2007 bp), a mobile extrinsic genetic element that is carried on a genomic island called staphylococcal cassette chromosome mec (SCCmec) [3]. According to the International Working Group on the Classification of Staphylococcal Cassette Chromosome Elements (IWG-SCC), eleven genotypes of MRSA have been identified based on the type of SCCmec [4]. SCCmec types I-III are generally detected in hospital acquired MRSA (HA-MRSA), which are the strains reported to cause hospital associated infections and outbreaks [5]. Other SCCmec types (IV, V or VII) are more frequently detected in community acquired MRSA (CA-MRSA), which cause infections in otherwise healthy individuals who had not been previously hospitalized [5]. However, CA-MRSA strains

*Correspondence: kalkharsah@iau.edu.sa
[2] Department of Microbiology, College of Medicine, Imam Abdulrahman Bin Faisal University (IAU), P.O. Box 1982, Dammam 31441, Saudi Arabia
Full list of author information is available at the end of the article

are increasingly reported in hospitals causing health-care associated infections [6]. Data from clinical and epidemiologic studies provide convincing indication that attribute the increased virulence of CA-MRSA over the HA-MRSA to the *lukF-PV* and *lukS-PV* (PVL) genes, which make the Panton–Valentine leukocidin (PVL) [7]. PVL causes cell lysis and is considered as a genetic symbol for CA-MRSA strains [8], however, PVL positive HA-MRSA has been reported in different studies [7].

MRSA strains could be also grouped into biologically meaningful groups called clonal complexes (CC) based on sequencing fragments from seven housekeeping genes in a method called multi locus sequence typing (MLST) [9]. CC showed geographically distinct distribution. For example, sequence types (ST) such as ST5 and ST8, belonging to CC5 and CC8 respectively, are commonly found in the United States and Japan, whereas strains belonging to the clonal complexes CC22 are more commonly found in Europe and Australia [10]. The ST80 (CC80) strain has been detected widely in the Middle East [11].

Hospitalization appears to present a patient with a major risk of infection with *S. aureus*. However, studies have shown that about one-fifth to one-third of the population carry *S. aureus* in their nose and about 2–3% of people carry MRSA [12]. In health care workers, this percentage increases to approximately 5% [13]. *S. aureus* carriers are another major risk factor and source of infection. The transmission of MRSA in hospitals and community needs to be better understood to determine the prevalence and peculiarity of circulating MRSA. Studies conducted in European hospitals on MRSA carriers have shown large variations in genetic diversity and in the prevalence of MRSA strains [14, 15]. Screening and identification of hospitalized MRSA carriers will result in a more effective control of MRSA.

In the current study, we have characterized MRSA strains isolated from carriers or infected individuals from the Eastern Province of Saudi Arabia and compared their genotypes and antibiotic susceptibility patterns. A better understanding of the circulating MRSA strains will result in a greater control and management of the disease.

Methods

Study design and bacterial isolates

A cross-sectional study was conducted from January 2010 to September 2011 at King Fahd hospital of the University (KFHU) in Al-Khobar in the Eastern Province of Saudi Arabia. A total of 106 MRSA isolates were collected from the microbiology laboratory of the hospital during the period of the study. All of these isolates were identified using standard microbiology procedures were confirmed using Vitek II (biomerieux, France). The isolates were confirmed for their resistance to oxacillin and cefoxitin using the disc diffusion method as described below. Clinical and demographic data were collected from patients' medical records.

Ethical approval for the study was obtained from the Institutional Review Board at the University of Dammam (IRB-2013-08-023).

Antimicrobial susceptibility testing

Twenty-four antibiotics were used in disc diffusion method on Mueller–Hinton agar (Oxoid, Hampshire, England) according to the Clinical Laboratory Standard Institute [16]. All antibiotic discs were purchased from Oxoid (Oxoid, Hampshire, England). Vancomycin susceptibility testing was performed by the E test strips (AB Biodisk, Sweden) [16].

Molecular genotyping

Extraction of DNA

Bacterial DNA was extracted using Qiagen DNA extraction kit (Qiagen, Hilden, Germany) according to the manufacturer's instructions. Extracted DNA was stored at − 80 °C till the time of analysis.

Detection of mecA and pvl genes

A multiplex PCR previously developed by Al-Talib et al. [17] was used to identify methicillin-resistant *Staphylococcus* by detecting the *mecA* gene. Additionally this multiplex PCR detects the presence of *lukS* gene of the Panton–Valentine leukocidin. To identify the genus *Staphylococcus* and to discriminate *S. aureus* from coagulase negative staphylococci, the primer-cocktail comprised primers targeting the 16S rRNA gene and the *femA* gene, respectively [17]. The internal control primers, originally included in Al-Talib protocol, were not included in our master mix. A laboratory isolate previously known to be positive for *mecA* and *PVL* genes was used as positive control. A water negative control was used with each run.

Detection of other staphylococcal virulence toxins

Two sets of primers were used in two multiplex PCR reactions (A and B) for detection of the staphylococcal enterotoxins genes A to E, toxic shock syndrome toxin 1 (tsst-1), and exfoliative toxins A and B according to Mehrotra et al. [18].

SCCmec typing

We followed a multiplex PCR protocol developed by Ghaznavi-Rad et al. for SCCmec genotyping [19]. The method uses nine pairs of primers to detect the SCCmec genotypes (I–III, IVa–IVd, IVh, and V) in addition to primers for *S. aureus* identification and detection of methicillin resistance *mecA* gene [19]. The PCR program was followed as described by Ghaznavi-Rad et al. [19]. The PCR product was run on 1.8% metaphor agarose (Lonza, Rockland, USA) at 25 V overnight in 0.5 × TBE buffer for good separation and size-based discrimination of the DNA bands.

MLST genotyping and sequence analysis

The multi locus sequence typing (MLST) protocol for *S. aureus* was followed according to the instructions on the MLST.net website (http://saureus.beta.mlst.net/). The allelic profile of each isolate was obtained and compared to the database to obtain the sequence type (ST). eBurst algorithm (http://saureus.beta.mlst.net/#eBURST) was used to categorize MLST into groups and clonal complexes (CC).

Data analysis

Statistical analysis was performed using SPSS version 23 and OpenEpi software. Phylogenetic tree of the STs was performed by eBurst.

Results

The 106 MRSA isolates included in this study were obtained from 39 females (36.8%) and 67 males (63.2%) with an average age of 27.1 years (Table 1). Fifty-one strains (48.1%) were isolated from infection sites, including wound (16%), abscess (14.2%), skin and tissue infections (5.7%), and lower respiratory tract infections (4.7%). MRSA strains isolated from ear, eye and throat infections were less frequent (1.9% each). One strain was isolated from cerebrospinal fluid (0.94%) and one from a patient with a urinary tract infection (0.94%). Fifty-five strains (51.9%) were isolated from colonization sites such as nose (40.6%), throat (6.6%), axilla (2.8%) and groin (1.9%). MRSA strains isolated from colonization sites were isolated from Patients hospitalized for diseases not related to MRSA infection. The detection of MRSA in these patients was performed as a part of infection control policy which placed patients suspected or confirmed to be MRSA positive under contact isolation until decolonization is proven after successful prophylactic nasal mupirocin ointment and chlorhexidine body wash therapy. There was no statistically significant correlation between MRSA isolation from infection or colonization sites on the basis of age, duration of hospitalization, ICU admission, or outcome of treatment (Table 1).

All MRSA isolates were positive for *mecA*, *femA*, and *sa442* genes. The most frequently detected SCCmec genotype was SCCmec-IV (77.3%) followed by SCCmec-V (13.2%), and III (9.4%). Further subtyping of SCCmec-IV revealed that subtypes IVa and IVc are the only subtypes prevalent among the isolates (41.5 and 58.5%, respectively) (Table 2). SCCmec-IVa genotype was more frequently found in MRSA isolated from the carriers compared to infected individuals (p value 0.002, OR 3.84) (Table 2).

MLST genotyping of the MRSA isolates showed that ST80 is the most frequently encountered genotype in our study (34.9%) followed by ST22 (10.4%) (Table 2 and

Table 1 Frequency of MRSA isolates from carrier colonization sites and infection sites with demographic and clinical data

	Carrier (n = 55)	Infection (n = 51)	p value	OR (95% CI)
Gender				
Male	32	35	0.27	0.64 (0.28–1.42)
Female	23	16		
Age (years)[a]				
≤ 30	34	32	0.9	0.96 (0.43–2.12)
> 30	20	18		
ICU admission[b]				
Yes	51	48	0.67	0.53 (0.02–7.21)
No	2	1		
Duration of hospitalization (days)				
≤ 7	24	20	0.65	1.12 (0.55–2.63)
> 7	31	31		
Treatment outcome[c]				
Discharged rescreened negative	26	27	0.36	0.58 (0.17–1.84)
Discharged rescreened positive	10	6		

[a] One sample from each group has no data

[b] Two samples from each group have no data

[c] 37 patients discharged without further screen

Table 2 Molecular characterization of MRSA isolates from infection sites and carrier colonization sites

	Genotype	Carrier (55)	Infection (51)	p value	OR (95% CI)
SCCmec	III	3	7	0.17	0.37 (0.07–1.48)
	IVa	25	9	0.002	3.84 (1.59–9.81)
	IVc	21	27	0.13	0.55 (0.25–1.20)
	V	6	8	0.49	0.66 (0.20–2.1)
MLST[a]	CC1 (ST1, ST772)	5	8	0.30	0.53 (0.15–1.76)
	CC5 (ST5, ST149)	4	5	0.64	0.71 (0.16–2.96)
	CC6 (ST6)	6	0	0.02	Undefined
	CC8 (ST8,ST239, ST241)	3	8	0.091	0.31 (0.06–1.19)
	CC22 (ST22)	10	1	0.01	10.7 (1.70–242)
	CC30 (ST30)	0	2	0.23	Undefined
	CC45 (ST46)	2	0	0.27	Undefined
	CC80 (ST80,ST1440)[b]	21	23	0.43	0.73 (0.33–1.59)
	CC88 (ST88)	3	2	0.76	1.38 (0.20–12)
	CC97 (ST97)	1	1	0.95	0.91 (0.02–36.08)
PVL	Pos	26	36	0.02	0.38 (0.17–0.84)
	Neg	29	15		
sea	Pos	16	22	0.14	0.54 (0.24–1.22)
	Neg	39	29		
seb	Pos	7	1	0.04	7.18 (1.06–168.6)
	Neg	48	50		
sec	Pos	0	0	NA	NA
	Neg	55	51		
sed	Pos	3	0	NA	NA
	Neg	52	51		
see	Pos	11	6	0.26	1.86 (0.63–5.88)
	Neg	44	45		
eta	Pos	0	0	NA	NA
	Neg	55	51		
etb	Pos	0	0	NA	NA
	Neg	55	53		
tst	Pos	8	7	0.91	1.07 (0.35–3.34)
	Neg	47	44		
Average vancomycin MIC		0.81	1.26	0.021[$]	(0.35–0.55)

sea, seb, sec, sed, and see staphylococcal enterotoxin A, B, C, D, and E

eta and etb exfoliative toxin A and B

tst toxic shock toxin

[a] One of the isolates in infection group was a singleton in eBurst and could not be allocated to any CC

[b] Includes also the 4 new STs from 6 samples according to eBurst

[$] p value (two-tailed) from Hartley's f test for equality of variance

Fig. 1). ST6 and ST22 were more frequently detected in the carrier group than the infection group (p value = 0.02 and 0.01, respectively) (Table 2). Other MLST genotypes, such as ST30, ST1930, ST239 and ST241 were more frequently detected among the infected patients but were statistically not significant (Table 2).

Toxic shock syndrome toxin 1 (TSST-1) was present in 14.2% of the isolates. Staphylococcal enterotoxin A (SEA) was the most frequently detected enterotoxin (35.8%) (Table 2). SEB was significantly more prevalent among the carrier group compared to the infection group (p value 0.04) (Table 2).

Panton-Valentine leucocidin (PVL) was positive in 58.5% (62/106) of the total MRSA isolates. It was more frequently detected in the infection group of MRSA isolates (70.6%) compared to the carrier group isolates (47.3%) (p value 0.02, Table 2). However, when analyzing the prevalence of PVL among the MRSA isolates from

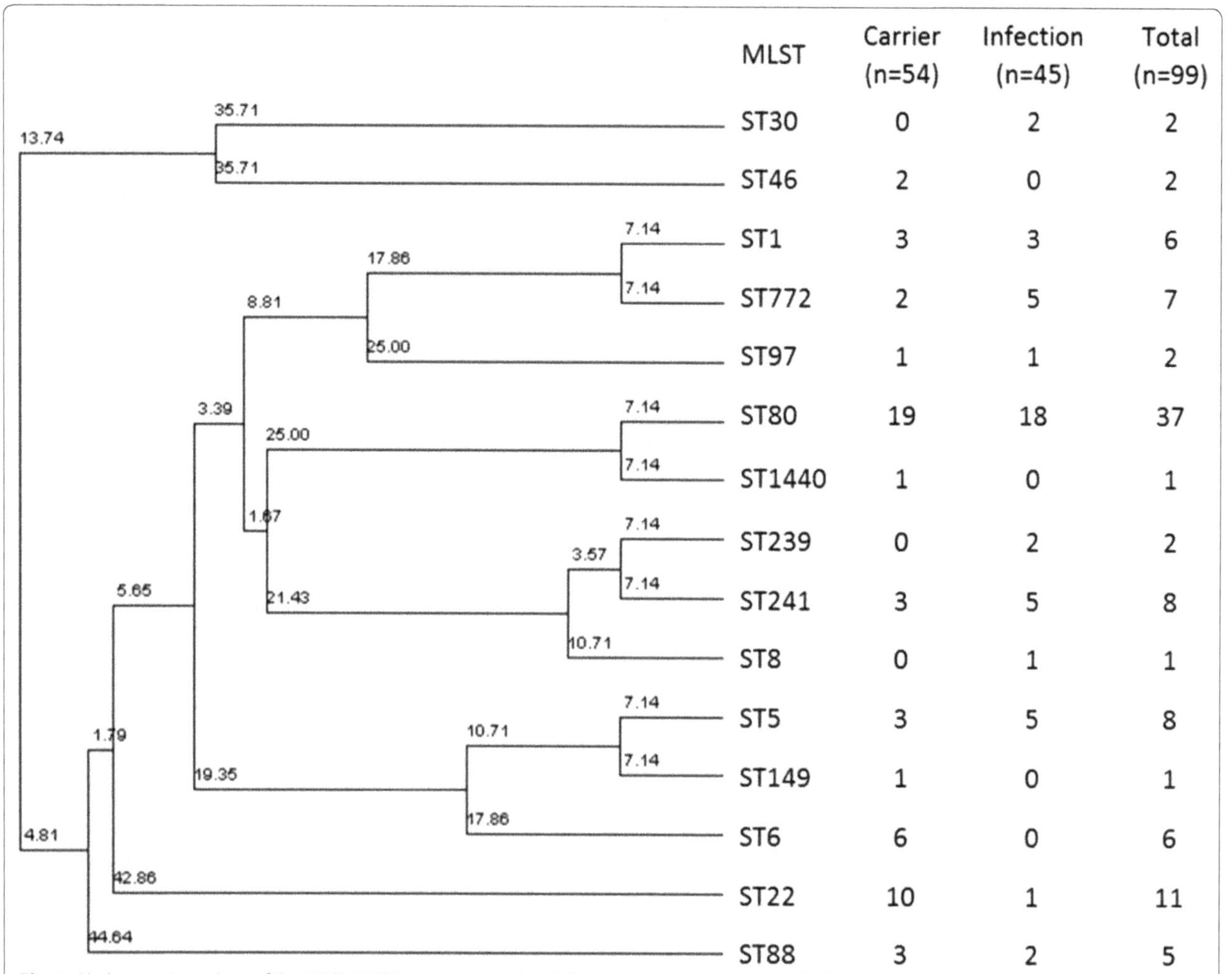

Fig. 1 Phylogenetic analysis of the MRSA MLST-genotypes and their frequency among carrier and infection groups. 7 new types are not included in the analysis

Table 3 Prevalence of PVL among the MRSA isolates from infection sites

	CA-MRSA[a] (n = 32)	HA-MRSA[a] (n = 19)	p value	OR (95% CI)
PVL				
Pos	24	12	0.4	1.7 (0.49–6.1)
Neg	8	7		

[a] According to our hospital infection control policy, the CDC classification of MRSA was used to classify MRSA as CA or HA

infection sites only based on whether these isolates are CA or HA-MRSA, PVL was more frequently detected in the CA-MRSA isolates but this difference was not statistically significant (Table 3).

Clonal complex 80 (CC80) was the most frequent clonal complex detected in the study (41.51%) (Table 4) followed by CC1 (12.26%), CC8 and CC22 (10.38% each), CC5 (8.49%), CC6 (5.66%), CC88 (4.71%). CC30, CC45, and CC97 were the least frequent isolates in the study (1.89% each) (Table 4). One new isolate was not possible to classify into any of the clonal complexes (0.94%) and seem to constitute singleton. Most of the clonal complexes harbored SCCmec type IV (IVa or IVc). SCCmec in ST239 and ST241 (CC8) was of type III only (Table 4).

All MRSA isolates were sensitive to vancomycin, however, MRSA strains isolated from infection sites had significantly higher minimum inhibitory concentrations (MIC) compared to strains isolated from carrier colonization sites (p value 0.021) (Table 2). There was no other significant difference in the antibiotic susceptibility pattern between MRSA isolates from infection sites and carrier colonization sites (Table 5). PVL was not associated with any antibiotic susceptibility pattern.

Table 4 Affiliation of MRSA isolates MLST, SCCmec, PVL, and TST to clonal complexes

CC	MLST	SCCmec	PVL	TST	Carrier	Infection	Total
CC1	ST1	IVa	Neg	Neg	3	2	5
		IVc	Pos	Neg	0	1	1
	ST772	IVa	Pos	Neg	0	1	1
		V	Pos	Neg	2	4	6
CC5	ST5	IVc	Neg	Pos	0	2	2
			Pos	Neg	1	1	2
		V	Neg	Neg	2	0	2
			Pos	Neg	0	2	2
	ST149	IVa	Neg	Neg	1	0	1
CC6	ST6	IVa	Neg	Neg	6	0	6
CC8	ST8	IVa	Pos	Neg	0	1	1
	ST239	III	Neg	Neg	0	2	2
	ST241	III	Neg	Neg	3	5	8
CC22	ST22	IVa	Neg	Pos	7	1	8
			Pos	Neg	1	0	1
		IVc	Pos	Neg	2	0	2
CC30	ST30	IVa	Pos	Pos	0	1	1
		IVc	Pos	Neg	0	1	1
CC45	ST46	IVc	Neg	Neg	2	0	2
CC80	ST80	IVa	Neg	Neg	3	0	3
			Pos	Neg	1	0	1
		IVc	Neg	Neg	1	0	1
			Pos	Pos	0	2	2
			Pos	Neg	13	15	28
		V	Pos	Neg	1	1	2
	ST1440	IVc	Pos	Neg	1	0	1
CC88	ST88	IVa	Neg	Neg	0	1	1
			Pos	Pos	1	0	1
			Pos	Neg	2	1	3
CC97	ST97	V	Neg	Neg	1	1	2

Five new MLST alleles from seven samples were identified in this study (Table 6). The isolates were obtained from scalp abscess, endotracheal aspirate, breast abscess, skin swab (cellulitis), urine, wound swab and one sample from nasal swab (Table 6). These alleles produced new sequence types (STs) that have not been previously described in the MLST database. All except one were PVL positive and harbored the SCCmec-IV (Table 6).

Discussion

Extensive knowledge of the circulating MRSA strains is an important prerequisite for control and surveillance measures. Little is known about the genetic diversity of MRSA in the Middle East and the Gulf area. The Arabian Gulf countries attract a wide range of working manpower from different countries, which in turn enriches the microbial diversity in these countries. In the current study we characterized the MRSA isolates from the Eastern Province in Saudi Arabia and compared the molecular types of these isolates from infection sites and from carrier colonization sites.

We did not find difference between the two groups regarding duration of hospitalization. Other studies have reported that MRSA infection prolongs the duration of hospitalization [20]. However, the type of infections in our study comprises mainly skin infections (abscess and wound) which do not necessarily require hospitalization. Interestingly, we found some molecular types confined to either the carrier or infection sites.

The most frequently detected SCCmec was type IV (IVa and IVc), which is in line with a previous study from the same region [21]. Type IV SCCmec is typically detected in MRSA isolates from samples outside hospitals [4, 5]. In our study SCCmec type IV strains were equally detected in carriers and from infection sites (Table 2). SCCmec subtype IVa was significantly associated with strains

Table 5 Frequency of antibiotic resistance among the isolated strains

Antibiotic	Carrier (n = 55)	Infection (n = 51)	p value	Odds ratio (CI 95%)
Amikacin	7 (12.7%)	10 (19.6%)	0.35	0.60 (0.20–1.74)
Azithromycin	26 (47.3%)	27 (52.9%)	0.57	0.80 (0.37–1.72)
Cefoxitin	55 (100%)	51 (100%)	NA	NA
Chloramphenicol	53 (96.4%)	49 (96.1%)	0.94	1.08 (0.11–10.71)
Ciprofloxacin	27 (49.1%)	31 (60.8%)	0.24	0.62 (0.29–1.36)
Clindamycin	3 (5.5%)	5 (0.1%)	0.43	0.53 (0.10–2.44)
Doxycycline	21 (38.2%)	19 (37.3%)	0.92	1.04 (0.47–2.3)
Erythromycin	43 (78.2%)	40 (78.4%)	0.98	0.99 (0.38–2.52)
Fosfomycin	3 (5.5%)	1 (0.02%)	0.41	2.86 (0.29–77.36)
Fusidic acid	55 (100%)	51 (100%)	NA	NA
Gentamycin	5 (9.1%)	10 (19.6%)	0.13	0.41 (0.12–1.30)
Kanamycin	38 (69.1%)	41 (80.4%)	0.19	0.55 (0.22–1.34)
Levofloxacin	8 (14.5%)	10 (19.6%)	0.50	0.70 (0.24–1.97)
Linezolid	0 (0%)	0 (0%)	NA	NA
Oflоxcacin	7 (12.7%)	9 (17.6%)	0.50	0.68 (0.22–2.03)
Oxacillin	55 (100%)	51 (100%)	NA	NA
Vancomycin	0 (0%)	0 (0%)	NA	NA
Quinu_Dalfo	9 (16.4%)	5 (0.1%)	0.34	1.79 (0.56–6.31)
Rifampicin	2 (3.6%)	1 (0.02%)	0.66	1.88 (0.14–56.7)
Sulphamethoxazol	3 (5.5%)	2 (0.04%)	0.74	1.41 (0.20–12.27)
Teicoplanin	53 (96.4%)	50 (98%)	0.66	0.53 (0.02–7.19)
Tetracycline	36 (65.5%)	36 (70.6%)	0.58	0.79 (0.34–1.81)
Tigecycline	53 (96.4%)	46 (90.2%)	0.23	2.85 (0.54–22.1)
Tobramycin	4 (7.3%)	7 (13.7%)	0.30	0.50 (0.12–1.83)

Table 6 Characteristics of the new ST alleles found in the study

MLST genes							CC	SSCmec	PVL	Type of sample
arcC	*aroE*	*glpF*	*gmk*	*pta*	*tpi*	*yqil*				
1	3	1	14	4	51	10	80	IVc	Pos	Scalp abscess
1	3	1	14	New	51	10	80	IVc	Pos	Endotracheal aspirate
1	New	1	14	11	51	10	80	IVc	Pos	Nasal swab
1	New	1	14	11	51	10	80	IVc	Pos	Breast abscess
1	New	1	14	11	51	10	80	IVc	Pos	Skin swab (cellulitis)
3	New	1	1	4	4	3	ND	IVa	Neg	Urine
1	3	1	14	11	New	10	80	IVc	Pos	Wound swab

ND not determined, *Pos* positive, *Neg* negative

isolated from carrier colonization sites. Sccmec type V, which is commonly associated with CA-MRSA infections [5], was equally detected in isolates from carriers and infection sites in our study. Similarly the sequence types ST6 and ST22 (except for one case) were only detected in MRSA isolates from carriers in our study.

PVL was highly prevalent among our isolates (56.5%), an observation which has been reported elsewhere [21, 22]. However, other studies reported a lower prevalence (8–12%) [23, 24]. Moreover, PVL was significantly associated with MRSA strains isolated from infection sites compared to carriers. Among MRSA isolates from infection sites, PVL was more frequently found in CA-MRSA, which is consistent with the literature [25]. Nonetheless, our study found that a large number of HA-MRSA isolates from infection sites harbor PVL (63.1%). This indicates that PVL-positive strains are invading hospitals and causing infections, which is in line with previous reports

[26]. Despite the controversial role of PVL as virulence factor in MRSA pathogenesis [27, 28], it seems to play an important role in the successful evolutionary fitness of these strains [15]. Therefore, special control and clearance measure should be directed toward PVL-positive MRSA. Four MRSA strains were found to be simultaneously positive for both PVL and TSST-1 genes in our study, which is otherwise uncommon [29]. One of the four isolates was obtained from a patient with severe necrotizing pneumonia that required ventilation and developed sepsis and one isolate was obtained from deep cutaneous abscess. The other two isolates came from surgical wound infection and colonization sites. A similar finding has also been reported in the Middle East and other countries [29–32].

The most commonly identified clonal complex in our study was the CC80-MRSA-IV. This has been previously reported in several countries in the Middle East and North Africa and has also been reported from Riyadh in the central region of Saudi Arabia [11, 21, 22, 33–37]. This could indicate that it is the most common MRSA strain circulating in Saudi Arabia. This clone represents the European CA-MRSA clone. The spread of this clone in the Middle East and North Africa and the presence of sporadic cases in Europe suggest that this clone was introduced to Europe through migration from both the Middle East and North Africa. CC80-MRSA-IV isolates are usually PVL positive. However, PVL negative clones have been sporadically reported [11, 21, 35, 38, 39]. Four of the CC80-MRSA-IV isolates in our study were PVL negative. Since it has been suggested that PVL provides fitness to this isolate, in addition to the presence of this isolate in small numbers, it could be assumed that they are sporadic deletion variants. ST1440-IV was detected in only one sample in the present study. This isolate is very rare and has only been reported in Tunisia [40]. ST80-MRSA-V was identified in two cases in our study. This genotype has not been reported previously and seems to be a new isolate as all reported ST80 strains harbor the SCCmec genotype IV.

Two sequence types (ST1 and ST772) belonging to CC1 were identified in our study. Most ST1 strains were PVL negative and harbored SCCmec-IV, which may resemble the West Australian strain WA MRSA-1. The rest were PVL-positive strain, which may resemble the USA400 strain. ST772-MRSA-V is usually more distinct from the other CC1 isolates and is known as the Bengal Bay clone. This strain is more prevalent in India [41] and was also detected in many European countries, where it was linked to transmission associated with migration to these countries [42]. Similarly, the detection of this strain in Saudi Arabia could be explained by the presence of the large number of Indian workers in the country. The detection of ST772-MRSA-IV has not been previously reported and it was isolated from one case in our study.

The UK-MRSA-15 strain, which is also called Barnim Epidemic strain (C22-MRSA-IV PVL-negative), was detected in 7.5% of our isolates and was found more frequently among carriers. Similar to other reports, it differs from the UK-MRSA-15 strain in that it is positive for the *tst1* gene and has the SSC-IVa [22]. The other PVL-positive strain was detected in three cases and was confined to the carrier group. This strain has been reported in many other countries, including the neighboring United Arab Emirates [15].

Contrary to other studies from Riyadh in Saudi Arabia [21, 22], ST241-MRSA-III PVL-negative strain was the most frequently detected isolate belonging to CC8, which indicates interregional variation in the distribution of these strains. This isolate has been reported in Kuwait, Tunisia, Taiwan and Poland [43–46]. The other CC8 strains were the ST239-MRSA-III and the USA300 (ST8-MRSA-IV PVL-positive) were previously reported from Riyadh region [21, 22].

Similar to previous reports from Saudi Arabia, PVL-negative and positive CC5 strains harboring the SCCmec IV or V were identified in our study [21, 22]. These strains were isolated also in Qatar, Tunisia and Egypt [24, 44, 47, 48]. One sample in our study has genotypes similar to the Maltese strain (CC 5/ST149) [49].

All the CC6 isolates were detected in the carrier group and they were also reported previously in Riyadh and the United Arab Emirate [15, 22], which indicates that it is an established strain in the region.

Other clonal complexes such as CC30, CC45 and CC97 were isolated from 1.9% of the cases each. ST30-MRSA-IV PVL-positive resembles the US1100 (southwest pacific clone) and is widespread in Europe and the Gulf region [15, 50]. Interestingly, CC45-MSSA strains were previously detected in Saudi Arabia from nasal colonization carriers [51]. Therefore, it is possible that this strain has acquired the mecA gene and transformed to MRSA. CC45-MRSA-IV was also reported previously in one case from Riyadh in Saudi Arabia [21] and one case from Hong Kong. Similarly, the CC97-MRSA-V was sporadically reported from many countries, including the Middle Eastern region [15].

The phenomenon of vancomycin MIC creep was described by Wang et al. and confirmed by several reports worldwide [52]. In MRSA strains, high vancomycin MICs, which still lay within the susceptible range (≥ 1.0), was linked with poor clinical outcome and higher mortality [53]. In our cohort, isolates originating from infected sites, but not colonization sites, exhibited high MICs to vancomycin raising a concern of clinical efficacy of the drug as monotherapy in this case. The method used to measure the MIC, E test, may have contributed to the increased MICs values [54]. However, a recent meta-analysis by van Hal et al. has shown that despite the methodology applied, these MICs close to the break point of 2.0, such as the isolates representing infected sites in this study, carry poor prognosis irrespective of the infection site [55]. Appropriate alternatives in such circumstances include daptomycin in cases of bacteremia and Linezolid in pneumonias.

Five new sequence types from seven samples are reported in this study (Table 6). All except one were isolated from infection sites. They belong to CC80 according to the eBust website. Due to the diversity of nationalities working and living in the Gulf region, further studies should be conducted on MRSA to reveal and monitor the emergence of new strains.

Conclusions

A highly diverse population of MRSA isolates is reported from both carriers and patients' infection sites in our study from the Eastern Province in Saudi Arabia. Some of the isolate types were more prevalent among the carriers more than the infection sites. Therefore, screening and control measures should consider the polyclonal nature of the problem. A good understanding of the genetic spectrum of the MRSA isolates and its prevalence in the population calls for continuous surveillance and clearance measures. With SCCmec type IV being most prevalent; this suggests a community origin of most MRSA strains which is also supported by low resistance rates to clindamycin and sulfonamides. Therefore very well designed surveillance and intervention strategies, in particular restricting antimicrobial use, should be implemented to prevent emergence and control spread of MRSA in the community.

Abbreviations

MRSA: methicillin resistant *Staphylococcus aureus*; *S. aureus*: *Staphylococcus aureus*; PBP2a: penicillin binding protein 2a; mecA gene: methicillin resistance gene; SCCmec: staphylococcal cassette chromosome mec; HA-MRSA: hospital acquired MRSA; CA-MRSA: community acquired MRSA; lukF-PV: leukocidin gene subunit F; lukS-PV: leukocidin gene subunit S; PVL: Panton–Valentine leukocidin; CC: clonal complexes; MLST: multi locus sequence typing; ST: sequence types; femA: factor essential for mecA; PCR: polymerase chain reaction; ICU: intensive care unit; MIC: minimum inhibitory concentration.

Authors' contributions

KRA: overall study design, raising fund, experimental design, and manuscript writing and editing. SR: experimental work and manuscript writing. FA: analysis of MLST sequences. AA: collection of bacterial isolates, collection of demographic data, and manuscript reading and editing. AD: collection of bacterial isolates. AKA: manuscript writing and editing. All authors read and approved the final manuscript.

Author details

[1] Department of Epidemic Diseases Research, Institute for Research and Medical Consultations (IRMC), Imam Abdulrahman Bin Faisal University (IAU), P.O. Box 1982, Dammam 31441, Saudi Arabia. [2] Department of Microbiology, College of Medicine, Imam Abdulrahman Bin Faisal University (IAU), P.O. Box 1982, Dammam 31441, Saudi Arabia. [3] Department of Biochemistry, College of Medicine, Imam Abdulrahman Bin Faisal University (IAU), P.O. Box 1982, Dammam 31441, Saudi Arabia.

Acknowledgements

The authors are grateful to Mr. Nestor Recella, Mrs. Janaika Yu Logan and the technical staff in the diagnostic microbiology laboratory (KFHU) for their technical assistance. The authors acknowledge the use of the *S. aureus* MLST database which is located at Imperial College London. This work is funded by the Deanship for Scientific Research at the University of Dammam (Project Number: 2013229).

Competing interests

The authors declare that they have no competing interests.

Funding

This work was funded by the Deanship for Scientific Research at the University of Dammam for Khaled R. Alkharsah (Project Number 2013229). The role of the funding body was financial support for the study and had no role in design of the study and collection, analysis, and interpretation of data and in writing the manuscript.

Informed consent

Not applicable.

References

1. Conner-Kerr TA, Sullivan PK, Gaillard J, Franklin ME, Jones RM. The effects of ultraviolet radiation on antibiotic-resistant bacteria in vitro. Ostomy Wound Manag. 1998;44(10):50–6.
2. Chambers HF, Deleo FR. Waves of resistance: *Staphylococcus aureus* in the antibiotic era. Nat Rev Microbiol. 2009;7(9):629–41.
3. Wong H, Louie L, Lo RY, Simor AE. Characterization of *Staphylococcus aureus* isolates with a partial or complete absence of staphylococcal cassette chromosome elements. J Clin Microbiol. 2010;48(10):3525–31.
4. Liu J, Chen D, Peters BM, Li L, Li B, Xu Z, Shirliff ME. Staphylococcal chromosomal cassettes mec (SCCmec): a mobile genetic element in methicillin-resistant *Staphylococcus aureus*. Microb Pathog. 2016;101:56–67.
5. David MZ, Daum RS. Community-associated methicillin-resistant *Staphylococcus aureus*: epidemiology and clinical consequences of an emerging epidemic. Clin Microbiol Rev. 2010;23(3):616–87.
6. Seybold U, Kourbatova EV, Johnson JG, Halvosa SJ, Wang YF, King MD, Ray SM, Blumberg HM. Emergence of community-associated methicillin-resistant *Staphylococcus aureus* USA300 genotype as a major cause of health care—associated blood stream infections. Clin Infect Dis. 2006;42(5):647–56.
7. Boyle-Vavra S, Daum RS. Community-acquired methicillin-resistant *Staphylococcus aureus*: the role of Panton–Valentine leukocidin. Lab Investig J Tech Methods Pathol. 2007;87(1):3–9.
8. Deresinski S. Methicillin-resistant *Staphylococcus aureus*: an evolutionary, epidemiologic, and therapeutic odyssey. Clin Infect Dis. 2005;40(4):562–73.
9. Enright MC, Day NP, Davies CE, Peacock SJ, Spratt BG. Multilocus sequence typing for characterization of methicillin-resistant and methicillin-susceptible clones of *Staphylococcus aureus*. J Clin Microbiol. 2000;38(3):1008–15.
10. Otto M. MRSA virulence and spread. Cell Microbiol. 2012;14(10):1513–21.
11. Tokajian S. New epidemiology of *Staphylococcus aureus* infections in the Middle East. Clin Microbiol Infect. 2014;20(7):624–8.
12. Chen CJ, Wang SC, Chang HY, Huang YC. Longitudinal analysis of methicillin-resistant and methicillin-susceptible *Staphylococcus aureus* carriage in healthy adolescents. J Clin Microbiol. 2013;51(8):2508–14.
13. Dulon M, Peters C, Schablon A, Nienhaus A. MRSA carriage among healthcare workers in non-outbreak settings in Europe and the United States: a systematic review. BMC Infect Dis. 2014;14:363.

14. Dulon M, Haamann F, Peters C, Schablon A, Nienhaus A. MRSA prevalence in European healthcare settings: a review. BMC Infect Dis. 2011;11:138.
15. Monecke S, Coombs G, Shore AC, Coleman DC, Akpaka P, Borg M, Chow H, Ip M, Jatzwauk L, Jonas D, et al. A field guide to pandemic, epidemic and sporadic clones of methicillin-resistant *Staphylococcus aureus*. PLoS ONE. 2011;6(4):e17936.
16. CLSI. Performance standards for antimicrobial susceptibility testing; eighteenth informational supplement. In CLSI document M100-S26. Wayne: CLSI; 2016.
17. Al-Talib H, Yean CY, Al-Khateeb A, Hassan H, Singh KK, Al-Jashamy K, Ravichandran M. A pentaplex PCR assay for the rapid detection of methicillin-resistant *Staphylococcus aureus* and Panton–Valentine Leucocidin. BMC Microbiol. 2009;9:113.
18. Mehrotra M, Wang G, Johnson WM. Multiplex PCR for detection of genes for *Staphylococcus aureus* enterotoxins, exfoliative toxins, toxic shock syndrome toxin 1, and methicillin resistance. J Clin Microbiol. 2000;38(3):1032–5.
19. Ghaznavi-Rad E, Nor Shamsudin M, Sekawi Z, van Belkum A, Neela V. A simplified multiplex PCR assay for fast and easy discrimination of globally distributed staphylococcal cassette chromosome mec types in meticillin-resistant *Staphylococcus aureus*. J Med Microbiol. 2010;59(Pt 10):1135–9.
20. Rasmussen RV, Fowler VG Jr, Skov R, Bruun NE. Future challenges and treatment of *Staphylococcus aureus* bacteremia with emphasis on MRSA. Future Microbiol. 2011;6(1):43–56.
21. Monecke S, Skakni L, Hasan R, Ruppelt A, Ghazal SS, Hakawi A, Slickers P, Ehricht R. Characterisation of MRSA strains isolated from patients in a hospital in Riyadh, Kingdom of Saudi Arabia. BMC Microbiol. 2012;12:146.
22. Senok A, Ehricht R, Monecke S, Al-Saedan R, Somily A. Molecular characterization of methicillin-resistant *Staphylococcus aureus* in nosocomial infections in a tertiary-care facility: emergence of new clonal complexes in Saudi Arabia. New Microbes New Infect. 2016;14:13–8.
23. Moussa I, Shibl AM. Molecular characterization of methicillin-resistant *Staphylococcus aureus* recovered from outpatient clinics in Riyadh, Saudi Arabia. Saudi Med J. 2009;30(5):611–7.
24. Abou Shady HM, Bakr AE, Hashad ME, Alzohairy MA. *Staphylococcus aureus* nasal carriage among outpatients attending primary health care centers: a comparative study of two cities in Saudi Arabia and Egypt. Braz J Infect Dis. 2015;19(1):68–76.
25. Vandenesch F, Naimi T, Enright MC, Lina G, Nimmo GR, Heffernan H, Liassine N, Bes M, Greenland T, Reverdy ME, et al. Community-acquired methicillin-resistant *Staphylococcus aureus* carrying Panton–Valentine leukocidin genes: worldwide emergence. Emerg Infect Dis. 2003;9(8):978–84.
26. Bukharie HA. Increasing threat of community-acquired methicillin-resistant *Staphylococcus aureus*. Am J Med Sci. 2010;340(5):378–81.
27. Bae IG, Tonthat GT, Stryjewski ME, Rude TH, Reilly LF, Barriere SL, Genter FC, Corey GR, Fowler VG Jr. Presence of genes encoding the Panton–Valentine leukocidin exotoxin is not the primary determinant of outcome in patients with complicated skin and skin structure infections due to methicillin-resistant *Staphylococcus aureus*: results of a multinational trial. J Clin Microbiol. 2009;47(12):3952–7.
28. Otto M. A MRSA-terious enemy among us: end of the PVL controversy? Nat Med. 2011;17(2):169–70.
29. Li Z, Stevens DL, Hamilton SM, Parimon T, Ma Y, Kearns AM, Ellis RW, Bryant AE. Fatal *S. aureus* hemorrhagic pneumonia: genetic analysis of a unique clinical isolate producing both PVL and TSST-1. PLoS ONE. 2011;6(11):e27246.
30. Al-Bakri AG, Al-Hadithi H, Kasabri V, Othman G, Kriegeskorte A, Becker K. The epidemiology and molecular characterization of methicillin-resistant staphylococci sampled from a healthy Jordanian population. Epidemiol Infect. 2013;141(11):2384–91.
31. Harastani HH, Tokajian ST. Community-associated methicillin-resistant *Staphylococcus aureus* clonal complex 80 type IV (CC80-MRSA-IV) isolated from the Middle East: a heterogeneous expanding clonal lineage. PLoS ONE. 2014;9(7):e103715.
32. Holmes A, Ganner M, McGuane S, Pitt TL, Cookson BD, Kearns AM. *Staphylococcus aureus* isolates carrying Panton–Valentine leucocidin genes in England and Wales: frequency, characterization, and association with clinical disease. J Clin Microbiol. 2005;43(5):2384–90.
33. Tokajian ST, Khalil PA, Jabbour D, Rizk M, Farah MJ, Hashwa FA, Araj GF. Molecular characterization of *Staphylococcus aureus* in Lebanon. Epidemiol Infect. 2010;138(5):707–12.
34. Enany S, Yaoita E, Yoshida Y, Enany M, Yamamoto T. Molecular characterization of Panton–Valentine leukocidin-positive community-acquired methicillin-resistant *Staphylococcus aureus* isolates in Egypt. Microbiol Res. 2010;165(2):152–62.
35. Udo EE, Sarkhoo E. The dissemination of ST80-SCCmec-IV community-associated methicillin resistant *Staphylococcus aureus* clone in Kuwait hospitals. Ann Clin Microbiol Antimicrob. 2010;9:31.
36. Bekkhoucha SN, Cady A, Gautier P, Itim F, Donnio PY. A portrait of *Staphylococcus aureus* from the other side of the Mediterranean Sea: molecular characteristics of isolates from Western Algeria. Eur J Clin Microbiol Infect Dis. 2009;28(5):553–5.
37. Ben Nejma M, Mastouri M, Jrad BB, Nour M. Characterization of ST80 Panton–Valentine leukocidin-positive community-acquired methicillin-resistant *Staphylococcus aureus* clone in Tunisia. Diagn Microbiol Infect Dis. 2013;77(1):20–4.
38. Djoudi F, Bonura C, Benallaoua S, Touati A, Touati D, Aleo A, Cala C, Fasciana T, Mammina C. Panton–Valentine leukocidin positive sequence type 80 methicillin-resistant *Staphylococcus aureus* carrying a staphylococcal cassette chromosome mec type IVc is dominant in neonates and children in an Algiers hospital. New Microbiol. 2013;36(1):49–55.
39. Tristan A, Bes M, Meugnier H, Lina G, Bozdogan B, Courvalin P, Reverdy ME, Enright MC, Vandenesch F, Etienne J. Global distribution of Panton–Valentine leukocidin—positive methicillin-resistant *Staphylococcus aureus*, 2006. Emerg Infect Dis. 2007;13(4):594–600.
40. Mariem BJ, Ito T, Zhang M, Jin J, Li S, Ilhem BB, Adnan H, Han X, Hiramatsu K. Molecular characterization of methicillin-resistant Panton–Valentine leukocidin positive *staphylococcus aureus* clones disseminating in Tunisian hospitals and in the community. BMC Microbiol. 2013;13:2.
41. D'Souza N, Rodrigues C, Mehta A. Molecular characterization of methicillin-resistant *Staphylococcus aureus* with emergence of epidemic clones of sequence type (ST) 22 and ST 772 in Mumbai, India. J Clin Microbiol. 2010;48(5):1806–11.
42. Huh K, Chung DR. Changing epidemiology of community-associated methicillin-resistant *Staphylococcus aureus* in the Asia-Pacific region. Expert Rev Anti Infect Ther. 2016;14(11):1007–22.
43. Boswihi SS, Udo EE, Al-Sweih N. Shifts in the clonal distribution of methicillin-resistant *Staphylococcus aureus* in Kuwait Hospitals: 1992–2010. PLoS ONE. 2016;11(9):e0162744.
44. Elhani D, Gharsa H, Kalai D, Lozano C, Gomez P, Boutheina J, Aouni M, Barguellil F, Torres C, Ben Slama K. Clonal lineages detected amongst tetracycline-resistant meticillin-resistant *Staphylococcus aureus* isolates of a Tunisian hospital, with detection of lineage ST398. J Med Microbiol. 2015;64(6):623–9.
45. Wang WY, Chiueh TS, Sun JR, Tsao SM, Lu JJ. Molecular typing and phenotype characterization of methicillin-resistant *Staphylococcus aureus* isolates from blood in Taiwan. PLoS ONE. 2012;7(1):e30394.
46. Mlynarczyk A, Szymanek-Majchrzak K, Grzybowska W, Durlik M, Deborska-Materkowska D, Paczek L, Chmura A, Swoboda-Kopec E, Tyski S, Mlynarczyk G. Molecular and phenotypic characteristics of methicillin-resistant *Staphylococcus aureus* strains isolated from hospitalized patients in transplantation wards. Transplant Proc. 2014;46(8):2579–82.
47. El-Mahdy TS, El-Ahmady M, Goering RV. Molecular characterization of methicillin-resistant *Staphylococcus aureus* isolated over a 2-year period in a Qatari hospital from multinational patients. Clin Microbiol Infect. 2014;20(2):169–73.
48. Kechrid A, Perez-Vazquez M, Smaoui H, Hariga D, Rodriguez-Banos M, Vindel A, Baquero F, Canton R, Del Campo R. Molecular analysis of community-acquired methicillin-susceptible and resistant *Staphylococcus aureus* isolates recovered from bacteraemic and osteomyelitis infections in children from Tunisia. Clin Microbiol Infect. 2011;17(7):1020–6.
49. Scicluna EA, Shore AC, Thurmer A, Ehricht R, Slickers P, Borg MA, Coleman DC, Monecke S. Characterisation of MRSA from Malta and the description of a Maltese epidemic MRSA strain. Eur J Clin Microbiol Infect Dis. 2010;29(2):163–70.
50. Monecke S, Gavier-Widen D, Hotzel H, Peters M, Guenther S, Lazaris A, Loncaric I, Muller E, Reissig A, Ruppelt-Lorz A, et al. Diversity of *Staphylococcus aureus* isolates in European wildlife. PLoS ONE. 2016;11(12):e0168433.
51. Sarkar A, Raji A, Garaween G, Soge O, Rey-Ladino J, Al-Kattan W, Shibl A,

Senok A. Antimicrobial resistance and virulence markers in methicillin sensitive *Staphylococcus aureus* isolates associated with nasal colonization. Microb Pathog. 2016;93:8–12.
52. Wang G, Hindler JF, Ward KW, Bruckner DA. Increased vancomycin MICs for *Staphylococcus aureus* clinical isolates from a university hospital during a 5-year period. J Clin Microbiol. 2006;44(11):3883–6.
53. Hidayat LK, Hsu DI, Quist R, Shriner KA, Wong-Beringer A. High-dose vancomycin therapy for methicillin-resistant *Staphylococcus aureus* infections: efficacy and toxicity. Arch Intern Med. 2006;166(19):2138–44.
54. Prakash V, Lewis JS 2nd, Jorgensen JH. Vancomycin MICs for methicillin-resistant *Staphylococcus aureus* isolates differ based upon the susceptibility test method used. Antimicrob Agents Chemother. 2008;52(12):4528.
55. van Hal SJ, Lodise TP, Paterson DL. The clinical significance of vancomycin minimum inhibitory concentration in *Staphylococcus aureus* infections: a systematic review and meta-analysis. Clin Infect Diseases. 2012;54(6):755–71.

25

Detection of urinary *Chlamydia trachomatis*, *Mycoplasma genitalium* and human papilloma virus in the first trimester of pregnancy by PCR method

Monireh Rahimkhani[1*], A. Mordadi[2] and M. Gilanpour[3]

Abstract

Background: Miscarriage and preterm delivery are the most important challenges of pregnancy. Different bacterial and viral infection may cause miscarriage and preterm delivery. Among bacterial factors, *Mycoplasma genitalium* and *Chlamydia trachomatis* have the most important role and human papilloma virus (HPV) is the leading viral factor in this regard.

Methods: First void urine samples were collected from 119 pregnant women who visited health centers for routine first-trimester screening (12–14 weeks gestation). About 10 ml of the sample was centrifuged at 3000×*g* for 20 min and 1–2 ml of the sediment was transferred to sterile microfuges and stored at − 20 °C until analysis. DNA extraction was conducted using A101211 kits imported by Pars Tous Biotechnology Company. The following commercial kits, imported by Pars Tous Biotechnology, were used for PCR.

Results: There is no significant association between urinary isolation of *C. trachomatis* and miscarriage (P = 0.93) and there is no significant association between urinary isolation of *M. genitalium* and miscarriage (P = 0.80). Regarding HPV, since all urine samples were PCR-negative, comparison was not possible. *C. trachomatis* was isolated from the urine samples of 6.72% of the pregnant women who underwent first-trimester screening in health centers using PCR. Previous studies reported a mean chlamydia isolation rate of 3% from urine specimens collected from pregnant women in general. *T* test showed no significant difference between the two groups (P = 0.10). Based on present study the mycoplasma isolation rate was 17.65% using PCR. Previous studies reported a mean mycoplasma isolation rate of 10% from urine specimens collected from pregnant women in general. T-test showed a significant difference between the two groups (P = 0.03).

Discussion: First void urine samples in pregnant women may be an appropriate sample for detection of *C. trachomatis* and *M. genitalium*; however, it is not a good method for HPV isolation therefore vaginal or cervical discharge specimens should be used instead for detection of HPV.

Keywords: Pregnant women, Miscarriage, *Chlamydia trachomatis*, *Mycoplasma genitalium*, Human papilloma virus, Urine sample

*Correspondence: rrahimkhani@sina.tums.ac.ir
[1] Department of Lab Medical Sciences, Faculty of Allied Medical Sciences, Tehran University of Medical Sciences, Tehran, Iran
Full list of author information is available at the end of the article

Importance

In the present study, we decided to investigate three major causes of STDs that also cause miscarriage in the first trimester in a number of pregnant women. Since cervical swabbing is invasive and dangerous and is not accepted by pregnant women, first void urine specimens were used in this study. Among bacterial agents, *Chlamydia trachomatis* and *Mycoplasma genitalium*, and among viral agents, HPV, have a major role in miscarriage. These agents were surveyed in present research.

Background

Miscarriage is one of the greatest risks threatening the life of the mother and fetus. Different bacterial, viral, and parasitic factors can cause miscarriage. Statistics suggest that more than 90% of miscarriages are related to an infectious or inflammatory factor in the placenta or amniotic fluid [1]. Among bacterial agents, *Chlamydia trachomatis* and *Mycoplasma genitalium*, and among viral agents, human papilloma virus (HPV), have a major role in miscarriage.

Chlamydia trachomatis is an obligate intracellular, nonmotile, Gram-negative bacterium in the family Chlamydiaceae. Because it is an intracellular parasite, it does not grow on bacteriologic cultures, and cellular cultures are used for its isolation and reproduction. *Chlamydia trachomatis* is the major cause of trachoma but it can also cause miscarriage, fetal anomaly, endometritis, preterm delivery, and stillbirth. Since this bacterium is not easy to culture and serological methods have a rather low accuracy, molecular methods like PCR are used to detect it.

Mycoplasma genitalium is a Gram-negative, pleomorphic, nonmotile bacterium lacking a cell wall. It requires special media for growth and reproduction. It is a leading cause of miscarriage in pregnant women. Since mycoplasmas are difficult to grow and colonies grow after 3–7 days even on special media, it is rarely possible to isolate the bacterium from clinical specimens; therefore, other diagnostic methods are used. One of these methods is serological tests that are not very reliable and false positive results and cross-reaction are frequent in these tests. Therefore, molecular methods like PCR are used for detection. Similar to chlamydia, the samples used to detect mycoplasma include cervical swabs and amniotic fluid, placenta, and urine samples. Urine is least dangerous sample in pregnant women.

HPV is a DNA virus and causes reproductive tract infection in men and women. The relationship between the genome of this virus and cervical cancer was proved years ago; however, few studies have investigated the association between HPV infection and spontaneous abortion, which have shown non-significant associations [2, 3].

Similar to mycoplasma and chlamydia, the samples used for detection of HPV include swab specimens sampled from the cervix and urine.

In the present study, we decided to investigate three major causes of sexually transmitted disease (STDs) that also cause miscarriage in the first trimester in a number of pregnant women. Since cervical swabbing is invasive and dangerous and is not accepted by pregnant women, early urine specimens were used in this study.

Methods

Considering a precision of 7% to detect the difference and a prevalence of 2.8% for *C. trachomatis*, 10% for *M. genitalium*, and 8.4% for HPV, the sample size was estimated 119, 61, and 66, respectively. Finally, the largest sample size was considered for the study by this formula:

$$n' = \frac{NZ^2P(1-P)}{d^2(N-1)+Z^2P(1-P)}.$$

In this study, urine samples were collected from 119 pregnant women who visited Almahdi Clinic Center in south of Tehran for routine first-trimester screening (12–14 weeks gestation). Almahdi Clinic is under the supervision of the Tehran University of Medical Sciences. The sampling duration time was October 2016 to August 2017. Approvals of the Ethics Committees of all patients participating in the study were obtained (IR.TUMS.REC.1395-2322) The subjects first completed a questionnaire and gave informed consent. Then, urine specimens were collected. First void urine is the best urine sampling method for PCR to detect *C. trachomatis*, *M. genitalium*, and HPV. The subjects were requested no to pass urine for 4 h before sampling and then their first-catch urine was collected in sterile containers. About 10 ml of the sample was centrifuged at 3000×*g* for 20 min and 1–2 ml of the sediment was transferred to sterile microfuges and stored at − 20 °C until analysis.

DNA extraction was conducted using A101211 kits imported by Pars Tous Biotechnology Company. After extraction, DNA samples were stored at − 70 °C until PCR was done.

The following commercial kits, imported by Pars Tous Biotechnology, were used for PCR.

HPV PCR kit with code number A101032.

This PCR amplification kit includes all necessary PCR amplification reagents, capable of amplifying a wide spectrum of HPV types and a house keeping gene as internal control. The most well-known and clinically important HPV are detectable with this kit, including type 6, 11,

16, 18, 26, 31, 32, 33, 34, 35, 42, 45, 51, 52, 53, 55, 56, 58, 59, 61, 66, 67, 68, 69, 70, 73, PAP 155, PAP291, X4. Viral DNA present in positive samples is specifically amplified by using primers complementary to viral sequences.

Mycoplasma genitalium PCR kit with code number A101112. This PCR amplification kit includes all necessary PCR amplification reagents with an exception of mineral oil. The *M. genitalium* PCR kit is a qualitative analysis test, using a DNA amplification technique for direct detection of *M. genitalium* DNA. Bacterial DNA present in positive samples is specifically amplified by using primers complementary to bacterial sequences. Each kit offered Pars Tous's optimal buffer system which will enhance amplification specificity with a detection limit of ~ 2 copies per reaction.

Chlamydia trachomatis nested PCR kit with code number A101122 is a qualitative analysis test, using a DNA amplification technique for direct detection of *C. trachomatis* DNA. Bacterial DNA present in positive samples is specifically amplified by using primers complementary to bacterial sequences. Each kit offered Pars Tous's optimal buffer system which will enhance amplification specificity.

Results

In this study, urine samples were collected from 119 pregnant women with mean age 29 years old who visited health centers for routine first-trimester screening (12–14 weeks gestation). The subjects first completed a questionnaire and gave informed consent. Then, urine specimens were collected and have detected *C. trachomatis, M. genitalium*, and HPV with PCR method.

The frequency distribution of abortion, preterm labor, multiple pregnancies history, number of pregnancies and methods of contraception in pregnant women studied are shown in Tables 1 and 2, respectively.

Statistical analyses showed no significant relationship between the variables assessed in the questionnaire, including history of preterm delivery, number of pregnancies, history of multiple pregnancy, contraception method and urinary isolation of chlamydia and mycoplasma.

The number of positive *M. genitalium, C. trachomatis* and HPV in urine samples with PCR method is shown in Table 3.

Table 2 Frequency distribution of variables, number of pregnancies and methods of contraception in pregnant women studied

Variables	Number (%)
Pregnancy number	
1	35 (29.41)
2	47 (39.50)
3	28 (23.53)
4	7 (5.88)
5	2 (1.68)
Pregnancy prevention method	
Natural	85 (71.43)
Condom	12 (10.08)
LD	12 (10.08)
IUD	8 (6.72)
Injection	2 (1.68)

The statistical analysis between urinary isolation of *C. trachomatis* and *M. genitalium* and miscarriage is shown in Tables 4 and 5, respectively.

According to Table 4, we found no significant association between urinary isolation of *C. trachomatis* and miscarriage ($P = 0.93$) and according to Table 5, we found no significant association between urinary isolation of *M. genitalium* and miscarriage ($P = 0.80$). Regarding HPV, since all urine samples were PCR-negative, comparison was not possible.

According to the present study, chlamydia was isolated from the urine samples of 6.72% of the pregnant women who underwent first-trimester screening in health centers using PCR. Previous studies reported a mean chlamydia isolation rate of 3% from urine specimens collected from pregnant women in general. T-test showed no significant difference between the two groups ($P = 0.10$).

In our study, the mycoplasma isolation rate was 17.65% using PCR. Previous studies reported a mean mycoplasma isolation rate of 10% from urine specimens collected from pregnant women in general. T-test showed a significant difference between the two groups ($P = 0.03$).

The pictures gel electrophoresis of PCR products of *C. trachomatis* and *M. genitalium* is shown in Figs. 1 and 2, respectively

Figure 3 is about the DNA quality.

Table 1 Frequency distribution of abortion, preterm labor and multiple pregnancies history in pregnant women

Variable	Abortion history			Premature delivery		Multiple pregnancy		Total
	Non	One	More	No	Yes	No	Yes	
Number (%)	88 (73.95)	25 (21.01)	6 (5.04)	116 (97.48)	3 (2.52)	116 (97.48)	3 (2.52)	119

Table 3 **The urinary isolation of *M. genitalium*, *C. trachomatis* and HPV in pregnant women by PCR method**

Microorganism isolated	Positive (%)	Negative (%)	Total
M. genitalium	21 (17.65)	98 (82.35)	119
C. trachomatis	8 (6.72)	111 (93.28)	119
HPV	0 (0)	119 (100)	119

Table 4 **The statistical analysis between urinary isolation of *C. trachomatis* and miscarriage in pregnant women**

Variables	Chlamydia infection		
Abortion	Positive	Negative	P-value
	Number (%)	Number (%)	
No	6 (75)	82 (73.87)	
Yes	2 (25)	29 (26.13)	0.93

Table 5 **The statistical analysis between urinary isolation of *M. genitalium* and miscarriage in pregnant women**

Variables	Mycoplasma infection		
Abortion	Positive	Negative	P-value
	Number (%)	Number (%)	
No	15 (71.43)	73 (74.49)	
Yes	6 (28.57)	25 (25.51)	0.80

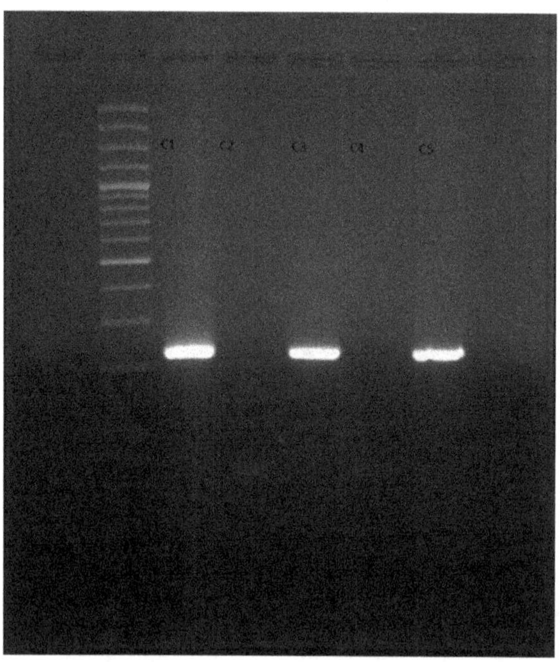

Fig. 1 Gel electrophoresis of PCR products of *Chlamydia trachomatis* (*C1* control positive, *C2* control negative, *C3–5* urine samples)

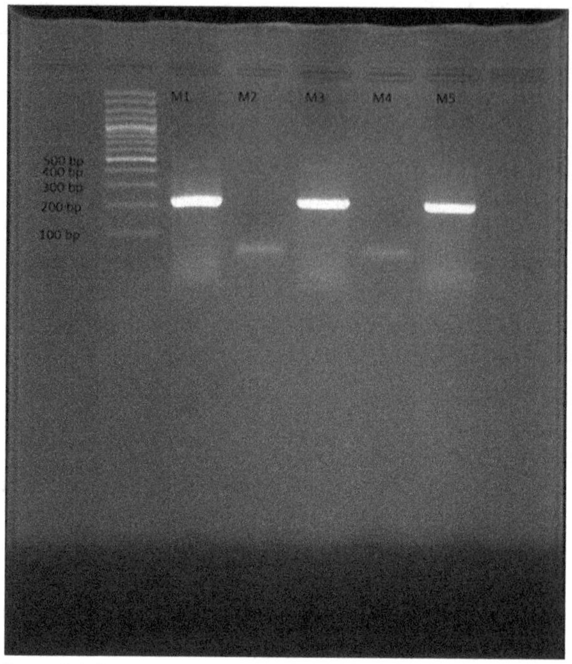

Fig. 2 Gel electrophoresis of PCR products of *Mycoplasma genitalium* (*M1* control positive, *M2* control negative, *M3–5* urine samples)

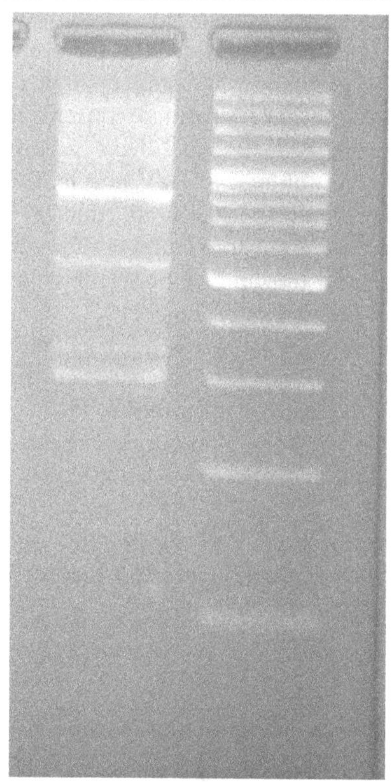

Fig. 3 DNA quality

Discussion

Miscarriage and preterm delivery are the most important challenges of pregnancy. Different bacterial and viral infection may cause miscarriage and preterm delivery [4]. Among bacterial factors, *M. genitalium* and *C. trachomatis* have the most important role and HPV is the leading viral factor in this regard [1].

All the above agents are colonized in the vaginal either symptomatically or asymptomatically. If symptomatic, the person seeks treatment. What is important is a woman in whom these agents are colonized in the vagina and the patient is asymptomatic. These women are at increased risk of preterm delivery or miscarriage if they become pregnant [1, 2, 5]

According to a study in Samoa, 239 women aged 18–29 years were evaluated for *C. trachomatis* infection using PCR. The results showed that 36% of the women were infected that were mostly 18–24 years. Urine samples were used in this study [6]. A retrospective study on 590 women between 2010 and 2014 showed that 11 and 6.9% of the women were infected with HPV and *C. trachomatis*, respectively [7]. Researchers in Switzerland compared 146 pregnant women with preterm delivery with 261 women with term delivery. The results of PCR showed a significantly higher rate of *C. trachomatis* infection in women with preterm delivery [8]. In the USA, about 3–6% of the women below 25 years who look healthy have *C. trachomatis* infection. In general, the percentage of *C. trachomatis* infection is different in different countries; for example, 3.9% in England, 6% in Finland, 17% in France, 9% in Poland, and 6.5–22% in Iran. In a study in 2016, *C. trachomatis* DNA was detected on the endocervical swabs of 17.43% of the subjects [9]. A similar study in Iran showed the colonization rate of *C. trachomatis* is 2.8% in pregnant women. The rate is reported to be about 4.8% in the urine of pregnant women with a history of miscarriage or infertility [10, 11].

Numerous studies have investigated *M. genitalium*. The colonization rate of mycoplasma is 12–50% in pregnancy but the prevalence of mycoplasma is even higher in women with a history of miscarriage. A colonization rate of about 84% was reported in a study in Malaysia.

A similar study in China showed that the colonization rate of *Mycoplasma hominis* was about 27.6 and 10% in women with a history of miscarriage and normal women, respectively. According to a study in Iran, mycoplasma is colonized in 10% of the pregnant women [10]. A similar study showed a colonization rate of 21–45% for mycoplasma in women [12].

As for HPV, studies have shown that the DNA of this virus can be detected in the vaginal swabs of 30–45% of women using PCR. In another study, HPV was isolated from vaginal swabs of 5.5–65% of the subjects, depending on the geographical region, using PCR. In a study in Poland, HPV was isolated from the vaginal specimens of 35.14% of pregnant women using PCR [13, 14]. Another study reported an isolation rate of 36%. A study in Brazil, HPV DNA was detected in the vaginal samples of 25.3% of pregnant women and 13% of non-pregnant women using PCR, which showed a significant difference [14]. The results of a study in Iran showed that of 2577 healthy women, HPV DNA was isolated from 8.4% of vaginal specimens using PCR [15].

The results of a study by Ducancelle et al. showed that HPV was isolated from the 42 and 49% of the urine and cervical discharge samples of 230 women, respectively. In this study, real time PCR was used to detect HPV. The women participating in this study were not pregnant, so there was no risk of miscarriage. The isolation rate of the two sampling methods had a significant correlation [16]. In a similar study, the correlation of HPV isolation from cervical discharge specimens (45%) and urine samples (37%) using real time PCR was about (93%) [17]. Tamim et al. assessed *C. trachomatis* and HPV in cervical discharge and urine specimens (2–4 h after urinary retention) using PCR [18].

Vanessa et al. investigated the prevalence of mycoplasma in the urine samples of 82 women with a history of miscarriage and 34 pregnant women 22 weeks gestation and reported similar results [19]. Jensen et al. reported that urine specimens are better than urogenital swabs for detection of mycoplasma and chlamydia using PCR [20].

About antibiotic treatment of genital infections with *C. trachomatis* fortunately investigations has shown the clinical strains of *C. trachomatis* with macrolide or fluoroquinolone resistance would be uncommon, and azithromycin or fluoroquinolone regimens could be recommended as treatments for chlamydial infections [21].

Although in genital infections caused by *M. genitalium* based on Anderson et al. investigation, the clinical observation of increasing treatment failure indicating antibiotic resistance has been confirmed by molecular testing. Fluoroquinolone mutation screening was performed on 86 (74.8%) of the 115 samples, of which 20 (23.3%) samples had a mutation or mutations associated with increased resistance. This study shows the increasing antibiotic resistance and the need for appropriate guidelines to treat at-risk patients [22].

The most common sampling method is vaginal and cervical sampling to detect the above bacterial and viral agents, which required the use of speculum. Since this sampling method is invasive and may cause miscarriage, less invasive methods should be used. In recent years, the results of studies isolating these bacterial and viral agents from first void urine have been promising. In this method, the patient should not void for at least 4 h, and then first-catch urine is collected a sterile container for urine culture.

In our study, first void urine was used to detect the above bacterial and viral agents that play a role in miscarriage and preterm delivery. One hundred and nineteen pregnant women (11–14 weeks gestation) who underwent first-trimester screening in health centers were recruited. After completing the questionnaire and obtaining informed consent, the subjects were given urine collection containers to collect their urine. Urine samples were centrifuged for 20 min and DNA was extracted from the sediment. PCR was done on the samples to detect *M. genitalium, C. trachomatis,* and HPV. According to the results, chlamydia was isolated from the urine specimens of 6.78% of the pregnant women. Previous studies reported a mean chlamydial isolation rate of 3% from urine specimens collected from pregnant women in general. T-test showed no significant difference between the two groups ($P=0.10$). According to the above results, the isolation rate of chlamydia from urine specimens of pregnant women was more than two times higher than vaginal and cervical discharge specimens because previous studies showed an isolation rate of 3% for *C. trachomatis* from vaginal and cervical discharge specimens. Therefore, urine is an appropriate sample for detection of *C. trachomatis* because its collection is non-invasive and offers a higher isolation rate.

According to our results, the mycoplasma isolation rate was 17.8% using PCR. Previous studies reported a mean mycoplasma isolation rate of 10% from urine specimens collected from pregnant women in general. T-test showed a significant difference between the two groups ($P=0.03$).

The 10% prevalence of mycoplasma in the pregnant women was based on cervical or vaginal specimens, which is an invasive sampling method in pregnant women and is not well accepted. We used urine samples in our study and found a higher isolation rate than vaginal and cervical discharge specimens. Therefore, first void urine may yield better results.

We found no significant relationship between the isolation rate of mycoplasma and chlamydia using PCR and the history of miscarriage. Since HPV was not isolated from any of the urine specimens, statistical analysis was not possible. HPV was isolated from 8.4% of vaginal and cervical discharge specimens of pregnant women; therefore, it may be concluded that urine is not a good sample for HPV detection and cervical or vaginal specimens should be used to detect these viral agent.

All 119 women were followed up until delivery. Three cases of preterm delivery were noted, of whom two were positive for mycoplasma and one was positive for both mycoplasma and chlamydia. Statistical analysis showed a significant difference in preterm delivery between women who were positive for one of the above agents and women who were negative.

In general, the aim of the present study was to isolate three important causes of septic abortion, i.e., *C. trachomatis, M. genitalium,* and HPV, from urine specimens of pregnant women in the first trimester. According to the results, first void may be an appropriate sample for detection of *C. trachomatis* and *M. genitalium*; however, urine is not a good sample for HPV isolation and vaginal or cervical discharge specimens should be used instead. Regarding mycoplasma, urine specimens are even better than vaginal and cervical specimens considering the higher isolation rate.

Abbreviations

M. genitalium: *Mycoplasma genitalium*; *C. trachomatis*: *Chlamydia trachomatis*; HPV: Human papilloma virus; STD: Sexually transmitted diseases.

Authors' contributions

Monireh Rahimkhani (50%), Alireza Mordadi (35%), Maryam Gilanpour (15%). All authors read and approved the final manuscript.

Author details

[1] Department of Lab Medical Sciences, Faculty of Allied Medical Sciences, Tehran University of Medical Sciences, Tehran, Iran. [2] Department of Epidemiology, Pasteur Institute, Tehran, Iran. [3] Almahdi Kheyrieh Clinics, Tehran, Iran.

Acknowledgements

The authors thank all staff in Almahdi Clinic, especially Dr. Mohammad Zayandeh who had corporated in sampling from pregnant women and also We appreciate the Research Vice-chancellor of the Tehran University of Medical Sciences for funding the Research Project Code Number 94-04-31-30491.

Competing interests

The authors declare that they have no competing interests.

Funding

Not applicable.

References

1. Doyle RM, Alber DG, Jones HE, Harris K, Fitzgerald F, Peebles D, Klein N. Term and preterm labour are associated with distinct microbial community structures in placental membranes which are independent of mode of delivery. Placenta. 2014;35(12):1099–101.
2. Conde-Ferráez L, de May AAC, Carrillo-Martínez JR, Ayora-Talavera G, del Refugio González-Losa M. Human papillomavirus infection and spontaneous abortion: a case–control study performed in Mexico. Eur J Obstet Gynecol Reprod Biol. 2013;170(2):468–73.

3. Skoczyński M, Goździcka-Józefiak A, Kwaśniewska A. Prevalence of human papillomavirus in spontaneously aborted products of conception. Acta Obstet Gynecol Scand. 2011;90(12):1402–5.
4. Rahimkhani M, Khavari-Daneshvar H, Sharifian R. Asymptomatic bacteriuria and pyuria in pregnancy. Acta Med Iran. 2008;46(5):409–12.
5. Rahimkhani M, Mordadi A, Varmazyar S, Tavakoli A. Evaluation of urinary Interleukin-8 levels in patients with spinal cord injury. Recent Pat Antiinfect Drug Discov. 2015;9(2):144–9.
6. Walsh MS, Hope E, Isaia L, Righarts A, Niupulusu T, Temese SV, Iosefa-Siitia L, Auvaa L, Tapelu SA, Motu MF. Prevalence of *Chlamydia trachomatis* infection in Samoan women aged 18 to 29 and assessment of possible risk factors: a community-based study. Trans R Soc Trop Med Hyg. 2015;109(4):245–51.
7. Depuydt CE, Verstraete L, Berth M, Beert J, Bogers J-P, Salembier G, Vereecken AJ, Bosmans E. Human papillomavirus positivity in women undergoing intrauterine insemination has a negative effect on pregnancy rates. Gynecol Obstet Investig. 2016;81(1):41–6.
8. Baud D, Goy G, Vasilevsky S, Osterheld M-C, Roth-Kleiner M, Croxatto A, Greub G. Roles of bovine *Waddlia chondrophila* and *Chlamydia trachomatis* in human preterm birth. N Microbes N Infect. 2015;3:41–5.
9. Ahmadi A, Khodabandehloo M, Ramazanzadeh R, Farhadifar F, Roshani D, Ghaderi E, Farhangi N. The relationship between *Chlamydia trachomatis* genital infection and spontaneous abortion. J Reprod Infertil. 2016;17(2):110.
10. Dehghan Marvast L, Aflatoonian A, Talebi A, Eley A, Pacey A. Relationship between *Chlamydia trachomatis* and *Mycoplasma genitalium* infection and pregnancy rate and outcome in Iranian infertile couples. Andrologia. 2017. https://doi.org/10.1111/and.12747.
11. Ahmadi MH, Mirsalehian A, Bahador A. Association of *Chlamydia trachomatis* with infertility and clinical manifestations: a systematic review and meta-analysis of case–control studies. Infect Dis (Lond). 2016;48(7):517–23.
12. Vosooghi S, Kheirkhah B, Karimi NA, Reza MT. A review of the role of Mycoplasma infections in humans infertility. NCMBJ. 2012;2:9–20 **(Persian)**.
13. Medeiros LR, de Ethur ABM, Hilgert JB, Zanini RR, Berwanger O, Bozzetti MC, Mylius LC. Vertical transmission of the human papillomavirus: a systematic quantitative review. Cad Saúde Pública. 2005;21(4):1006–15.
14. Salcedo MM, Damin AP, Agnes G, Pessini SA, El Beitune P, Alexandre CO. Prevalence of human papillomavirus infection in pregnant versus non-pregnant women in Brazil. Arch Gynecol Obstet. 2015;292(6):1273–8.
15. Jalilvand S, Shoja Z, Nourijelyani K, Tohidi HR, Hamkar R. Meta-analysis of type-specific human papillomavirus prevalence in Iranian women with normal cytology, precancerous cervical lesions and invasive cervical cancer: implications for screening and vaccination. J Med Virol. 2015;87(2):287–95.
16. Ducancelle A, Legrand M, Pivert A, Veillon P, Le Guillou-Guillemette H, De Brux M, Beby-Defaux A, Agius G, Hantz S, Alain S, Catala L, Descamps P, Postec E, Caly H, Charles-Pétillon F, Labrousse F, Lunel F, Payan C. Interest of human papillomavirus DNA quantification and genotyping in paired cervical and urine samples to detect cervical lesions. Arch Gynecol Obstet. 2014;290(2):299–308.
17. Payan C, Ducancelle A, Aboubaker MH, Caer J, Tapia M, Chauvin A, Peyronnet D, le Hen E, Arab Z, Legrand MC. Human papillomavirus quantification in urine and cervical samples by using the Mx4000 and LightCycler general real-time PCR systems. J Clin Microbiol. 2007;45(3):897–901.
18. Tamim H, Finan RR, Sharida HE, Rashid M, Almawi WY. Cervicovaginal coinfections with human papillomavirus and *Chlamydia trachomatis*. Diagn Microbiol Infect Dis. 2002;43(4):277–81.
19. Short VL, Jensen JS, Nelson DB, Murray PJ, Ness RB, Haggerty CL. *Mycoplasma genitalium* among young, urban pregnant women. Infect Dis Obstet Gynecol. 2010. https://doi.org/10.1155/2010/984760.
20. Jensen JS, Björnelius E, Dohn B, Lidbrink P. Comparison of first void urine and urogenital swab specimens for detection of *Mycoplasma genitalium* and *Chlamydia trachomatis* by polymerase chain reaction in patients attending a sexually transmitted disease clinic. Sex Transm Dis. 2004;31(8):499–507.
21. Deguchi T, Hatazaki K, Ito S, Kondo H, Horie K, Nakane K, Mizutani K, Tsuchiya T, Yasuda M, Yokoi S, Nakano M. Macrolide and fluoroquinolone resistance is uncommon in clinical strains of *Chlamydia trachomatis*. J Infect Chemother. 2018. https://doi.org/10.1016/j.jiac.2018.03.007 **(Epub ahead of print)**.
22. Anderson T, Coughlan E, Werno A. *Mycoplasma genitalium* macrolide and fluoroquinolone resistance detection and clinical implications in a selected cohort in New Zealand. J Clin Microbiol. 2017;55(11):3242–8.

Coagulase gene polymorphism, enterotoxigenecity, biofilm production, and antibiotic resistance in *Staphylococcus aureus* isolated from bovine raw milk in North West India

Vishnu Sharma[1], Sanjita Sharma[1*], Dinesh Kumar Dahiya[1], Aarif Khan[1], Manisha Mathur[1] and Aayushi Sharma[2]

Abstract

Background: *Staphylococcus aureus* is the predominant bacterium responsible for various diseases in animals and humans. Preventive strategies could be better implemented by understanding the prevalence, genetic patterns, and the presence of enterotoxin and biofilm-producing genes along with the antibiotic susceptibility of this organism. This study was conducted in Rajasthan, the northwestern state of India, holding the largest population of cattle that makes it the second largest milk producer in India and no such prior information is available on these aspects.

Methods: A total of 368 individual quarter bovine raw milk samples were collected from 13 districts of Rajasthan, and screened for the presence of *S. aureus*. Microbiological and molecular approaches were followed for bacterial identification. Genetic diversity was determined by polymerase chain reaction-restriction fragment length polymorphism (PCR–RFLP) of coagulase gene (*coa*), whereas enterotoxin and biofilm-producing genes were studied by PCR analysis. Antibiotic strips were employed to study the antibiotic resistance among strains.

Results: In all, 73 *S. aureus* strains were obtained from 368 bovine raw milk samples out of that only 30 showed the presence of *coa*. Nine types of *coa* patterns ranging from 730 to 1130 bp were observed among these isolates. PCR–RFLP of *coa* distinguished the isolates into 15 genotypic patterns, of which patterns I, IV, V, and VI were predominant. Of the isolates, 30% were positive for *sec*, 10% for *sea*, and 3.3% for *seb*; these genes are responsible for enterotoxin production, whereas all isolates were found positive for *ica*AD and *eno*. The prevalence rates of other biofilm-producing genes *fnb*A, *clf*B, *ebp*S, *sas*G, *fnbB*, *sas*C, *cna*, *bap*, *fib* and, *bbp* were 97, 93, 90, 80, 80, 77, 53, 27, 10, and 6.6%, respectively. Twenty-seven (90%) strains were multidrug resistant, of which 15 were methicillin resistant. Maximum sensitivity was reported for kanamycin and it could be considered as a drug of choice for controlling *S. aureus* mediated cattle infections in the studied regions.

Conclusions: Overall, these strains could cause several diseases to humans, insisting the need for developing a stricter hygiene program for improving milking practices and animal health.

Keywords: *Staphylococcus aureus*, Coagulase gene polymorphism, RFLP, Biofilm, Enterotoxin, Antibiotic susceptibility

*Correspondence: drsanjitas@gmail.com
[1] Advanced Milk Testing Research Laboratory, Postgraduate Institute of Veterinary Education and Research, Rajasthan University of Veterinary and Animal Sciences at Bikaner, B-2 Bypass, Shiprapath, Mansarovar, Jaipur 302020, Rajasthan, India
Full list of author information is available at the end of the article

Background

The dairy sector in India has grown substantially over the years, making India the world's largest producer of milk [1], and Rajasthan, the northwestern state of India, has the largest number of cattle that makes it the second largest milk producer in India [2]. However, the yield of animals within the state is not satisfactory due to various production diseases and is understood as the major factor responsible for economic losses to the dairy industry in India [3, 4].

Subclinical mastitis (SCM) with no sign of inflammation is more severe than clinical forms and is responsible for a huge loss to the dairy industry [5, 6]. *Staphylococcus aureus* is a part of the normal gut microbiota [7] but is also a predominant microorganism implicated in clinical mastitis and SCM [8] and is difficult to eliminate. The pathogenic strains of *S. aureus* are generally coagulase positive and reported to cause illness in their host around the world [9]. From the infected udders, *S. aureus* directly passes into the raw milk and affects the quality of milk and makes the milk less suitable for further product formulations (e.g., cheese, paneer [a soft, white cheese]). In India, 85% of total milk produced is handled by the noncommercial sector [1]. Therefore, the direct consumption and transformation of such milk into traditional dairy foods increase the chances of associated infections because of improper storage and transportation facilities. The hygiene present in dairies and the literacy of handlers about safe milk production in Rajasthan are below satisfactory level [10]. For the effective control measures of *S. aureus*, its genetic characterization is necessary [11, 12]. Coagulase gene (*coa*) typing has been proven to be the most successful method to discriminate isolates at the strain level, recovered from different regions, mainly because of simple, accurate, and reproducible results obtained with this technique over other methods [13–15].

Multiple virulence factors have been suspected for the pathogenicity of *S. aureus*, among which the production of enterotoxins and toxic shock syndrome toxin–1 and the ability to form biofilms are important and worrisome for the food industry [16, 17]. Staphylococcal enterotoxins (SEs) are heat-stable; therefore, they may retain their biological activity even after pasteurization and various processing steps. An accidental ingestion of SEs causes several gastrointestinal disorders in the host [18].

Biofilm-producing *S. aureus* strains, especially the enterotoxigenic and antibiotic-resistant ones, are the major cause of several persistent bacterial diseases in the livestock sector, including mastitis [19]. During biofilm formation, initially, the bacteria adhere to each other by polysaccharide intercellular adhesion (PIA) and then propagate. The PIA is under the control of the *icaADBC* operon, and the strains possessing this gene cluster have been reported as strong biofilm producers [20]. In addition, several other surface markers have been reported to play a crucial role in biofilm formation, specifically called as microbial surface components recognizing adhesive matrix molecules (MSCRAMMs) such as collagen-binding protein (Cna) and elastin-binding protein (Ebps). The formation of biofilm also provides a shielding effect to the bacterium from antibiotic attacks.

To tackle *S. aureus*-mediated infections, antibiotics are used by veterinary professionals but their therapeutic outcomes are nearly insignificant because of the stubborn nature of the pathogen [21]. The frequent use of antibiotics leads to the evolution of antibiotic-resistance genes in *S. aureus* that can be easily transferred among healthier commensals and to other animals and humans by close interactions [9]. Studying the response of *S. aureus* to different relevant antibiotics gives the present drug resistance scenario from a region and the measure of associated risk factors. In addition, it may also help in selecting a more effective drug from a veterinary clinical point of view.

Therefore, the aims of this study were to check the prevalence of *S. aureus* from bovine raw milk samples and determine the genetic heterogeneity, virulence potential, and antimicrobial susceptibility of *S. aureus* from different regions of Rajasthan. These tasks were performed to generate useful information for field veterinarians and policy makers to form strategies for controlling *S. aureus*-mediated infections and ultimately improving the quality of milk.

Methods

Milk sampling and microbiological analysis

From May 2014 to November 2015, 368 individual quarter bovine raw milk samples were collected from 13 districts of Rajasthan, India (Fig. 1). The samples were randomly taken from clinically healthy animals. The samples were collected from different dairy herds, and before sampling, the teats of animals were cleaned with cotton balls soaked with 70% alcohol and the first few milliliters of milk were discarded. The samples were maintained at 4 °C before processing in a laboratory. The samples were serially diluted in 2% peptone water, and 100 μL of each sample was poured onto *S. aureus* chromogenic agar plates (HiMedia Laboratories, Mumbai, India) containing polymyxin B (50 unit/mL). After 24-h of incubation at 37 °C, *Staphylococcus* colonies showing blue-green color from each sample were transferred to brain heart infusion (BHI) broth. The chromogenic mixture present in the medium is specifically cleaved by *S. aureus* to produce blue-green colonies, which are clearly visible against the opaque background. For reconfirmation, the cultures were streaked on

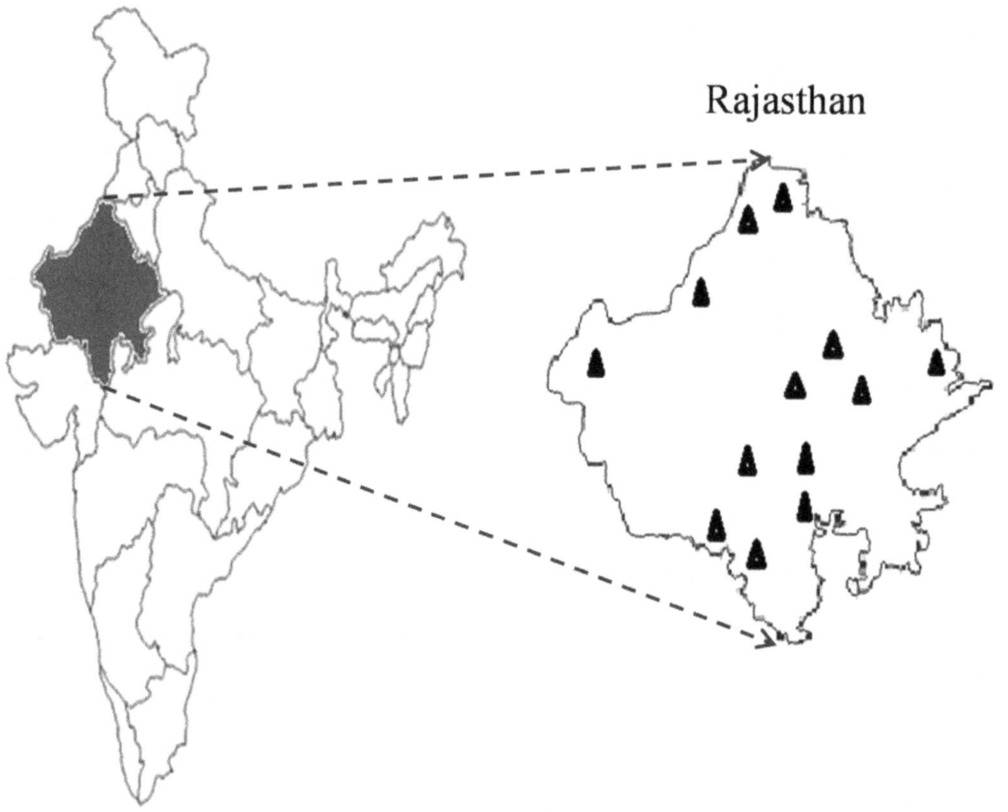

Fig. 1 Map of Rajasthan India showing the districts from where sampling was carried out

Mannitol salt agar and Baird Parker agar plates (Himedia Laboratories). Next, the colonies were examined for morphology after Gram staining and were confirmed using the API Staph kit (bioMeriux, Marcy-l'Etoile, France). Confirmed *S. aureus* colonies were examined for coagulase activity by tube plasma agglutination test. The presumptively identified *S. aureus* colonies were maintained at −80 °C in glycerol stocks for further analysis. A single colony was picked per positive sample and used to determine the prevalence rate among different samples. The isolates were coded conforming to their origin.

DNA extraction and purification

Genomic DNA was extracted from a freshly grown culture in BHI broth by using a modified method [22]. Briefly, 2 mL of overnight grown culture was centrifuged at 12,000×*g* for 10 min to form pellets. Afterwards, the pellets were resuspended in 200 μL of sucrose EDTA Tris (SET) buffer containing lysostaphin (100 μg/mL; Sigma, St. Louis, Missouri, USA) and lysozyme (100 μg/mL; Amersco, Solon, USA) for 1 h at 37 °C. The remaining procedure was similar as described elsewhere [22]. The extracted DNA was examined for purity and concentration using a microplate reader at 260 nm and thereafter stored at −20 °C.

All conventionally identified *S. aureus* were ascertained by species-specific primers (F 5′-CCATGTGTAGCGG TGAAATG-3′ and R 5′-TAAGGTTCTTCGCGTTG CTT-3′) obtained from the 16S rRNA region of *S. aureus* (GenBank accession number: KF993676.1) by using Primer 3 plus software. A 25-μL PCR reaction mixture consisting of 12.5 μL of 2X DreamTaq Green PCR Master Mix (Thermo Scientific, Mumbai, India), 0.5 μM of each primer, and 1 μL of template DNA was prepared and performed in a SureCycler 8800 Thermal Cycler (Agilent Technologies, New Delhi, India). Following program was used for PCR cycles: 2 min at 95 °C, followed by 35 cycles of 30 s at 95 °C, 45 s at 57 °C, and 60 s at 72 °C with a final extension of 10 min at 72 °C. A PCR product of approximately 306 bp signifies the presence of *S. aureus* isolates.

Using an earlier protocol, *coa* was identified in the *S. aureus* isolates [23]. The amplified products were electrophoresed on 2.0% agarose gel at 100 V for 1 h and photographed in a gel documentation system (BioRad Laboratories, Gurgaon, India). A suitable ladder was used as the size marker during electrophoresis.

Restriction enzyme digestion of PCR-amplified *coa* product

Of the PCR-amplified *coa* product, 10 μL was mixed with 17 μL of nuclease-free water, 2 μL of buffer Tango, and 1 μL of *Alu*I (Thermo Scientific) and incubated at 37 °C for 1 h for digestion. The digested products were resolved on 2.0% agarose gel and examined in a gel documentation system. A 100–1500-bp ladder (Promega, Wisconsin, USA) was used as the size marker for analyzing the digested *coa* fragments.

The generated Coa-RFLP patterns were analyzed by the BioNumerics (version 7.6) software package (Applied Maths, Sint-Martens-Latem, Belgium). A dendrogram was prepared by using the Dice-coefficient and the unweighted pair group method with arithmetic averages as the cluster analysis method.

Reproducibility testing

PCR reproducibility was analyzed by testing five isolates for five consecutive days. The PCR–RFLP reproducibility of *coa* was determined by digesting four products twice with the *Alu*I enzyme.

Calculating numerical index of discrimination

A numerical index equation was used to determine the discriminatory power of the typing method as described previously [24]. The following formula was used:

$$D = 1 - \frac{1}{N(N-1)} \sum_{j=1}^{s} nj(nj-1)$$

where D = discriminatory index, s = total number of different types, nj = number of isolates representing each type, and N = total number of isolates in the sample population.

Detection of enterotoxin and biofilm genes

The amplification of the genes coding for enterotoxins and biofilm production (Table 1) was performed using the multiplex PCR method [25, 26].

Determination of minimum inhibitory concentration

The minimum inhibitory concentration (MIC) of all *S. aureus* isolates was determined using E-strips as per the manufacturer's instructions after adjusting their OD to McFarland 0.5 as disclosed previously [27]. The results obtained were analyzed according to CLSI guidelines [28]. The MIC E-strips (0.016–256 μg/mL) (HiMedia Laboratories) were used for susceptibility observation. The antimicrobials used were according to the information collected from the field veterinarians and practicing clinicians. *S. aureus* ATCC 29213 was used as the reference strain for quality control. Methicillin-resistant *S. aureus* (MRSA)-positive strains were further confirmed on HiCrome MeReSa Agar (HiMedia Laboratories) and validated by the amplification of *mec*A by PCR [29].

Results

Out of 368 bovine raw milk samples, *S. aureus* contamination was present in 73 (19.84%) samples (Table 2) as revealed by media plating analysis. All 73 isolates were found as *S. aureus* in API analysis. Out of the 73 isolates, 30 (41.1%) showed coagulase activity and were further confirmed as *S. aureus* by PCR. Furthermore, all these phenotypically coagulase-positive *S. aureus* scored positive for *coa* during PCR analysis (Fig. 2). Nine types of *coa* patterns ranging from 730 to 1130 bp were observed (Table 3), and the sizes, 820 and 920 bp, were the most predominantly noticed product sizes, accounting altogether for 67% of the total *coa*-positive isolates (Table 3). Twenty-seven isolates depicted one PCR band while three isolates (15, 17, and 19) depicted double bands (Fig. 2). The polymorphism in *coa* was studied by RFLP (Fig. 3), where fifteen (I–XV) RFLP patterns (Table 3 and Fig. 4) were observed. RFLP patterns I, IV, V, and VI were the dominant patterns being noticed in three (10%), three (10%), six (20%), and four (13.3%) isolates, respectively (Table 3). The isolates with the most predominant pattern (V) displayed two DNA fragments of 540 and 260 bp. The isolates with pattern VI had DNA fragments of 565 and 270 bp. The isolates with patterns I and IV had DNA fragments of 430 and 260 bp and 528 and 250 bp, respectively. Rest all other remaining patterns were shown by a single (II, VII, X, XI, XII, and XIV) or two (VIII, IX, and XIII) isolates. The reproducibility of the PCR products and *coa* PCR–RFLP was demonstrated with 100% of the repeatedly tested isolates; however, the results showed some variations in the intensity of bands.

The discriminatory index for the *Alu*I RFLP method was about 0.80, indicating a fair discriminatory power of this method for typing *S. aureus*. Further RFLP analysis classified the 30 *S. aureus* strains into five major clusters designated as A, B, C, D, and E (Fig. 4). The dendrogram depicted that cluster A was 40% similar to other clusters (B-D) and was composed of isolates obtained from eight regions. Cluster B was 52% identical with clusters C to E and was composed of isolates obtained from three regions. Similarly, cluster C with approximately 82% identity with clusters D and E included isolates from four regions. Cluster D was composed of five isolates obtained from two regions. The remaining cluster E was composed of only one isolate that was derived from a totally different region.

Of the analyzed enterotoxin genes, 30% isolates were positive for *sec*, 10% for *sea*, and 3.3% for *seb* (Table 4). No isolate was detected harboring the remaining enterotoxin genes.

Table 1 Primers used for detection of *S. aureus* enterotoxin and biofilm genes

Gene	Primer sequence (5′–3′)	Product size (bp)	Multiplex PCR set
sea[a]	GGTTATCAATGTGCGGGTGG CGGCACTTTTTTCTCTTCGG	102	A
seb[a]	GTATGGTGGTGTAACTGAGC CCAAATAGTGACGAGTTAGG	164	A
sec[a]	AGATGAAGTAGTTGATGTGTATGG CACACTTTTAGAATCAACCG	451	A
sed[a]	CCAATAATAGGAGAAAATAAAAG ATTGGTATTTTTTTTCGTTC	278	A
see[a]	AGGTTTTTTCACAGGTCATCC CTTTTTTTTCTTCGGTCAATC	209	A
eta[a]	GCAGGTGTTGATTTAGCATT AGATGTCCCTATTTTTGCTG	93	B
etb[a]	ACAAGCAAAAGAATACAGCG GTTTTTGGCTGCTTCTCTTG	226	B
tst[a]	ACCCCTGTTCCCTTATCATC TTTTCAGTATTTGTAACGCC	326	B
bap[b]	GAGCCAAGACAAAGGTGAAG GTAGCCATAGCACGGAACAT	873	
bbp[b]	CTTAGCAGTTCAACAGGGTG TTGGCTTTATTGTGATGGTC	1662	
cna[b]	CGATAACATCTGGGAATAAA ATAGTCTCCACTAGGCAACG	716	
clfA[b]	AGTACCAAATGAGGCTGTTC AAATGCTACTTCGTTGTCCC	796	
clfB[b]	CACTTACTTTACCGCTACTTTC AACGAGCAATACCACTACAACAG	968	
ebpS[b]	GGTGAACCTGAACCGTAG CTGGCAAGGCGAATAACT	661	
eno[b]	GTCGTGCATTAGTACCATCAGG TTTCCAACCATCCCAGTCG	812	
fib[b]	AGATGCGAGCGAAGGGTA TAAACGAAACTAAGTTGACTGC	347	
fnbpA[b]	TCCGCCGAACAACATACC TCAAGCACAAGGACCAAT	952	
fnbpB[b]	TCTGCGTTATGAGGATTT ACAGTAGAGGAAAGTGGG	452	
icaAD[b]	TGGCTACTGGGATACTGATA TGGAAATGCGACAAGAACTA	520	
icaBC[b]	GCCTATCCTTATGGCTTGA TGGAATCCGTCCCATCTC	182	
sasC[b]	AGAATGAAGTCCGATAGAGT AATCATACAGATGGCAATAC	936	
sasG[b]	TATCAACACTTCCGTAACCTTC CGTCAGTCACTCATAACGCAGA	159	

[a] Represents the enterotoxin genes while [b] depicts the biofilm genes

Regarding biofilm-encoding genes, all isolates typed 100% positive for *ica*AD, *ica*BC, and *eno* (Table 5). The prevalence rates of *fnb*A, *clf*B, *ebp*S, *sas*G, *fnbB, sas*C, *cna, bap, fib,* and *bbp* were 97, 93, 90, 80, 80, 53, 77, 27, 10, and 6.6%, respectively. Low prevalence was noticed for *clf*A (3.3%) as only one isolate was found positive for this gene.

Antibiotic susceptibility test revealed that 27 (90%) isolates were resistant to penicillin, 23 (77%) to ampicillin, 17 (57%) to amikacin, 15 (50%) to oxacillin, 12 (40%) to ciprofloxacin, 9 (30%) to azithromycin, and 7 (23%) to piperacillin (Table 6). Five (17%) isolates showed resistance to linezolid and tetracycline; 3 (10%) to gatifloxacin and rifampicin; 2 (7%) to ceftazidime, chloramphenicol, and norfloxacin; and 1 (3%) to gentamicin, teicoplanin, and vancomycin (Table 6). Intermediate resistance to amikacin, azithromycin, ceftazidime, ceftriaxone, chloramphenicol, ciprofloxacin, gatifloxacin, gentamicin,

Table 2 Details of samples contaminated with *S. aureus* and their prevalence

Sampling districts/ regions	No. of raw milk samples collected	No. of positive samples (% prevalence)
Ajmer	28	4 (1.09)
Bharatpur	28	7 (1.90)
Bhilwara	28	3 (0.82)
Bikaner	28	2 (0.54)
Chittorgarh	28	4 (1.09)
Hanumangarh	28	7 (1.90)
Jaipur	30	5 (1.36)
Mount Abu	28	8 (2.17)
Pali	28	6 (1.63)
Sirohi	30	13 (3.53)
Sikar	28	5 (1.36)
Shri-Ganganagar	28	6 (1.63)
Udaipur	28	3 (0.82)
Total	368	73 (19.84)

teicoplanin, and vancomycin was shown by 1 (3%), 1 (3%), 2 (7%), 3 (10%), 2 (7%), 4 (13%), 3 (10%), 1 (3%), 1 (3%), and 3 (10%) isolates, respectively. Twenty-seven (90%) of the strains tested showed multiple drug resistance (complete or intermediate) to three or more antibiotics. All isolates were completely (100%) sensitive to kanamycin. Additionally, 15 strains were resistant to oxacillin, penicillin, and ampicillin along with other antibiotics and were considered as MRSA strains [9]. All 15 strains further showed their presence on MeReSa Agar and found positive for *mecA* (Fig. 5).

Discussion

In this study, the prevalence, genetic patterns, pathogenic potential, and antibiotic susceptibility of *S. aureus* recovered from 13 districts of Rajasthan, India, were discussed. Our results indicated that 19.84% of milk samples were positive for *S. aureus*, and to the best of our knowledge, this is the first comprehensive study from Rajasthan. Similar findings concerning the prevalence of *S. aureus* in bovine raw milk samples were reported from different sub-parts of India; however, the prevalence rate varied greatly among the studies [30–36]. Of note, moderate prevalence was reported in the present study. We posit that inadequate hygiene and inferior management practices facilitate the entry of microorganisms to udders and concomitantly the shedding of microorganisms into milk.

The phenotypic method is not sufficient for categorizing between coagulase-positive and -negative *S. aureus*

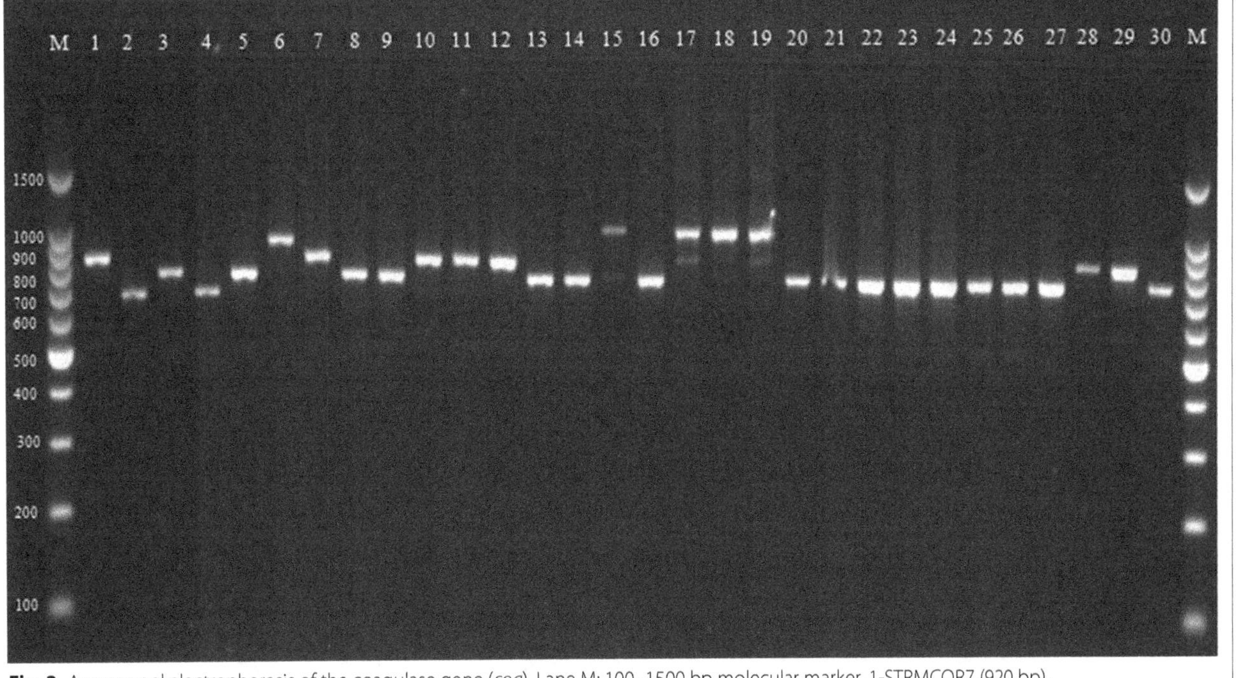

Fig. 2 Agarose gel electrophoresis of the coagulase gene (*coa*). Lane M; 100–1500 bp molecular marker, 1-STRMCOR7 (920 bp), 2-STRMPL47(730 bp), 3-STRMSH56 (820 bp), 4-STRMBHL57 (750 bp), 5-STRMSH58 (820 bp), 6-STRMHMO59 (1060 bp), 7-STRMUDZ70 (920 bp), 8-STRMSH73 (820 bp), 9-STRMSH74 (820 bp), 10-STRMHMO79 (920 bp), 11-STRMSH37 (920 bp), 12-STRMSH42 (920p), 13-STRMMA11 (820 bp), 14-STRMMA20 (820p), 15-STRMUDZ2 (1130 bp) 16-STRMMA3 (820 bp), 17-STRMSGNR64 (1130 bp), 18-STRMSGNR19 (1130 bp), 19-STRMUDZ6 (1130 bp), 20-STRMBKN5 (820 bp), 21-STRMSK96 (820 bp), 22-STRMSK98 (820 bp), 23-STRMSK100 (820 bp), 24-STRMBP11 (820 bp), 25-STRMB12 (820 bp), 26-STRMJ102 (820 bp), 27-STRMJ3 (820 bp), 28-STRMP23 (920 bp), 29-STRMSGNR9 (880 bp), 30-STAJM33 (800 bp)

Table 3 Genotype distributions of *S. aureus* cultures obtained from different regions of Rajasthan and their RFLP patterns

Coa gene PCR product (bp)	RFLP pattern	n	Isolate name	Isolated region	Genotype code/ distinct RFLP pattern
730	430-260	1	STRMPL47	PL; Pali	I
750	620	1	STRMBHL57	BHL; Bhilwara	II
800	420-240	1	STAJM33	AJM; Ajmer	III
820	528-250	3	STRMBP12, STRMJ102, STRMJ3	BP; Bharatpur, J; Jaipur	IV
820	540-260	6	STRMMA20, STRMMA3, STRMSK96, STRMSK 98, STRMSK100, STRMBP11	SH; Sirohi MA; Mount abu, SK; Sikar, BP; Bharatpur	V
820	565-270	4	STRMSH56, STRMSH58, STRMSH73, STRMSH74	SH; Sirohi	VI
820	430-260	1	STRMMA11	MA; Mount abu	I
820	440-360	1	STRMBKN5	BKN; Bikaner	VII
880	420-330	1	STRMSGNR9	SGNR; Shri-Ganganagar	VIII
920	440-260-170	2	STRMSH37, STRMSH42	SH; Sirohi	IX
920	420-330	1	STRMPL23	PL: Pali	VIII
920	462-373	1	STRMHMO79	HMO; Hanumangarh	X
920	425-260	1	STRMCOR7	COR; Chittorgarh	I
940	452-273-186	1	STRMUDZ70	UDZ; Udaipur	XI
1060	540-350	1	STRMHMO59	HMO; Hanumangarh	XII
1130	445-360-170	2	STRMSGNR19, STRMUDZ6	SGNR; Shri-Ganganagar, UDZ; Udaipur	XIII
1130	452-370-175	1	STRMSGNR64	SGNR; Shri-Ganganagar	XIV
1130	460-380-182	1	STRMUDZ2	UDZ; Udaipur	XV

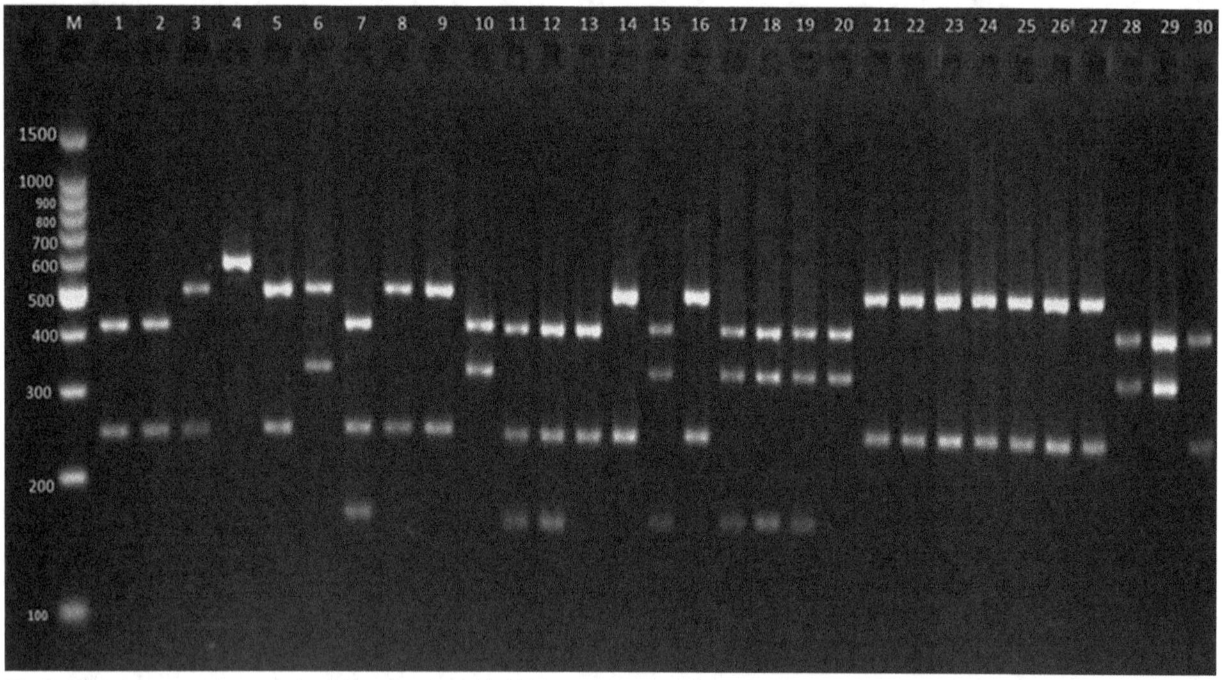

Fig. 3 RFLP of the coagulase gene (coa) after digestion with *AluI*. Lane M; 100–1500 bp molecular marker, 1-STRMCOR7, 2-STRMPL47, 3-STRMSH56, 4-STRMBHL57, 5-STRMSH58, 6-STRMHMO59, 7-STRMUDZ70, 8-STRMSH73, 9-STRMSH74, 10-STRMHMO79, 11-STRMSH37, 12-STRMSH42, 13-STRMMA11, 14-STRMMA20, 15-STRMUDZ2, 16-STRMMA3, 17-STRMSGNR64, 18-STRMSGNR19, 19-STRMUDZ6, 20-STRMBKN5, 21-STRMSK96, 22-STRMSK98, 23-STRMSK100, 24-STRMBP11, 25-STRMB12, 26-STRMJ102, 27-STRMJ3, 28-STRMP23, 29-STRMSGNR9, 30-STAJM33

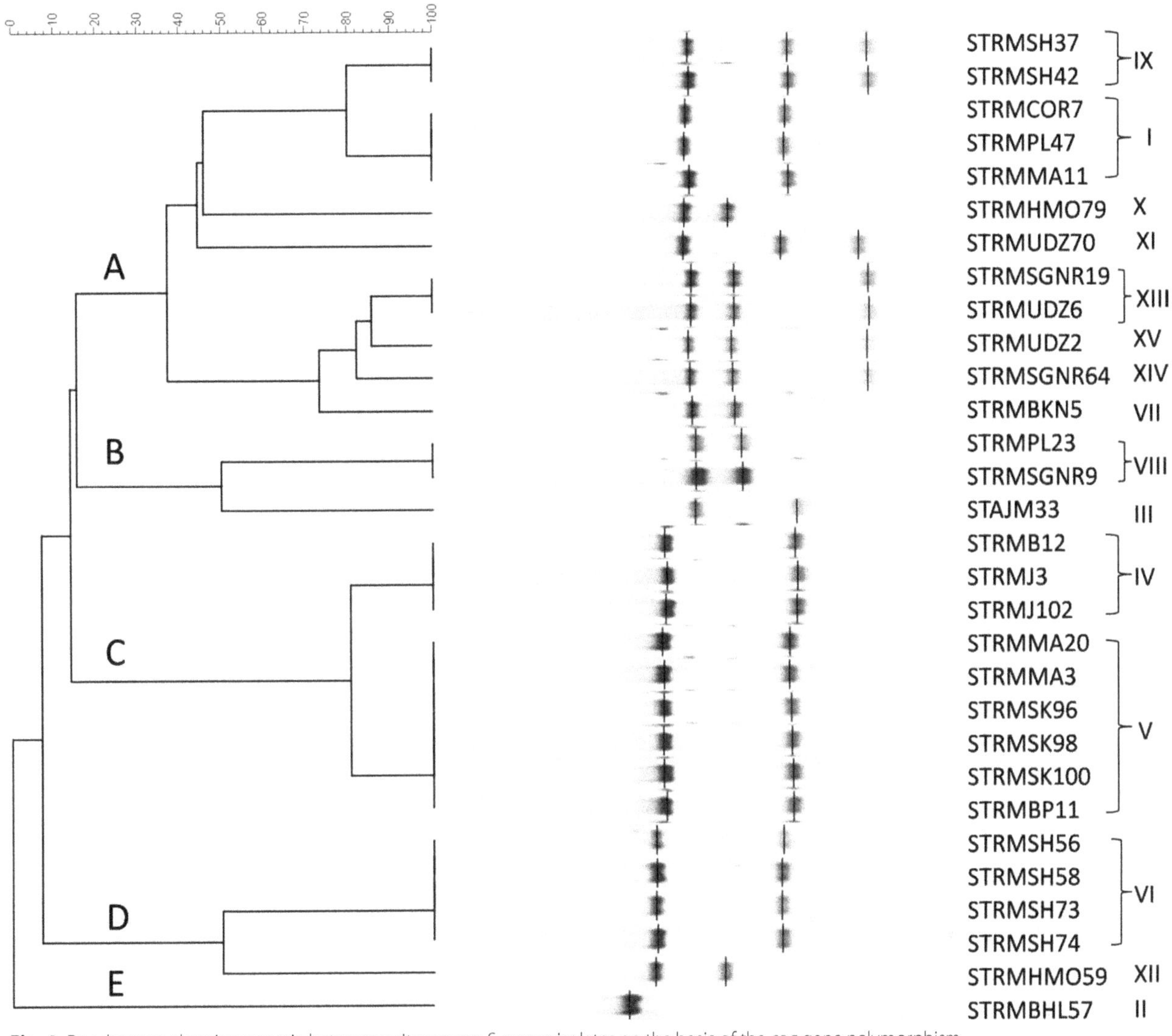

Fig. 4 Dendrogram showing genetic heterogeneity among *S. aureus* isolates on the basis of the *coa* gene polymorphism

isolates [37]. Therefore, we examined the isolates for the *coa* presence by PCR. Nine *coa* PCR types were obtained, signifying considerable variation among the *S. aureus* types and this finding is in agreement with others [14, 23, 38]. The precise reason for this high rate of polymorphism observed among the strains is debatable. However, because of the presence of a series of 81-bp tandem repeats in the 3′-end region of *coa*, the high rate of polymorphism possibly alters the antigenic properties of the gene. Therefore, the gene's conformity is possibly recognized as the topmost reason behind the failure in the action of neutralizing antibodies [39]. A double band for *coa* was also visualized among three isolates, indicating the existence of distinct allelic forms of *coa*. The appropriate reason behind this distinct *coa* pattern is linked to the production of more than one immunologic form of the coagulase protein by some *S. aureus* isolates [23], although this pattern is rarely observed and only a few authors have reported it [38, 40].

In the present study, the digestion of the different *coa* amplicons with *Alu*I reveals considerable genetic variability as it classifies them into 15 patterns. The findings are similar to those of others [14, 23, 41] who found a considerable degree of variability in *coa* RFLP patterns after digestion with the same enzyme, although the sizes of PCR products obtained here were almost different from those in earlier studies. Besides, the typing method opted for the discrimination was found full-proof as it displayed a fairly good discriminatory power, i.e., of 0.80 and is supported by the findings of Sarvari et al. [15] who

Table 4 Results of enterotoxins genes in *S. aureus* isolates

Isolates (n = 30)	*sea*	*seb*	*sec*	*sed*	*see*	*eta*	*etb*	*tst*
STRMPL47	–	+	–	–	–	–	–	–
STRMPL23	–	–	–	–	–	–	–	–
STRMBHL57	+	–	+	–	–	–	–	–
STAJM33	–	–	–	–	–	–	–	–
STRMSH56	–	–	+	–	–	–	–	–
STRMSH58	–	–	–	–	–	–	–	–
STRMSH73	–	–	–	–	–	–	–	–
STRMSH74	–	–	+	–	–	–	–	–
STRMSH37	–	–	–	–	–	–	–	–
STRMSH42	–	–	–	–	–	–	–	–
STRMMA20	–	–	–	–	–	–	–	–
STRMMA3	–	–	–	–	–	–	–	–
STRMMA11	–	–	+	–	–	–	–	–
STRMSK96	–	–	–	–	–	–	–	–
STRMSK 98	–	–	–	–	–	–	–	–
STRMSK100	–	–	–	–	–	–	–	–
STRMBP11	+	–	+	–	–	–	–	–
STRMBP12	–	–	–	–	–	–	–	–
STRMJ102	–	–	–	–	–	–	–	–
STRMJ3	–	–	–	–	–	–	–	–
STRMBKN5	–	–	+	–	–	–	–	–
STRMSGNR9	–	–	–	–	–	–	–	–
STRMSGNR19	–	–	–	–	–	–	–	–
STRMSGNR64	+	–	+	–	–	–	–	–
STRMCOR7	–	–	–	–	–	–	–	–
STRMHMO79	–	–	–	–	–	–	–	–
STRMHMO59	–	–	+	–	–	–	–	–
STRMUDZ70	–	–	+	–	–	–	–	–
STRMUDZ2	–	–	–	–	–	–	–	–
STRMUDZ6	–	–	–	–	–	–	–	–
Occurrence (%)	10	3.3	30	0	0	0	0	0

obtained a discriminatory index of 0.82 among *S. aureus* isolates.

As mentioned earlier, the study segregated all 30 *S. aureus* isolates into five clusters (A–E), among which patterns I, IV, V, and VI were predominant. Most patterns belonged to clusters A and C. This indicates weak to no heterogeneity in the *Alu*I recognition sites among the isolates of these predominant patterns. Momtaz et al. [14] found that out of 42 *coa*-positive *S. aureus* isolates, 31 (73.8%) belonged to genotype pattern I and 11 (26%) to II. Likewise, in another study [39], pattern I was found predominant. These findings support our results and justify that in a particular geographical region a predominant genotype is present because of prevailing favorable environmental conditions. Besides, the internal resistance of strains toward the host immune system also substantially plays an important role in the strain's dominance. The predominant isolates from a region have possibly evolved mechanisms to bypass the host phagocytosis than the isolates with rare genotypes [42, 43]. Furthermore, the existence of a similar RFLP pattern for intra-regional strains in genotypes, I, IV, V, VI, VIII, IX, and XIII suggests the possibility of transmission of some strains from one region to another during the transportation of milk.

Next, we tested all isolates for enterotoxin-producing genes and none of them from Ajmer, Jaipur, and Chittorgarh regions scored positive for these genes. In our study, the genes for toxins (*sed, see, eta, etb,* and *tst*) were not amplified in any of the 30 isolates. Enterotoxins contribute to the pathogenesis of *S. aureus* by modulating immunity and susceptibility to antibiotics resulting in the onset of many diseases [44]. The reports concerning

Table 5 Results of adhesion genes typed in *S. aureus* isolates

Isolates (n = 30)	*ica*AD	*ica*BC	*clf*B	*clf*A	*fnb*A	*fnb*B	*ebpS*	*eno*	*fib*	*sas*G	*sas*C	*bbp*	*bap*	*cna*
STRMPL47	+	+	+	−	+	+	+	+	−	−	−	−	−	−
STRMPL23	+	+	+	−	+	+	+	+	−	+	−	−	−	+
STRMBHL57	+	+	+	−	+	+	+	+	+	+	+	+	+	+
STAJM33	+	+	+	−	+	+	+	+	−	+	−	−	−	−
STRMSH56	+	+	+	−	+	+	+	+	−	+	+	−	−	+
STRMSH58	+	+	+	−	+	+	+	+	−	+	+	−	−	+
STRMSH73	+	+	+	−	+	+	+	+	−	+	−	−	−	+
STRMSH74	+	+	+	−	+	+	+	+	−	+	+	−	+	+
STRMSH37	+	+	+	−	+	+	+	+	−	+	+	−	−	+
STRMSH42	+	+	+	−	+	−	−	+	−	+	−	−	−	−
STRMMA20	+	+	+	−	+	+	+	+	−	+	−	−	−	+
STRMMA3	+	+	+	−	+	−	+	+	−	−	−	−	−	−
STRMMA11	+	+	+	−	+	+	+	+	−	+	+	−	−	+
STRMSK96	+	+	+	−	+	+	+	+	−	+	+	−	−	+
STRMSK 98	+	+	+	−	+	+	+	+	−	+	−	−	−	+
STRMSK100	+	+	+	−	+	+	+	+	−	+	+	−	−	+
STRMBP11	+	+	+	+	+	+	+	+	+	+	+	+	+	+
STRMBP12	+	+	+	−	+	+	+	+	−	+	+	−	+	+
STRMJ102	+	+	−	−	−	−	−	+	−	−	−	−	−	−
STRMJ3	+	+	+	−	+	+	+	+	−	+	+	−	−	+
STRMBKN5	+	+	+	−	+	−	+	+	−	+	−	−	−	+
STRMSGNR9	+	+	+	−	+	+	+	+	+	+	+	−	+	+
STRMSGNR19	+	+	+	−	+	+	+	+	−	+	+	−	+	+
STRMSGNR64	+	+	+	−	+	−	+	+	−	−	−	−	−	+
STRMCOR7	+	+	+	−	+	+	+	+	−	+	+	−	−	+
STRMHMO79	+	+	+	−	+	+	+	+	−	+	+	−	+	+
STRMHMO59	+	+	−	−	+	−	−	+	−	−	−	−	−	−
STRMUDZ70	+	+	+	−	+	+	+	+	−	+	−	−	−	+
STRMUDZ2	+	+	+	−	+	+	+	+	−	+	+	−	+	+
STRMUDZ6	+	+	+	−	+	+	+	+	−	−	−	−	−	−
Occurrence (%)	100	100	93	3.3	97	80	90	100	10	80	53	6.6	27	77

the presence of enterotoxin-producing genes (*sea*, *seb*, *sec*, *sed*, and *see*) among *S. aureus* strains isolated from milk of animals with bovine mastitis concur with our findings [44]. Here, we did not find the presence of *eta* and *etb* exfoliative genes, and these results are in agreement with previous studies [11, 44, 45], which inferred that *S. aureus* strains isolated from animals with mastitis were rarely found positive for exfoliative toxins. Similarly, the presence of *tsst–1* was not observed in any isolate, although its prevalence in isolates from cattle with mastitis was reported in conjunction with *sec* and *sed* [44].

Most information about the ability of *S. aureus* to form biofilms is restricted to the isolates recovered from clinical studies or medical devices, and insufficient information is available for bovine milk-derived isolates. Therefore, we studied MSCRAMM genes to understand their prevalence. The products of these genes aid the bacterium to adhere to the host components and produce biofilm. Previous studies on MSCRAMM genes in *Enterococcus faecium*, *S. saprophyticus*, and *S. aureus* mention that instead of their active role in biofilm development, some gene products are also involved in pathogenesis. Here, a great diversity in the presence of biofilm-producing genes was observed among the isolates recovered from different regions. The complete dominance was observed for *icaAD* and *eno* responsible for polysaccharide intracellular adhesion and laminin-binding proteins that have a crucial role in bovine mastitis pathogenesis [46]. These findings are in agreement with previous studies [26, 45, 47] that reported higher prevalence rates for these genes. *fnb*A and *fnb*B that are usually associated with invasive diseases [48] were also

Table 6 Antibiotic susceptibility patterns of *S. aureus* isolates

Isolates (n = 30)	Antibiotics																			
	Ami-kacin	Amox-yclav	Ampi-cillin	Azithro-mycin	Cef-tazi-dime	Cef-triax-one	Chlo-ram-phen-icol	Cipro-floxa-cin	Gati-floxa-cin	Gen-tamicin	Kana-mycin	Line-zolid	Nor-floxa-cin	Oxa-cillin	Peni-cillin	Piper-acillin	Rifampcin	Teico-planin	Tetra-cyclin	Vanco-mycin
STRMPL47	R	R	S	S	S	S	S	R	S	S	S	R	S	S	R	R	S	S	S	I
STRMPL23	S	S	R	S	S	S	S	S	S	S	S	S	S	S	R	S	R	S	S	S
STRMBHL57	I	R	R	S	S	S	S	S	S	S	S	R	S	S	R	R	S	S	S	S
STAJM33	R	R	R	S	S	S	S	I	S	R	S	S	S	S	R	R	S	S	S	S
STRMSH56	R	S	R	S	S	S	S	I	I	S	S	S	S	S	R	R	S	S	S	S
STRMSH58	S	S	S	S	S	S	S	S	S	S	S	S	S	S	R	R	S	S	S	S
STRMSH73	R	S	R	R	S	S	S	R	S	S	S	R	S	S	R	S	S	S	S	S
STRMSH74	R	S	R	S	R	S	S	R	S	S	S	S	S	R	R	S	S	S	R	R
STRMSH37	R	S	R	S	S	S	R	S	S	S	S	S	S	R	R	S	S	S	R	S
STRMSH42	S	S	S	S	S	S	S	S	R	S	S	S	S	S	R	S	S	S	S	S
STRMMA20	R	S	R	S	S	S	S	R	R	S	S	S	S	R	R	S	S	S	S	S
STRMMA3	R	S	R	R	I	S	S	R	S	S	S	S	S	R	R	S	S	R	S	S
STRMMA11	R	S	R	R	S	S	S	I	S	S	S	S	S	R	R	S	S	S	S	S
STRMSK96	S	S	S	S	S	S	S	R	S	S	S	S	S	S	R	S	S	I	S	S
STRMSK 98	R	S	R	R	S	S	S	R	S	S	S	S	S	R	R	S	S	S	S	S
STRMSK100	R	S	R	I	S	I	S	R	S	S	S	S	R	S	R	S	S	S	S	S
STRMBP11	R	S	R	S	S	S	S	S	S	S	S	R	R	R	R	S	S	S	S	S
STRMBP12	R	R	R	R	R	S	I	R	I	S	S	S	S	R	R	S	S	S	S	S
STRMJ102	R	S	S	S	S	S	R	R	S	S	S	S	S	S	S	R	S	S	S	I
STRMJ3	R	S	R	R	I	I	S	I	S	S	S	S	S	R	R	S	S	S	R	S
STRMBKN5	R	S	R	R	S	S	S	S	S	S	S	S	S	R	R	S	S	S	S	S
STRMSGNR9	S	S	R	R	S	S	S	S	S	S	S	S	S	S	S	S	S	S	R	S
STRMSGNR19	S	S	R	S	S	I	S	S	S	S	S	S	S	R	R	S	S	S	S	S
STRMSGNR64	S	S	R	S	S	S	S	S	S	S	S	R	S	R	R	S	R	S	S	S
STRMCOR7	S	R	R	S	S	S	S	S	I	S	S	S	S	R	R	S	S	S	S	S
STRMHMO59	R	S	S	S	S	S	S	R	S	I	S	S	S	S	R	S	S	S	S	S
STRMHMO79	S	R	R	S	S	S	S	S	S	S	S	S	S	S	R	S	R	S	S	I
STRMUDZ70	S	R	S	S	S	S	S	S	S	S	S	S	S	S	S	S	S	S	S	S
STRMUDZ2	S	S	R	S	S	S	I	R	R	S	S	S	S	R	R	S	S	S	R	S
STRMUDZ6	S	R	R	R	S	S	S	S	S	S	S	S	S	R	R	R	S	S	S	S
Sensitive	12	22	07	20	26	27	26	14	24	28	30	25	28	15	03	23	27	28	25	26
Intermediate	01	0	0	01	02	03	02	04	03	01	0	0	0	0	0	0	0	01	0	03
Resistant	17	08	23	09	02	0	02	12	03	01	0	05	02	15	27	07	03	01	05	01

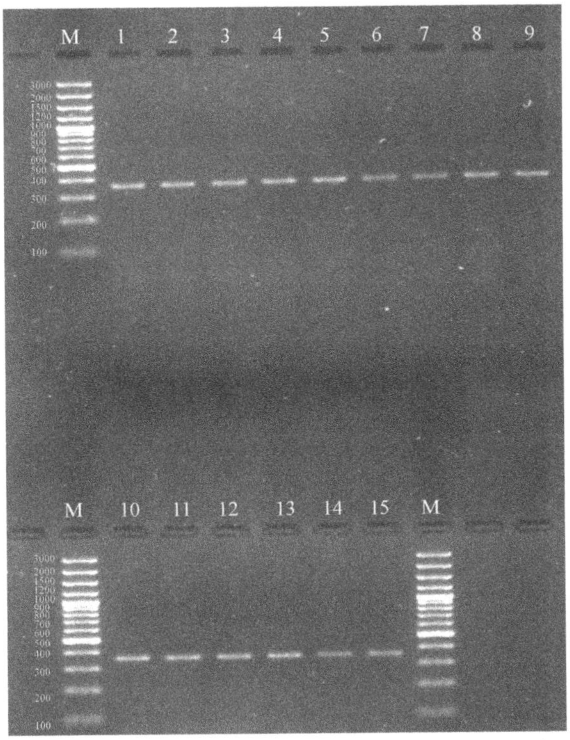

Fig. 5 Agarose gel photograph showing the MRSA positive samples. Lane M; 100–3000 bp molecular marker, 1-STRMSH74, 2-STRMSH37, 3-STRMMA20, 4-STRMMA3, 5-STRMMA11, 6-STRMSK98, 7-STRMBP11, 8-STRMBP12, 9-STRMJ3, 10-STRMBKN5, 11-STRMSGNR19, 12-STRMSGNR64, 13-STRMUDZ2, 14-STRMUDZ2, 15-STRMUDZ6

found abundantly (97 and 80%, respectively) among the isolates in this study; these rates are comparable to those in other studies [20, 26]. Similarly, *clfB* encoding an Fn-binding protein that facilitates *S. aureus* to establish nasal colonization [49] was also present in most (93%) strains. Proteins EbpS, SasG, and SasC, which play a considerable role in maintaining cell density, biofilm accumulation, and intercellular adhesion, were present in 90, 80, and 53% of isolates, respectively. These findings are comparable and in complete agreement with the findings of Tang et al. [26] who noticed a high prevalence of these genes. Another collagen-binding protein, Cna, which has been associated with virulence potential in rabbit models [48], was identified in 77% of isolates; this value is comparably higher than that reported by Pereyra et al. [50] but lower than others [20, 26]. Gene *bbp*, which is often found in the clinical strains of *S. aureus* and linked with bone infections, was only typed in a few (6.6%) isolates. The result is in accordance with the findings of Kot et al. [51] and Puacz et al. [52] who detected the presence of *bbp* in a few isolates of mastitis origin. Gene *bap*, whose protein was probably the first protein elucidated to have a role in biofilm formation in *S. aureus* and associated with chronic bovine mastitis, was present in 7% of isolates. This finding is consistent with the observations of Darwish and Asfour [45], who observed the presence of *bap* in 2.5 and 4.4% of *S. aureus* and coagulase-negative *S. aureus* isolates, respectively. Another gene *fib*, elucidated to have a crucial role in binding to extracellular matrix fibrinogen, was also detected in 10% of isolates. This finding is different from the findings of Pereyra et al. [50] and Zuniga et al. [53] who reported a higher prevalence of 90 and 71.7%, respectively. Altogether, our results suggest that most strains had the biofilm-forming ability, which may facilitate in establishing intramammary gland infections in cattle. Moreover, this property varies from strain to strain and depends on the genetic composition and geographical evolution.

In the present study, the observed antibiotic resistance level was relatively high (90%) and two strains (STRMSH74 and STRMBP12) from Sirohi and Bharatpur, respectively, were found to be most resistant. MRSA-positive strains were observed from each area except for Pali, Bhilwara, and Hanumangarh; this finding is in agreement with studies reporting varied MRSA prevalence in bovine milk [9, 43, 54]. No similarities in resistance patterns were observed among the strains from different regions except for one strain each from Jaipur (STRMJ3) and Bikaner (STRMBKN5). The inconsistencies in the resistance profile observed might be due to the excessive, indiscriminate use of a particular antibiotic in each geographical region for combating infections. This fact was established by similar findings in studies undertaken in the United States and European countries, where a lower resistance profile among *S. aureus* isolates was noticed because of stricter use of antibiotics in veterinary practice [54]. In Rajasthan, β-lactams, macrolides, aminopenicillins, cephalosporins, aminoglycosides, fluoroquinolones, tetracyclines, and amphenicols are frequently used in veterinary clinical practices. However, resistance toward the less commonly used antibiotics such as vancomycin, teicoplanin, and rifampicin in veterinary practice is not fully understood. This is possibly due to the contamination from human handlers [18], as strains with rare and high antibiogram patterns were generally isolated from hospital settings because of a high antimicrobial pressure [54]. Earlier, vancomycin-resistant enterococci strains were isolated from tertiary care hospitals in Rajasthan [55, 56], and it was proved that the gene cluster VanA was transferable from *E. faecalis* to *S. aureus* [57]. Similarly, teicoplanin-resistant *S. aureus* strains were reported from a hospital in Jaipur, Rajasthan [57]. Thus, considerable attention is needed for treating the vancomycin-resistant MRSA-induced infection. Based on our results, all strains were sensitive to kanamycin, and it could be the drug of choice to treat *S. aureus* mediated infections.

Overall, our results clearly indicate that bovine raw milk samples collected from different regions of Rajasthan were contaminated with coagulase-positive strains of *S. aureus*. Considerable variability in *coa* was observed, and genotypes I, IV, V, and VI were predominant. The close similarity in the RFLP pattern among the isolates of different regions suggested the transmission of isolates from one place to another by various means. The presence of enterotoxin and biofilm-producing genes among these strains poses a potential public health risk, as these strains may be implicated in milk-borne intoxications. Furthermore, the presence of multidrug-resistant and MRSA strains indicates the improper use of antibiotics for mastitis control and is a growing health concern globally. However, all strains were found susceptible to kanamycin, and it can be referred to as a drug of choice in case of mastitis infections in the regions included in the study. The information generated here might be useful for concerned veterinarians in improving cattle health and designing strategies for better and safe milk production. This will not only lower the risk of associated food poisoning but also prevent the spread of antibiotic resistance in the regions. Future research is warranted to establish the relationship between the presence of these strains in milk and their ability to cause infections in humans.

Authors' contributions

SS and VS provide the financial support, proof-read the manuscript. DKD conceived the idea and wrote the manuscript and proof-read it. AK, MM and AS perform the experiments and help in proof-reading. All authors read and approved the final manuscript.

Author details

[1] Advanced Milk Testing Research Laboratory, Postgraduate Institute of Veterinary Education and Research, Rajasthan University of Veterinary and Animal Sciences at Bikaner, B-2 Bypass, Shiprapath, Mansarovar, Jaipur 302020, Rajasthan, India. [2] Sawai Man Singh Medical College, Jaipur 302004, Rajasthan, India.

Acknowledgements

This study was supported by Rashtriya Krishi Vikas Yojana (RKVY), Government of Rajasthan, India.

Competing interests

The authors declare that they have no competing interests.

Funding

We did not receive any specific funding for conducting this research.

References

1. FAO. A report on milk and milk products. Food and agricultural organization, United States. 2013. www.milkproduction.com/Library/Editorial-articles/FAO-Food-Outlook-Nov-2013—Milk-and-Milk-products/.
2. Ministry of Agricultural. State/UT-wise estimates of Milk Production, Government of India. 2015. https://data.gov.in/catalog/stateut-wise-estimates-milk-production.
3. Reshi AA, Husain I, Bhat S, Rehman MU, Razak R, Bilal S, Mir MR. Bovine mastitis as an evolving disease and its impact on the dairy industry. Int J Curr Res Rev. 2015;7(5):48–55.
4. Motwani KT. Mastitis in dairy cattle in India. In Social Science Research Network. 2011. doi:10.2139/ssrn.1798382.
5. Kader M, Samad M, Saha S, Taleb M. Prevalence and etiology of subclinical mastitis with antibiotic sensitivity to isolated organisms among milch cows in Bangladesh. Indian J Dairy Sci. 2002;55(4):218–23.
6. Seegers H, Fourichon C, Beaudeau F. Production effects related to mastitis and mastitis economics in dairy cattle herds. Vet Res. 2003;34(5):475–91.
7. Dahiya DK, Renuka MP, Puniya M, Shandilya UK, Dhewa T, Kumar N, Kumar S, Puniya AK, Shukla P. Gut microbiota modulation and its relationship with obesity using prebiotic fibers and probiotics: a review. Front Microbiol. 2017;8:563.
8. Sahu B, Mukherjee R, Kumar A, Kumar A, Sahu J. Prevalence of coagulase gene positive *Staphylococcus aureus* bovine mastitis in three distinct geoclimatic regions of India. Buffalo Bull. 2014;33(2):208–14.
9. Daka D, Yihdego D. Antibiotic-resistance *Staphylococcus aureus* isolated from cow's milk in the Hawassa area, South Ethiopia. Ann Clin Microbiol Antimicrob. 2012;11(1):26.
10. Sharma S, Sharma V, Dahiya DK, Khan A, Mathur M, Sharma A. Prevalence, virulence potential, and antibiotic susceptibility profile of *Listeria monocytogenes* isolated from bovine raw milk samples obtained from Rajasthan, India. Foodborne Pathog Dis. 2017;14(3):132–40.
11. Salasia SIO, Lammler C. Comparative studies on pheno-and genotypic properties of *Staphylococcus aureus* isolated from bovine subclinical mastitis in central Java in Indonesia and Hesse in Germany. J Vet Sci. 2004;5(2):103–9.
12. Omuse G, Zyl KN, Hoek K, Abdulgader S, Kariuki S, Whitelaw A, Revathi G. Molecular characterization of *Staphylococcus aureus* isolates from various healthcare institutions in Nairobi, Kenya: a cross sectional study. Ann Clin Microbiol Antimicrob. 2016;15(1):51.
13. Acosta A, Guelfer E, Ruiz A, Mota RA, Uffo O, Gomes-Filho MA, Barbosa SBP. Molecular subtyping of *Staphylococcus aureus* isolated from bovine mastitis in Pernambuco State, Brazil. Comp Clin Path. 2014;23(4):1037–41.
14. Momtaz H, Tajbakhsh E, Rahimi E, Momeni M. Coagulase gene polymorphism of *Staphylococcus aureus* isolated from clinical and sub-clinical bovine mastitis in Isfahan and Chaharmahal va Bakhtiari provinces of Iran. Comp Clin Path. 2011;20(5):519–22.
15. Sarvari J, Bazargani A, Kandekar-Ghahraman MR, Nazari-Alam A, Motamedifar M. Molecular typing of methicillin-resistant and methicillin-susceptible *Staphylococcus aureus* isolates from Shiraz teaching hospitals by PCR-RFLP of coagulase gene. Iran J Microbiol. 2014;6(4):246–52.
16. Oliver SP, Jayarao BM, Almeida RA. Foodborne pathogens in milk and the dairy farm environment: food safety and public health implications. Foodborne Pathog Dis. 2005;2(2):115–29.
17. Srey S, Jahid IK, Ha S-D. Biofilm formation in food industries: a food safety concern. Food Control. 2013;31(2):572–85.
18. Al-Ashmawy MA, Sallam KI, Abd-Elghany SM, Elhadidy M, Tamura T. Prevalence, molecular characterization, and antimicrobial susceptibility of methicillin-resistant *Staphylococcus aureus* isolated from milk and dairy products. Foodborne Pathog Dis. 2016;13(3):156–62.
19. Fox L, Zadoks R, Gaskins C. Biofilm production by *Staphylococcus aureus* associated with intramammary infection. Vet Microbiol. 2005;107(3):295–9.
20. Tang J, Chen J, Li H, Zeng P, Li J. Characterization of adhesin genes, staphylococcal nuclease, hemolysis, and biofilm formation among *Staphylococcus aureus* strains isolated from different sources. Foodborne Pathog Dis. 2013;10(9):757–63.
21. J-p Li, H-j Zhou. Yuan L, He T, Hu S-h. Prevalence, genetic diversity, and antimicrobial susceptibility profiles of *Staphylococcus aureus* isolated from bovine mastitis in Zhejiang Province, China. J Zhejiang Univ Sci B. 2009;10(10):753–60.
22. Dahiya DK, Puniya AK. Isolation, molecular characterization and screening of indigenous lactobacilli for their abilities to produce bioactive conjugated linoleic acid (CLA). J Food Sci. 2017;54(3):792–801.
23. Goh SH, Byrne S, Zhang J, Chow A. Molecular typing of *Staphylococcus aureus* on the basis of coagulase gene polymorphisms. J Clin Microbiol. 1992;30(7):1642–5.

24. Hunter PR, Gaston MA. Numerical index of the discriminatory ability of typing systems: an application of Simpson's index of diversity. J Clin Microbiol. 1988;26(11):2465–6.
25. Mehrotra M, Wang G, Johnson WM. Multiplex PCR for detection of genes for *Staphylococcus aureus* enterotoxins, exfoliative toxins, toxic shock syndrome toxin 1, and methicillin resistance. J Clin Microbiol. 2000;38(3):1032–5.
26. Tang J, Chen J, Liu J, Zhang R, Yang R, Chen L. Effects of different cultivation conditions on *Staphylococcus aureus* biofilm formation and diversity of adhesin genes. J Food Saf. 2012;32(2):210–8.
27. Dahiya DK, Puniya AK. Evaluation of survival, free radical scavenging and human enterocyte adherence potential of lactobacilli with anti-obesity and anti-inflammatory cla isomer-producing attributes. J Food Process Preserv. 2015;39(6):2866–77.
28. CLSI. M100-S25 performance standards for antimicrobial susceptibility testing; Twenty-fifth informational supplement; 2015.
29. Stegger A, Andersen P, Kearns A, Pichon B, Holmes M, Edwards G, Laurent F, Teale C, Skov R, Larsen A. Rapid detection, differentiation and typing of methicillin-resistant Staphylococcus aureus harbouring either mecA or the new mecA homologue mecALGA251. Clin Microbiol Infect. 2012;18(4):395.
30. Lingathurai S, Vellathurai P. Bacteriological quality and safety of raw cow milk in Madurai. South India. Webmed Cent Microbiol. 2013;1:1–10.
31. Sadashiv S, Kaliwal B. Antibiotic resistance of *Staphyloccocus aureus* and Coagulase negative Staphylococci (CNS) isolated from bovine mastitis in the region of North Karnataka, India. World J Pharm Res. 2013;3:571–86.
32. Sharma S, Khan A, Dahiya DK, Jain J, Sharma V. Prevalence, identification and drug resistance pattern of *Staphylococcus aureus* and *Escherichia coli* isolated from raw milk samples of jaipur city of Rajasthan. J Pure Appl Microbiol. 2015;9(1):341–8.
33. Sudhanthiramani S, Swetha CS, Bharathy S. Prevalence of antibiotic resistant *Staphylococcus aureus* from raw milk samples collected from the local vendors in the region of Tirupathi, India. Vet world. 2015;8(4):478–81.
34. Kumar R, Prasad A. Detection of *E. coli* and *Staphylococcus* in milk and milk products in and around Pantnagar. Pak J Nutr. 2010;1(3):151–2.
35. Thaker H, Brahmbhatt M, Nayak J, Thaker HC. Isolation and identification of *Staphylococcus aureus* from milk and milk products and their drug resistance patterns in Anand, Gujarat. Vet World. 2013;6(1):10–3.
36. Vieira-da-Motta O, Folly MM, Sakyiama CCH. Detection of different *Staphylococcus aureus* strains in bovine milk from subclinical mastitis using PCR and routine techniques. Braz J Microbiol. 2001;32(1):27–31.
37. da Silva ER, da Silva N. Coagulase gene typing of *Staphylococcus aureus* isolated from cows with mastitis in southeastern Brazil. Can J Vet Res. 2005;69(4):260–4.
38. Saei HD, Ahmadi M, Mardani K, Batavani R. Molecular typing of *Staphylococcus aureus* isolated from bovine mastitis based on polymorphism of the coagulase gene in the north west of Iran. Vet Microbiol. 2009;137(1):202–6.
39. Schwarzkopf A, Karch H. Genetic variation in *Staphylococcus aureus* coagulase genes: potential and limits for use as epidemiological marker. J Clin Microbiol. 1994;32(10):2407–12.
40. Ishino K, Tsuchizaki N, Ishikawa J, Hotta K. Usefulness of PCR-restriction fragment length polymorphism typing of the coagulase gene to discriminate arbekacin-resistant methicillin-resistant *Staphylococcus aureus* strains. J Clin Microbiol. 2007;45(2):607–9.
41. Abdulghany HM, Khairy RM. The Frequency of methicillin-resistant *Staphylococcus aureus* and coagulase gene polymorphism in Egypt. Int J Bacteriol. 2014;2014:1–6.
42. Moon J, Lee A, Kang H, Lee E, Joo Y, Park YH, Kim M, Koo H. Antibiogram and coagulase diversity in staphylococcal enterotoxin-producing *Staphylococcus aureus* from bovine mastitis. J Dairy Sci. 2007;90(4):1716–24.
43. Kumar R, Yadav B, Singh R. Antibiotic resistance and pathogenicity factors in *Staphylococcus aureus* isolated from mastitic Sahiwal cattle. J Biosci. 2011;36(1):175–88.
44. El-Sayed A, Alber J, Lammler C, Jager S, Woter W, Vázquez H. Comparative study on genotypic properties of *Staphylococcus aureus* isolated from clinical and subclinical mastitis in Mexico. Vet Mex. 2006;37(2):165–79.
45. Darwish SF, Asfour HA. Investigation of biofilm forming ability in *Staphylococci* causing bovine mastitis using phenotypic and genotypic assays. Sci World J. 2013;2013:1–9.
46. Raza A, Muhammad G, Sharif S, Atta A. Biofilm producing *Staphylococcus aureus* and bovine mastitis: a review. Mol Microbiol Res. 2013;3(1):1–8.
47. Salgado-Ruiz T, Rodríguez A, Gutiérrez D, Martínez B, García P, Espinoza-Ortega A, Martínez-Campos A, Lagunas-Bernabé S, Vicente F, Arriaga-Jordán C. Molecular characterization and antimicrobial susceptibility of *Staphylococcus aureus* from small-scale dairy systems in the highlands of Central México. Dairy Sci Technol. 2015;95(2):181–96.
48. Mulcahy ME, Geoghegan JA, Monk IR, O'Keeffe KM, Walsh EJ, Foster TJ, McLoughlin RM. Nasal colonisation by *Staphylococcus aureus* depends upon clumping factor B binding to the squamous epithelial cell envelope protein loricrin. PLoS Pathog. 2012;8(12):e1003092.
49. Nakakido M, Aikawa C, Nakagawa I, Tsumoto K. The staphylococcal elastin-binding protein regulates zinc-dependent growth/biofilm formation. J Biochem. 2014;156(3):155–62.
50. Pereyra EA, Picech F, Renna MS, Baravalle C, Andreotti CS, Russi R, Calvinho LF, Diez C, Dallard BE. Detection of *Staphylococcus aureus* adhesion and biofilm-producing genes and their expression during internalization in bovine mammary epithelial cells. Vet Microbiol. 2016;183:69–77.
51. Kot B, Szweda P, Frankowska-Maciejewska A, Piechota M, Wolska K. Virulence gene profiles in *Staphylococcus aureus* isolated from cows with subclinical mastitis in eastern Poland. J Dairy Res. 2016;83(2):228–35.
52. Puacz E, Ilczyszyn WM, Kosecka M, Buda A, Dudziak W, Polakowska K, Panz T, Białecka A, Kasprowicz A, Lisowski A. Clustering of *Staphylococcus aureus* bovine mastitis strains from regions of Central-Eastern Poland based on their biochemical and genetic characteristics. Pol J Vet Sci. 2015;18(2):333–42.
53. Zuniga E, Melville PA, Saidenberg AB, Laes MA, Gonsales FF, Salaberry SR, Gregori F, Brandao PE, Santos FG, Lincopan NE. Occurrence of genes coding for MSCRAMM and biofilm-associated protein Bap in *Staphylococcus* spp. isolated from bovine subclinical mastitis and relationship with somatic cell counts. Microb Pathog. 2015;89:1–6.
54. Li L, Zhou L, Wang L, Xue H, Zhao X. Characterization of methicillin-resistant and-susceptible staphylococcal isolates from bovine milk in Northwestern China. PLoS ONE. 2015;10(3):e0116699.
55. Atray D, Sharma A, Atray M. Prevalence of *enterococci* and its antibiotic resistance in various clinical samples at tertiary care hospital in Southern Rajasthan, India. Int J Res Med Sci. 2017;4(8):3413–6.
56. Sood S, Gupta R. Antibiotic resistance pattern of community acquired uropathogens at a tertiary care hospital in Jaipur, Rajasthan. Indian J Comm Med. 2012;37(1):39–44.
57. Sharma KD, Saini RP, Karthik L. Current trends of antibiotic resistance in clinical isolates of *Staphylococcus aureus*. Front Biol. 2014;9(4):287–90.

Influence of borderline cefepime MIC on the outcome of cefepime-susceptible *Pseudomonas aeruginosa* bacteremia treated with a maximal cefepime dose

Ting-Yi Su[1], Jung-Jr Ye[1], Chien-Chang Yang[1], Ching-Tai Huang[1], Ju-Hsin Chia[2,3] and Ming-Hsun Lee[1*]

Abstract

Background: We assessed the influence of current cefepime minimal inhibitory concentration (MIC) breakpoints and the maximal cefepime dose on treatment outcomes in patients with bacteremia caused by cefepime-susceptible *Pseudomonas aeruginosa*.

Methods: Adult patients hospitalized between July 2010 and June 2014 with a positive blood culture for cefepime-susceptible *P. aeruginosa* and receipt of cefepime as the primary therapy throughout the course were reviewed. Cefepime Etest® MICs and clinical outcomes for *P. aeruginosa* bacteremia were reviewed to identify the MIC breakpoint influencing treatment outcomes.

Results: Of the 90 patients enrolled, 49 (54.4%) were male (mean age = 66.8 years). The mean Acute Physiology and Chronic Health Evaluation II score was 22.01. Sixty patients (66.7%) received a maximal cefepime dose, and the 30-day crude mortality rate was 36.7%. MIC_{90} of cefepime for *P. aeruginosa* was 8 mg/L. The cumulative survival rate at 30 days revealed that a lower cefepime MIC (<4 mg/L) for *P. aeruginosa* was associated with a higher survival rate than a higher MIC (≥4 mg/L) (72.6% vs. 23.5%, $p < 0.0001$). A cefepime MIC of ≥4 mg/L and age were independent risk factors for mortality, whereas the maximal cefepime dose was the independent protective factor. The use of a maximal cefepime dose did not improve the outcomes of patients with *P. aeruginosa* bacteremia at a MIC of ≥4 mg/L.

Conclusions: A cefepime MIC of 4 mg/L may predict an unfavorable outcome among patients with serious infections caused by *P. aeruginosa*, even the MICs still within the CLSI susceptibility breakpoint.

Keywords: *Pseudomonas aeruginosa*, Bacteremia, Cefepime, Minimal inhibitory concentrations, Maximal cefepime dose

Background

Pseudomonas aeruginosa is a leading cause of nosocomial infections [1, 2], which are often life threatening [3]. Recently, actual minimal inhibitory concentrations (MICs) of fluoroquinolones [4], extended-spectrum penicillins [5], and carbapenems [6] have predicted patient outcomes more accurately than did the categorical classification of MICs as susceptible, intermediate, and resistant. Cefepime is a fourth-generation cephalosporin with a broad-spectrum antibacterial activity; it has been widely used since its approval for clinical use in 1997 [7]. According to the Clinical and Laboratory Standards Institute (CLSI) criteria of 2016 [8], the susceptible range of cefepime MIC was ≤8 mg/L. However, the mortality

*Correspondence: drharrylee@gmail.com
[1] Division of Infectious Diseases, Department of Internal Medicine, Chang Gung Memorial Hospital at Linkou, Chang Gung University College of Medicine, 5 Fu-Shin Street, Gueishan 333, Taoyuan, Taiwan
Full list of author information is available at the end of the article

rates of patients infected with gram-negative organisms treated with cefepime increased with increasing MICs [9]. Therefore, the primary aim of this study was to determine the predictive value of cefepime MICs on the therapeutic outcomes in patients with cefepime-susceptible *P. aeruginosa* bacteremia and to evaluate if the current cefepime breakpoints for *P. aeruginosa* require revision.

The present recommended cefepime dosage may be suboptimal for the treatment of infections caused by *P. aeruginosa* strains with a higher cefepime MIC value [10, 11], and therapy with a higher cefepime dose was associated with a lower mortality rate in patients with gram-negative bacilli (GNB) infections [12] and requirement of the intensive care [13, 14]. The secondary aim of this study was to evaluate whether the maximal cefepime dose could improve clinical outcomes in patients with cefepime-susceptible *P. aeruginosa* bacteremia.

Methods

Setting

This retrospective study was conducted at the Chang Gung Memorial Hospital (CGMH), Linkou, Northern Taiwan, a 3715-bed university-affiliated tertiary-care medical center with 308 intensive care unit (ICU) beds. All clinical specimens were processed using computer-assisted microbiology laboratory databases at a central microbiology laboratory. This study was approved by the Institutional Review Board of the CGMH (103-3354B).

Study design and patients

In this retrospective study, 586 patients admitted to CGMH from July 2010 to June 2014 with an unduplicated monomicrobial blood culture positive for cefepime-susceptible *P. aeruginosa* and a clinical syndrome suggestive of systemic infection were reviewed. The additional inclusion criteria are as follows: age ≥18 years, clear medical records, cefepime as the first-line therapy within 48 h of bacteremia onset and monotherapy against GNB throughout the treatment. Patients who met any of the following criteria were not eligible for the study: no receipt of cefepime therapy, receipt of cefepime <3 days, combination therapy with other antimicrobials against GNB including aminoglycosides, anti-pseudomonal β-lactams or anti-pseudomonal fluoroquinolones, and inadequate clinical information from the medical records. In this study, none of the patients had received cefepime more than 3 days initially, and then received other antibiotics instead. Finally, ninety patients were enrolled in this study (Fig. 1).

Microbiology

Blood cultures were processed in the clinical microbiology laboratory by using an automated blood culture system (BACTEC 9240 system; Becton–Dickinson Diagnostic Instrument Systems, Sparks, MD, USA). Before June 2013, *P. aeruginosa* isolates were identified on the basis of the following properties: aerobic GNB on Gram staining with glucose nonfermentation, positive oxidase test, blue–green or yellow–green fluorescent

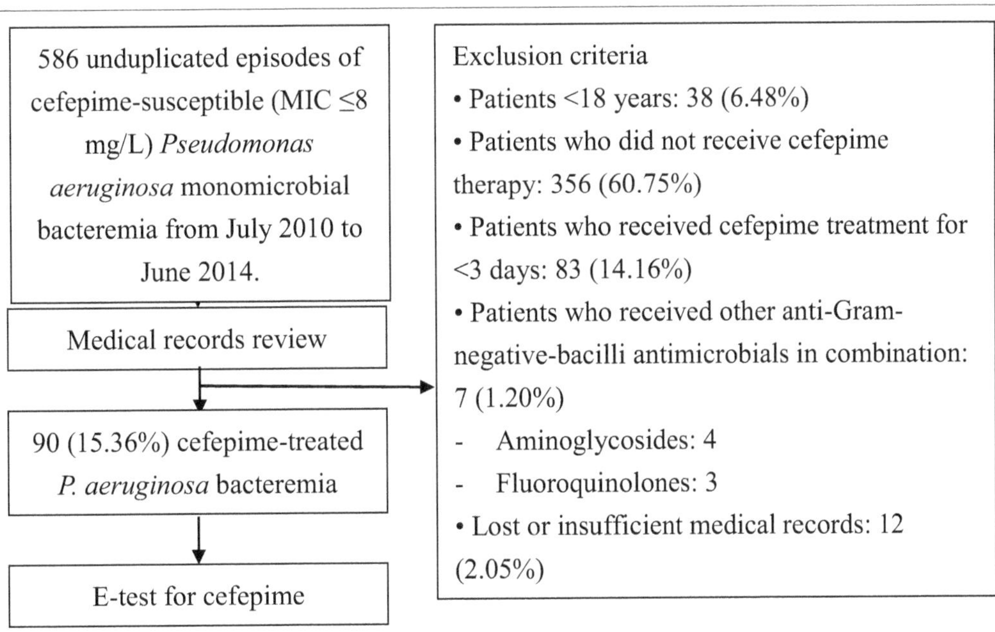

Fig. 1 Flow chart of the exclusion of patients with *Pseudomonas aeruginosa*

pigment production, and growth at 42 °C [15]. After June 2013, bacterial species were identified through matrix-assisted laser desorption ionization-time of flight (MALDI-TOF). *P. aeruginosa* blood isolates are routinely preserved at our clinical microbiology laboratory in skimmed milk at −70 °C until further use. All the *P. aeruginosa* blood isolates investigated in this study were selected from these stocks and tested to determine the cefepime MICs using Etest® strips (bioMerieux, Lyon, France) according to the manufacturer instructions. An isolate of *P. aeruginosa* was defined as cefepime susceptible, intermediate, or resistant if its MIC was ≤8, 16, or ≥32 mg/L, respectively [8]. *P. aeruginosa* ATCC 27853 was the control.

Data collection and definition

Demographic data, such as age, sex, concomitant diseases, and clinical characteristics, of patients with *P. aeruginosa* bacteremia were retrieved by reviewing inpatient medical records. Concomitant diseases included severe renal impairment (defined as chronic kidney disease stage 4, 5 and needed renal replacement therapy), diabetes mellitus, cerebral vascular accident, liver cirrhosis, chronic pulmonary disease, and malignancy. Central venous catheter (CVC) placement, ventilator use, ICU stay, and the time interval between hospitalization and occurrence of *P. aeruginosa* bacteremia were recorded. Disease severity scores were calculated using the Acute Physiology and Chronic Health Evaluation II (APACHE II) score on the day *P. aeruginosa* bacteremia occurred. All the patients had collected the following parameters, age, comorbidities, systolic and mean arterial blood pressure (mmHg), heart rate, respiratory rate, body temperature, initial Glasgow Coma Scale score, arterial blood gas analysis: pH, arterial oxygen tension (PaO_2), arterial carbon dioxide tension (pCO_2), laboratory data (white blood cell count, hematocrit, sodium, potassium, and creatinine). However, the following values, if missing, were considered normal: PaO_2, pH, and pCO_2. Severe sepsis were defined as sepsis plus evidence of organ dysfunction included either one criteria as bellowed: (1) arterial hypoxemia (PaO_2/fraction of inspiration O_2; FiO_2 <300), (2) acute oliguria (urine output <0.5 mL/kg per hour for at least 2 h despite adequate fluid resuscitation, (3) increase in creatinine >0.5 mg/dL, (4) coagulation abnormalities: international normalized ratio (INR) >1.5, activated partial thromboplastin time (aPTT) >60 s, platelets <100,000/μL, (5) hepatic dysfunction (elevated bilirubin), (6) paralytic ileus, and (7) decreased capillary refill or skin mottling. Septic shock was defined as sepsis with hypotension refractory to fluid resuscitation or hyperlactatemia. Neutropenia was defined as absolute neutrophil count of $<0.5 \times 10^9$/L.

The sources of bacteremia determined from medical records, imaging studies, surgical findings, and microbiological evidences were categorized into lower respiratory and urinary tracts, skin and skin structure, central catheter-associated bloodstream infection (CABSI), and intra-abdominal infections. If no source was identified, the infection was categorized as primary bacteremia.

Treatment and outcomes

The dosage and dosing frequency of cefepime were reviewed from patient medical records. Cefepime was infused over 30 min. Creatinine clearance (CL_{CR}) was calculated on the date of first dose of cefepime was given. CL_{CR} was calculated using an adjusted Cockcroft–Gault equation that excluded patient weight [CL_{CR} = (140 − age)/serum creatinine concentration]; the result was multiplied by 0.85 for female patients. The maximal cefepime dose adjusted by CL_{CR} was defined as 2 g every 8 h, 2 g every 12 h, 2 g every 24 h, and 1 g every 24 h, while CL_{CR} was ≥50, 30–49, 10–29, and <10 mL/min, respectively [10]. Patients receiving above CL_{CR}-adjusted dosing regimens throughout the course of cefepime treatment were defined as using the maximal cefepime dose. Clinical outcomes were assessed using the 30-day crude mortality.

Statistical analyses

All statistical analyses were performed using the Statistical Package for Social Sciences for Windows (version 18.0; SPSS Inc., Chicago, IL, USA). Categorical variables were compared using the χ^2 or Fisher exact tests, as appropriate; continuous variables were compared using the Mann–Whitney *U* test. Variables with $p < 0.1$ in the univariate analysis were included in a multiple logistic regression model using the backward stepwise method for identifying the risk factors for the 30-day sepsis-related mortality. Adjusted odds ratios (ORs) and 95% confidence intervals (CIs) were calculated. The survival curve was plotted by means of the Kaplan–Meier method, and the log rank test was used to compare univariate survival distribution. All tests were two-tailed, and $p < 0.05$ was considered significant.

Results

Patient enrollment and their clinical characteristics

A total of 586 unduplicated cefepime-susceptible *P. aeruginosa* blood isolates from 586 patients were identified. On the basis of our inclusion criteria, 496 patients were excluded because of age <18 years, no receipt of cefepime therapy or cefepime use <3 days, or receipt of combination therapy with other anti-GNB antimicrobials. Ninety patients with individual unduplicated *P. aeruginosa* blood isolates were enrolled (Fig. 1). Patient demographics and clinical characteristics are listed in Table 1. Of the 90 patients, 49 (54.4%) were male with a mean age of 66.8 years. The most common concomitant disease was solid organ malignancy (43.3%), followed by diabetes mellitus (32.2%), and chronic kidney disease stage IV and above (31.1%). Time between hospital admission and occurrence of *P. aeruginosa* bacteremia ranged from 0 to 252 days with a mean interval of 23.2 days.

Table 1 Clinical characteristics of 90 patients with cefepime-susceptible *Pseudomonas aeruginosa* monomicrobial bacteremia receiving cefepime monotherapy

Variables	Value[a]
Demographic parameters	
Age, year	66.8 (14.6)
Male gender	49 (54.4)
Concomitant diseases	
Diabetes mellitus	29 (32.2)
Severe renal impairment	28 (31.1)
Liver cirrhosis	10 (11.1)
Chronic pulmonary disease	8 (8.9)
Cerebral vascular accident	19 (21.1)
Solid organ malignancy	39 (43.3)
Haematological malignancy	16 (17.8)
Autoimmune disease	5 (5.6)
Clinical conditions	
Time interval between admission and occurrence of bacteremia, day	23.2 (36.3)
Central venous catheter use	68 (75.6)
Patients' severity	
APACHE II score	22.07 (6.0)
Ventilator use	23 (25.6)
Intensive care unit stay	29 (32.2)
Severe sepsis or septic shock	21 (23.3)
Neutropenia	18 (20.0)
Source of bacteremia	
Primary bacteremia	38 (42.2)
Lower respiratory tract	27 (30)
Urinary tract	7 (7.8)
Skin and skin structure	2 (2.2)
Central catheter associated blood stream infection	12 (13.3)
Intra-abdominal infection	10 (11.1)
Treatment	
Use of maximum cefepime dose	60 (66.7)
Treatment duration	16.4 (7.031)
Remove catheter or operation	8 (8.9)
Outcome	
30-day crude mortality	33 (36.7)

APACHE II score Acute Physiology and Chronic Health Evaluation II score

[a] Categorical data: number (%) of patients; continuous data are expressed as mean (standard deviation)

Sixty-eight patients (75.6%) had received a CVC placement, 23 (25.6%) ever used a ventilator, 29 (32.2%) had ICU stay, 21 (23.3%) had severe sepsis or septic shock, and 18 (20%) had neutropenia. The mean APACHE II score was 22.01. Thirty-eight patients (38.8%) had primary bacteremia and the remaining 52 (61.2%) had identified sources of bacteremia. One case had vertebral osteomyelitis. The most common source of bacteremia was lower respiratory tract infection (27/52, 51.9%), followed by CABSI (12/52, 23.1%).

Treatment and outcomes

Sixty patients (66.7%) used the maximal cefepime dose. The treatment duration varied from 3 to 30 days with a mean duration of 16.4 days, and the 30-day crude mortality rate was 36.7%. Besides, none of the studied cases had reported the adverse effects including neurotoxicity during cefepime use.

MIC versus mortality

Figure 2 depicts the relationship between MICs and mortality rates. Cefepime MIC_{50} and MIC_{90} for *P. aeruginosa* were 1 and 8 mg/L, respectively. The lower MICs (0.5, 0.75, and 1 mg/L) were associated with the lower mortality rates (0, 15.8, and 36.4%, respectively). The mortality rate extended to 42.9 and 100% at the MICs of 4 and >4 mg/L, respectively.

Risk factors for 30-day mortality of *P. aeruginosa* bacteremia

The cumulative survival rate at 30 days revealed that a lower cefepime MIC (<4 mg/L) for *P. aeruginosa* was associated with a significantly higher survival rate than a higher MIC (≥4 mg/L) (72.6% versus 23.5%, $p < 0.0001$) (Fig. 3).

The factors associated with the 30-day mortality in univariate analysis (Table 2) included older ages (71.5 ± 12.7 vs. 64.1 ± 15.1 years, $p = 0.028$), a longer time interval between the dates of admission and positive blood cultures (31.8 ± 34.6 vs. 18.3 ± 33.6 days, $p = 0.02$), a longer ICU stay (54.5% vs. 19.3%, $p = 0.001$), more episodes of severe sepsis or septic shock (36.4% vs. 15.8%, $p = 0.038$), more respiratory tract infections (48.5% vs. 19.3%, $p = 0.004$), a higher cefepime MIC (≥4 mg/L) (76.5% vs. 27.4%, $p < 0.001$), and fewer instances of maximal cefepime dose use (48.5% vs. 78.9%, $p = 0.003$). The mortality rate of patients with a cefepime MIC of ≥4 mg/L for *P. aeruginosa* was 76.5%, which was higher than those with a MIC of <4 mg/L (27.4%).

Those factors associated with the 30-day mortality in univariate analysis and APACHE II score were entered into multivariate analysis (Table 3), and the result showed that MIC ≥4 mg/L (adjusted OR 5.111;

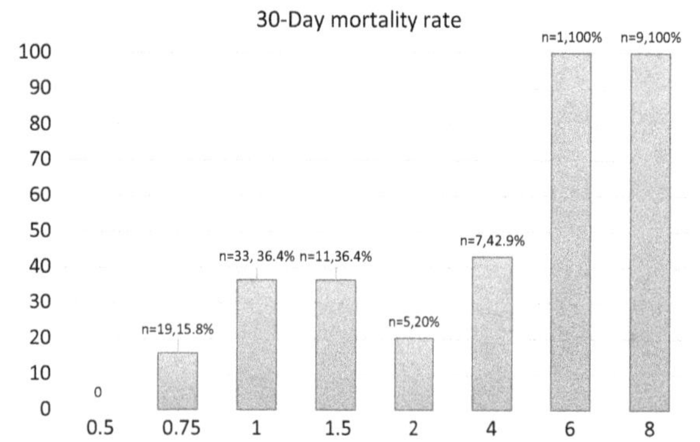

Fig. 2 Cefepime minimal inhibitory concentrations versus rate of mortality. *n* numbers, presented as the blood isolate number and the following is mortality rate, *MIC* minimal inhibitory concentration (mg/L)

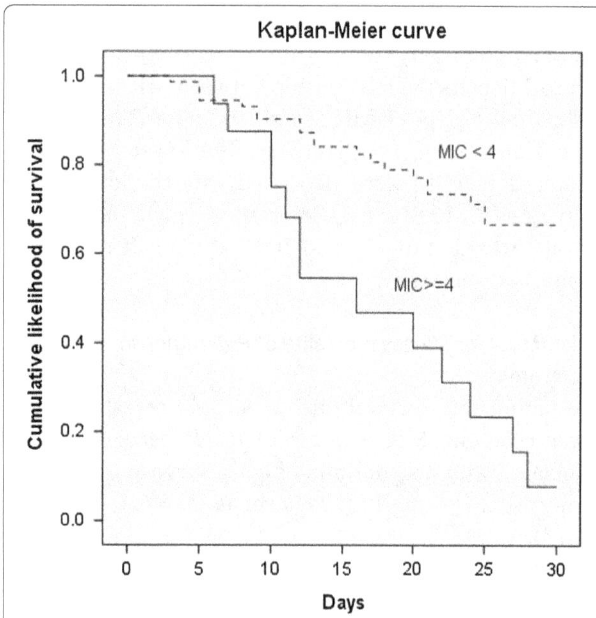

Fig. 3 Kaplan-Meier survival curve in patients with cefepime-susceptible *Pseudomonas aeruginosa* bacteremia. Comparison of the cumulative survival between cefepime minimal inhibitory concentration (MIC) <4 and ≥4 mg/L ($p < 0.0001$)

95% CI 1.090–23.974; $p = 0.039$) and age (adjusted OR 1.065; 95% CI 1.011–1.122; $p = 0.023$) were the independent risk factors for the 30-day mortality. Maximal cefepime dose usage was an independent protecting factor (adjusted OR 0.271; 95% CI 0.08–0.889; $p = 0.031$).

Relationship between MIC and the maximal dose of cefepime

Seventy-three patients had *P. aeruginosa* blood isolates with a cefepime MIC of <4 mg/L. Among them, compared with the survived, the deceased had fewer patients receiving a maximal dose of cefepime (50.0% vs. 81.1%, $p = 0.008$), more solid organ malignancy (65% vs 35.8%, $p = 0.025$) and a shorter treatment duration (14.0 ± 7.0 vs. 17. 8 ± 6.6 days, $p = 0.048$). In the multivariate analysis, use of the maximal cefepime dose was the only protecting factor for mortality (adjusted OR 0.244; 95% CI 0.077–0.771; $p = 0.016$). This protection was not found among patients with a MIC of ≥4 mg/L for *P. aeruginosa*. When the MIC was ≥4 mg/L, the mortality rate of patients using the maximal cefepime dose was 75% (6 of 8 patients), which is similar to those using a lower dose of cefepime (7 of 9 patients, 77.8%, $p = 1.000$). For those patients receiving a maximal dose of cefepime (n = 60), patients with a cefepime MIC of ≥4 mg/L for *P. aeruginosa* had a higher 30-day crude mortality rate than those with a MIC of <4 mg/L (33.3% vs. 4.4%, $p = 0.008$).

Discussion

According to our review of relevant literature, our study is the first one to provide clinical data demonstrating that treatment of cefepime-susceptible *P. aeruginosa* bacteremia with a maximal dose of cefepime improved the outcomes of patients with a lower cefepime MIC for *P. aeruginosa*. Besides, the current CLSI criteria for cefepime susceptibility did not predict clinical outcomes appropriately in this study. The 30-day crude mortality rate was 36.7% and the mortality rate was higher at the group of patients with a MIC of ≥4 mg/L for *P. aeruginosa* than those with a MIC of <4 mg/L (76.5% vs. 27.4%). Cefepime MIC ≥4 mg/L influenced patient outcomes independently, whereas using a maximal dose of cefepime in patients with various degrees of renal function was the only independent protecting factor for mortality. In addition, using the maximal dose of cefepime significantly decreased the mortality rate at patients with a MIC of <4 mg/L for *P. aeruginosa*. However, the protective effect vanished at a MIC of ≥4 mg/L. Our results revealed that using the maximal cefepime dose could improve patient outcomes at a lower MIC level. In this study, the antibiotic susceptibility testing was performed using Etest, not broth microdilution (BMD) methods, which is the CLSI criteria based on. However, Etest results generally have correlated well with MICs generated by BMD method [16]. Thus, the current CLSI criteria for cefepime susceptibility breakpoint of ≤8 mg/L may be reevaluated for severe *P. aeruginosa* infections.

In optimal situations, antibiotic susceptibility breakpoints are determined by integrating various microbiologic, pharmacokinetic/pharmacodynamic (PK/PD), and clinical data. However, after antibiotics were released commercially, new mechanisms of antibiotic resistance developed and probably affected the efficacy

Table 2 Univariate analyses of risk factors for 30-day crude mortality of cefepime-susceptible *Pseudomonas aeruginosa* bacteremia treated with cefepime

Variables	Deceased[a] $n = 33$	Survived[a] $n = 57$	Univariate p
Demographic parameters			
Age, year	71.5 (12.7)	64.1 (15.1)	0.028
Male gender	21 (63.6)	28 (49.1)	0.183
Concomitant diseases			
Diabetes mellitus	9 (27.3)	20 (35.1)	0.445
Severe renal impairment	13 (39.4)	15 (26.3)	0.197
Liver cirrhosis	4 (12.1)	6 (10.5)	1.000
Chronic pulmonary disease	4 (12.1)	4 (7.0)	0.458
Cerebral vascular accident	8 (24.2)	11 (19.3)	0.580
Solid organ malignancy	17 (51.5)	22 (38.6)	0.233
Haematological malignancy	4 (12.1)	12 (21.1)	0.394
Autoimmune disease	2 (6.1)	3 (5.3)	1.000
Clinical conditions			
Time interval between admission and occurrence of bacteremia, day	31.8 (34.6)	18.3 (33.6)	0.019
Central venous catheter use	27 (81.8)	41 (71.9)	0.293
Patients' severity			
APACHE II score	23.9 (5.5)	21.0 (6.1)	0.091
Intensive care unit stay	18 (54.5)	11 (19.3)	0.001
Severe sepsis or septic shock	12 (36.4)	9 (15.8)	0.038
Neutropenia	7 (21.2)	11 (19.3)	0.827
Source of bacteremia			
Primary bacteremia	11 (33.3)	27 (47.4)	0.194
Lower respiratory tract	16 (48.5)	11 (19.3)	0.004
Urinary tract	1 (3.0)	6 (10.5)	0.416
Skin and skin structure	1 (3.0)	1 (1.8)	1.000
CABSI	3 (9.1)	9 (15.8)	0.524
Intra-abdominal site	5 (15.2)	5 (8.8)	0.488
Microbiology			
MIC $\geq$4 mg/L	13 (39.4)	4 (7.0)	<0.001
Treatment			
Use of maximum cefepime dose	15 (45.5)	45 (78.9)	0.001
Treatment duration	14.7 (7.2)	17.5 (6.8)	0.062
Remove catheter or operation	2 (6.1)	6 (10.5)	0.705

APACHE II score Acute Physiology and Chronic Health Evaluation II score, *CABSI* central catheter associated blood stream infection, *MIC* minimal inhibitory concentration

[a] Categorical data: number (%) of patients; continuous data are expressed as mean (standard deviation)

of antibiotics. Falagas et al. [17] described that high MICs of GNB, particularly in *Salmonella enterica* and *P. aeruginosa* infections, within the currently accepted "susceptible" range were associated with worse outcomes. Several studies have revealed that high piperacillin MICs are associated with increasing mortality rates and microbiological treatment failure. This led to lowering of the CLSI recommendation of the breakpoint of piperacillin against *P. aeruginosa* from $\leq$64 to $\leq$16 mg/L [5, 18, 19]. Worse outcomes related to high MICs were also found on carbapenem use for patients with either bloodstream [6] or lower respiratory tract infections [20]. Patients with levofloxacin-treated gram-negative bloodstream infections, who have elevated levofloxacin MICs but are nevertheless categorized as susceptible, had worse outcomes than those infected with gram-negative organisms, which had lower MICs [4]. Cefepime was inferior to carbapenems in treating patients with bacteremia caused by cefepime-susceptible extended-spectrum ß-lactamase producing strains. The mortality

Table 3 Multivariate analyses of risk factors for 30-day crude mortality of cefepime-susceptible *Pseudomonas aeruginosa* bacteremia treated with cefepime

Variables	*p*	OR	95% CI
MIC ≥4 mg/L	0.039	5.111	1.090–23.974
Use of maximum cefepime dose	0.031	0.271	0.082–0.889
Age, year	0.023	1.065	1.011–1.122
Lower respiratory tract infections	0.056	4.008	0.967–16.621
APACHE II score	0.824	0.986	0.869–1.119
Intensive care unit stay[a]	0.146	2.945	0.687–12.619
Severe sepsis or septic shock[a]	0.210	2.609	0.582–11.706
Time interval between admission and occurrence of bacteremia	0.861	1.002	0.983–1.021
Treatment duration	0.063	0.923	0.848–1.004

All variables with $p < 0.1$ in univariate analysis were included in a multivariate regression model using the backward stepwise method

OR odds ratio, *CI* confidence interval, *MIC* minimal inhibitory concentration

[a] The factors of intensive care unit stay and severe sepsis or septic shock had strongly correlation (correlation coefficient 0.9), however, single factor with either intensive care unit stay or severe sepsis and septic shock were still remained insignificantly in the multivariate analyses model (factor with intensive care unit only: adjusted OR 3.127, 95% CI 0.746–13.111, $p = 0.119$; factor with severe sepsis or septic shock only: adjusted OR 2.813, 95% CI 0.647–12.226, $p = 0.168$)

rate increased significantly because cefepime MICs increased ($p = 0.004$) [21]. Compared with a cefepime MIC of ≤4 mg/L for *P. aeruginosa*, patients with a MIC of 8 mg/L had a significantly higher mortality rate (66.7% versus 20.8%, $p = 0.01$) regardless of the cefepime dosage [9].

Studies have demonstrated that free or nonprotein-bound drug concentration over the MIC of the organism (fT > MIC) is the ideal predictor for bactericidal and microbiologic response for β-lactams. A larger fT > MIC (50–70%) is required for the maximal activity against gram-negative organisms [22]. However, several studies have now assessed the PK/PD profile of cefepime and support a change in cefepime dose or breakpoints for susceptibility. Crandon et al. [10] revealed that at the CLSI MIC breakpoint of cefepime susceptibility for *P. aeruginosa* (≤8 mg/L), a dose of only 2 g every 8 h has a ≥82% likelihood of achieving at least 60% fT > MIC in patients with normal renal function. At this MIC (≤8 mg/L), the dose of 1 or 2 g every 12 h for immunocompetent patients with severe *P. aeruginosa* infections has a target attainment rate of only 47.7 or 65.8%, respectively. Another PK/PD study of cefepime revealed that when $C_{67\%}$ >MIC was used as the pharmacodynamic target, a dose of 2 g every 12 h had a more than 80% likelihood of achieving the optimal target with an MIC of up to 4 mg/L, whereas a dose of 2 g every 24 h can probably achieve a target attainment rate of up to 80% only when the MICs were ≤2 mg/L [11]. The aforementioned studies explain the failure of achieving pharmacodynamics and the possible microbiological failure in cefepime-treated *P. aeruginosa* infections with a high cefepime MIC. In addition, they revealed the influence of different cefepime dosages on pharmacodynamics.

Alves et al. [12] demonstrated that treatment with cefepime at a dose of 2 g every 8 h over a 30-min infusion was associated with significantly lower hospital mortality rates in patients with GNB bloodstream infection compared with the usual dosage regimens, such as 1 or 2 g every 12 h and 1 g every 8 h. Moreover, they included 113 patients with *Escherichia coli* (62, 54.9%) and *P. aeruginosa* (19, 16.8%) infections. The median MIC of all GNB was 0.0625 mg/L, and most (78.8%) MICs were ≤0.25 mg/L; MIC_{90} was 2 mg/L. High-dose cefepime therapy was associated with lower mortality rates in patients with GNB infection, including GNB with a low cefepime MIC.

Our study has the limitations for being a retrospective design with the treatment decisions dependent on the physicians' judgments and the hospital antimicrobial stewardship program [23]. However, some study results suggested E test provides equal or more clear and accurate results in clinical set-up [24, 25]. Furthermore, the mechanisms for increasing cefepime MICs in *P. aeruginosa* isolates remain unclear. Additional investigations concerning the resistance are thus necessary.

Conclusions

In summary, our data showed that patients treated with cefepime for cefepime-susceptible *P. aeruginosa* bloodstream infections had a worse outcome while the isolates had a higher MIC value that was still within the susceptible category. Use of a higher cefepime dose in cases with a MIC of <4 mg/L for *P. aeruginosa* improved patient outcomes. Mortality rate increased in patients with a higher cefepime MIC (≥4 mg/L) for *P. aeruginosa* even with a maximal cefepime dose. Thus, when using cefepime to treat serious *P. aeruginosa* infections, the current CLSI cefepime MIC of 8 mg/L as the susceptibility breakpoint may not predict the clinical outcome well.

Abbreviations

APACHE II: Acute Physiology and Chronic Health Evaluation II; aPTT: activated partial thromboplastin time; BMD: broth microdilution; CABSI: central catheter-associated bloodstream infection; CGMH: Chang Gung Memorial Hospital; CIs: confidence intervals; CL_{CR}: creatinine clearance; CLSI: Clinical and Laboratory Standards Institute; CVC: central venous catheter; GNB: gram-negative bacilli; FiO_2: fraction of inspiration O_2; ICU: intensive care unit; INR: international normalized ratio; MALDI-TOF: matrix-assisted laser desorption ionization-time of flight; MICs: minimal inhibitory concentrations; ORs: odds ratios; PaO_2: arterial oxygen tension; pCO_2: arterial carbon dioxide tension; PK/PD: pharmacokinetic/pharmacodynamic.

Authors' contributions

TYS made substantial contributions to concept and design, acquisition of data, analysis, interpretation of data and drafted the manuscript. JJY participated in the design of the study, drafted of article and critical revision. CCY and CTH participated in the design of the study and drafted of article. JHC made substantial contributions to acquisition of data, analysis, and interpretation of data. MHL is the corresponding author and made substantial contributions to concept and design, acquisition of data, analysis, interpretation of data and responsible to all the training sessions. All authors read and approved the final manuscript.

Author details

[1] Division of Infectious Diseases, Department of Internal Medicine, Chang Gung Memorial Hospital at Linkou, Chang Gung University College of Medicine, 5 Fu-Shin Street, Gueishan 333, Taoyuan, Taiwan. [2] Department of Laboratory Medicine, Chang Gung Memorial Hospital at Linkou, Taoyuan, Taiwan. [3] Department of Medical Biotechnology and Laboratory Science, Chang Gung University, Taoyuan, Taiwan.

Acknowledgements

We wish to thank Department of Laboratory Medicine, Chang Gung Memorial Hospital at Linkou for laboratory support and data analysis.

Competing interests

The authors declare that they have no competing interests.

References

1. Eliopoulos GM, Cosgrove SE, Carmeli Y. The impact of antimicrobial resistance on health and economic outcomes. Clin Infect Dis. 2003;36:1433–7.
2. Gaynes RP, Edwards JR. The impact of antimicrobial-resistant, health care-associated infections on mortality in the United States. Clin Infect Dis. 2008;47:927–30.
3. Hirsch EB, Cottreau JM, Chang K-T, Caeiro J-P, Johnson ML, Tam VH. A model to predict mortality following *Pseudomonas aeruginosa* bacteremia. Diagn Microbiol Infect Dis. 2012;72:97–102.
4. DeFife R, Scheetz MH, Feinglass JM, Postelnick MJ, Scarsi KK. Effect of differences in MIC values on clinical outcomes in patients with bloodstream infections caused by gram-negative organisms treated with levofloxacin. Antimicrob Agents Chemother. 2009;53:1074–9.
5. Tam VH, Gamez EA, Weston JS, Gerard LN, LaRocco MT, Caeiro JP, et al. Outcomes of bacteremia due to *Pseudomonas aeruginosa* with reduced susceptibility to piperacillin–tazobactam: implications on the appropriateness of the resistance breakpoint. Clin Infect Dis. 2008;46:862–7.
6. Esterly JS, Wagner J, McLaughlin MM, Postelnick MJ, Qi C, Scheetz MH. Evaluation of clinical outcomes in patients with bloodstream infections due to gram-negative bacteria according to carbapenem MIC stratification. Antimicrob Agents Chemother. 2012;56:4885–90.
7. Endimiani A, Perez F, Bonomo RA. Cefepime: a reappraisal in an era of increasing antimicrobial resistance. Expert Rev Anti Infect Ther. 2008;6:805–24.
8. Clinical and Laboratory Standards Institute. Performance standards for antimicrobial susceptibility testing; twenty-fourth informational supplement M100-S26 2016 USA.
9. Bhat SV, Peleg AY, Lodise TP, Shutt KA, Capitano B, Potoski BA, et al. Failure of current cefepime breakpoints to predict clinical outcomes of bacteremia caused by gram-negative organisms. Antimicrob Agents Chemother. 2007;51:4390–5.
10. Crandon JL, Bulik CC, Kuti JL, Nicolau DP. Clinical pharmacodynamics of cefepime in patients infected with *Pseudomonas aeruginosa*. Antimicrob Agents Chemother. 2010;54:1111–6.
11. Tam VH, McKinnon PS, Akins RL, Drusano GL, Rybak MJ. Pharmacokinetics and pharmacodynamics of cefepime in patients with various degrees of renal function. Antimicrob Agents Chemother. 2003;47:1853–61.
12. Alves MD, Ribeiro VB, Tessari JP, Mattiello F, De Bacco G, Luz DI, et al. Effect of cefepime dose on mortality of patients with gram-negative bacterial bloodstream infections: a prospective cohort study. J Antimicrob Chemother. 2014;69:1681–7.
13. Nicasio AM, Eagye KJ, Nicolau DP, Shore E, Palter M, Pepe J, et al. Pharmacodynamic-based clinical pathway for empiric antibiotic choice in patients with ventilator-associated pneumonia. J Crit Care. 2010;25:69–77.
14. Roos JF, Bulitta J, Lipman J, Kirkpatrick CMJ. Pharmacokinetic–pharmacodynamic rationale for cefepime dosing regimens in intensive care units. J Antimicrob Chemother. 2006;58:987–93.
15. Gaby WL, Hadley C. Practical laboratory test for the identification of *Pseudomonas aeruginosa*. J Bacteriol. 1957;74:356–8.
16. Jorgensen JH, Ferraro MJ. antimicrobial susceptibility testing: a review of general principles and contemporary practices. Clin Infect Dis. 2009;49:1749–55.
17. Falagas ME, Tansarli GS, Rafailidis PI, Kapaskelis A, Vardakas KZ. Impact of antibiotic MIC on infection outcome in patients with susceptible gram-negative bacteria: a systematic review and meta-analysis. Antimicrob Agents Chemother. 2012;56:4214–22.
18. Tamma PD, Turnbull AE, Milstone AM, Hsu AJ, Carroll KC, Cosgrove SE. Does the piperacillin minimum inhibitory concentration for *Pseudomonas aeruginosa* influence clinical outcomes of children with pseudomonal bacteremia? Clin Infect Dis. 2012;55:799–806.
19. Yamagishi Y, Terada M, Ohki E, Miura Y, Umemura T, Mikamo H. Investigation of the clinical breakpoints of piperacillin–tazobactam against infections caused by *Pseudomonas aeruginosa*. J Infect Chemother. 2012;18:127–9.
20. Drusano GL, Lode H, Edwards JR. Meropenem: clinical response in relation to in vitro susceptibility. Clin Microbiol Infect. 2000;6:185–94.
21. Lee NY, Lee CC, Huang WH, Tsui KC, Hsueh PR, Ko WC. Cefepime therapy for monomicrobial bacteremia caused by cefepime-susceptible extended-spectrum beta-lactamase-producing Enterobacteriaceae: MIC matters. Clin Infect Dis. 2013;56:488–95.
22. Craig WA. Pharmacokinetic/pharmacodynamic parameters: rationale for antibacterial dosing of mice and men. Clin Infect Dis. 1998;26:1–12.
23. Wang HY, Chiu CH, Huang CT, Cheng CW, Lin YJ, Hsu YJ, et al. Blood culture-guided de-escalation of empirical antimicrobial regimen for critical patients in an online antimicrobial stewardship programme. Int J Antimicrob Agents. 2014;44:520–7.
24. Rajkumari N, Mathur P, Bhardwaj N, Gupta G, Dahiya R, Behera B, et al. Resistance pattern of mupirocin in methicillin-resistant *Staphylococcus aureus* in trauma patients and comparison between disc diffusion and E-test for better detection of resistance in low resource countries. J Lab Physicians. 2014;6:91–5.
25. Ogbolu DO, Terry-Alli OA, Daini OA, Olabiyi FA, Igharo EA. Comparison of E-test with other conventional susceptibility testing methods for ciprofloxacin and gentamicin against gram negative enteric bacilli. Afr J Med Med Sci. 2012;41:135–40.

28

An evaluation of multidrug-resistant *Escherichia coli* isolates in urinary tract infections from Aguascalientes, Mexico

Flor Y. Ramírez-Castillo[1], Adriana C. Moreno-Flores[1], Francisco J. Avelar-González[2], Francisco Márquez-Díaz[3], Josée Harel[4] and Alma L. Guerrero-Barrera[1*]

Abstract

Background: Uropathogenic *Escherichia coli* (UPEC) are one of the main bacteria causing urinary tract infections (UTIs). The rates of UPEC with high resistance towards antibiotics and multidrug-resistant bacteria have increased dramatically in recent years and could difficult the treatment.

Methods: The aim of the study was to determine multidrug-resistant bacteria, antibiotic resistance profile, virulence traits, and genetic background of 110 *E. coli* isolated from community (79 isolates) and hospital-acquired (31 isolates) urinary tract infections. The plasmid-mediated quinolone resistance genes presence was also investigated. A subset of 18 isolates with a quinolone-resistance phenotype was examined for common virulence genes encoded in diarrheagenic and extra-intestinal pathogenic *E. coli* by a specific *E. coli* microarray.

Results: Female children were the group most affected by UTIs, which were mainly community-acquired. Resistance to trimethoprim–sulfamethoxazole, ampicillin, and ampicillin–sulbactam was most prevalent. A frequent occurrence of resistance toward ciprofloxacin (47.3%), levofloxacin (43.6%) and cephalosporins (27.6%) was observed. In addition, 63% of the strains were multidrug-resistant (MDR). Almost all the fluoroquinolone (FQ)-resistant strains showed MDR-phenotype. Isolates from male patients were associated to FQ-resistant and MDR-phenotype. Moreover, hospital-acquired infections were correlated to third generation cephalosporin and nitrofurantoin resistance and the presence of *kpsMTII* gene. Overall, *fimH* (71.8%) and *fyuA* (68.2%), had the highest prevalence as virulence genes among isolates. However, the profile of virulence genes displayed a great diversity, which included the presence of genes related to diarrheagenic *E. coli*. Out of 110 isolates, 25 isolates (22.7%) were positive to *qnrA*, 23 (20.9%) to *qnrB*, 7 (6.4%) to *qnrS1*, 7 (6.4%) to *aac(6')Ib-cr*, 5 (4.5%) to *qnrD*, and 1 (0.9%) to *qnrC* genes. A total of 12.7% of the isolates harbored $bla_{CTX\text{-}M}$ genes, with $bla_{CTX\text{-}M\text{-}15}$ being the most prevalent.

Conclusions: Urinary tract infection due to *E. coli* may be difficult to treat empirically due to high resistance to commonly used antibiotics. Continuous surveillance of multidrug resistant organisms and patterns of drug resistance are needed in order to prevent treatment failure and reduce selective pressure. These findings may help choosing more suitable treatments of UTI patients in this region of Mexico.

Keywords: Urinary tract infection, Multidrug-resistant, Fluoroquinolone-resistant, Plasmid-mediated quinolone resistance (PMQR), CTX-M

*Correspondence: alguerre@correo.uaa.mx
[1] Laboratorio de Biología Celular y Tisular, Departamento de Morfología, Universidad Autónoma de Aguascalientes, Av. Universidad 940, Col. Cd. Universitaria, 20131 Aguascalientes, Mexico
Full list of author information is available at the end of the article

Background

Escherichia coli is an important cause of extra-intestinal infections, enteric disease, and systemic infections in humans and animals. Uropathogenic *Escherichia coli* (UPEC), one of the members of the extra-intestinal pathogenic *E. coli* (ExPEC) is a predominant pathogen causing urinary tract infections (UTIs) [1]. UPEC is one of the main causes of community (80–90%) and nosocomial-acquired UTIs (30–50%) [2]. These strains harbor a variety of virulence factors that allow them to establish an infection, including adhesins, toxins, host defense avoidance mechanisms and multiple iron acquisition systems [3].

UTIs are one of the most common bacterial infections worldwide. It has been estimated that 150 million UTIs occur per year worldwide [4]. ExPEC strains are responsible for an estimated 40,000 deaths and at least $2.6 billion of expenses in healthcare treatment in the United States alone [5]. In Mexico, 3'648,784 cases were reported on 2015 [6]. Although these infections are treatable, the increasingly accelerated rates or multi-drug resistant organisms (MDRO) lead to complication, treatment failure and increased rates of mortality and morbidity [7].

The enhanced prevalence and global spread of extended-spectrum beta-lactamase (ESBL) genes [8] such as CTX-M enzymes that are associated to multidrug-resistant (MDR) phenotypes and fluoroquinolones resistance, has become a major concern [9, 10]. Quinolones are broad-spectrum antibiotics and very important in the treatment of a wide range of diseases, especially urinary tract infections. Quinolone resistance is mainly caused by chromosomal mutations in the quinolone resistance-determining region (QRDR) of gyrase (*gyrA* and *gyrB*) and topoisomerase (*parC* and *parE*) genes, but also is caused by plasmid-mediated quinolone resistance (PMQR) which include: the pentapeptide repeat family Qnr proteins (QnrA, QnrB, QnrS, QnrC and QnrD) [11], the variant of the aminoglycoside-acetyltransferase modifying enzyme, AAC(6′)-Ib-cr [12], and the efflux pumps QepA and OqxAB [13–15]. Although PMQR genes confer only low-level of resistance to quinolones [16] they could spread horizontally among *Enterobacteria* and facilitate the selection of resistant mutants as well as the selection of additional resistance mechanisms, enabling bacteria to become fully resistant [8, 17].

The emergence of MDR *E. coli* causing urinary tract infections with high virulence potential is alarming. In Mexico, a high rate of resistance against quinolones has been observed in environmental, diarrheagenic [18], and pediatric clinical isolates [19]. MDR phenotype of UPEC has also been shown [20, 21]. However, lack of sufficient data on virulence spectrum and MDR-UPEC isolates from community and hospital infections hinders the infections control and management efforts. The aim of this study was to determine the occurrence of MDR-phenotype, antibiotic resistance profile, virulence traits, and genetic background of *E. coli* isolates from community and hospital-acquired UTIs from Mexico.

Methods

Escherichia coli isolation

This study was conducted on a total of one hundred and ten urine cultures collected from patients suspected to have an UTI (urine samples contained bacterial counts to $\geq 10^5$ CFU/ml) and sought attention in the Centenario Hospital Miguel Hidalgo, in Aguascalientes, Mexico during the period June to November 2012. Patient's ages ranged from neonatal to 91 years. Only one non-duplicated *E. coli* isolate per culture was considered. Patients from whom *E. coli* was isolated at least 48 h after admission were considered to have a hospital-acquired infection, all other infections were considered to be community-acquired [22]. To isolate *E. coli*, serial decimal dilutions of the sample were prepared in 0.85% NaCl, and were used to inoculate MacConkey agar plates which were incubated overnight at 37 °C. All the isolates were screened by PCR for the *uidA* gene as confirmation (Table 1). The *E. coli* isolates were stored at − 80 °C in Luria–Bertani broth and 20% (vol/vol) glycerol.

Antimicrobial susceptibility test

Susceptibility to antimicrobial agents was determined by the agar dilution method as recommended by the standards of Clinical Laboratory Standards Institute [23]. The following antimicrobial agents were tested: ampicillin, ampicillin–sulbactam, amoxicillin–clavulanic acid, piperacillin–tazobactam, cefazolin, cefotaxime, ceftazidime, ceftriaxone, cefepime, amikacin, gentamicin, tobramycin, netilmicin, imipenem, ertapenem, trimethoprim–sulfamethoxazole, ciprofloxacin, levofloxacin and norfloxacin. *E. coli* ATCC 25922 was included in each assay as a negative control.

Determination of phylo-groups

Phylo-grouping was determined by PCR as previously described by Clermont et al. [24]. *E. coli* strains H10407 (phylo-group A), E22 (phylo-group B1), CFT073 (phylo-group B2), ECOR 70 (phylo-group C), O42 (phylo-group D), EDL933 (phylo-group E) and ECOR 36 (phylo-group F), were taken as positive controls. Water was used as negative control. All strains controls were kindly provided by Laboratoire de référence pour *Escherichia coli*, EcL, Faculté de Médecine Vétérinaire, Université de Montréal.

Table 1 Oligonucleotides used in this study

Oligonucleotide name	Target gene	Oligonucleotide 5′→3′	Amplification product (bp)	References
E. coli marker				
uidA-forward	*uidA*	ATGTGCTGTGCCTGAACC	450	[60]
uidA-reverse		ATTGTTTGCCTCCCTGCTG		
Virulence genes for extra-intestinal pathogenic *E. coli*				
papC-forward	*papC*	GACGGCTGTACTGCAGGGTGTGGCG	350	[61]
papC-reverse		ATATCCTTTCTGCAGGGATGCAATA		
SfaSf	*sfaS*	GTGGATACGACGATTACTGTG	240	[62]
SfaSr		CCGCCAGCATTCCCTGTATTC		
Afaf	*afa/dra*	GGCAGAGGGCCGGCAACAGGC	592	[62]
Afar		CCCGTAACGCGCCAGCATCTC		
FyuAf	*fyuA*	TGATTAACCCCGCGACGGGAA	880	[62]
FyuAr		CGCAGTAGGCACGATGTTGTA		
yfcV-forward	*yfcV*	ACATGGAGACCACGTTCACC	292	[63]
yfcV-reverse		GTAATCTGGAATGTGGTCAGG		
Vat-forward	*vat*	TCAGGACACGTTCAGGCATTCAGT	1100	[63]
Vat-reverse		GGCCAGAACATTTGCTCCCTTGTT		
KpsMIIf	*kpsMT II*	GCGCATTTGCTGATACTGTTG	272	[62]
KpsMIIr		CATCCAGACGATAAGCATGAGCA		
Quinolone resistance genes				
gyrA11753	*gyrA*	GTATAACGCATTGCCGC	251	[64]
gyrA12004		TGCCAGATGTCCGAGAT		
EC-PAR-A	*parC*	CTGAATGCCAGCGCCAAATT	189	[65]
EC-PAR-B		GCGAACGATTTCGGATCGTC		
qnrA-forward	*qnrA*	TCAGCAAGAGGATTTCTCA	605	[66]
qnrA-reverse		GGCAGCACTATTACTCCCA		
qnrB-forward	*qnrB*	GATCGTGAAAGCCAGAAAGG	469	[12]
qnrB-reverse		ACGATGCCTGGTAGTTGTCC		
qnrS-forward	*qnrS*	ACGACATTCGTCAACTGCAA	417	[12]
qnrS-reverse		TAAATTGGCACCCTGTAGGC		
qnrC-forward	*qnrC*	GGGTTGTACATTTATTGAATC	447	[64]
qnrC-reverse		TCCACTTTACGAGGTTCT		
qnrD-forward	*qnrD*	CGAGATCAATTTACGGGGAATA	582	[27]
qnrD-reverse		AACAAGCTGAAGCGCCTG		
qepA-forward	*qepA*	CTGCAGGTACTGCGTCATG	403	[67]
qepA-reverse		CGTGTTGCTGGAGTTCTTC		
aac-forward	*acc-(6′)-Ib*	TTGCGATGCTCTATGAGTGGCTA	482	[26]
aac-reverse		CTCGAATGCCTGGCGTGTTT		
Beta-lactamase resistant genes				
blaTEM-forward	bla_{TEM}	GAGTATTCAACATTTTCGT	857	[30]
blaTEM-reverse		ACCAATGCTTAATCAGTGA		
blaSHV-forward	bla_{SHV}	TCGCCTGTGTATTATCTCCC	768	[30]
blaSHV-reverse		CGCAGATAAATCACCACAATG		
blaOXA-1-forward	bla_{OXA-1}	GCAGCGCCAGTGCATCAAC	198	[30]
blaOXA-1-reverse		CCGCATCAAATGCCATAAGTG		
blaOXA-7-forward	$bla_{OXA-7,-9}$	AGTTCTCTGCCGAAGCC	591	[30]
blaOXA-7-reverse		TCTCAACCCAACCAACCC		
blaPSE-4-forward	bla_{PSE-4}	CTGCTCGTATAGGTGTTTCC	705	[30]
blaPSE-4-reverse		TCGCATCATTTCGCTCTTC		

Table 1 (continued)

Oligonucleotide name	Target gene	Oligonucleotide 5′→3′	Amplification product (bp)	References
blaCTX-M-3-f	$bla_{CTX-M-3}$	AATCACTGCGTCAGTTCAC	701	[30]
blaCTX-M-3-r		TTTATCCCCCACAACCCAG		
blaCTX-M-forward	bla_{CTX-M}	AAGGCGTTTTGACAGACTATT	920	This study
blaCTX-M-reverse		GGTGACGATTTTAGCCGC		

Table 2 PCR control strains used in this study

Control strain	Positive gene (s)
J53pMG252	*qnrA*
J53pMG298	*qnrB*
J53pMG306	*qnrS*
Salmonella SA20042859	*aac(6′)-Ib*
CFT073	*uidA, papC, fyuA, chuA, kpsMTII, yfcV*
J96	*sfaS*
UTI89	*vat*
R455	bla_{OXA-1}
R6 K	bla_{TEM}
HB101	bla_{SHV}
pMG202	$bla_{OXA-7,-9}$
pMON711	bla_{PSE-4}
CCRI-2167	bla_{CTX-M}

Detection of virulence factors

Escherichia coli isolates from urinary tract infections were screened for the presence of commonly detected UPEC virulence genes including: *fyuA, fimH, sfaS, afa/dra, papC, agn43, yfcV, vat, hlyA, cnf1*and *kpsMTII.* Primers and controls used in this study are listed in Tables 1 and 2.

Characterization of resistance genes and mutations

Screening for plasmid mediated quinolone resistance (PMQR) genes, including *qnrA, qnrB, qnrS, qnrC, qnrD, qepA*, and *acc(6′)-lb* genes was performed as previously described [13, 25–28]. The *qnrC, qnrD* and *aac (6′)-Ib cr* variants were identified sequencing the PCR products. The quinolone resistance determining regions (QRDR) of *gyrA* and *parC* genes were amplified and sequenced on both strands and predicted peptide sequences were compared to the corresponding gene from the MG1655 genome as described by Namboodiri et al. [29]. Beta-lactams genes detection including bla_{TEM}, bla_{SHV}, bla_{OXA}, bla_{PSE} and bla_{CTX-M} were carried out by PCR amplification using specific primers [30]. Amplicons from all of the bla_{CTX-M} positive isolates were sequenced. The nucleotide sequences obtained were aligned and further analyzed by comparison to sequences from a catalogue of beta-lactamases (http://www.lahey.org/studies/).

DNA microarray analysis

Microarray hybridizations were performed using *E. coli* maxivirulence version 3.1 microarray as previously described [31]. It allows the detection of 348 virulence genes and 98 antibiotic resistance genes and variants. DNA extraction and hybridizations were performed as described previously [32]. Each isolate was assigned to a specific *E. coli* pathotype according to its virulence gene profile and based on the classification published in previous papers [31, 33].

Statistical analysis

Categorical variables were compared using Pearson's Chi square or Fisher's exact test as appropriate. Continuous variables were compared using Mann–Whitney U test (STATISTICA V. 10, StatSoft, United States). p values less than 0.05 were considered statistically significant.

Results

Patient demographics

During the period of study, females (86 samples, 78.2%) were the most affected group of patients ($p<0.05$) as compared to males (24 samples, 21.8%). Most of the UTIs were detected in community obtained samples (79 samples, 71.8%). Thirty-one samples were recovered from hospital-acquired infections (28.2%). *E. coli* isolated from female patients were correlated with community-acquired UTIs ($p=0.0297$). No differences among the prevalence of *E. coli* isolated from male patients among community- and hospital-acquired infections were found (54.2% vs 45.8%, respectively). Maximum number of cases was found in female children in the age group of 2–10 years (34 samples, 39%, $p=0.0372$, Table 3).

Antibiotic resistance and MDR profiles in *E. coli* isolates

High frequencies of resistance were observed toward trimethoprim–sulfamethoxazole (72.7%), ampicillin (70.9%), ampicillin–sulbactam (55.5%), piperacillin–tazobactam (55.5%), ciprofloxacin (47.3%), and levofloxacin (43.6%). From the twenty different antibiotic tested,

Table 3 Patients with urinary tract infections, n (%)

Age group	All patients, $n=110$ (%)	Male, $n=24$ (%)	Female, $n=86$ (%)	*p	Hospital-acquired, $n=31$ (%)	Community-acquired, $n=79$ (%)	*p
0–1	17 (15.5)	6 (25.0)	11 (12.8)	0.1434	5 (16.1)	12 (15.2)	0.9024
2–10	38 (34.5)	4 (16.7)	34 (39.5)	*0.0372*	9 (29.0)	29 (36.7)	0.4462
11–20	12 (10.9)	1 (4.2)	11 (12.8)	0.2308	2 (6.5)	10 (12.7)	0.3475
21–30	7 (6.4)	2 (8.3)	5 (5.8)	0.6548	1 (3.2)	6 (7.6)	0.3983
31–40	6 (5.5)	1 (4.2)	5 (5.8)	0.7533	1 (3.2)	5 (6.3)	0.5191
41–50	5 (4.5)	0 (0.0)	5 (5.8)	0.2266	1 (3.2)	4 (5.1)	0.6772
51–60	6 (5.5)	2 (8.3)	4 (4.7)	0.4824	3 (9.7)	3 (3.8)	0.2218
61–70	7 (6.4)	3 (12.5)	4 (4.7)	0.1636	3 (9.7)	4 (5.1)	0.3724
>71	12 (10.9)	5 (20.8)	7 (8.1)	0.0777	6 (19.4)	6 (7.6)	0.0751

* Italic number shown statistical significant values

all isolates were susceptible to carbapenems (ertapenem and imipenem, Table 4). Eighty-seven percent of the isolates were resistant to at least one antimicrobial agent, and 63.3% (70 isolates) were multidrug-resistant (MDR). MDR isolates were resistant to ampicillin (85.7%), trimethoprim–sulfamethoxazole (84.3%), ampicillin–sulbactam (77.1%), piperacillin–tazobactam (77.1%) and ciprofloxacin (70%, Table 4). A total of 94.2% (49/52 isolates) of FQ-resistant strains showed MDR-phenotype. A similar distribution of FQ-resistant isolates was found in the same at hospital as community-acquired infections, except for norfloxacin, which was

Table 4 Antibiotic and multidrug resistance of the UPEC's isolates, n (%)

Antibiotics	Total isolates, $n=110$ (%)	MDR, $n=70$ (%)	Male, $n=24$ (%)	Female, $n=86$ (%)	*p	Hospital-acquired, $n=31$ (%)	Community-acquired, $n=79$ (%)	*p
Amikacin	11 (10.0)	11 (15.9)	4 (16.7)	7 (8.1)		1 (3.2)	10 (12.7)	
Gentamicin	31 (28.2)	29 (41.4)	11 (45.8)	20 (23.3)	0.0297	10 (32.3)	21 (26.6)	
Tobramycin	21 (19.1)	21 (30.0)	10 (41.7)	11 (12.8)	0.0015	9 (29.0)	12 (15.2)	
Netilmicin	6 (5.5)	5 (7.1)	2 (8.3)	4 (4.7)		2 (6.5)	4 (5.1)	
Ampicillin	78 (70.9)	60 (85.7)	20 (83.3)	58 (67.4)		24 (77.4)	54 (68.4)	
Ampicillin–sulbactam	61 (55.5)	54 (77.1)	15 (62.5)	46 (53.5)		18 (58.1)	43 (54.4)	
Amoxicillin–clavulanic acid	26 (23.6)	23 (32.9)	5 (20.8)	21 (24.4)		6 (19.4)	20 (25.3)	
Piperacillin–tazobactam	61 (55.5)	54 (77.1)	15 (62.5)	46 (53.5)		18 (58.1)	43 (54.4)	
Cefazolin	46 (41.8)	45 (64.3)	15 (62.5)	31 (36.0)	0.0202	16 (51.6)	30 (38.0)	
Cefotaxime	20 (18.2)	20 (28.6)	5 (20.8)	15 (17.4)		6 (19.4)	14 (17.7)	
Ceftazidime	27 (24.5)	27 (38.6)	13 (54.2)	14 (16.3)	0.0001	12 (38.7)	15 (19.0)	0.0306
Ceftriaxone	30 (27.3)	30 (42.9)	14 (58.3)	16 (18.6)	0.0001	13 (41.9)	17 (21.5)	0.0305
Cefepime	29 (26.4)	29 (41.4)	14 (58.3)	15 (17.4)	0.0001	12 (38.7)	17 (21.5)	
Trimethoprim–sulfamethoxazole	80 (72.7)	59 (84.3)	18 (75.0)	62 (72.1)		24 (77.4)	56 (70.9)	
Ciprofloxacin	52 (47.3)	49 (70.0)	17 (70.8)	35 (40.7)	0.0089	15 (48.4)	37 (46.8)	
Levofloxacin	48 (43.6)	45 (64.3)	16 (66.7)	32 (37.2)	0.0314	13 (41.9)	35 (44.3)	
Norfloxacin	18 (16.4)	18 (25.7)	3 (12.5)	15 (17.4)		2 (6.5)	16 (20.3)	
Nitrofurantoin	14 (12.7)	12 (17.1)	5 (20.8)	9 (10.5)		4 (12.9)	10 (12.7)	0.0002
Ertapenem	0 (0.0)	0 (0.0)	0 (0.0)	0 (0.0)		0 (0.0)	0 (0.0)	
Imipenem	0 (0.0)	0 (0.0)	0 (0.0)	0 (0.0)		0 (0.0)	0 (0.0)	

* Only statistical significant values are shown

higher among community-acquired infections (20.3% vs 6.5%, Table 4). Distribution of ciprofloxacin and levofloxacin resistance was significantly higher among male than female gender (70.8, 66.7%, $p=0.0089$, 0.0314 vs 40.7, 37.2%, respectively, Table 4).

Co-resistance phenotype between cephalosporins and beta-lactams towards fluoroquinolones was frequently observed [(amoxicillin–clavulanic acid ($p=0.0004$), cefazolin ($p=0.0299$), cefotaxime ($p=0.0001$), ceftriaxone ($p=0.0002$) and, cefepime ($p=0.0015$)]. Trimethoprim–sulfamethoxazole and cephalosporins [cefotaxime ($p=0.0232$) and ceftazidime ($p=0.0001$)] also showed a co-resistance.

Overall, hospital-acquired isolates were slightly more resistant than community-acquired isolates (33.1% vs 28.7%, respectively). Both hospital and community-acquired isolates showed higher resistance towards ampicillin (77.4% vs 68.4%) and trimethoprim–sulfamethoxazole (77.4% vs 70.9%). UPEC isolates from hospital-acquired infections were associated to ceftazidime ($p=0.0306$), ceftriaxone ($p=0.0305$), and nitrofurantoin ($p=0.0002$) resistance phenotype (Table 4). MDR-phenotype was equally distributed among community-acquired (64.5%) and hospital-acquired (61.3%) isolates. Moreover, MDR-phenotype was associated to male infections (83.33%, $p=0.02329$). MDR-phenotype (69.6%) as well as the FQ-resistant phenotype (69.6%, p=0.0008) was also prevalent among older adults (> 60 years old).

Phylogenetic characterization, virulence genes, and their association to MDR-phenotype

All seven phylogenetic lineages (A, B1, B2, C, D, E and F) and cryptic clades were found on the 110 urinary *E. coli* isolates. The phylo-groups D (23.6%) and A (19.1%) were the most commonly found, followed by B1 (15.5%), C (13.6%), B2 (11.8%), F (10%), cryptic clades (5.5%) and phylo-group E (0.9%). The different phylo-groups and cryptic clades were distributed in both hospital and community settings, except the phylo-group E which was only distributed in the hospital-acquired infections. MDR strains were distributed into all phylogenetic-groups: 26% (16/70) to A, 17.1% (12/70) to D, 15.7% (11/70) to B1, 12.9% (9/70) to C, 11.4% (8/70) to B2 and F, and 6.7% (5/70) to cryptic clades. Phylo-group D was significantly associated to MDR-phenotype ($p=0.0339$) as well as FQ-resistant phenotype (26%, $p=0.0173$). Phylo-groups B2 and D were more common among community-acquired isolates (18.2, 9.1%) than hospital-acquired isolates (5.5, 2.7%), as well as in females (20.9, 7.3%) than in males (4.5, 2.7%) but not significantly associations were found.

Overall, *fimH* (71.8%), *fyuA* (68.2%), and *agn43* (54.5%) were the virulence genes with the highest distributions among isolates, while *afa/dra* (8.2%) and *cnf1* (2.7%) had the lowest. Others virulence genes tested had the following distribution: *chuA*, 49.1%; *papC*, 42.7%; *kpsMTII*, 37.3%; *vat*, 20%; *yfcV*, 20%; *sfaS* 10%, and *hlyA*, 9.1% (Table 5). Isolates from hospital-acquired infections presented slightly more prevalence of virulence genes than community-acquired infections (35.2% vs 30.2%). Prevalence of *fyuA* (71.0% vs 67.1%), *papC* (48.4% vs 40.5%), *yfcV* (25.8% vs 55.7%), *hlyA* (12.9% vs 7.6%), *cnf1* (3.2% vs 2.5%), *kpsMTII* (58.1% vs 29.1%) and *chuA* (51.6% vs 48.1%) were higher among UPEC isolated from hospital-acquired than community-acquired infections. However, only the *kpsMTII* was significantly associated with hospital-acquired isolates (58.1% vs 29.1%, $p=0.0047$, Table 5).

Table 5 Distribution of virulence genes among UPEC strains, n (%)

Virulence genes	Total isolates, $n=110$ (%)	MDR, $n=70$ (%)	Male, $n=24$ (%)	Female, $n=86$ (%)	*p	Hospital-acquired, $n=31$ (%)	Community-acquired, $n=79$ (%)	*p
fyuA	75 (68.2)	46 (65.7)	14 (58.3)	61 (70.9)		22 (71.0)	53 (67.1)	
fimH	79 (71.8)	51 (72.9)	20 (83.3)	59 (68.6)		21 (67.7)	58 (73.4)	
sfaS	11 (10)	6 (8.6)	2 (8.3)	9 (10.5)		2 (6.5)	9 (11.4)	
afa/dra	9 (8.2)	5 (7.1)	0 (0.0)	9 (10.5)		2 (6.5)	7 (8.9)	
papC	47 (42.7)	27 (38.6)	12 (50.0)	35 (40.7)		15 (48.4)	32 (40.5)	
agn43	60 (54.5)	39 (55.7)	14 (58.3)	46 (53.5)		16 (51.6)	44 (55.7)	
yfcV	22 (20)	15 (21.4)	10 (41.7)	12 (14.0)	0.0026	8 (25.8)	14 (17.7)	
vat	22 (20)	13 (18.3)	7 (29.2)	15 (17.4)		6 (19.4)	16 (20.3)	
hlyA	10 (9.1)	7 (10.0)	4 (16.7)	6 (7.0)		4 (12.9)	6 (7.6)	
cnf1	3 (2.7)	2 (2.9)	1 (4.2)	2 (2.3)		1 (3.2)	2 (2.5)	
kpsMTII	41 (37.3)	25 (35.7)	9 (37.5)	32 (37.2)		18 (58.1)	23 (29.1)	0.0047
chuA	54 (49.1)	32 (45.7)	11 (45.8)	43 (50.0)		16 (51.6)	38 (48.1)	

* Only statistical significant values are shown

Comparing male vs female patients, isolates from females had a higher mean of virulence genes compared those isolates from male origin (21.5% vs 7.9%, respectively). Moreover, the *yfcV* was significantly more associated to male infections (41.7%, $p=0.0026$). The presence of the *chuA* gene was associated to UPEC isolated from children ($p=0.0483$). Furthermore, the presence of *vat* was associated to UPEC isolates from adults ($p=0.0153$).

Virulence genes *fimH* (72.9%), *fyuA* (65.7%), *agn43* (55.7%) and *chuA* (45.7%, Table 5), were highly distributed among MDR strains. However none virulence genes were significantly associated to MDR-phenotype or FQ-resistant isolates. Nevertheless, *fimH* (69.2%), *fyuA* (67.3%) and *chuA* (57.7%) were highly distributed among FQ-resistant bacteria.

Identification of virulence, and antimicrobial resistance genes by microarray analysis

Microarray analysis was done on 18 *E. coli* isolates belonging to the phylo-groups B2, D and F. Overall, 145 virulence and 40 antimicrobial resistance genes among the 315 and 82 genes and variants investigated were detected at least once in one or more of the isolates. The total number of virulence genes per isolate ranged from 18 to 63 genes. The median number of the virulence genes per isolate was 35. Microarray hybridizations demonstrated that all the *E. coli* isolates tested possessed virulence genes related to a pathotype including ExPEC and diarrheagenic *E. coli* (DEC). The total number of antimicrobial resistance genes per isolate ranged from 0 to 21 genes with a median number of 6.5 genes. Since the microarray carries a large set of virulence factors, numerous incomplete ExPEC that would normally be missed in a PCR-based assay were found. Thus, various unusual gene combinations were discovered, such as ExPEC pathogenic profiles with assorted EPEC genes coding for the type III secretion system 2 proteins ErpJ and SpaS (gene *eprJ* and *epaS*, respectively). Moreover, detection of virulence (mean 39.0 ± 16.9) and antimicrobial resistance (mean 9.0 ± 1.9) genes were higher on hospital-acquired UTIs isolates compared to community-acquired infections (Table 6). Higher frequency of virulence genes was found among isolates retrieved from females compared to those from males (36.25 ± 17.04

Table 6 Virulence and antimicrobial resistance genes detected by microarray analysis exclusively among *E. coli* B2, D and F isolates from UTIs patients

	Type of infection	
	Hospital-acquired ($n=4$)	Community-acquired ($n=14$)
Virulence genes (mean)	39	32
Antimicrobial resistance genes (mean)	9	6
Phylo-groups	B2 ($n=2$) and D ($n=2$)	B2 ($n=9$), D ($n=3$) and F ($n=2$)
Virulence genes function		
Resistance	bla_{TEM}, bla_{OXA-1}, bla_{PSE-1}, $bla_{CTX-M-15}$, bla_{CMY-2}, *mphA*, *ant(3″)-Ia (aadA1)*, *aac(3)-IIa (aacC2)*, *tet(A)*, *tet(B)*, *tet(30)*, *tet(R)*, *sulI sulII*, *qnrA*, *aac(6′)-Ib-cr*, class 1 integron	bla_{TEM}, bla_{OXA-1}, bla_{OXA-9}, bla_{PSE-1}, $bla_{CTX-M-15}$, $bla_{CTX-M-12}$, $bla_{OXY/K1}$, *ant(3″)-Ia (aadA1)*, *aac(3)-IIa (aacC2)*, *aac(3)-IV*, *aph(3′)-Ia (aphA1)*, *aph(3′)-IIa (aphA2)*, *aph3 (strA)*, *dhfrI*, *dhfrVII*, *catI*, *sulI*, *sulII*, *tet(A)*, *tet(B)*, *tet(30)*, *mphA*, class 1 integron, class 2 integron
Adhesins	*afaD, afaD8, afaE1, afaE2, afaE5, bfpA, fimC, ibeB, csgA, csgE, f165(1)A, fimA, fimH, iha, lpfA(O113), papA(10), papA(11), papA(16), papA(8), papC, papGI2, fitA, sfaHII, sfaD*	*afaE1, afaE2, afaE5, cofA, lpfA2, fimC, csgA, csgE, csuA, F17b-A, F17d-A, facA, lpfA1, fimA, iha, lpfA(O113), lpfA, papA(8), papA(9), papA(10), papA(12), papA(13), papA(15), papA(40), papA(48), papC, papGII, papGIV, fitA, sfaHII, sfaA*
Colcins and microsins	*cvaC, mchB*	*cda, ce1a, cib, cvaC, mcbA.*
Toxins	*Sat*	*astA, astA(2), cdtB-4, cnf1, sat*
Iron acquisition or transport system	*chuA, fepC, fyuA, iroN, iroN(2), irp1, irp2, iucD, iutA, iutA(2), iutA(UPEC), sitA, sitD*	*chuA, fepC, fimH, fyuA, iroN(2), irp1, irp2, iucD, iutA, iutA(2), iutA(UPEC), sitA, sitD*
Capsular and somatic antigens	*kpsMTII, neuC*	*kpsMTII, neuA, neuC*
Locus of enterocyte effacement (LEE)	*eae(delta)*	*eae(lambda), espG, esta1*
ETT2 elements	*eivG, eprJ*	*eivG, eprJ, epaS*
Haemolysins and hemagglutinins	*hlyA, hlyE, hra1*	*bmaE, hlyA, hlyE, hra1.*
Various functions	*agn43, capU, ccdB, deoK, fliC, gad, iss, iss(3), malX, ompA, ompT, ompT(2), senB, traT*	*agn43, capU, ccdB, ibeA, ibeB, deoK, eaf, fliC, fliC(H7), gad, invX, iss, iss(3), malX, ompA, ompT, ompT(2), senB, traT*
Newly recognized or putative *E. coli* virulence genes	*artJ, b1121, b1432, gimB(orf1), mviM, mviN, shf, usp, virK*	*artJ, b1121, mviM, mviN, set, shf, usp, virK*

mean vs 31.66 ± 13.00 mean, respectively), as well as those isolates from children vs adults (36.58 ± 7.4 mean vs 26.6 ± 16.39 mean, respectively). In addition, antimicrobial resistance genes were also detected on higher ratios among isolates retrieved from males compared to those from females (7.88 ± 5.53 mean vs 4.0 ± 3.03 mean, respectively); a similar situation was observed when strains isolates from children vs those from adults were compared (14.60 ± 5.79 mean vs 4.4 ± 2.60 mean, respectively). Interestingly, the maximum number of antimicrobial resistance genes was found among UPEC isolates from children.

Distribution of plasmid-mediated quinolone resistance genes, and ESBL genes

Overall, 22% of the isolates were positive for *qnrA* (25 isolates), 20.9% (23 isolates) to *qnrB*, 6.4% (7 isolates) to *qnrS1*, 0.9% (1 isolates) to *qnrC*, 4.5% (5 isolates) to *qnrD*, and 6.4% (7 isolates) to *aac(6′)-Ib-cr* (Table 7). None isolates were positive to *qepA* gene. Isolates were taken to sequencing to obtain information on the QRDRs of the *gyrA* and *parC* genes, respectively. The sequencing results for the QRDR of *gyrA* and *parC* are summarized in Table 8. Only one isolate tested had no mutations in the QRDRs of *gyrA* and *parC* since was sensitive to ciprofloxacin (CIP), levofloxacin (LEV), and norfloxacin (NOR). The double mutations in Ser-83 → Leu and Asp-87 → Tyr or Asp-87 → Asn substitution in *gyrA* were present in 92% of the strain tested. Ser-80 → Ile substitution in *parC* were found in 92% of the isolates tested, which also were resistant to both ciprofloxacin and levofloxacin. The substitution Thr-66 → Ser (1 strain, CIP-resistant, LEV-resistant), Thr-66 → Asn (1 strain, CIP-resistant, LEV-resistant), and Thr-66 → Tyr (2 strains, CIP-resistant, LEV-resistant) were also found in *parC*. Other substitutions in *parC* as Glu-84 → Val (2 strains, CIP-resistant, LEV-resistant) and Glu-84 → Ala were also detected. Interestingly, one strain (isolated UEc 76) which was resistant to ciprofloxacin, levofloxacin and norfloxacin, belonging to B2 phylo-group and blaCTX-M-containing, also carried the double mutations in Ser-83 → Leu and Asp-87 → Asn substitution in *gyrA* and the triple mutation in *parC* Ser-80 → Ile, Thr-66 → Tyr and Glu-84 → Val.

ESBL genes were investigated through microarray and PCR assay. A total of 27 isolates (24.5%) suspected as cephalosporinase producers showed positive PCRs for $bla_{CTX\text{-}M}$ (12.7%/14 isolates), bla_{TEM} (18.2%/20 isoaltes), bla_{PSE} (2.7%/3 isoaltes), and bla_{OXA} (9.1%/10 isolates). Sequencing of the $bla_{CTX\text{-}M}$ amplicons identified the presence of $bla_{CTX\text{-}M\text{-}15}$ in 7.2% of the strains (8 isolates), $bla_{CTX\text{-}M\text{-}12}$ in 4.5% (5 isolates), $bla_{CTX\text{-}M\text{-}3}$ in 1.8% (2 isolates), and $bla_{CTX\text{-}M\text{-}14}$ in 1.8% (2 isolates). Furthermore, $bla_{ROB\text{-}1}$, $bla_{SHV\text{-}37}$, and $bla_{CMY\text{-}2}$ genes, were identified in one isolate (0.9%) through the microarray assay.

Overall $bla_{CTX\text{-}M}$ genes and PMQR genes as well as mutation in QRDR were found in both community- and hospital-acquired infections as well as in male and female genders. The PMQR *qnrA* (21.4%), and *qnrB* (18.6%), were highly distributed on MDR-phenotype (Table 7). Isolates from males had higher prevalence of *aac(6′)-Ib*-cr gene compare to female isolates (16.6% vs 3.5%, $p = 0.0194$). Quinolone-resistance isolates also presented higher prevalence to $bla_{CTX\text{-}M}$ compared to quinolone-sensitive phenotype isolates (21% vs 5.2%, $p = 0.012$).

Discussion

In accordance with global trends, our results reveal higher prevalence of urinary tract infections in female patients than in males [7, 34–36]. The emergence of high rates of antibiotic resistance and MDR-phenotype from urinary tract infections related bacteria becomes a public health concern worldwide. In this study, more than 70% of the isolates showed resistance to trimethoprim–sulfamethoxazole (TMP–SXT) that is recommended as a first choice for UTI treatment [36]. Previous

Table 7 Distributions of PMQR and blaCTX-M genes among UPEC, n (%)

Virulence genes	Total isolates, $n = 110$ (%)	MDR, $n = 70$ (%)	Male, $n = 24$ (%)	Female, $n = 86$ (%)	*p	Hospital-acquired, $n = 31$ (%)	Community-acquired, $n = 79$ (%)
qnrA	25 (22.7)	15 (21.4)	7 (29.2)	18 (20.9)		9 (29.0)	16 (20.3)
qnrB	23 (20.9)	13 (18.6)	6 (25.0)	17 (19.8)		10 (32.3)	13 (16.5)
qnrS	7 (6.4)	3 (4.3)	3 (12.5)	4 (4.7)		2 (6.5)	5 (6.3)
qnrC	1 (0.9)	0 (0.0)	0 (0.0)	1 (1.2)		0 (0.0)	1 (1.3)
qnrD	5 (4.5)	4 (5.7)	1 (4.2)	4 (4.7)		3 (9.7)	2 (2.5)
aac(6′)-Ib-cr	7 (6.4)	4 (5.7)	4 (16.6)	3 (3.5)	0.0194	2 (6.5)	5 (6.3)
$bla_{CTX\text{-}M}$	14 (12.4)	11 (15.7)	5 (20.8)	9 (10.5)		4 (12.9)	10 (12.7)

* Only statistical significant values are shown

Table 8 Characterization of UTI isolates

Strain	Resistance profile	Phylo-group	PMQR genes	QRDR mutations		β-lactamase-resistance-genes	Other resistant genes	Integron
				ΔGyrA	ΔParC			
UEc 11	AMP, SXT	B2		NA	NA	*bla*$_{TEM}$	*ant(3″)-Ia (aadA1), aph3 (strA), dhfrI, sulI, tet(B)*	Class 2 integron
UEc 22	AMP, SAM, AMC, CFZ, SXT, CIP, LEV, NOR	B2		S83→L D87→N	S80→I T66→N	*bla*$_{TEM}$	*tet(B)*	
UEc 23	AMP, SAM, CFZ, CTZ, CAZ, CRO, FEP, SXT, CIP, LEV	F	*aac(6′)-Ib-cr*	NA	NA		*aac(3)-IIa (aacC2)*	Class 1 integron
UEc 27	GEN, AMP, SAM, AMC, SXT, CIP, LEV	B2		S83→L D87→N	S80→I E84→V	*bla*$_{PSE-1}$	*sulI, tet(A)*	
UEc 30	GEN, SAM, AMC, SXT	B2		NA	NA	*bla*$_{OXA-1}$	*ant(3″)-Ia (aadA1), tet(A), tet(30), tet®, sulI*	Class 1 integron
UEc 58	AMP, SXT, CIP, LEV	B2		S83→L D87→N G114→S	S80→I	*bla*$_{TEM}$	*dhfrVII, sulII, tet(B), aph3 (strA), mphA*	
UEc 65	AMP, CFZ, CAZ, CRO, FEP, CIP, LEV	D		S83→L D87→N G114→S	S80→I	*bla*$_{CTX-M-15}$ *bla*$_{TEM}$	*aac(3)-IIa (aacC2), dhfrVII, mphA, sulI, tet(B)*	Class 1 integron
UEc 69	AMP, SXT, NIT	B2	*qnrA*	NA	NA	*bla*$_{TEM}$	*sulII*	
UEc 75	AMK, GEN, AMP, SAM, AMC, TZP, CFZ, CTX, CRO, FEPCIP, LEV, NOR	B2	*qnrA*	S83→L D87→N	S80→I T66→Y	*bla*$_{OXY/K1}$, *bla*$_{TEM}$	*aac(3)-IIa (aacC2), aph(3′)-Ia (aphA1), aph(3′)-IIa (aphA2), aph3 (strA), sulI, sulII, tet(A), tet(B)*	
UEc 76	CFZ, CAZ, CRO, FEP, CIP, LEV	B2		S83→L D87→N	S80→I T66→Y E84→V	*bla*$_{CTX-M-15}$ *bla*$_{OXA-1}$	*tet(A), tet(30)*	
UEc 84	GEN, TOB, AMP, SAM, TZP, CFZ, CTX, CAZ, CRO, FEP, SXT, CIP, LEV	D	*aac(6′)-Ib-cr*	S83→L D87→N	S80→I	*bla*$_{CTX-M-15}$, *bla*$_{OXA-1}$ *bla*$_{TEM}$ *bla*$_{PSE-4}$	*tet(30), mphA*	
UEc 99	AMP, SXT	B2	*qnrA*	None	None	*bla*$_{CTX-M-12}$, *bla*$_{OXA-9}$, *bla*$_{TEM}$	*aac(3)-IV, aac(3)-IIa (aacC2), aph3 (strA), catI, sulI, sulII*	Class 1 integron
UEc 102	AMP, CFZ, CAZ, CRO, FEP, SXT, CIP, LEV	B2		S83→L D87→N G114→S	S80→I	*bla*$_{TEM}$	*aph(3′)-Ia (aphA1), sulII*	
UEc 104	AMP, SXT	D	*qnrA, aac(6′)-Ib-cr*	NA	NA	*bla*$_{CMY-2}$, *bla*$_{CTX-M-12}$, *bla*$_{OXA-1}$	*aac(3)-IIa (aacC2), sulI, tet(B), mphA*	Class 1 integron
UEc 107		F		NA	NA			
UEc 108	AMP	D	*qnrA*	NA	NA	*bla*$_{TEM}$	*sulI*	Class 1 integron
UEc 109	AMP, SAM	D	*aac(6′)-Ib-cr*	NA	NA	*bla*$_{TEM}$	*sulII*	
UEc 110	GEN, TOB, AMP, SAM, CTX, SXT, CIP, NIT	B2		NA	NA		*aac(3)-IIa (aacC2), tet(B)*	Class 1 integron

AMK Amikacin, *GEN* gentamicin, *TOB* tobramycin, *NET* netilmicin, *AMP* ampicillin, *SAM* ampicillin–sulbactam, *AMC* amoxicillin–clavulanic acid, *TZP* piperacillin–tazobactam, *CFZ* cefazolin, *CTX* cefotaxime, *CAZ* ceftazidime, *CRO* ceftriaxone, *FEP* cefepime; *SXT* trimethoprim–sulfamethoxazole, *CIP* ciprofloxacin, *LEV* levofloxacin, *NOR* norfloxacin, *NIT* nitrofurantoin, *ETP* ertapenem, *IPM* imipenem, *PMQR* plasmid-mediated quinolone resistance genes, *QRDR* quinolone resistance-determining region, *NA* not analyzed

studies reported similar results [20, 36]. In agreement with Bouchillon et al. [34] in this study, UPEC isolates presented more than 40% resistance to ciprofloxacin and levofloxacin antibiotics. Moreover, resistance rates to antimicrobial drugs were higher in isolates from male than in those from female patients [37]. Interestingly, fluoroquinolones are widely used for the treatment of UTIs in male patients [36, 38]. It is possible that male infections may be more difficult to eradicate because of the higher rates of antibiotic resistance observed in strains isolated from males, which may lead to recurrent infections. These observations were similar to previous papers [35, 36, 39]. Susceptibility analysis of isolates to antibiotics prior to treatment choice is recommended.

Multidrug-resistant strain prevalence (63.3%) was higher in this work than in other study from Mexico, which reported only 16.4% of MDR strains [21]. While work of Paniagua-Contreras et al. [20], showed 97% of MDR strains. It is well known that susceptibility patterns may vary in different geographical regions and can be change over time [36]. In addition, an unexpected result was found, as the percentage of resistance to the antibiotics tested and MDR-phenotype were similar in hospital and community-acquired infections, indicating an important reservoir of resistance in both settings [34]. This could be due to household use of antibiotics before 2010, which would were acquired without prescription then. Moreover, resistance to cephalosporin and nitrofurantoin was associated to hospital-acquired infections. Co-resistance with fluoroquinolones and TMP–SXT was also observed in both hospital and community.

As detected by Ochoa et al. [21], phylo-group D, an important phylo-group in pathogenic ExPEC was associated to MDR-phenotype. Additionally, FQ-resistant strains were correlated to phylo-group D strains. Strains from hospital-acquired infections exhibited a greater number of virulence genes than those from community. In addition, *E. coli* isolates from hospital-acquired UTIs are correlated to the presence of *kpsMTII* gene that has been associated to pyelonephritis, a more severe infection of the upper urinary tract [40]. In agreement with other studies [20, 41], our results showed an important frequency of *fyuA*-encoding yersiniabactin receptor and, *fimH* encoding type 1 fimbrial adhesion.

Detailed analysis of a strains subset using microarrays, revealed that some of them from both, hospital- and community-acquired infections carried virulence related genes of enteroaggregative and diffusely adherent *E. coli* (EAEC and DAEC), including *capU* (cap locus protein, hexosyltransferasa), *deoK* (deoxyribokinase), *shf* (putative virulence factor, plasmid pAA2, similar to *Shigella flexneri* Shf), *virK* (similar to *Shigella flexneri* virulence protein VirK, plasmid pAA2) and *astA* gene (EAEC heat-stable enterotoxin 1). This was also reported in previous works [42–45], which noticed that EAEC virulence related genes were among the most frequent markers of diarrheagenic *E. coli* reported in ExPEC strains. The *deoK* operon is frequently associated with strains isolated from infected urine and blood and is part of a large genetic island carrying genes contributing to the strain intrinsic virulence and/or adaptive properties [43]. These strains, by acquiring the pAA plasmid, could become a potential diarrheal agent [42].

Another finding was the presence of enteropathogenic *E. coli* (EPEC) related genes on five UPEC isolates. These genes included the *eae* (coding for intimin, a protein involved in attaching and effacing lesions), as well as virulence related genes such as *espG* (protein secreted by the type III secretion system and translocated into host epithelial cells), *eprJ* (*E. coli* type III secretion system 2 protein ErpJ), *epaS* (*E. coli* type III secretion system 2 protein EpaS), and *eivG* (*E. coli* type III secretion system 2 protein EivG) [3, 46]. T3SS genes are not common in UPEC isolates, however genes encoding components of T3SS have been found [47, 48]. These unusual gene combinations illustrate genome plasticity displayed by UPEC strains that may result in new hybrids pathotypes [45, 49, 50].

In this study, UPEC strains carrying PMQR genes associated to quinolones resistance including *qnrA*, *qnrB*, *qnrS*, *qnrC* and *qnrD* as well as *aac(6′)-Ib-cr* were detected. The most common PMQR-genes identified were *qnrA* and *qnrB*, which is in contrast to previous studies were *aac(6′)-Ib-cr* gene detection was more frequent on ExPEC isolates [19, 51]. Moreover, *qnrA* and *qnrB* were frequently found as a part of MDR-phenotype. *qnrD* gene was found in 4.5% of the isolates. Previous papers reported *qnrD* in bacteria isolated from rooks [51], pigs [15] and humans clinical isolates of *Salmonella enterica* serovar Kentucky, serovar Bovismorbificans, *Proteus mirabilis* and *Morganella morganii* [52, 53], as well as in *E. coli* from dogs [54]. In accordance to others studies [19, 55, 56], *qepA* was not identified. Although PMQR genes provide a low level of FQ-resistance, they have been reported to favor the selection of additional chromosome-encoded resistance mechanism [57]. In our study, QRDR mutations in *gyrA* and *parC* were prevalent in community-acquired infections (89% vs 11%). Overall, mutations in QRDR were equally present among isolates from males and females patients.

In our study, ESBL genes $bla_{CTX\text{-}M}$ ($bla_{CTX\text{-}M\text{-}15}$, $bla_{CTX\text{-}M\text{-}14}$, $bla_{CTX\text{-}M\text{-}12}$, and $bla_{CTX\text{-}M\text{-}3}$), bla_{TEM}, bla_{PSE}, and bla_{OXA} were detected. For the isolates carrying resistance genes, ESBL genes such as TEM, SHV and CTX-M, are the most widespread and frequently detected in *E. coli* [9]. In addition, CTX-M-15 is quite common in Mexico [58, 59].

Conclusions

Our study describes significant antimicrobial resistance in *E. coli* UTI isolates from hospital and community in Mexico. Diverse genotypes and phenotypes including multidrug-resistance, fluoroquinolone resistance and carriage of virulence genes related to several enteropathogenic *E. coli* were found among UPEC isolates. Thus, continuous surveillance for antimicrobial resistance of UPEC is needed in order to prevent treatment failure and to improve the strategies to mitigate the occurrence of antibiotic resistance organisms and ensure the best treatment to UTI patients. This study highlights the importance of antimicrobial resistance of virulent *E. coli* from urinary tract infection in Mexico.

Abbreviations

UTIs: urinary tract infections; MDR: multiple drug resistance; ExPEC: extra-intestinal pathogenic *E. coli*; ESBL: extended-spectrum beta-lactamase; QRQR: quinolone resistance-determining region; FQ-phenotype: fluoroquinolone resistance phenotype.

Authors' contributions

All authors contributed towards the study concept, data analysis and revising of the paper and agreed to be accountable for all aspects of the work. All authors read and approved the final manuscript.

Author details

[1] Laboratorio de Biología Celular y Tisular, Departamento de Morfología, Universidad Autónoma de Aguascalientes, Av. Universidad 940, Col. Cd. Universitaria, 20131 Aguascalientes, Mexico. [2] Laboratorio de Ciencias Ambientales, Departamento de Fisiología y Farmacología, Universidad Autónoma de Aguascalientes, Av. Universidad 940, Col. Cd. Universitaria, 20131 Aguascalientes, Mexico. [3] Departamento de Infectología, Centenario Hospital Miguel Hidalgo, Galeana Sur 495, Obraje, 20000 Aguascalientes, Mexico. [4] Département de pathologie et microbiologie, Centre de Recherche en Infectologíe Porcine et Aviaire, Faculté de Médecine Vétérinaire, Université de Montréal, 3200, rue Sicott, Saint-Hyacinthe, Montreal, QC J2S 2M2, Canada.

Acknowledgements

We thank for the technical assistance to Fabiola Galindo Guerrero and Nayeli Amalinalli Pulido Hornedo. We also acknowledge the collaboration and help of the technician support of the clinical laboratory of the Centenario Hospital Miguel Hidalgo at Aguascalientes, Mexico. We thank to M.Sc. Philippe Garneau and Ph.D. Ricardo Oropeza for profiting the paper. We are thankful to Laboratoire de référence pour *Escherichia coli* (EcL), of the Faculté de médecine vétérinaire of the Université de Montréal for kindly provide the controls for the phylo-group assay. We are gratefully acknowledge the fie grate support of the Natural Sciences and Engineering Research Council of Canada (RGPIN–25120) and from—Fonds de la recherché du Québec en Nature et Technologies (Centre de recherché en infectiologie porcine et avicole, CRIPA—Regroupements stratégiques RS-170946) to J. H. (RGPIN–25120) and from the DFAIT Canada's Emerging leaders in the Americas program. Authors contributed on this article are: Alma Lilian (AL) Guerrero Barrera; Flor Yazmín (FY) Ramírez Castillo; Adriana Cecilia (AC) Moreno Flores; Francisco Javier (FJ) Avelar González; Francisco (F) Márquez Díaz; Josée (J) Harel.

Competing interests

The authors declare that they have no competing interests.

Funding

Not applicable.

References

1. Struelens MJ, Denis O, Rodriguez-Villalobos H. Microbiology of nosocomial infections: progress and challenges. Microbes Infect. 2004;6(11):1043–8.
2. Kucheria R, Dasgupta P, Sacks SH, Khan MS, Sheerin NS. Urinary tract infections: new insights into a common problem. Postgrad Med J. 2005;81(952):83–6.
3. Kaper JB, Nataro JP, Mobley HL. Pathogenic *Escherichia coli*. Nat Rev Microbiol. 2004;2(2):123–40.
4. Stamm WE, Norrby SR. Urinary tract infections: disease panorama and challenges. J Infect Dis. 2001;183(Suppl 1):S1–4.
5. Russo TA, Johnson JR. Medical and economic impact of extraintestinal infections due to *Escherichia coli*: focus on an increasingly important endemic problem. Microbes Infect. 2003;5(5):449–56.
6. SINAVE/DGE/Salud. Boletín Epidemiológico. Sistema Nacional de Vigilancia Epidemiológica. Sistema Único de informaicón. Dirección General de Epidemiología. 2016;33(46):semana 46.
7. Dehbanipour R, Rastaghi S, Sedighi M, Maleki N, Faghri J. High prevalence of multidrug-resistance uropathogenic *Escherichia coli* strains, Isfahan, Iran. J Nat Sci Biol Med. 2016;7(1):22–6.
8. Liu BT, Yang QE, Li L, Sun J, Liao XP, Fang LX, Yang SS, Deng H, Liu YH. Dissemination and characterization of plasmids carrying *oqxAB-bla*$_{CTX-M}$ genes in *Escherichia coli* isolates from food-producing animals. PLoS ONE. 2013;8(9):e73947.
9. Pitout JD, Laupland KB. Extended-spectrum beta-lactamase-producing Enterobacteriaceae: an emerging public-health concern. Lancet Infect Dis. 2008;8(3):159–66.
10. Urban C, Mariano N, Bradford PA, Tuckman M, Segal-Maurer S, Wehbeh W, Grenner L, Colon-Urban R, Johnston B, Johnson JR, et al. Identification of CTX-M beta-lactamases in *Escherichia coli* from hospitalized patients and residents of long-term care facilities. Diagn Microbiol Infect Dis. 2010;66(4):402–6.
11. Martinez-Martinez L, Pascual A, Jacoby GA. Quinolone resistance from a transferable plasmid. Lancet. 1998;351(9105):797–9.
12. Robicsek A, Strahilevitz J, Sahm DF, Jacoby GA, Hooper DC. *qnr* prevalence in ceftazidime-resistant Enterobacteriaceae isolates from the United States. Antimicrob Agents Chemother. 2006;50(8):2872–4.
13. Perichon B, Courvalin P, Galimand M. Transferable resistance to aminoglycosides by methylation of G1405 in 16S rRNA and to hydrophilic fluoroquinolones by QepA-mediated efflux in *Escherichia coli*. Antimicrob Agents Chemother. 2007;51(7):2464–9.
14. Hansen LH, Johannesen E, Burmolle M, Sorensen AH, Sorensen SJ. Plasmid-encoded multidrug efflux pump conferring resistance to olaquindox in *Escherichia coli*. Antimicrob Agents Chemother. 2004;48(9):3332–7.
15. Zhao J, Chen Z, Chen S, Deng Y, Liu Y, Tian W, Huang X, Wu C, Sun Y, Sun Y, et al. Prevalence and dissemination of *oqxAB* in *Escherichia coli* isolates from animals, farmworkers, and the environment. Antimicrob Agents Chemother. 2010;54(10):4219–24.
16. Poirel L, Cattoir V, Nordmann P. Plasmid-mediated quinolone resistance; interactions between human, animal, and environmental ecologies. Front Microbiol. 2012;3:24.
17. Andres P, Lucero C, Soler-Bistue A, Guerriero L, Albornoz E, Tran T, Zorreguieta A, Group P, Galas M, Corso A, et al. Differential distribution of plasmid-mediated quinolone resistance genes in clinical enterobacteria with unusual phenotypes of quinolone susceptibility from Argentina. Antimicrob Agents Chemother. 2013;57(6):2467–75.
18. Amabile-Cuevas CF, Arredondo-Garcia JL, Cruz A, Rosas I. Fluoroquinolone resistance in clinical and environmental isolates of *Escherichia coli* in Mexico City. J Appl Microbiol. 2010;108(1):158–62.
19. Silva-Sanchez J, Cruz-Trujillo E, Barrios H, Reyna-Flores F, Sanchez-Perez A, Bacterial Resistance C, Garza-Ramos U. Characterization of plasmid-mediated quinolone resistance (PMQR) genes in extended-spectrum beta-lactamase-producing Enterobacteriaceae pediatric clinical isolates in Mexico. PLoS ONE. 2013;8(10):e77968.
20. Paniagua-Contreras GL, Monroy-Perez E, Rodriguez-Moctezuma JR, Dominguez-Trejo P, Vaca-Paniagua F, Vaca S. Virulence factors, antibiotic resistance phenotypes and O-serogroups of *Escherichia coli* strains isolated from community-acquired urinary tract infection patients in Mexico. J Microbiol Immunol Infect. 2017;50(4):478–85.
21. Ochoa SA, Cruz-Cordova A, Luna-Pineda VM, Reyes-Grajeda JP, Cazares-Dominguez V, Escalona G, Sepulveda-Gonzalez ME, Lopez-Montiel F, Arellano-Galindo J, Lopez-Martinez B, et al. Multidrug- and extensively drug-resistant uropathogenic *Escherichia coli* clinical strains: phylogenetic groups widely associated with integrons maintain high genetic diversity. Front Microbiol. 2016;7:2042.
22. Sotto A, De Boever CM, Fabbro-Peray P, Gouby A, Sirot D, Jourdan J. Risk factors for antibiotic-resistant *Escherichia coli* isolated from hospitalized patients with urinary tract infections: a prospective study. J Clin Microbiol. 2001;39(2):438–44.

23. Standards NCCL, National Committee for Clinical Laboratory Standards. Performance standards for antimicrobial susceptibility testing; Twenty-Second Informational Supplement: M100-S22. National Committee for Clinical Laboratory Standards: Wayne; 2012.
24. Clermont O, Christenson JK, Denamur E, Gordon DM. The Clermont *Escherichia coli* phylo-typing method revisited: improvement of specificity and detection of new phylo-groups. Environ Microbiol Rep. 2013;5(1):58–65.
25. Jacoby GA, Chow N, Waites KB. Prevalence of plasmid-mediated quinolone resistance. Antimicrob Agents Chemother. 2003;47(2):559–62.
26. Park CH, Robicsek A, Jacoby GA, Sahm D, Hooper DC. Prevalence in the United States of *aac(6')-Ib-cr* encoding a ciprofloxacin-modifying enzyme. Antimicrob Agents Chemother. 2006;50(11):3953–5.
27. Cavaco LM, Hasman H, Xia S, Aarestrup FM. *qnrD*, a novel gene conferring transferable quinolone resistance in *Salmonella enterica* serovar Kentucky and Bovismorbificans strains of human origin. Antimicrob Agents Chemother. 2009;53(2):603–8.
28. Wang M, Guo Q, Xu X, Wang X, Ye X, Wu S, Hooper DC, Wang M. New plasmid-mediated quinolone resistance gene, *qnrC*, found in a clinical isolate of *Proteus mirabilis*. Antimicrob Agents Chemother. 2009;53(5):1892–7.
29. Namboodiri SS, Opintan JA, Lijek RS, Newman MJ, Okeke IN. Quinolone resistance in *Escherichia coli* from Accra Ghana. BMC Microbiol. 2011;11:44.
30. Maynard C, Fairbrother JM, Bekal S, Sanschagrin F, Levesque RC, Brousseau R, Masson L, Lariviere S, Harel J. Antimicrobial resistance genes in enterotoxigenic *Escherichia coli* O149:K91 isolates obtained over a 23-year period from pigs. Antimicrob Agents Chemother. 2003;47(10):3214–21.
31. Jakobsen L, Garneau P, Kurbasic A, Bruant G, Stegger M, Harel J, Jensen KS, Brousseau R, Hammerum AM, Frimodt-Moller N. Microarray-based detection of extended virulence and antimicrobial resistance gene profiles in phylogroup B2 *Escherichia coli* of human, meat and animal origin. J Med Microbiol. 2011;60(10):1502–11.
32. Bruant G, Maynard C, Bekal S, Gaucher I, Masson L, Brousseau R, Harell J. Development and validation of an oligonucleotide microarray for detection of multiple virulence and antimicrobial resistance genes in *Escherichia coli*. Appl Environ Microbiol. 2006;72(5):3780–4.
33. Bonnet C, Diarrassouba F, Brousseau R, Masson L, Topp E, Diarra MS. Pathotype and antibiotic resistance gene distributions of *Escherichia coli* isolates from broiler chickens raised on antimicrobial-supplemented Diets. Appl Environ Microbiol. 2009;75(22):6955–62.
34. Bouchillon S, Hoban DJ, Badal R, Hawser S. Fluoroquinolone resistance among gram-negative urinary tract pathogens: global smart program results, 2009–2010. Open Microbiol J. 2012;6:74–8.
35. Tabasi M, Asadi Karam MR, Habibi M, Yekaninejad MS, Bouzari S. Phenotypic assays to determine virulence factors of uropathogenic *Escherichia coli* (UPEC) isolates and their correlation with antibiotic resistance rattern. Osong Public Health Res Perspect. 2015;6(4):261–8.
36. Ali I, Rafaque S, Ahmed S, Malik JI, Dasti P. Prevalence of multi-drug resistant uropathogenic *Escherichia coli* in Potohar region of Pakistan. Asian Pac J Trop Biomed. 2016;6(1):60–6.
37. Linhares I, Raposo T, Rodrigues A, Almeida A. Frequency and antimicrobial resistance patterns of bacteria implicated in community urinary tract infections: a ten-year surveillance study (2000–2009). BMC Infect Dis. 2013;13:19.
38. Wagenlehner FM, Weidner W, Naber KG. Therapy for prostatitis, with emphasis on bacterial prostatitis. Expert Opin Pharmacother. 2007;8(11):1667–74.
39. Ibrahim ME, Bilal NE, Hamid ME. Increased multi-drug resistant *Escherichia coli* from hospitals in Khartoum state, Sudan. Afr Health Sci. 2012;12(3):368–75.
40. Lavigne JP, Bruyere F, Bernard L, Combescure C, Ronco E, Lanotte P, Coloby P, Thibault M, Cariou G, Desplaces N, et al. Resistance and virulence potential of uropathogenic *Escherichia coli* strains isolated from patients hospitalized in urology departments: a French prospective multicentre study. J Med Microbiol. 2016;65(6):530–7.
41. Tarchouna M, Ferjani A, Ben-Selma W, Boukadida J. Distribution of uropathogenic virulence genes in *Escherichia coli* isolated from patients with urinary tract infection. Int J Infect Dis. 2013;17(6):e450–3.
42. Abe CM, Salvador FA, Falsetti IN, Vieira MA, Blanco J, Blanco JE, Blanco M, Machado AM, Elias WP, Hernandes RT, et al. Uropathogenic *Escherichia coli* (UPEC) strains may carry virulence properties of diarrhoeagenic *E. coli*. FEMS Immunol Med Microbiol. 2008;52(3):397–406.
43. Martinez-Jehanne V, Pichon C, du Merle L, Poupel O, Cayet N, Bouchier C, Le Bouguenec C. Role of the vpe carbohydrate permease in *Escherichia coli* urovirulence and fitness in vivo. Infect Immun. 2012;80(8):2655–66.
44. Toval F, Kohler CD, Vogel U, Wagenlehner F, Mellmann A, Fruth A, Schmidt MA, Karch H, Bielaszewska M, Dobrindt U. Characterization of *Escherichia coli* isolates from hospital inpatients or outpatients with urinary tract infection. J Clin Microbiol. 2014;52(2):407–18.
45. Lara FB, Nery DR, de Oliveira PM, Araujo ML, Carvalho FR, Messias-Silva LC, Ferreira LB, Faria-Junior C, Pereira AL. Virulence markers and phylogenetic analysis of *Escherichia coli* strains with hybrid EAEC/UPEC genotypes recovered from sporadic cases of extraintestinal infections. Front Microbiol. 2017;8:146.
46. Zhou M, Guo Z, Duan Q, Hardwidge PR, Zhu G. *Escherichia coli* type III secretion system 2: a new kind of T3SS? Vet Res. 2014;45:32.
47. Miyazaki J, Ba-Thein W, Kumao T, Akaza H, Hayashi H. Identification of a type III secretion system in uropathogenic *Escherichia coli*. FEMS Microbiol Lett. 2002;212(2):221–8.
48. Subashchandrabose S, Hazen TH, Rasko DA, Mobley HL. Draft genome sequences of five recent human uropathogenic *Escherichia coli* isolates. Pathog Dis. 2013;69(1):66–70.
49. Bekal S, Brousseau R, Masson L, Prefontaine G, Fairbrother J, Harel J. Rapid identification of *Escherichia coli* pathotypes by virulence gene detection with DNA microarrays. J Clin Microbiol. 2003;41(5):2113–25.
50. Hamelin K, Bruant G, El-Shaarawi A, Hill S, Edge TA, Bekal S, Fairbrother JM, Harel J, Maynard C, Masson L, et al. A virulence and antimicrobial resistance DNA microarray detects a high frequency of virulence genes in *Escherichia coli* isolates from Great Lakes recreational waters. Appl Environ Microbiol. 2006;72(6):4200–6.
51. Röderova M, Halova D, Papousek I, Dolejska M, Masarikova M, Hanulik V, Pudova V, Broz P, Htoutou-Sedlakova M, Sauer P, et al. Characteristics of quinolone resistance in *Escherichia coli* isolates from humans, animals, and the environment in the Czech Republic. Front Microbiol. 2016;7:2147.
52. Seija V, Medina-Presentado JC, Bado I, Papa-Ezdra R, Batista N, Gutierrez C, Guirado M, Vidal M, Nin M, Vignoli R. Sepsis caused by New Delhi metallo-β-lactamase (blaNDM-1) and qnrD-producing *Morganella morganii*, treated successfully with fosfomycin and meropenem: case report and literature review. Int J Infect Dis. 2015;30:20–6.
53. Szabó O, Gulyás D, Szabó N, Kristóf K, Kocsis B, Szabó D. Plasmid-mediated quinolone resistance determinants in Enterobacteriaceae from urine clinical samples. Acta Microbiol Immunol Hung. 2018;23:1–11.
54. Liu X, Liu H, Li Y, Hao C. High prevalence of β-lactamase and plasmid-mediated quinolone resistance genes in extended-spectrum cephalosporin-resistant *Escherichia coli* from Dogs in Shaanxi, China. Front Microbiol. 2016;16(7):1843.
55. Garcia-Fulgueiras V, Bado I, Mota MI, Robino L, Cordeiro NF, Varela A, Algorta G, Gutkind G, Ayala JA, Vignoli R. Extended-spectrum beta-lactamases and plasmid-mediated quinolone resistance in enterobacterial clinical isolates in the paediatric hospital of Uruguay. J Antimicrob Chemother. 2011;66(8):1725–9.
56. Han C, Yang Y, Wang M, Wang A, Lu Q, Xu X, Wang C, Liu L, Deng Q, Shen X. The prevalence of plasmid-mediated quinolone resistance determinants among clinical isolates of ESBL or AmpC-producing *Escherichia coli* from Chinese pediatric patients. Microbiol Immunol. 2010;54(3):123–8.
57. Wang M, Tran JH, Jacoby GA, Zhang Y, Wang F, Hooper DC. Plasmid-mediated quinolone resistance in clinical isolates of *Escherichia coli* from Shanghai, China. Antimicrob Agents Chemother. 2003;47(7):2242–8.
58. Garza-Gonzalez E, Mendoza Ibarra SI, Llaca-Diaz JM, Gonzalez GM. Molecular characterization and antimicrobial susceptibility of extended-spectrum {beta}-lactamase-producing Enterobacteriaceae isolates at a tertiary-care centre in Monterrey, Mexico. J Med Microbiol. 2011;60(Pt 1):84–90.
59. Merida-Vieyra J, De Colsa A, Calderon Castaneda Y, Arzate Barbosa P, Aquino Andrade A. First report of froup CTX-M-9 extended spectrum beta-lactamases in *Escherichia coli* isolates from pediatric patients in Mexico. PLoS ONE. 2016;11(12):e0168608.
60. Ramirez Castillo FY, Avelar Gonzalez FJ, Garneau P, Marquez Diaz F, Guerrero Barrera AL, Harel J. Presence of multi-drug resistant pathogenic *Escherichia coli* in the San Pedro River located in the State of Aguascalientes, Mexico. Front Microbiol. 2013;4:147.

61. Blanco M, Blanco JE, Alonso MP, Mora A, Balsalobre C, Munoa F, Juarez A, Blanco J. Detection of *pap*, *sfa* and *afa* adhesin-encoding operons in uropathogenic *Escherichia coli* strains: relationship with expression of adhesins and production of toxins. Res Microbiol. 1997;148(9):745–55.
62. Johnson JR, Stell AL. Extended virulence genotypes of *Escherichia coli* strains from patients with urosepsis in relation to phylogeny and host compromise. J Infect Dis. 2000;181(1):261–72.
63. Spurbeck RR, Dinh PC Jr, Walk ST, Stapleton AE, Hooton TM, Nolan LK, Kim KS, Johnson JR, Mobley HL. *Escherichia coli* isolates that carry *vat*, *fyuA*, *chuA*, and *yfcV* efficiently colonize the urinary tract. Infect Immun. 2012;80(12):4115–22.
64. Wang H, Dzink-Fox JL, Chen M, Levy SB. Genetic characterization of highly fluoroquinolone-resistant clinical *Escherichia coli* strains from China: role of *acrR* mutations. Antimicrob Agents Chemother. 2001;45(5):1515–21.
65. Deguchi T, Yasuda M, Nakano M, Ozeki S, Kanematsu E, Nishino Y, Ishihara S, Kawada Y. Detection of mutations in the *gyrA* and *parC* genes in quinolone-resistant clinical isolates of *Enterobacter cloacae*. J Antimicrob Chemother. 1997;40(4):543–9.
66. Maynard C, Bekal S, Sanschagrin F, Levesque RC, Brousseau R, Masson L, Lariviere S, Harel J. Heterogeneity among virulence and antimicrobial resistance gene profiles of extraintestinal *Escherichia coli* isolates of animal and human origin. J Clin Microbiol. 2004;42(12):5444–52.
67. Cattoir V, Poirel L, Nordmann P. Plasmid-mediated quinolone resistance pump QepA2 in an *Escherichia coli* isolate from France. Antimicrob Agents Chemother. 2008;52(10):3801–4.

Permissions

 Every chapter published in this book has been scrutinized by our experts. Their significance has been extensively debated. The topics covered herein carry significant findings which will fuel the growth of the discipline. They may even be implemented as practical applications or may be referred to as a beginning point for another development.

The contributors of this book come from diverse backgrounds, making this book a truly international effort. This book will bring forth new frontiers with its revolutionizing research information and detailed analysis of the nascent developments around the world.

We would like to thank all the contributing authors for lending their expertise to make the book truly unique. They have played a crucial role in the development of this book. Without their invaluable contributions this book wouldn't have been possible. They have made vital efforts to compile up to date information on the varied aspects of this subject to make this book a valuable addition to the collection of many professionals and students.

This book was conceptualized with the vision of imparting up-to-date information and advanced data in this field. To ensure the same, a matchless editorial board was set up. Every individual on the board went through rigorous rounds of assessment to prove their worth. After which they invested a large part of their time researching and compiling the most relevant data for our readers.

The editorial board has been involved in producing this book since its inception. They have spent rigorous hours researching and exploring the diverse topics which have resulted in the successful publishing of this book. They have passed on their knowledge of decades through this book. To expedite this challenging task, the publisher supported the team at every step. A small team of assistant editors was also appointed to further simplify the editing procedure and attain best results for the readers.

Apart from the editorial board, the designing team has also invested a significant amount of their time in understanding the subject and creating the most relevant covers. They scrutinized every image to scout for the most suitable representation of the subject and create an appropriate cover for the book.

The publishing team has been an ardent support to the editorial, designing and production team. Their endless efforts to recruit the best for this project, has resulted in the accomplishment of this book. They are a veteran in the field of academics and their pool of knowledge is as vast as their experience in printing. Their expertise and guidance has proved useful at every step. Their uncompromising quality standards have made this book an exceptional effort. Their encouragement from time to time has been an inspiration for everyone.

The publisher and the editorial board hope that this book will prove to be a valuable piece of knowledge for researchers, students, practitioners and scholars across the globe.

List of Contributors

Ayodele T. Adesoji
Department of Biological Sciences, Federal University Dutsin-Ma, Dutsin-Ma, Katsina State, Nigeria

Adeniyi A. Ogunjobi
Department of Microbiology, University of Ibadan, Ibadan, Nigeria

Isaac O. Olatoye
Department of Veterinary Public Health and Preventive Medicine, University of Ibadan, Ibadan, Oyo State, Nigeria
Paul G. Allen School for Global Animal Health, Washington State University, Pullman, WA, USA

Birson Ingti, Deepjyoti Paul, Anand Prakash Maurya and Amitabha Bhattacharjee
Department of Microbiology, Assam University, Silchar 788011, India

Debadatta Dhar Chanda and Atanu Chakravarty
Department of Microbiology, Silchar Medical College and Hospital, Silchar 788014, India

Debajyoti Bora
Department of Statistics, Dibrugarh University, Dibrugarh, India

Behsan Hemmatinezhad
Graduated Student of Veterinary Medicine, College of Veterinary Medicine, Islamic Azad University, Shahrekord, Iran

Hassan Momtaz
Department of Microbiology, College of Basic Sciences, Islamic Azad University, Shahrekord, Iran

Ebrahim Rahimi
Department of Food Hygiene and Public Health, College of Veterinary Medicine, Islamic Azad University, Shahrekord, Iran

Neriman Aksu
Department of Microbiology, Ankara Numune Training and Research Hospital, Talatpaşa Bulvarı No:5 Altındağ, 06100 Ankara, Turkey

Irmak Baran
Department of Microbiology, Ankara Numune Training and Research Hospital, Talatpaşa Bulvarı No:5 Altındağ, 06100 Ankara, Turkey
Esat Caddesi 101/3 Küçükesat, 06660 Ankara, Turkey

Marion Chazel, Dominique Terru and Nicolas Bouzinbi
Département de Bactériologie-Virologie, CHRU Montpellier, Montpellier, France

Hélène Marchandin
Département de Bactériologie-Virologie, CHRU Montpellier, Montpellier, France
UMR 5119 ECOSYM, Equipe Pathogènes et Environnements, Laboratoire Bactériologie, U.F.R. des Sciences Pharmaceutiques et Biologiques, Montpellier, France

Christian Carrière and Sylvain Godreuil
Département de Bactériologie-Virologie, CHRU Montpellier, Montpellier, France
Department of Bacteriology-Virology, INSERM U1058 "Pathogenesis and Control of Chronic Infections", Université Montpellier-EFS, CHU Arnaud de Villeneuve 371 avenue Université Montpellier, Montpellier, France

Nicolas Keck
Laboratoire Départemental Vétérinaire de l'Hérault, Montpellier, France

Michael Ponsoda, Véronique Jacomo and Gilles Panteix
Laboratoire Biomnis, Lyon, France

Jérôme Solassol
Université Montpellier, Montpellier, France
Department of Biopathology, CHRU Montpellier, Montpellier, France
Department of Clinical Oncoproteomic, Montpellier Cancer Institute, Montpellier, France

Anne-Laure Bañuls and Marc Choisy
MIVEGEC (Laboratoire Maladies Infectieuses et Vecteurs, Ecologie, Génétique, Evolution et Contrôle), UMR CNRS 5290/IRD 224, Université de Montpellier, Montpellier, France

Alexandra Aubry
Centre National de Référence des Mycobactéries et de la Résistance aux Antituberculeux, Paris, France
Laboratoire de Bactériologie-Hygiène Paris, AP-HP, Hôpital Pitié-Salpêtrière, 75013 Paris, France
Centre for Immunology and Microbial Infections, team 13, Sorbonne Universités, UPMC Univ Paris 06, U1135, 75013 Paris, France
13 INSERM, U1135, Paris, France

Kazım Sahin and Aziz Ramazan Dilek
Department of Microbiology, Medical Faculty, Recep Tayyip Erdogan University, Islampasa mah., 53000 Rize, Turkey

Ayse Tekin
Department of Infectious Diseases, Cengiz Gökcek Women and Obstetrics Hospital, Osmangazi mah., 27010 Gaziantep, Turkey

Sule Ozdas
Department of Molecular Biology and Genetics, Medical Faculty, Istanbul Bilim University, Buyukdere cad., No: 120, Esentepe-Sisli-Istanbul, Turkey

Demet Akin
Department of Pharmacology, Medical Faculty, Istanbul Bilim University, Buyukdere cad., No: 120, 34394 Esentepe-Sisli-Istanbul, Turkey

Hande Yapislar
Department of Physiology, Medical Faculty, Istanbul Bilim University, Buyukdere cad., No: 120, 34394 Esentepe-Sisli-Istanbul, Turkey

Emine Sonmez
Department of Infectious Diseases, Medical Faculty, Recep Tayyip Erdogan University, Islampasa mah., 53000 Rize, Turkey

Eszter J. Tóth, Mónika Homa, Gábor Nagy and Tamás Papp
MTA-SZTE "Lendület" Fungal Pathogenicity Mechanisms Research Group, Hungarian Academy of Sciences, University of Szeged, Közép fasor 52, Szeged 6726, Hungary
Department of Microbiology, Faculty of Science and Informatics, University of Szeged, Közép fasor 52, Szeged 6726, Hungary

Csaba Vágvölgyi
Department of Microbiology, Faculty of Science and Informatics, University of Szeged, Közép fasor 52, Szeged 6726, Hungary

Géza R. Nagy, Zsuzsanna Bata-Csörgő and Lajos Kemény
Department of Dermatology and Allergology, Albert Szent-Györgyi Medical
Centre, University of Szeged, Szeged, Hungary

Marianna Ábrók, Ildikó É. Kiss and Edit Urbán
Institute of Clinical Microbiology, Albert Szent-Györgyi Medical Centre, University of Szeged, Szeged, Hungary

Amit Gupta and Mike Almond
Southend University Hospital, Prittlewell Chase, Westcliff-on-Sea SS0 0RY, UK

Nada Elhag
Southend University Hospital, Prittlewell Chase, Westcliff-on-Sea SS0 0RY, UK
Antimicrobial Resistance and Healthcare Associated Infections (AMRHAI) Reference Unit, Public Health England, London NW9 5EQ, UK

Julie Logan
Antimicrobial Resistance and Healthcare Associated Infections (AMRHAI) Reference Unit, Public Health England, London NW9 5EQ, UK

Xiao-hong Xu, Ying-ping Cao and Bin Li
Department of Clinical Laboratory, Fujian Medical University Union Hospital, 29# Xinquan Road, Fuzhou 350001, Fujian, China

Qing-wen He, Fang-jun Lan and Zhi-yun Wu
Department of Clinical Laboratory, Fujian Medical University Union Hospital, 29# Xinquan Road, Fuzhou 350001, Fujian, China
The Union Clinical Medical College of Fujian Medical University, Fuzhou 350004, Fujian, China

Zhi-chang Zhao
Department of Pharmacy, Fujian Medical University, Union Hospital, Fuzhou 350001, Fujian, China

S. M. Hijazi
Department of Pharmaceutical Sciences (Pharmaceutical Microbiology), Faculty of Pharmacy, Beirut Arab University, Beirut, Lebanon

K. H. Abd El Galil
Department of Pharmaceutical Sciences (Pharmaceutical Microbiology), Faculty of Pharmacy, Beirut Arab University, Beirut, Lebanon
Department of Pharmaceutical Microbiology, Faculty of Pharmacy, Mansoura University, Mansoura, Egypt

M. A. Fawzi
Department of Pharmaceutical Microbiology, Faculty of Pharmacy, Alexandria University, Alexandria, Egypt

F. M. Ali
Department of Microbiology and Immunology, Infection Control, Faculty of Medicine, Ain Shams University, Cairo, Egypt

Mahoko Ikeda, Yuka Yagihara, Keita Tatsuno, Shu Okugawa and Kyoji Moriya
Department of Infection Control and Prevention, Faculty of Medicine, The University of Tokyo, 7-3-1 Hongo, Bunkyo, Tokyo 113-8655, Japan

Mitsuhiro Okazaki
Department of Medical Technology, School of Health Sciences, Tokyo University of Technology, 5-23-22 Nishikamata, Ota, Tokyo 144-8535, Japan

Kamelia Osman and Ahmed Orabi
Department of Microbiology, Faculty of Veterinary Medicine, Cairo University, Giza, Egypt

Avelino Alvarez-Ordóñez
Department of Food Hygiene and Technology and Institute of Food Science and Technology, University of León, León, Spain

Lorena Ruiz
Department of Nutrition, Bromatology and Food Technology, Universidad Complutense de Madrid, Madrid, Spain

Jihan Badr and Alaa Saad
Department of Poultry Diseases, Animal Health Research, Institute, Giza, Egypt

Fatma ElHofy
Department of Bacteriology, Immunology and Mycology, Faculty of Veterinary Medicine, Benha University, Moushtohor, Egypt

Khalid S. Al-Maary and Ihab M. I. Moussa
Department of Botany and Microbiology, College of Science, King Saud University, Riyadh, Kingdom of Saudi Arabia

Ashgan M. Hessain
Department of Health Science, College of Applied Studies and Community Service, King Saud University, Riyadh, Kingdom of Saudi Arabia

Mohamed Elhadidy
Department of Bacteriology, Mycology and Immunology, Faculty of Veterinary Medicine, Mansoura University, Mansoura 35516, Egypt
Foodborne Pathogens, Scientific Institute of Public Health, Juliette Wytsmanstraat 14, 1050 Brussels, Belgium

George Tetz
TGV-Laboratories LLC, 303 5th avenue, # 2012, New York, NY 10016, USA

Daria Vikina and Victor Tetz
Institute of Human Microbiology, New York, NY 10016, USA

Nadezhda K. Fursova, Eugeny I. Astashkin, Anastasia I. Knyazeva, Nikolay N. Kartsev, Ekaterina S. Leonova, Nikolay V. Volozhantsev, Edward A. Svetoch and Ivan A. Dyatlov
State Research Center for Applied Microbiology and Biotechnology, Obolensk, 142279 Moscow Region, Russia

Olga N. Ershova, Irina A. Alexandrova, Natalia V. Kurdyumova and Svetlana Yu. Sazikina
The Burdenko Neurosurgery Institute, Moscow 125047, Russia

P. T. Fowoyo
Biosciences Department, Salem University, Kogi State, Nigeria

S. T. Ogunbanwo
Microbiology Department, University of Ibadan, Ibadan, Oyo State, Nigeria

Li Cheng, Xiao-Li Cao, Zhi-Feng Zhang, Ming-zhe Ning, Xue-Jing Xu, Wanqing Zhou, Jun-Hao Chen, Jin-hua Zhang, Han Shen and Kui Zhang
Department of Laboratory Medicine, Nanjing Drum Tower Hospital, The Affiliated Hospital of Nanjing University Medical School, Zhongshan Road, 321#, Gulou District, Nanjing, Jiangsu, People's Republic of China

M. Smiljanic, P. Ahmad-Nejad and B. Ghebremedhin
Center for Clinical and Translational Research, Institute for Medical Laboratory Diagnostics, HELIOS University Clinic Wuppertal; Witten/ Herdecke University, Heusnerstr. 40, 42283 Wuppertal, Germany

M. Kaase
Department of Medical Microbiology, Ruhr-University Bochum, Bochum, Germany
Department of Infection Control, University Medical Center Göttingen, Göttingen, Germany

Tetsuya Yumoto, Hiromichi Naito, Hiromi Ihoriya, Kohei Tsukahara and Atsunori Nakao
Advanced Emergency and Critical Care Medical Center, Okayama University Hospital, 2-5-1 Shikata-cho, Kita-ku, Okayama-shi, Okayama 700-8558, Japan

Tomoyuki Ota and Toshiyuki Watanabe
Department of Plastic and Reconstructive Surgery, Okayama University Graduate School of Medicine, Dentistry and Pharmaceutical Sciences, 2-5-1 Shikata-cho, Kita-ku, Okayama-shi, Okayama 700-8558, Japan

Na Du, Shumin Liu, Min Niu, Yong Duan, Shuangmeng Zhang, Jing Yao, Jian Mao, Ran Chen and Yan Du
Department of Clinical Laboratory, the First Affiliated Hospital of Kunming Medical University, Yunnan Institute of Laboratory Diagnosis, Yunnan Key Laboratory of Laboratory Medicine, No. 295, Xichang Road, Wuhua, Kunming Yunnan, China

Menyfah Q. Alanazi
Clinical Pharmacy Practice, Drug Policy and Economics Center, King Abdulaziz Medical City, Ministry of National Guard, Health Affairs, Riyadh 22490, Saudi Arabia

Fulwah Y. Alqahtani and Fadilah S. Aleanizy
Department of PharmaceUTIscs, College of Pharmacy, King Saud University, Riyadh 22452, Saudi Arabia

Mamadou Alpha Diallo, Khadim Diongue, Mame Cheikh Seck, Mouhamadou Ndiaye, Younouss Diedhiou, Tolla Ndiaye, Yaye Die Ndiaye, Aida Sadikh Badiane and Daouda Ndiaye
Laboratory of Parasitology and Mycology, Cheikh Anta Diop University, Avenue Cheikh Anta Diop, BP 5005 Fann, Dakar, Senegal

Ibrahima Diallo
Malaria Control Program (NMCP), Rue Aimé Césaire, Fann Résidence, Dakar, Senegal

Xiao-Ping Chen, Wen-Ge Li, Hao Zheng, Jie Che and Yuan Wu
State Key Laboratory for Infectious Disease Prevention and Control, Collaborative Innovation Center for Diagnosis and Treatment of Infectious Diseases, National Institute for Communicable Disease Control and Prevention, Chinese Center for Disease Control and Prevention, Beijing 102206, China

Jin-Xing Lu
State Key Laboratory for Infectious Disease Prevention and Control, Collaborative Innovation Center for Diagnosis and Treatment of Infectious Diseases, National Institute for Communicable Disease Control and Prevention, Chinese Center for Disease Control and Prevention, Beijing 102206, China
Changbai Road 155, ChangPing, Beijing 102206, China

Hai-Yan Du, Li Zhang and Lei Zhang
Microbiology Laboratory, Fu Xing Hospital, Capital Medical University, Beijing 100038, China

Shu-Mei Liu
Microbiology Laboratory, Fu Xing Hospital, Capital Medical University, Beijing 100038, China
FuXingMenWai Road 20, XiCheng, Beijing 100038, China

Saeam Shin, Min-Jeong Park and Wonkeun Song
Department of Laboratory Medicine, Hallym University College of Medicine, Seoul, South Korea

Seok Hoon Jeong, Hyukmin Lee and Jun Sung Hong
Department of Laboratory Medicine and Research Institute for Antimicrobial Resistance, Yonsei University College of Medicine, Seoul, South Korea

Suriya Rehman and Fatimah Alkhamis
Department of Epidemic Diseases Research, Institute for Research and Medical Consultations (IRMC), Imam Abdulrahman Bin Faisal University (IAU), Dammam 31441, Saudi Arabia

Khaled R. Alkharsah
Department of Epidemic Diseases Research, Institute for Research and Medical Consultations (IRMC), Imam Abdulrahman Bin Faisal University (IAU), Dammam 31441, Saudi Arabia
Department of Microbiology College of Medicine, Imam Abdulrahman Bin Faisal University (IAU), Dammam 31441, Saudi Arabia

Amani Alnimr and Asim Diab
Department of Microbiology College of Medicine, Imam Abdulrahman Bin Faisal University (IAU), Dammam 31441, Saudi Arabia

Amein K. Al-Ali
Department of Biochemistry, College of Medicine, Imam Abdulrahman Bin Faisal University (IAU), Dammam 31441, Saudi Arabia

Monireh Rahimkhani
Department of Lab Medical Sciences, Faculty of Allied Medical Sciences, Tehran University of Medical Sciences, Tehran, Iran

A. Mordadi
Department of Epidemiology, Pasteur Institute, Tehran, Iran

M. Gilanpour
Almahdi Kheyrieh Clinics, Tehran, Iran

Vishnu Sharma, Sanjita Sharma, Dinesh Kumar Dahiya, Aarif Khan and Manisha Mathur
Advanced Milk Testing Research Laboratory, Postgraduate Institute of Veterinary Education and Research, Rajasthan University of Veterinary and Animal Sciences at Bikaner, B-2 Bypass, Shiprapath, Mansarovar, Jaipur 302020, Rajasthan, India

Aayushi Sharma
Sawai Man Singh Medical College, Jaipur 302004, Rajasthan, India

Ting-Yi Su, Jung-Jr Ye, Chien-Chang Yang, Ching-Tai Huang and Ming-Hsun Lee
Division of Infectious Diseases, Department of Internal Medicine, Chang Gung Memorial Hospital at Linkou, Chang Gung University College of Medicine, 5 Fu-Shin Street, Gueishan 333, Taoyuan, Taiwan

Ju-Hsin Chia
Department of Laboratory Medicine, Chang Gung Memorial Hospital at Linkou, Taoyuan, Taiwan
Department of Medical Biotechnology and Laboratory Science, Chang Gung University, Taoyuan, Taiwan

Flor Y. Ramírez-Castillo, Adriana C. Moreno-Flores and Alma L. Guerrero-Barrera
Laboratorio de Biología Celular y Tisular, Departamento de Morfología, Universidad Autónoma de Aguascalientes, Av. Universidad 940, Col. Cd

Francisco J. Avelar-González
Laboratorio de Ciencias Ambientales, Departamento de Fisiología y Farmacología, Universidad Autónoma de Aguascalientes, Av. Universidad 940, Col. Cd. Universitaria, 20131 Aguascalientes, Mexico

Francisco Márquez-Díaz
Departamento de Infectología, Centenario Hospital Miguel Hidalgo, Galeana Sur 495, Obraje, 20000 Aguascalientes, Mexico

Josée Harel
Département de pathologie et microbiologie, Centre de Recherche en Infectologíe Porcine et Aviaire, Faculté de Médecine Vétérinaire, Université de Montréal, 3200, rue Sicott, Saint-Hyacinthe, Montreal, QC J2S 2M2, Canada

Index

www.ingramcontent.com/pod-product-compliance
Lightning Source LLC
LaVergne TN
LVHW080737210926
848485LV00003B/572